Emergency Procedures and Techniques

FOURTH EDITION

Emergency Procedures and Techniques

FOURTH EDITION

Robert R. Simon, M.D.
Professor and Chairman
Department of Emergency Medicine
Cook County Hospital—Rush Medical College
Chairman, Department of Emergency Medicine
Provident Hopital
Chicago, Illinois

Barry E. Brenner, M.D., Ph.D.
Professor, Emergency and Internal Medicine
Chairman, Department of Emergency Medicine
University of Arkansas for Medical Services
Little Rock, Arkansas

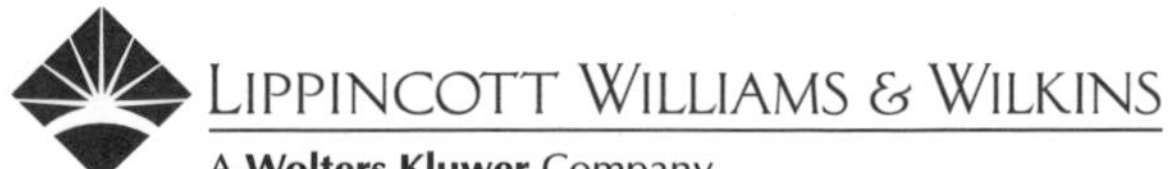
LIPPINCOTT WILLIAMS & WILKINS
A **Wolters Kluwer** Company
Philadelphia • Baltimore • New York • London
Buenos Aires • Hong Kong • Sydney • Tokyo

Acquisitions Editor: Anne M. Sydor
Developmental Editor: Selina M. Bush
Production Editor: Allison L. Risko
Manufacturing Manager: Colin Warnock
Cover Designer: LWW Desktop Division, NY
Compositor: Maryland Composition Company, Inc.
Printer: Edwards Brothers

530 Walnut Street
Philadelphia, PA 19106 USA
LWW.com

Printed in the USA

First Edition, 1982
Second Edition, 1987
Third Edition, 1994

Library of Congress Cataloging-in-Publication Data

Emergency procedures and techniques / editors, Robert R. Simon, Barry E. Brenner.– 4th ed.
p. ; cm
Rev. ed. of: Emergency procedures and techniques / Robert R. Simon, Barry E. Brenner. 3rd ed. c1994.
Includes bibliographical references and index.
ISBN 0-7817-2699-9 (alk. paper)
1. Emergency medicine. I. Simon, Robert R. (Robert Rutha) II. Brenner, Barry E. III. Simon, Robert R. (Robert Rutha). Emergency procedures and techniques.
[DNLM: 1. Emergencies. 2. Emergency Medicine–methods. WB 105 E5585 2001]
RC86.7 .S54 2001
616.02′5–dc21

2001038346

---

10 9 8 7 6 5 4 3 2 1

To my wife, Marilynn, and my sons, Adam, Timothy, and Jeremy, who give purpose to my life.
To my mother, an illiterate Lebanese villager who has contributed more than any other in both my personal development and the progression of my work.
R. R. S

To those who have taught me to maneuver patients in that fearful interface: the tightrope between life and death. To my teachers, honored parents, and cherished wife, Cherlyn, and children, Dovi and Moshe, Yehudeh Zev, Abraham, Aaron, Naphtoli, Rachel, Matthew, and Sara Rifka.
B. E. B.

Contents

1 / Abdominal Procedures

2 / Airway Procedures

3 / Anesthesia and Regional Blocks

4 / Cardiothoracic Procedures

5 / Neurosurgical Procedures

6 / Obstetric and Gynecologic Procedures

7 / Orthopedic Procedures

8 / Otolaryngologic and Ophthalmologic Procedures

9 / Common Dental Emergencies

10 / Plastic Surgery Principles and Techniques

11 / Urologic Procedures

12 / Vascular Procedures

Contributing Authors

Martin John Carey, MB, BCh, MPH
Assistant Professor/Residency Director
Emergency Medicine
University of Arkansas for Medical Sciences
Little Rock, Arkansas
Attending Physician
Emergency Medicine
University of Arkansas Medical Center
Little Rock, Arkansas
Chapter 11, *Urological Procedures*

Sylvie Desouza, MD
Emergency Medicine
New York Presbyterian Hospitals
Weill Medical College
Cornell University
New York, New York
The Brooklyn Hospital Center
Brooklyn, New York
Chapter 6, *Obstetric and Gynecologic Procedures*

Darren E. Flamik, MD, FACEP
Assistant Professor
Emergency Medicine
University of Arkansas for Medical Sciences
Little Rock, Arkansas
Attending Physician
Emergency Medicine
University of Arkansas Hospital
Little Rock, Arkansas
Chapter 8, *Otolaryngologic and Ophthalmologic Procedures*

Gregory S. Hall, MD
Assistant Professor
Emergency Medicine
Vice Chairman
Department of Emergency Medicine
University of Arkansas for Medical Sciences
Little Rock, Arkansas
Chapter 10, *Plastic Surgery Principals and Techniques (section on Pathophysiology and Basic Principals of Wound Healing)*

Christopher Don Melton, MD, FACEP
Assistant Professor
Emergency Medicine
University of Arkansas for Medical Sciences
Little Rock, Arkansas
Attending Physician
Emergency Medicine
University of Arkansas Hospital
Little Rock, Arkansas
Chapter 8, *Otolaryngologic and Ophthalmologic Procedures*

Philip L. Rice Jr., MD, FAAEM, FACEP
Department of Emergency Medicine
Brigham and Women's Hospital
Harvard University Medical School
Boston, Massachusetts
Chapter 4, *Cardiothoracic Procedures*

Kenneth Scott Whitlow, DO
Emergency Medicine
New York Presbyterian Hospitals
Weill Medical College
Cornell University
New York, New York
The Brooklyn Hospital Center
Brooklyn, New York
Chapter 6, *Obstetric and Gynecologic Procedures*

Anton Adolphus Wray, MD
New York Presbyterian Hospitals
Weill Medical College
Cornell University
New York, New York
Brooklyn Hospital Center
Brooklyn, New York
Chapter 5, *Neurosurgical Procedures*

Preface

Emergency medicine is a procedure-laden specialty whose procedures span many fields of medicine. This book, for almost 20 years, has described procedures performed under emergency circumstances. Tacit within the word "emergency" is the concept that time is of the essence. A deft emergency department practitioner needs efficient time management skills and needs to be highly competent in procedures, not only to be successful and avoid complications but also to perform the procedures quickly. Although this text was written primarily for emergency physicians, all physicians who deliver emergency care, including medical students, house officers, general internists, and critical care specialists, will find it useful.

Several manuals and texts on procedures and techniques have been published over the past two decades. Many of these texts offer a cookbook approach that gives an author's individual experience in performing a particular procedure. A few of these texts provide exhaustive treatments of the subject including the history, research, and complications associated with a procedure. While these texts are useful as references, the style and content of these books do not avail themselves for real-time use in a busy emergency department. We have extensively revised and updated the fourth edition to include new procedures and techniques, delete less effective ones, and supplement the text with our current understandings of complications and their remedies. Major revisions have been made to the chapters on Airway Procedures, Cardiothoracic Procedures, Otolaryngology, Ophthalmology, and Urologic Emergencies.

The purpose of this text is to provide the physician with an easy-to-use, step-by-step approach to procedures performed in an emergency department. Each procedure is divided into *Preparatory Steps* and *Procedural Steps.* Preparatory Steps discuss positioning the patient, prepping the patient, and other steps. Procedural Steps describe the actual procedure in detail, supplying ample illustrations of key points.

In addition, several unique features have been incorporated into the book using a special format for extra information needed at certain points during a procedure. CAUTION, NOTE, and AXIOM headline this information, separating it from the Procedural Steps and placing it in key positions to provide the reader with appropriate information at the right time. CAUTION appears with a discussion on how to avoid a particular complication. NOTE is used to give important information about alternative approaches, variations in anatomy, or positioning. AXIOM gives an applicable rule or law from which the procedure should not deviate (e.g., " . . . the amount of undermining necessary to close a laceration has been determined to be approximately double the width of the laceration at its widest point . . . "). Throughout the text, the CAUTIONs, NOTEs, and AXIOMs are capitalized and set off from the rest of the text so that the information can not be overlooked.

Finally, Preparatory Steps and Procedural Steps are followed by *Aftercare,* which discusses and summarizes treatment of the patient after a procedure is completed.

In most of the text, the format for discussing a particular procedure follows the routine that would be carried through in preparing and performing emergency procedures. We hope that by following the format in the book, it will enable a more organized approach to performing procedures in the emergency department. This format is as follows:

- Indications and contraindications for performing a procedure are listed.
- Equipment necessary for performing a procedure is described.
- The steps necessary for performing a procedure are divided into the three parts as described before: Preparatory Steps, Procedural Steps, and Aftercare.

Finally, possible complications resulting from a procedure are listed separately under Complications, usually accompanied by a detailed discussion and information on prevention.

The format of this book offers the reader a practical, procedural "toolkit" for "real time" emergency department use, without the "background filler" unnecessary for the actual performance of emergency procedures. The scholarship and academic approach in this book is succinct and oriented towards clinical practice. We have prepared it as a guide to procedures for actual use during a shift in the emergency department.

Acknowledgments

We would like to express our deepest appreciation to Susan Gilbert for the fine diagrams that are featured in this text. The senior author would like to give special thanks to Mishelle Taylor for her dedicated support in editing and typing the manuscript and for her careful and diligent search for errors.

1

Abdominal Procedures

NASOGASTRIC INTUBATION

Nasogastric intubation is one of the most common procedures performed in the emergency center. Ideally, the patient should be in a semiupright position. In the traumatized patient, however, this position may not be possible. The unconscious patient should have an endotracheal tube inserted before nasogastric intubation to decrease the chance of aspiration and to prevent gastric dilatation secondary to ileus (39). A number of techniques have been described to aid in inserting the nasogastric tube when difficulties are encountered in its passage. These are discussed in a separate section later.

INDICATIONS

There are numerous indications for nasogastric intubation, some of which are

1. Emptying of gastric contents (overdose, poisoning).
2. Presence of an ileus or mechanical obstruction.
3. Prevention of gastric dilatation and aspiration in patients with major trauma.
4. Rehydration in children with acute diarrhea and vomiting (46).

EQUIPMENT

Nasogastric tube
K-Y jelly

TECHNIQUE OF INSERTION

Preparatory Steps

1. Select the appropriate tube size: in the adult, a 16 French nasogastric tube usually can be inserted. In children, 12 French is the size usually selected.
2. Examine the nose and select the wider nares. Often patients have a deviation of the septum, making passage of the tube difficult on the narrower side.
3. Lubricate the tube well.

Procedural Steps

1. Insert the nasogastric tube along the floor of the nose directed posteriorly.

CAUTION

The tube should not be pointed superiorly when it is inserted; otherwise it may impinge on the turbinates, causing hemorrhage. In patients with severe facial and skull trauma, passage superiorly may lead to entrance of the tube intracranially (40, 45, 47, 95, 122, 123).

NOTE

The cribriform plate is easily fractured, and the dura in this area is quite thin and easily perforated by the nasogastric tube. Patients with significant facial and skull trauma may also have nasal, orbital floor, zygomatic, maxillary, or palatal fractures. In addition, these patients may have fractures of the cervical spine, frontal ethmoid, sphenoid sinuses, cribriform areas, or base of the skull. These fractures may be present with or without evidence of cerebrospinal fluid rhinorrhea (40, 45, 47, 105, 122, 123).

---

2. Pass the tube past the soft palate into the posterior pharynx. One can feel a "give" or decreased resistance once the tube has passed into the posterior pharynx in most patients. Most patients initially will feel like "gagging" once the tube is passed beyond this point.
3. Instruct the conscious patient who is not traumatized to hold a sip of water in the mouth and to swallow while the tube is being passed down the esophagus.

CAUTION

If the patient begins to cough during this passage, this indicates the tube has passed into the trachea. Withdraw the tube back into the posterior pharynx and repeat the procedure.

NOTE

Passage of the nasogastric tube may be impeded by anterior and posterior choanal deviation, esophageal narrowing, or narrowing of the esophagus secondary to an inflated endotracheal tube (70). Inadequate relaxation of the cricopharyngeus muscle, a striated muscle of the upper pharynx, also has been implicated as a cause of difficult passage of the tube (70).

---

4. Aspirate the gastric contents to confirm proper placement of the tube within the stomach. Alternatively, inject 20 to 30 mL of air, auscultating with a stethoscope over the left upper quadrant of the abdomen to ascertain proper placement.

NOTE

An alternate method to ensure proper positioning has been described by Fry (41). He injects 4 mL of water and 5 mL of air together down the tube while auscultating in the left upper quadrant. If the nasogastric tube is lying freely within the stomach, sounds can be heard on injection as well as aspiration. However, if the tube is lying within the cardiac sphincter or is kinked within the stomach, sounds will be heard only on injection. According to Fry, water and air should be used together because either element alone may enter and leave the stomach silently. This test can be used to confirm both position and patency of the tube should gastric suctioning suddenly produce no aspirate.

TECHNIQUES TO FACILITATE PASSAGE OF A NASOGASTRIC TUBE

1. Chill the tube in either cold tap water or ice cubes to make the tube stiffer and easier to pass (26, 87, 113, 119). This is especially helpful when the problem is coiling of the tube within the mouth.
2. Place two fingers in the mouth to hold the tube against the posterior pharyngeal wall while advancing the tube to prevent or detect coiling in the oral cavity (24, 105, 113).
3. Pass the nasogastric tube through an endotracheal tube previously positioned within the esophagus (18, 26, 92, 113, 119). Ogawa (49) introduced a technique that is quite useful in the difficult patient: lubricate an endotracheal tube and insert it orally into the esophagus (Fig. 1.1). Remove the connector on the endotracheal tube. Lubricate and insert a standard nasogastric tube

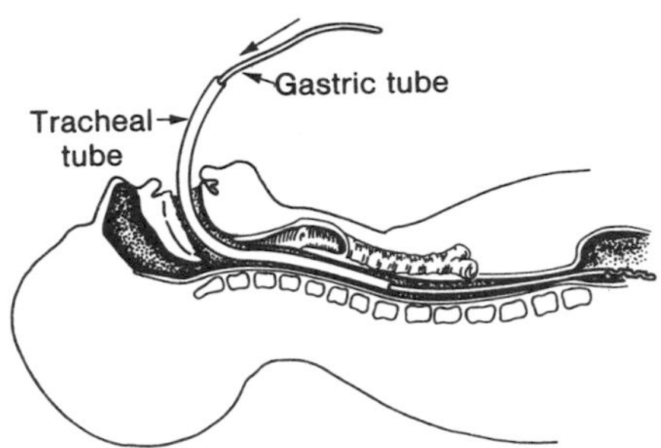

Figure 1.1. After the tracheal tube has been inserted perorally into the esophagus, insert the gastric tube through the tracheal tube and into the stomach. (From Ogawa H: A reliable technique for insertion of a gastric tube during operation. Surg Gynecol Obstet 132:498, 1971, with permission.)

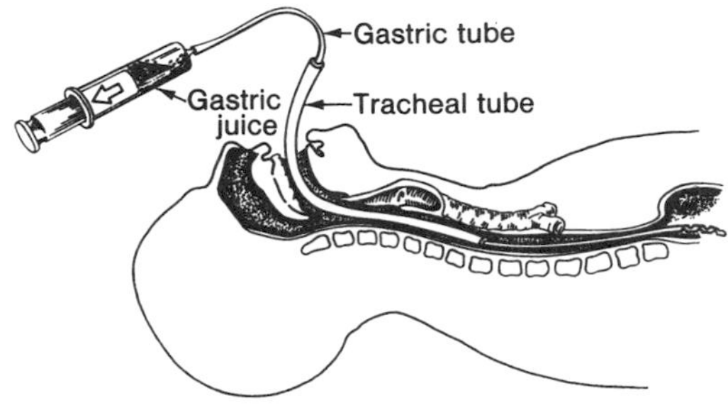

Figure 1.2. Verify that the inserted gastric tube is in the stomach by aspirating gastric juice through the nasogastric tube. (From Ogawa H: A reliable technique for insertion of a gastric tube during operation. Surg Gynecol Obstet 132:498, 1971, with permission.)

into the endotracheal tube (Fig. 1.1). Because the nasogastric tube follows the inside of the tracheal tube, no resistance is met, and it can be easily inserted into the stomach. When resistance is encountered distal to the endotracheal tube, pass the tracheal tube farther so that the nasogastric tube may be properly positioned. Passage of the nasogastric tube into the stomach should be ascertained either by the injection of air and auscultating over the epigastrium or by the aspiration of gastric contents (Fig. 1.2). Then withdraw the endotracheal tube, and leave the gastric tube in position (Fig. 1.3). After this, insert a small catheter with an outside diameter of approximately 3 to 5 mm or a suction tube nasally, and pull the tip out through the oral cavity and subsequently insert it into the gastric tube. Secure this attachment with a silk suture (Fig. 1.4). Then pull out the catheter through the nostril, and withdraw the gastric tube from the oral cavity into the nose in a retrograde fashion.

NOTE

A nasogastric tube encounters narrowing in the esophagus and resistance in passage at three sites. The first is located behind the cricoid cartilage of the larynx; the second is located behind the bifurcation of the bronchus where it crosses the aorta; and the third is at the lower end of the esophagus where it passes into the stomach. The distance of these narrowed areas from the incisors of the upper jaw in the average adult is 15, 25, and 40 cm, respectively (92). In most patients, difficulty in gastric tube insertion occurs when the tube becomes coiled in the oral cavity and fails to advance into the esophagus or when the tip is caught at the pharynx or larynx and does not advance farther.

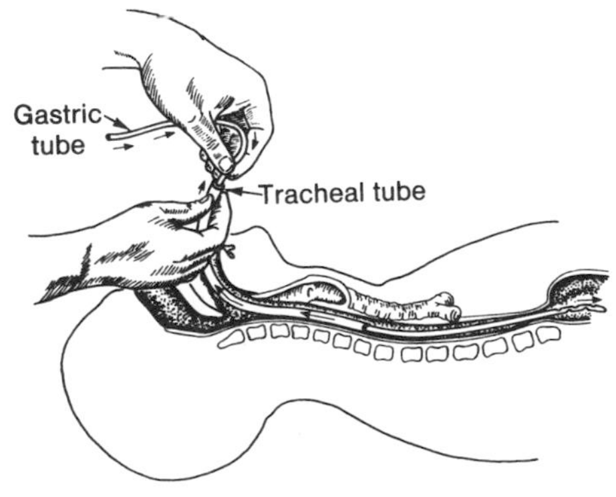

Figure 1.3. Remove the tracheal tube as shown. See text for details. (From Ogawa H: A reliable technique for insertion of a gastric tube during operation. Surg Gynecol Obstet 132:498, 1971, with permission.)

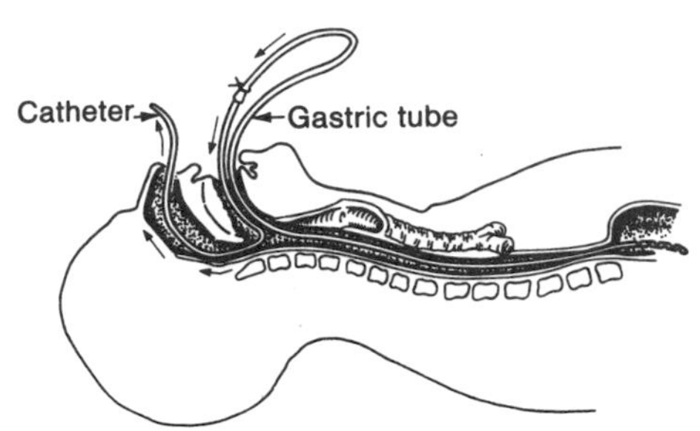

Figure 1.4. Connect the gastric tube to the catheter, which is inserted nasally, and pull the gastric tube in a retrograde fashion through the nose. (From Ogawa H: A reliable technique for insertion of a gastric tube during operation. Surg Gynecol Obstet 132:498, 1971, with permission.)

4. In patients in whom nasogastric tube insertion is difficult, we find it useful to squeeze into the patient's nostril a tube of 2% lidocaine jelly with a Toomey syringe. Insert the tip of the syringe into the patient's nostril, squeezing the nostril shut around the tip. Fill the nostril with the lidocaine jelly. The jelly will enter into the posterior pharynx and relax the posterior nasal constrictors, thus making nasogastric tube insertion much easier (34).
5. An alternate method has been described (87) for patients in whom the difficulty is at the narrowing in the esophagus posterior to the cricoid. In this situation, grasp the alae or wings of the thyroid cartilage between the thumb and index finger and lift anteriorly. Normally in the supine patient, the esophagus is collapsed because of gravity, and this maneuver opens the esophagus, allowing the tube to pass readily into the stomach. In one study, it was found that in those patients in whom passage was unsuccessful, the site of impingement of the tube was the periform sinuses in 46%, arytenoid cartilages in 25%, and the trachea in 21% (96). Lateral neck pressure was attempted, and it relieved 85% of the obstructions (96). Remember that vigorous palpation of the cricoid cartilage and adjacent structures may cause reflex bradycardia, and this should be avoided (87).
6. In patients in whom there is a disorder of esophageal motility or partial esophageal obstruction secondary to stricture, a technique has been described by Mahar (77) for the passage of nasogastric tube with the use of a bougie. Feed the tube to be passed either through the nares or perorally into the pharynx. Then feed a 20 to 25 French Maloney bougie (the bougie is a very firm catheter that, because of its stiffness, does not coil within the esophagus) orally into the hypopharynx with the fingers as a guide, and feed the nasogastric tube simultaneously into the esophagus. The bougie keeps the tube from curling in the esophagus. Occasionally this is not successful because of the extreme flexibility of the tube. This is especially true with the Sengstaken–Blakemore tube, which is extremely flexible (see "Sengstaken–Blakemore Balloon Tamponade," later). In this situation, pass a 0 chromic catgut suture through the most distal portion of the nasogastric tube, being careful not to perforate any balloons. Form a loop with the suture material and then place the bougie through the loop and pass it perorally into the stomach (Fig. 1.5). When the bougie is withdrawn, the loop releases the bougie without difficulty. When using this method, it is best to do the procedure under fluoroscopic control.
7. In small children, passage of a tube may be quite difficult. A technique described by Robinson and Cox (101) has been used successfully. Use a 7 or 8 French pediatric feeding tube in conjunction with a straight, stainless steel spring guide that is 145 cm long and 0.6 mm in diameter. First irrigate the pediatric feeding tube with normal saline, which serves as a lubricant between the

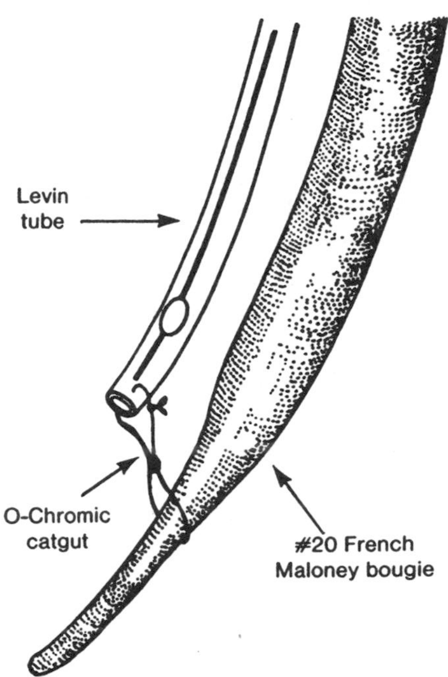

Figure 1.5. Pass a chromic suture through the Levine tube and loop it around the Maloney bougie, as shown. See discussion in the text. (From Mahar J: An aid in the passage of gastrointestinal tubes. Am J Surg 135:866, 1978, with permission.)

plastic and steel surfaces, and then insert the spring guidewire into the feeding tube, and advance the flexible tip of the guidewire to within 1 cm of the tip of the catheter. Next, introduce the catheter through the nose into the posterior pharynx where the tip of the catheter can be manipulated into the esophagus and gently threaded into the stomach. When the tube is properly positioned, as indicated by gastric aspiration or the injection of air accompanied by auscultation over the epigastrium, remove the spring guidewire. In situations in which one is uncertain of proper placement, obtain a radiograph with the guidewire in place because the wire is radiopaque.

8. In a difficult patient, place a nasogastric tube by using a fiberoptic bronchoscope and the Seldinger technique.

AFTERCARE

Secure the tube with tape to the nose by placing one loop of the tape around the tube and attaching the two distal ends of tape superiorly on the face or nose.

NOTE

A new method of stabilizing nasogastric tubes has been advocated to minimize the problem of decubitus ulcerations in the mucosa of the nose and pharynx in those patients who require prolonged nasogastric intubation (104). Tie a heavy thread around the tube and hold it to the skin of the nose and forehead with adhesive tape. The free part of the thread must be 3 or 4 cm long to allow short inward and outward movements of the tube during swallowing. In this way, pressure exerted on the tissues by the tube is alleviated periodically during swallowing, and erosions of the nasal mucosa are unlikely to occur.

COMPLICATIONS

1. **Ulceration of the mucosa.** The nasogastric tube can cause ulcerations at the site of the mucosa where the tube is positioned. This complication does occur with the double-lumen (Salem sump) tube, contrary to what is commonly believed (44).
2. **Sinusitis.** Sinusitis has been described in patients after nasogastric intubation for prolonged periods (22, 32, 52, 122, 123).
3. **Esophageal stricture** (22, 49, 52, 122, 123).
4. **Laryngeal obstruction** (22, 49, 52, 122, 123).
5. **Otitis media** (22, 49, 52, 122, 123).
6. **Rupture of esophageal varices** (22, 49, 52, 122, 123). A nasogastric tube may induce pressure necrosis of the esophageal variceal wall, resulting in significant bleeding. It is unclear how long one may leave a nasogastric tube

in place in the presence of esophageal varices.

7. **Rupture of the esophagus or stomach** (21, 49, 52, 122, 123).
8. **Inability to remove the tube.** The tube may coil or knot within the esophagus or stomach distal to a stricture, resulting in inability to remove the tube. When this occurs and is secondary to a stricture, dilatation may be necessary to facilitate removal of the tube.
9. **Tracheoesophageal fistula.** A nasogastric tube passed along with a rigid cuffed endotracheal tube can induce tracheoesophageal fistulas (107).
10. **Perforation of the esophagus.** A nasogastric tube pushed hard during insertion can cause perforation of the esophagus and penetration into the pleural cavity and may actually drained a pleural effusion (60). This complication maybe compounded by an enlarged heart that deviates the esophagus to the left (60).
11. **Insertion of the nasogastric tube into the submucosa of the posterior pharynx** (87, 108), which may result in pneumomediastinum and subcutaneous emphysema.
12. **Passage of the nasogastric tube intracranially.** In normal patients as well as in patients with maxillofacial trauma, nasogastric tubes have been placed intracranially, usually with fatal consequences. This complication has been described by numerous authors (40, 45, 47, 105, 122, 123). To prevent it, gently perform nasogastric intubation with a well-lubricated tube. In patients with maxillofacial trauma, pass the tube only under direct visualization or orally with the aid of a Magill forceps (40, 45, 70, 122). Direct the tube posteriorly and *not superiorly* (60, 70, 123). The initial aspiration through the tube followed by insufflation of air with concurrent auscultation over the epigastrium is recommended to ascertain proper positioning. Some authors suggested that a chest radiograph be obtained in all patients after nasogastric or orogastric intubation (52). When intracranial insertion does occur, take the patient to the operating room, where the nasogastric tube can be removed under direct vision, allowing the neurosurgeon to deal immediately with the complications, particularly bleeding. Start the patient on high doses of broad-spectrum antibiotics once this complication is recognized (45).
13. **Misplacement.** Pneumonia, perforation of a bronchus, pulmonary hemorrhage, and pneumothorax as well as bronchopleural fistula have all resulted from insertion into or through a bronchus.
14. **Nasal hemorrhage.** In patients who are taking anticoagulants or who have coagulopathies, tumors, or infections of the nares, pass the tube through the oral route (70). In patients with a gastrointestinal bleed that is secondary to a coagulopathy, especially cirrhotics, instill cocaine in the nostril before insertion of the nasogastric tube. This will shrink the nasal membrane and facilitate passage with less bleeding, which may be significant in such patients. In patients with a history of esophageal varices or coagulopathies, insert the tube by spontaneous passage during swallowing rather than forcing it down.

Clogged Feeding Tubes

Clogged feeding tubes can be unclogged by using pancreatic enzyme (79). To prepare the pancreatic enzyme solution, crush one tablet of Viokase and one tablet of sodium bicarbonate (325 mg) and dissolve this in 5 mL of warm water.

First, attempt injecting warm water into the tube and clamping it for 5 minutes. If the tube fails to clear, instill the pancreatic enzyme solution and then clamp the tube for another 5 minutes. Then flush this mixture by using a 50-mL syringe. In previous studies, no cases of tube perforation were reported (79).

FOREIGN BODIES IN THE ESOPHAGUS

The esophagus is a muscular tube and has three areas of narrowing: the upper esophageal sphincter, the area of crossover of the aortic arch, which is in the mid-esophageal region, and the lower esophageal sphincter. In these areas, the majority of entrapped esophageal foreign bodies are found (110). A thorough medical history will define the nature of the foreign body and its probable location. Respiratory symptoms suggest that the foreign body is entrapped in the hypopharynx, trachea, a Zenker's diverticulum, or pyriform sinus. Although this is true for adults, children may have had months of chronic, nonspecific respiratory symptoms after ingestion, leading to significant delay in diagnosis (72). Drooling in any patient indicates a complete esophageal obstruction. Radiographs of appropriate anatomic areas are mandatory, as they may provide clues about the nature of the foreign body, its current location, and any complications (9, 72). Computed tomography (CT) scan for fish or chicken bones has been found to be superior to plain films (110). Objects that are sharp have a high incidence of esophageal perforation, and endoscopy is needed not only to remove the objects but also to examine for resultant injuries. Elongated objects or objects longer than 6 cm in children or 13 cm in adults also should be promptly removed endoscopically, as they have a high incidence of penetration and entrapment in the small bowel. Button batteries in the esophagus should be considered true emergencies and should be removed promptly endoscopically (110).

Impacted bolus of meat is a treacherous clinical situation; if the patient cannot handle his or her saliva, then the bolus must be removed. If the patient can handle the saliva, removal may be delayed by a few hours, hoping that the bolus will pass. However, the bolus should not be allowed to remain in the esophagus for longer than 12 hours, as complications may develop (120).

Foreign bodies in the esophagus are often removed by esophagoscopy. This procedure can sometimes be avoided by using the technique described by Campbell et al. (22). This technique requires a fluoroscopy table and a 16 French Foley catheter. This technique was used to remove foreign bodies in 98 children with no complications. It avoids the use of endoscopy, which in children requires general anesthesia. Before passage of the catheter, spray the oropharynx with a small amount of local anesthetic. Most younger patients require sufficient immobilization, which can be done by wrapping the child in a sheet. Preinflating the balloon with contrast material facilitates later fluoroscopic identification by rendering the balloon slightly radiopaque. Insert the full catheter orally. After the tip of the catheter is passed just beyond the foreign body, inflate the balloon with contrast material. Before removing the catheter, place the patient in a prone oblique position, and turn the fluoroscopic table to a relatively steep head-down position. Then withdraw the catheter from the esophagus with moderate, steady traction, and the balloon pulls the foreign body ahead of it (35). With the aid of gravity, the foreign body is pulled from the esophagus and will normally fall out of the mouth, slide down the table, and spill onto the floor. If steady traction fails to dislodge the foreign body, then intravenous glucagon, 0.05 mg/kg, may be considered to induce sufficient esophageal relaxation to permit successful extraction. The patient must have no respiratory distress or evidence of perforation. A complete obstruction will make passage of the catheter impossible. Patients with underlying esophageal pathology are not candidates for this method of removal (8). If this measure fails, refer the patient to an endoscopist.

Other modalities to remove foreign bodies from the esophagus include pushing the foreign body into the stomach with a bougie. The administration of an enzyme to digest a bolus, such as papain (Adolph's meat tenderizer) and gas-forming pellets, cause major complications and thus should be avoided. Esophageal foreign-body complications include mucosal scratches or abrasions as well as life-threatening complications such as perforation. The complications increase as the entrapment of a foreign body exceeds 24 hours (110). Complications reported from esophageal foreign bodies include the following:

- Mucosal scratches and abrasions
- Esophageal necrosis (button batteries)
- Esophageal stricture
- Esophageal perforation

An occult esophageal foreign body may not be suspected as the cause of the symptoms until it is shown on chest radiograph or a barium swallow of the esophagus. Removal of blunt esophageal foreign bodies by balloon extraction under fluoroscopic control is a safe and expeditious procedure and is a good alternative to endoscopy. Although Foley catheter extraction is a fast and inexpensive way to remove a foreign body, esophagoscopy remains the safest method, particularly in infants and children (74).

Postprocedural Considerations

Once foreign-body extraction has been accomplished, one should always consider a perforation of the esophagus if it has been a difficult procedure, and immediately do radiograph contrast studies if this is suspected (120). Remember that in children, foreign bodies in the esophagus are a common problem. The longer the foreign body remains in the esophagus, the greater the incidence of respiratory symptoms including cough, fever, and congestion, which may mimic croup or an upper respiratory infection (72, 74).

GASTRIC LAVAGE FOR HEMORRHAGE INTO THE UPPER GASTROINTESTINAL TRACT

Several types of double-lumen tubes for gastric lavage after hemorrhage have been discussed in the literature (6, 68, 76, 111). Each of these tubes, however, has a number of problems, including increased overall outside diameter, causing discomfort, and small outflow lumens on the sides of the tubes, which limit the passage of larger blood clots. In contrast, a system devised by Atkenson and Nyhus (6) seems to be optimal in these patients. This system minimizes the discomfort to the patient and allows rapid evacuation of the large clots, because of its substantially larger outflow lumen size.

TECHNIQUE

Pass two single-lumen tubes nasally. One is a size 18 French, which functions as an inflow tube and is connected to a room-temperature normal saline lavage solution (83). In the method of Atkenson and Nyhus, an enema bucket functioned for this purpose (Fig. 1.6). Another nasogastric tube, a 24 French, functions as an outflow tube (53). This tube should have three side holes cut out, and insert it through the other nostril and connect it to an emptying bag with dependent drainage at the patient's bedside. Connect a Toomey syringe to the outflow tube through a wide connecter for aspiration should the outflow tube stop draining (Fig. 1.6). Irrigation begins when the inflow of room-temperature normal saline solution occurs and breaks up the blood clots, allowing rapid movement of the clots out of the outflow tube (83). A grossly bloody and clot-laden return through the outflow tube rapidly clears as bleeding is brought under control. When this clearing occurs, the inflow tube is switched off, and siphoning begins. In this phase, residual saline solution draining from the stomach may mix with hemorrhaging blood, causing the outflow to change from pink to red. This rate of color

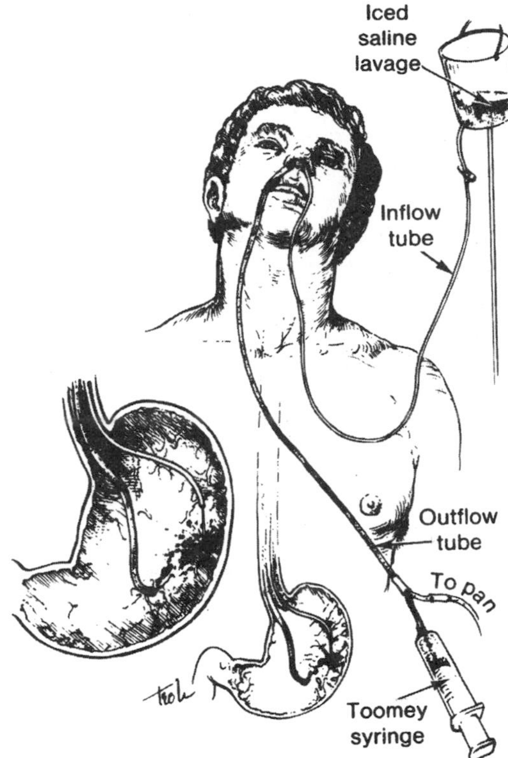

Figure 1.6. Flow of the iced saline solution occurs from the enema bucket, or iced saline lavage bag, through the inflow tube into the stomach. There, irrigation rates of up to 1 L/min break apart blood clots and prevent the collapse of the stomach around the outflow tube *(inset)*. The Toomey syringe is provided for the occasional clot that does not pass into and out of the outflow tube. (From Atkenson RJ, Nyhus LM: Gastric lavage for hemorrhage in the upper part of the gastrointestinal tract. Surg Gynecol Obstet 146:797, 1978, with permission.)

change is proportional to the rate of bleeding. If the outflow becomes red, the irrigation is started once again. This system requires much less nursing care than does the single-tube irrigation system that is commonly used. In the routine system, injections of 15-mL boluses and the frequently futile attempts to retrieve the injected fluid are avoided. In the system devised by Atkenson (4), nearly all the fluid is retrieved in the collecting system. Thus overdistention of the stomach, which may increase bleeding, is avoided.

NOTE

The effectiveness of Atkenson's water-sump irrigator is based on irrigation and simultaneous gravity drainage. Irrigation rates of up to 1 L/min can occur, breaking up clots and allowing gastric emptying. Outflow of clots and saline solution occurs at comparable rates. These rates never can be achieved by simple syringe irrigation or other techniques involving a single-lumen tube. With this technique, there is continuous irrigation of the stomach, avoiding the interruption of outflow by irrigating fluids in the conventional methods. There is no need for wall suction because the technique relies on the siphon principle and avoids adherence of the gastric mucosa to the portals of the nasogastric tube, which is a common problem obstructing outflow when wall suction is used.

It has been found that during lavage of the gastric contents, gentle palpation over the left upper quadrant to "massage" the stomach will achieve better mixing of the gastric contents with the lavage fluid and removal of these contents. This is particularly helpful with lavage for gastric emptying in an overdose patient (81).

SENGSTAKEN–BLAKEMORE BALLOON TAMPONADE

Portal hypertension is an increase in the portal vein pressure above the normal 5 to 10 mL of mercury. In the presence of portal hypertension, collateral venous circulation develops so as to decompress the high-pressure portal system into the low-pressure systemic circulation. Enlargement of hemorrhoidal plexuses and esophageal varices results from this collateralization. If esophageal variceal hemorrhage is untreated, the mortality rate is approximately 50% to 70% (98). In treated patients, 60% go on to have a second major bleed within 1 year. The goal in these patients is to identify and control the hemorrhage promptly and efficiently. Treatment options for acute variceal bleeding include vasopressin, which decreases portal venous pressure. Somatostatin, given in 250-mg boluses every 6 hours for 24 hours along with 250 mg for 48 hours, was shown to be an effective agent with the same degree of effectiveness as sclerotherapy in the short-term control of variceal bleeding with fewer side effects (83). Octreotide is a synthetic analogue of somatostatin with longer duration of action. Octreotide given as a continuous infusion at 25 mg per hour for 12 hours followed by subcutaneous injection of 100 mg every 6 hours was shown to be just as effective at short-term hemorrhage control as vasopressin with nitroglycerin, with fewer side effects (83). Sclerotherapy controls 80% to 90% of initial variceal bleeds, but rebleeding has occurred in anywhere from 2.9% to 66% at 2 years after sclerosis (98). "Balloon tamponade" is most useful today if bleeding continues despite pharmacologic therapy or sclerotherapy (98).

The Sengstaken–Blakemore tube is a triple-lumen tube that is used to control massive bleeding from esophageal varices. The three lumens are conduits for a gastric balloon, an esophageal balloon, and an accessory tube, essentially a simple nasogastric tube for drainage of gastric fluid. Since the introduction of this method for control of esophageal variceal bleeding, many articles have reported on the high incidence of complications, including death (28, 39). The complication rates reported range as high as 35% to 38% of cases, with death being reported in 22% and 18%, respectively (28). These complications are directly related to the tube itself. Other authors have reported a complication rate of 9.2% and have advocated the use of the balloon for control of variceal hemorrhage. One concluded that its use should be palliative and only for brief periods, pending definitive surgical intervention (28) when possible, although few such patients are acceptable candidates for surgery.

By far the most common method of inserting the tube is through the nose, similar to that used for insertion of a nasogastric tube. The size of the tube and the attached balloons make this difficult, even for those experienced in its use. Interestingly, those authors who use the nasal route also have the highest reported complication rates and fatalities (28, 39). The method advocated here is that of Pitcher (27, 100), whereby he reported the highest incidence of successful control of bleeding as well as the lowest incidence of complications by using the oral route.

INDICATION

Because of the high complication rate, the procedure should be reserved for those patients with proven unequivocal bleeding from esophageal varices in whom massive bleeding continues despite conservative therapy and/or in whom surgical intervention is impossible (28). Many physicians reserve use of the Sengstaken–Blakemore tube to patients with esophageal variceal hemorrhage who have been unresponsive to intravenous vasopressin.

EQUIPMENT

20 French Sengstaken–Blakemore tube (Davol, Inc., Providence, RI)
18 French plastic nasogastric tube and syringe
Two rubber-shod heavy surgical clamps
High-intermittent suction (Gomco)
Iced saline for irrigation
4 × 1/8-inch keyhole plywood retainer
1-inch adhesive tape
Mouthpiece
Manometer

TECHNIQUE

Preparatory Steps

1. Check the balloons for leaks.
2. Lubricate the tube well with viscous lidocaine (Xylocaine).
3. Anesthetize the pharynx with 10% cocaine solution in a spray.

4. Empty the stomach of blood clots and/or food before insertion of the tube (27, 100).
5. Refrigerate the tube to stiffen it and make it easier to pass (98).

NOTE

Nasogastric intubation is optimally performed after emergency endoscopy to verify whether bleeding is from esophageal varices. In this situation, the stomach is usually empty. If delay occurs between intubation and endoscopy and bleeding is brisk, lavage should be performed before intubation (100).

Procedural Steps

1. Place the patient in the left lateral decubitus position (100).
2. Insert the lubricated 20 French Sengstaken–Blakemore tube through the mouth until the gastric balloon is well within the stomach, usually by the 5-cm mark. When the stomach has been reached, blood can be aspirated. Instill 20 mL of air, and auscultate over the left upper quadrant to confirm that the tube is properly positioned (Fig. 1.7).
3. After the gastric tube is flushed with air, slowly inflatc thc gastric balloon with 250 to 275 mL of air while the clinician simultaneously auscultates over the epigastrium to ensure inflation of the gastric balloon and positioning of the gastric tube within the stomach and not the esophagus (100). One can usually auscultate the air being instilled into the balloon over the epigastrium.
4. Once the gastric balloon is inflated, double-clamp it with a rubber-shod heavy surgical clamp; apply firm traction manually at the mouth, and then connect the gastric-lumen inlet to high-intermittent suction (Gomco).

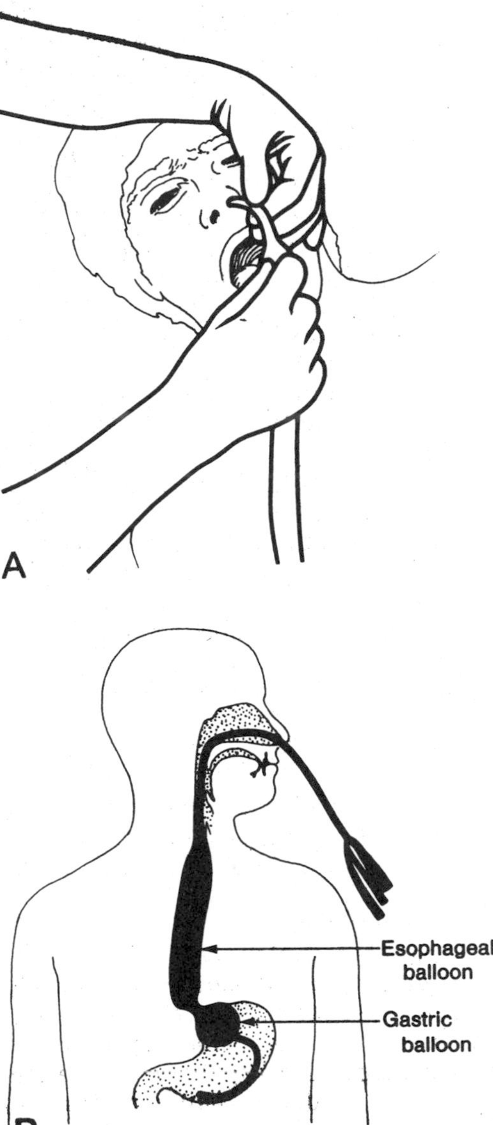

Figure 1.7. The placement of a Sengstaken–Blakemore tube. To pass the tube, fold the empty balloon around itself, and give the patient appropriate analgesia. *B:* The gastric and esophageal balloons are shown inflated in proper position. See text for details.

5. Lavage the stomach with copious amounts of room-temperature normal saline until the return is clear. If bleeding continues, inflate the esophageal balloon (83).

6. Inflate the esophageal balloon to a pressure of 25 to 45 mm Hg (this can be ascertained by using a simple manometer), with the lowest pressure that appears to control variceal bleeding, as determined by gastric lumen and accessory tube lavage (100). Double-clamp the esophageal lumen with a rubber-shod heavy surgical clamp, at the balloon pressure that stops the bleeding.
7. While maintaining firm traction on the Sengstaken–Blakemore tube, position a padded 4 × 1/8-inch keyhole plywood retainer around the tube at the angle of the mouth and hold it in place by strips of adhesive tape fixed to the retainer and tube. This maintains the traction on the gastric varices. Alternatively, use a catcher's mask or football helmet to secure the Sengstaken–Blakemore tube. The tube may easily be bitten through by an uncooperative, agitated patient (69). Insert a rubber mouthpiece and tape it into position with the retainer.
8. Switch suction on the accessory tube to low-intermittent.
9. After the esophageal balloon is inflated, insert a small nasogastric tube through the nose to check for bleeding proximal to the esophageal balloon and to remove secretions. The nasogastric tube usually extends from the top of the Sengstaken–Blakemore esophageal balloon to the mid-hypopharynx (100).
10. Continue inflation for 24 to 48 hours. Keep the head of the bed up to prevent hiccups and aspiration of vomitus.
11. Make subsequent radiographs to check the position of the balloon at 24-hour intervals or sooner, should the patient's status change because balloon displacement has been described (98).

NOTE

With this technique, variceal bleeding in up to 92% of patients can be safely controlled (100). Avoid overdistention of the gastric balloon by checking balloon pressure every 2 hours. If air is continually needed to maintain pressure, then suspect complications with the balloon. Check the balloon size with an anterior–posterior radiograph of the abdomen and add air only when there is a decrease in the balloon size by radiograph (89). Air is usually used for inflation of the balloon, even though some authors have used water. Water makes the tube heavy and increases the risk of pressure necrosis of the mucosa (69).

COMPLICATIONS

1. Completely empty the stomach to reduce pulmonary aspiration before passing the balloon.
2. **Difficult insertion.**
3. **Unintentional deflation or rupture** of one or both balloons.
4. **Inability to maintain constant traction** on the gastric or esophageal balloon as a result of improperly securing the catheter to the helmet or wood.
5. **Failure of the gastric balloon to deflate.** When this occurs, the tube may have to be cut to deflate the balloon.
6. **Persistent hiccups.**
7. **Cardiac arrhythmias.**
8. **Pulmonary edema** may occur as a result of pressure of the inflated esophageal and gastric balloons on mediastinal structures.
9. **Regurgitation and aspiration of gastric contents** during insertion and when the tube is in place. This can be prevented partially by placement of the nasogastric tube as indicated earlier.
10. **Dislodgement or herniation of the esophageal balloon,** causing airway obstruction (19, 28, 100). One must always keep a scissors at the bedside of a patient with a Sengstaken–Blakemore tube. If the esophageal balloon obstructs the airway, deflate it immediately by cutting the air inlet of the balloon.

11. **Pressure necrosis** at several levels along the tube: alae nasi (this is with nasal insertion of the tube), pharynx, esophagus, and stomach.
12. **Damage to the esophagus,** including laceration or rupture (19, 124).

ABDOMINAL STAB WOUND EXPLORATION

Abdominal stab wound exploration has been advocated by a number of authors (15, 115). Abdominal stab wound exploration combined with peritoneal lavage increases the diagnostic accuracy of peritoneal lavage. The incidence of negative laparotomies after peritoneal lavage when combined with local exploration to determine peritoneal penetration was 4% in one study involving 135 patients (114, 115, 118). Currently, a number of centers advocate observation in patients with abdominal stab wounds with or without penetration. In view of this, one may wonder why exploration of a stab wound to the abdomen is necessary. If the stab wound is explored, and penetration into the abdominal cavity is definitely ruled out, then the patient may be discharged from the emergency center with no further studies or observation necessary. In addition, wound exploration eliminates some patients with "an exaggerated response" to a superficial stab wound from going on to surgical intervention (103). When the stab wound penetrates the abdominal cavity, admit the patient to the hospital for observation and peritoneal lavage. In a number of cases, local exploration does not permit differentiation between penetration and non-penetration of the abdominal cavity; in this situation, observe the patient for signs of abdominal injury and perform peritoneal lavage (51).

TECHNIQUE

The technique of abdominal stab wound exploration is simple. With a no. 10 blade, extend the stab wound for 1 to 2 cm on each end (Fig. 1.8). Carefully dissect the stab wound through the fascia and the abdominal musculature and follow it to the abdominal fascia. If the fascia has been entered, then diagnose penetration into the abdominal cavity, and close the wound margins. To make exploration easier, insert an Angiocath into the stab wound before exploration, and inject a solution of methylene blue through the catheter (25). This may aid in visualizing the track of the stab wound and is preferred by us. Then close the stab wound primarily. In patients with grazing gunshot wounds to the abdomen in which peritoneal penetration is in question, use wound exploration in a similar fashion to ascertain penetration.

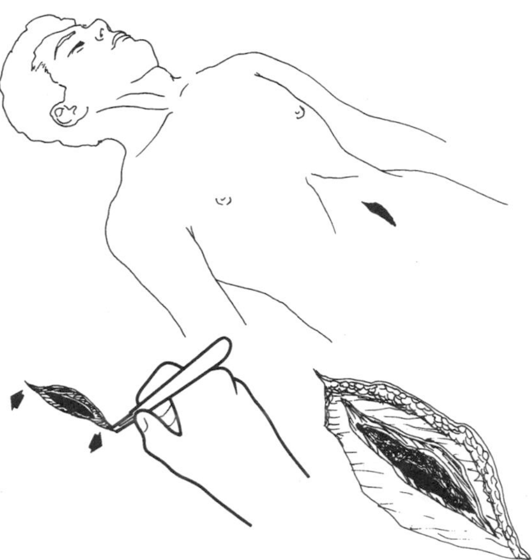

Figure 1.8. Abdominal stab wound exploration. See text for details.

PERITONEAL LAVAGE

To detect hemoperitoneum, peritoneal lavage is one of the most common procedures performed in the emergency center on the traumatized patient. Three techniques have been described in the literature, each of which has advantages and disadvantages, and all three are described and discussed here: insertion of the catheter through a midline incision, percutaneous insertion of a catheter, and insertion of the catheter through an infraumbilical incision (16). The accuracy of peritoneal lavage in detecting hemoperitoneum and the presence of significant abdominal injury has been reported variably by different authors. Some authors (3) have reported an accuracy rate of 97%, indicating significant intraabdominal injury, whereas others have reported a false-positive rate of 30% (107).

The problem that arises is deciding how much blood indicates a positive lavage. Olsen (93) divided patients with peritoneal lavage into three groups. In group 1, a strongly positive lavage indicating more than 25 mL of blood per liter of fluid was found to be associated with a 90% incidence of significant intraabdominal injury at laparotomy. In group 2, a negative lavage with no blood and no positive findings was associated with a very low incidence of significant intraabdominal injury. In group 3, lavage fluid that was weakly positive (eight drops to 15 mL of blood per liter) was associated with an incidence of significant intraabdominal injury of 32%. In interpreting the peritoneal lavage aspirate, place the intravenous tubing containing the returned lavage fluid over a newspaper. If the newspaper cannot be read through the tubing, this indicates a positive peritoneal lavage and correlates with a blood count of approximately 100,000 erythrocytes per milliliter of fluid. In addition, some authors reported that the presence of more than 500 leukocytes per milliliter of lavage fluid or the presence of more than 100 Somogyi units of amylase also is indicative of significant intraabdominal injury (99, 117). The significance of the white blood cell (WBC) count has been questioned by some. In one study, only 1 of 18 patients with more than 500 WBCs in the lavage fluid had significant intraabdominal injury (99).

INDICATIONS

A number of authors have verified the unreliability of physical examination in patients with blunt abdominal trauma in detecting significant intraabdominal injury. In one study, 40% of the patients who were thought to have surgically significant intraabdominal injury based on the initial physical examination were found to have no significant intraabdominal injury on laparotomy (71, 100). In this same study, there was a 6% incidence of false-negative examinations, believed to be due to the lack of release of intestinal contents into the peritoneal cavity, and only blood was present. Many patients with only blood in the peritoneal cavity have no findings on physical examination. It has been recommended that those patients who have a questionable peritoneal lavage should undergo abdominal ultrasound and arteriography (100). Any patient with significant abdominal injury who has abdominal pain, tenderness, rigidity, or distention should have peritoneal lavage (99). In a large series of more than 400 patients in which peritoneal lavage was performed in patients without evidence of abdominal injury but who had sustained significant trauma elsewhere, the following findings were reported (99): in patients with head injury with unconsciousness, 26% had positive peritoneal lavage; in those with unexplained hypotension, 42% had a positive lavage; in patients who had multiple-system injuries, 13% had a positive lavage. In this study, it was found that pelvic fractures and a decreasing hematocrit were not valid indications for peritoneal lavage (99). In children who sustained blunt abdominal injuries, physical examination has been documented to be very inexact. The indications for lavage in children are any evidence of abdominal signs or symptoms, altered sensorium, unexplained shock, major thoracic injuries, multiple-system injury, and major orthopedic injuries (such as a fractured pelvis, femur, or hip) (36).

Physical examination does not allow prompt and reliable assessment of intraabdominal injury from blunt trauma and was misleading in 45% of patients in one study (93). The role of peritoneal lavage for penetrating wounds of the abdomen has received little emphasis until recently, reflecting the former policy of exploring all patients with penetrating abdominal wounds (76). The incidence of organ injury in patients at Cook County Hospital (Chicago, Illinois) having sustained peritoneal penetration by a missile was 98.6% (76). At Detroit General Hospital (Detroit, Michigan), peritoneal lavage is performed in patients having sustained gunshot wounds of the abdomen in whom peritoneal penetration is questionable and in patients with hemothorax from stab or gunshot wounds to the lower thorax, especially the left side. In a recent study at Detroit General Hospital involving 135 patients with stab wounds to the lower chest and abdomen, it was concluded that chest wounds located between the two anterior axillary lines and below the fifth rib and all abdominal wounds are indications for peritoneal lavage, even when an abdominal examination is negative (115). With abdominal wounds, if the physical examination was negative and the stab wound was located between the two anterior axillary lines, local exploration of the stab wound was performed and was followed by peritoneal lavage if the exploration indicated peritoneal penetration. If the exploration revealed no penetration to the peritoneal cavity, the patient was observed. If the lavage was positive in those with penetration, the patient underwent surgery. In this study, 70% of patients were spared an unnecessary operation (115). The incidence of negative laparotomy was reduced to 4.0%, and it was concluded that the combination of local exploration and peritoneal lavage increased the diagnostic accuracy and decreased the incidence of negative laparotomies in patients with abdominal stab wounds (113). In another study involving 72 adults experiencing stab wounds in the abdomen that violated the anterior fascia, 11% of the patients underwent immediate celiotomy because of shock or peritonitis. Nine percent underwent celiotomy because previous extensive abdominal operations prohibited the use of paracentesis or a diagnostic peritoneal lavage (DPL), and 79% underwent paracentesis and DPL. In this series, approximately one third of the patients with fascial penetration had no injury found on exploratory celiotomy (103). Remember that a negative physical examination is associated with a 23% incidence of positive laparotomy in abdominal stab wounds (15). A negative lavage can occur with significant abdominal injuries that do not produce hemoperitoneum, including retroperitoneal injuries to the pancreas, great vessels, duodenum, and rectosigmoid and subcapsular injuries to the liver and spleen; even transection may not produce sufficient hemoperitoneum to cause a positive lavage (93).

Peritoneal lavage also has been used to diagnose acute pancreatitis in patients with a normal amylase level, because an elevated level will persist within the peritoneal fluid for 3 to 5 days after pancreatitis (81). Primary peritonitis also may be diagnosed by finding pneumococci or staphylococci. Intestinal flora and debris found on a Gram stain of the sediment of the lavage may signify perforation of the gastrointestinal tract (93).

CONTRAINDICATIONS

The following are contraindications to the use of peritoneal lavage:

1. Multiple previous abdominal operations (66).

NOTE

In the patient who has a midline scar in the infraumbilical region, make a midline incision above the umbilicus to introduce the catheter for a lavage. Alternatively, make an incision lateral to the rectus abdominis muscles, and introduce the catheter into the peritoneal cavity under direct vision to avoid adhesions. Make the supraumbilical incision approximately 3 to 4 cm above the umbilicus in the midline, by using the same technique as is described in the cutdown approach, with direct visualization of the peritoneum. When using an incision lateral to the rectus abdominis muscles, place the incision at the lateral border of the rectus abdominis muscle on the side selected (opposite the scar of the previous surgery, e.g., appendectomy). Here also, use a direct cutdown approach, with the same technique and length of incision as is described later.

---

2. Peritoneal lavage is contraindicated in the pregnant patient (97). It is unclear whether peritoneal lavage is contraindicated in the first trimester.
3. In the unstable patient requiring immediate surgical intervention, peritoneal lavage is not indicated (97).
4. Inability to catheterize bladder (here the cutdown approach is not contraindicated).
5. In patients with a coagulation defect, lavage is not contraindicated. In a large study involving 298 patients, it was found that the patients with a preexisting coagulopathy had the same incidence of false positives as did those patients without coagulopathy. The technique used was the open technique for lavage. Thus DPL does not mandate coagulation screening of any sort (10).

EQUIPMENT

The equipment necessary will depend on whether the incisional technique is used or the percutaneous puncture technique is selected.

Standard peritoneal dialysis catheter and trocar
20-mL syringe
Four mosquito hemostats
No. 11 blade
Suture material: 4-0 silk, 4-0 Vicryl, 5-0 nylon
Scissors
Adhesive tape
Local anesthetic: 1% lidocaine with epinephrine
Povidone–iodine (Betadine) solution for preparation
Shaver
5-mL syringe
18-gauge and 25-gauge 1.5-inch needles
Standard intravenous tubing with an extension tube
Needle holder
4 × 4-inch gauze pads

TECHNIQUE

Before this procedure is performed, when possible, make an upright or left lateral decubitus abdominal radiograph of the patient to exclude free air. During peritoneal lavage, introduced air may produce a false-positive finding of free air under the diaphragm. In this section, three techniques are described and discussed with regard to their advantages and disadvantages.

MIDLINE INCISION TECHNIQUE (3, 7, 11, 21, 23, 52, 56)

Preparatory Steps

1. Place the patient in the supine position.
2. Catheterize and empty the urinary bladder even if patient has voided.
3. Shave the area between the symphysis pubis and the umbilicus in the midline.
4. Prepare the shaved area with povidone–iodine solution and drape.
5. In the average adult, anesthetize an area 6 cm long, below the umbilicus in the midline. In the smaller patient, the area that should be anesthetized is one third of the distance between the umbilicus and the symphysis pubis. Extend the area of anesthesia approximately 3 cm.

Procedural Steps

1. Make a 3-cm vertical midline incision approximately 3 cm below the umbilicus. The incision must remain in the midline and should be carried down

to the linea alba. Ligate any bleeders encountered in the subcutaneous tissue. Place a self-retaining retractor as one carries the dissection down to the linea alba. In performing lavage with the open technique, one will commonly encounter muscle fibers that seem to cross the linea alba. If you are in the midline, go through these fibers and encounter the fascia of the linea alba. After going through the fascia, you will encounter a preperitoneal fat layer. Go through this top layer to reach the peritoneum. Remember that the preperitoneal fat layer will lie underneath the fascia. A common mistake is to think that this preperitoneal fat is intraperitoneal fat.

NOTE

This method offers the advantage of being able to visualize the peritoneum directly and to avoid perforation into a viscus by the trocar or catheter (3). In the patient who has had previous surgery in the lower abdomen, one can safely do the lavage through an upper midline incision 2 to 3 cm above the umbilicus (97).

---

2. After visualization of the peritoneum, pick up the fascia of the abdomen along the linea alba with two small hemostats (Fig. 1.9).
3. An assistant should lift up the hemostats; make a small 2-mm incision between the hemostats with a no. 11 blade. The peritoneum thus is visualized and opened.
4. Insert a standard peritoneal dialysis catheter through the incision, directing the catheter toward the pelvis until all the side holes are within the abdominal cavity (Fig. 1.10). Remove the trocar that comes with the catheter before insertion. Some authors prefer to direct the peritoneal dialysis catheter away from the midline so as to avoid the shallowest area of the abdomen (20).
5. Aspirate the catheter with a 20-mL syringe to ascertain whether there is any free blood in the abdominal cavity. If 20 mL of blood is withdrawn, the test is considered positive, and the procedure is concluded. If less than 20 mL of blood is withdrawn, infuse 1 L of Ringer's lactate solution through the catheter in the average adult. This infusion should be done rapidly.

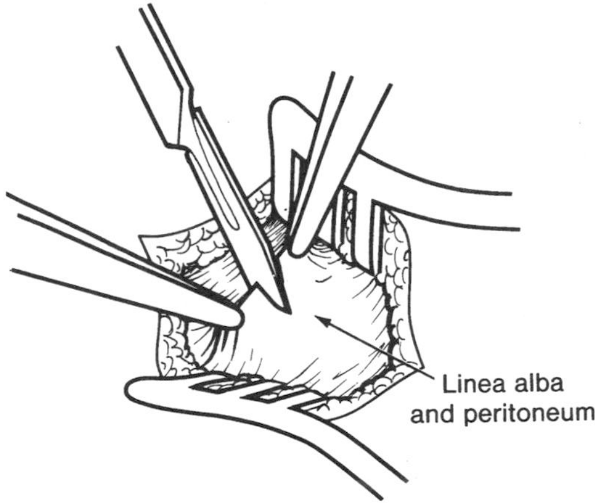

Figure 1.9. Make an incision between two hemostats that pick up the peritoneum and fascia as shown. See text for details.

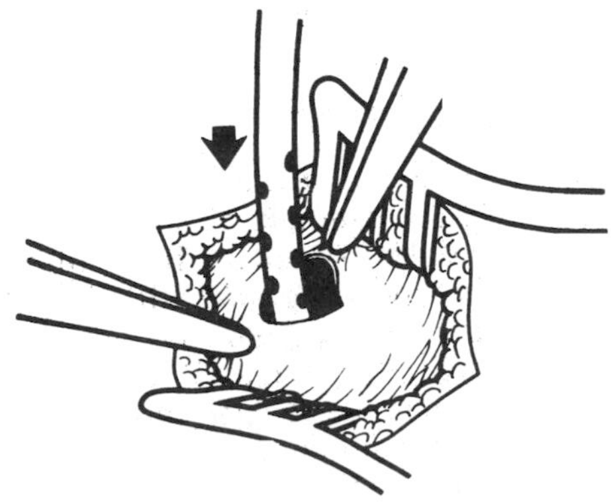

Figure 1.10. Pass a catheter through a 2-cm incision and direct it toward the pelvis. See text for details.

6. Shift the patient briefly from one side to the other as the clinical condition permits (36, 93, 97, 102).
7. Now place the infusion bottle on the floor to permit the fluid to return to the bottle. A positive lavage is defined as an inability to read a newspaper through the lavage fluid, which correlates with significant intraabdominal injury and allows early operative intervention (76). Usually, approximately 90% of the lavage fluid is recoverable (102).

NOTE

If the lavage is equivocal and signs and symptoms of abdominal injury are present, leave a catheter in place and suture the wound; repeat the lavage in 2 to 3 hours to determine whether it changes to a positive test (37). Send an aliquot of the lavage fluid for leukocyte count and amylase level as well as Gram stain of the sediment, if so desired (99).

Aftercare

1. Remove the catheter, and place a single suture of silk in the fascia of the abdominal wall.
2. Close the subcutaneous tissue and skin, and dress the wound.

Peritoneal Lavage in Children

In children, the preferred technique is the incisional method, using a small vertical infraumbilical midline incision approximately one third of the way between the umbilicus and the symphysis pubis. Sedate the child, and place the catheter in the peritoneal cavity under direct vision after dissection down to the peritoneum. After the bladder is empty, and following essentially the same procedures as described earlier, direct the catheter toward the pelvis. In a child, the test is considered positive if more than 10 mL of blood is returned before lavaging. If not, administer 15 to 20 mL of Ringer's lactate per kilogram of body weight into the peritoneal cavity (36, 37, 97). Turn the child gently from side to side if the condition permits, and perform the remainder of the examination similar to that in the adult.

NOTE

The criticism raised for the incisional method of peritoneal lavage is that this technique is essentially a minilaparotomy (65, 66). In addition, in the obese patient, the cutdown technique may be quite difficult, and significant bleeding may be encountered and may lead to a false-positive lavage (14).

PERCUTANEOUS TECHNIQUE (36, 37, 50, 60)

Preparatory Steps

1. Select a point in the lower midline approximately 2 to 3 cm below the umbilicus.
2. Decompress the urinary bladder in the routine fashion.
3. Cleanse the skin and prepare with iodinated antiseptic solution (povidone–iodine) after shaving a small area at the puncture site.
4. Raise a wheal with 1% lidocaine at the puncture site.

Procedural Steps

1. Make a stab wound in the skin with a no. 11 blade, and obtain hemostasis with local pressure.
2. Insert a standard peritoneal dialysis catheter attached to a trocar through the puncture site. The optimal method of inserting the catheter to avoid puncturing a viscus with the trocar is as follows:
   a. Rotate the trocar and advance it to the linea alba. A firm resistance will be felt at this point.

b. Place the index finger and thumb of the left hand around the trocar and catheter at the puncture site, holding it firmly (Fig. 1.11). Angulate the trocar at approximately 60 degrees inferiorly toward the pelvis.
c. Instruct the patient (if able) to raise his or her head, tensing the abdominal musculature and thus permitting easier introduction of the trocar.
d. With a back-and-forth rotary motion with the left hand and firm pressure on the trocar applied with the right hand, advance the trocar through the fascia. While this is done, the index finger and thumb of the left hand guard against passage of the trocar beyond the fascia and hold the trocar firmly, preventing further advancement once a "give" is felt and the trocar has entered into the peritoneal cavity.

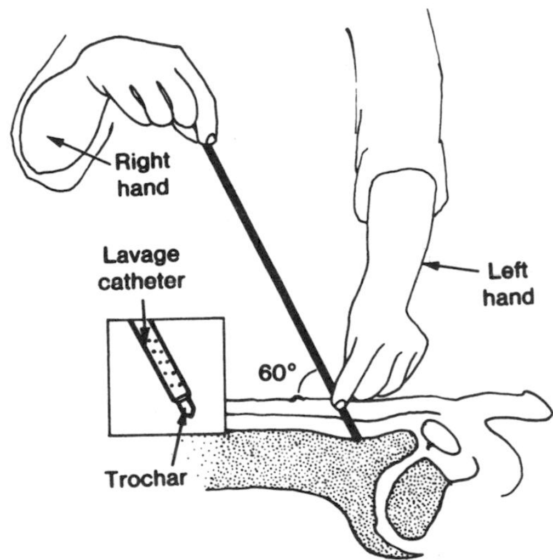

Figure 1.11. With the percutaneous approach, hold the trocar with the index finger and thumb of the left hand *(inset)* and resist the pressure applied by the right hand, thus preventing penetration too deeply into the peritoneal cavity. Apply a rotary motion by the right hand to pass the trocar. The angle of penetration is 60 degrees. After the trocar is inserted, pass the lavage catheter over it into the peritoneal cavity *(inset)*.

NOTE

With this technique of introducing the trocar, we have not had a single instance of viscus injury from the trocar. Most of the complications listed later are secondary to inadvertent advancement of the trocar too deeply into the peritoneal cavity as a result of "uncontrolled introduction."

---

3. Once the trocar has been introduced, advance the catheter into the peritoneal cavity over the trocar, and remove the trocar (Fig. 1.11, *inset*).
4. Aspirate for blood and, if none is present, introduce 1 L of saline over a 5- to 10-minute period, as indicated earlier (Fig. 1.12).
5. Turn the patient from side to side to disperse the fluid in the peritoneal cavity (93, 94, 116). This should not be done, however, in the presence of a pelvic fracture (116).
6. Place the bottle on the floor, and allow the abdominal cavity to drain into it. The criteria for a positive lavage are similar to those discussed earlier.

Umbilical Approach

NOTE

Most authors used either the percutaneous insertion technique in the midline or the incision methods already described. A number of complications have been reported with each of these two procedures. A technique has been described using an umbilical incision over the inferior portion of the umbilical ring. Fibrous changes within the vessels of the umbilical cord and urachus form a scar that draws against the superior circumference of the umbilical ring, and retraction

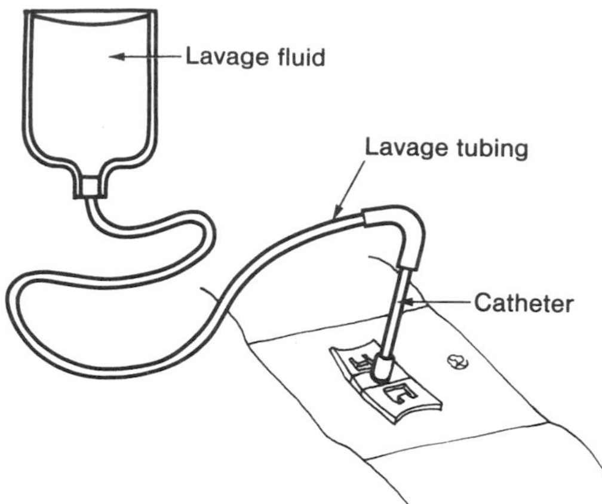

Figure 1.12. Then attach the lavage catheter to the tubing and the bag of lavage fluid, as shown.

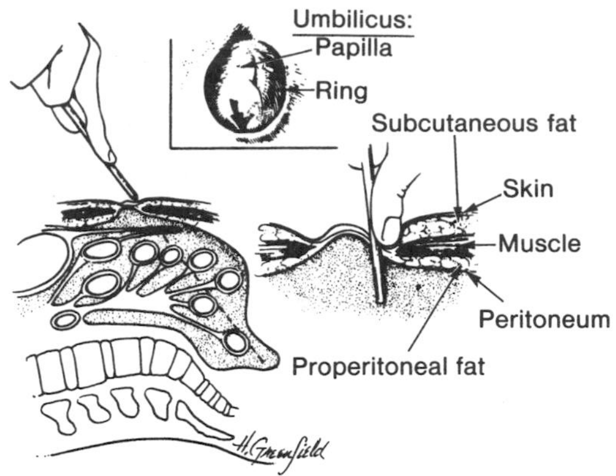

Figure 1.13. Technique of diagnostic peritoneal lavage performed by percutaneous insertion through the inferior portion of the umbilical ring. See text for details. *Inset* shows the anatomy of the umbilicus with the *arrow* demonstrating the precise location of the puncture. (From Slavin S: A new technique for diagnostic peritoneal lavage. Surg Gynecol Obstet 146:447, 1978, with permission.)

occurs around the umbilical vein. A similar scar forms inferiorly by fibrosis of the two arteries and urachus, which are likewise obliterated. The inferior adhesion is more dense and adherent than the superior one. A central papilla is surrounded by a circular bulge created by subcutaneous fat. Between these two areas lies a circular or elliptical depression that is free of subcutaneous fat; here the skin is quite thin and fused directly to the ring margins and is adherent to the underlying peritoneum (107).

TECHNIQUE

Decompress the urinary bladder and prepare and drape as in the routine fashion. Raise a skin wheal in the inferior portion of the umbilical ring. The area of incision is not infraumbilical but rather is in the inferior portion of the umbilical ring itself, which is formed by the umbilical papilla centrally in the umbilicus and a circular bulge made by the presence of subcutaneous fat (Fig. 1.13). Between these two areas is a depression of fat, and this is the ring over which the incision is made. Incise the ring with a no. 11 blade, and introduce a standard dialysis catheter, advancing the trocar grasped as indicated earlier to provide good control of the catheter and trocar. Once the catheter is inserted, remove the trocar immediately, and advance the catheter toward the pelvis. After aspirating for blood, instill 1 L of saline, and follow the same procedures as for the percutaneous method. Slavin (107) stated that in a small number of cases reported, there were no false positives or false negatives in the peritoneal lavage and no complications with this technique.

ALTERNATE TECHNIQUE

A method has been described using a sharp needle and a guidewire to introduce the catheter; this technique has been associated with a lower incidence of complications than the incidence with the standard percutaneous technique.

Make a 3-mm vertical skin incision with a no. 11 blade inferior to the umbilicus in the midline after adequate preparation and anesthesia. Make a 3-mm vertical skin incision with a no. 11 blade over the puncture side. Introduce an 18-gauge needle through the incision and carefully into the peritoneal cavity. Once the linea alba is penetrated, advance the needle an additional 2 to 3 mm, and introduce the floppy end of a guidewire through the needle. Once the guidewire moves freely within the abdominal cavity, introduce a 9 French catheter over the guidewire with a twisting and pushing motion so that it will penetrate the fascia. After this, remove the guidewire, and aspirate the catheter; if the aspiration is negative, introduce 1 L of fluid. The remainder of this procedure is similar to that described earlier (65, 66).

For a comparison between open and closed peritoneal lavage techniques, grossly positive lavages required a range of between 1 and 30 minutes to perform in the open group, whereas percutaneous DPL took between 1 and 12 minutes to perform (31). One potential disadvantage of the percutaneous method is that the return of fluid is usually slower and may be suboptimal (31).

COMPLICATIONS

The complication rate of peritoneal lavage varies from 1% to 6% (65). A number of complications have been reported in the literature.

1. **Bleeding within the rectus sheath** with a false-positive result (65, 107).
2. **Bleeding at the puncture site** with a false-positive result (107).
3. **Infusion of the lavage fluid into the abdominal wall** (80).
4. **Lack of fluid return.** This is not an uncommon problem. When only a portion of the fluid returns, one must analyze that portion that is obtained. The remainder will be absorbed by the peritoneum. When there is no fluid return, the catheter may be withdrawn slightly, or the patient may be turned, once again from side to side. This may result in return of lavage fluid into the drainage bag. Alternatively, the patient may be placed in 10 to 15 degrees of reverse Trendelenburg position, which may result in drainage through the catheter if the catheter has been placed in the pelvis. Finally, if none of these has worked, an additional 500 mL of fluid may be instilled, which may promote drainage through the catheter.
5. **Laceration of the mesenteric vessels, iliac artery, or vein** (65, 99, 107).
6. **Perforation of the small intestine or colon** (65, 99, 107). As the catheter and trocar pass through the abdominal wall, remove the trocar as soon as the peritoneum is pierced; otherwise, visceral or vessel perforation occurs.
7. **Inadvertent entry into the mesentery or retroperitoneal space** (14). This occurs more commonly with the percutaneous technique, as do any of the visceral or vessel injuries indicated earlier. This can be prevented by using the technique indicated earlier for introducing the trocar.
8. **Penetration of the bladder** (65, 107). Always empty the bladder before insertion of the catheter to prevent this complication. Inability to drain the bladder is a contraindication to this procedure.
9. **Incisional hernia** (65).
10. **Wound infection** (65).
11. **Wound separation** (65).

In a study undertaken to determine the accuracy of DPL for the evaluation of intraabdominal injury in patients with pelvic fractures after blunt trauma, DPL had a positive predictive value of 98% and a negative predictive value of 97% (86).

Because intraabdominal injuries and blunt trauma are frequently occult and can be fatal, early identification of the injury is critical for effective management (85). With the introduction of abdominal CT, the use of DPL in many institutions has been relegated to the assessment of hemodynamically unstable patients. Ultrasound was introduced as a diagnostic modality for blunt abdominal trauma

(33). In one study of 1,182 adult trauma patients, data presented demonstrated the advantages of DPL over CT in the evaluation of blunt abdominal trauma in patients with multiple injuries (11). Although CT has greatly enhanced the noninvasive evaluation of a blunt trauma patient, the speed, efficiency, and reduced cost of DPL continue to justify its use in the workup of patients with blunt abdominal trauma (11). In one study comparing DPL with CT, it was found that the evaluation with DPL required less time (41 minutes versus 2.5 hours) (84). There were no missed injuries in the DPL group; however, there were 7% of missed injuries in the abdominal CT group (85). The selective use of abdominal CT would have two beneficial effects. First, abdominal CT could identify those patients with a positive DPL who could be safely observed, and thus reduce the nontherapeutic celiotomy rate. Second, using abdominal CT only in patients with a positive screening DPL would reduce the overall use of a costly CT (85).

More recently, ultrasonography has been advocated as a modality. Sonography has advantages in that it is less costly, can be done at the bedside, and is readily available. It is also noninvasive (82). The use of sonography focuses on the detection of free fluid but includes an evaluation of parenchymal organs for injury. The sensitivity of ultrasonography in detecting free fluid in comparison with CT, DPL, and surgery is 63%. Specificity is 95% (82). In another study comparing abdominal ultrasound and DPL, it was found that the overall sensitivity and specificity of abdominal ultrasound were 82% and 99%, respectively (7). One must consider that there are no reported complications of ultrasonography, whereas DPL has a reported complication rate of approximately 1% (33). Another alternative approach in a patient with a positive DPL after blunt abdominal trauma is to use diagnostic laparoscopy. This is clearly less invasive than laparotomy, and with minor injuries such as grade I liver and splenic lacerations, a conservative approach can be adopted (7).

SIGMOIDOSCOPY

Sigmoidoscopic examination of the rectum and sigmoid colon is a very useful procedure that unfortunately is not used as often as it should be in the emergency center.

INDICATIONS

1. Sigmoid volvulus. In a patient with large bowel obstruction in whom one suspects sigmoid volvulus, sigmoidoscopy can be performed for both diagnostic and therapeutic purposes.
2. Gastrointestinal hemorrhage, when the nasogastric lavage does not demonstrate a cause proximally.
3. Laparotomy should be used only as a last resort for removal of a foreign body of the rectum (42).
4. Purulent or mucoid discharge from the anal canal.
5. Recurrent diarrhea lasting for several days.
6. Undifferentiated pain in the anoperineal region or lower abdomen.

CONTRAINDICATIONS

1. An uncooperative, agitated patient.
2. Patients with obstruction in the rectum prohibiting advancement of the sigmoidoscope.
3. Myocardial infarction is not an absolute contraindication to sigmoidoscopy and is considered useful in a medically stable patient with significant gastrointestinal bleeding (23).

EQUIPMENT

Sigmoidoscope and obturator. Sigmoidoscopes come in various sizes; usually the length is 25 cm

A long metal suction device

Cotton swabs on a long applicator

An insufflation bag and tubing to dilate the rectum

A good suction source such as a Venturi-type adapter that can be connected to a water faucet or other dependable, powerful suction apparatus

An electrical light source

TECHNIQUE

Preparatory Steps

1. Prepare the bowel. To empty the lower rectum, administer a nonirritating enema such as tap water 30 minutes to 1 hour before sigmoidoscopy is performed. Exercise caution in patients with colitis. In patients with sigmoid volvulus, severe gastrointestinal hemorrhage, or perianal abscess, preparation of the bowel is not necessary. In a trial comparing three methods of bowel preparation for a flexible sigmoidoscopy, a single hyper-phosphate enema 1 and then 2 hours before the procedure, preceded by a 290-mL bottle of magnesium citrate taken p.o. the night before, was found to enable the procedure to have a good to excellent result, with deeper insertion with procedures requiring a repeated performance (95).
2. Position the patient. When the procedure is performed at the bedside, the left lateral Sims' position is preferred with left knee flexed and right knee extended (Fig 1.14*A*). The pelvis should be at or beyond the edge of the table. Optimally the patient should be in Trendelenburg in the knee–chest position. A special table is available for this procedure, and the jackknife position is preferred when such a table is available in the emergency center (Fig. 1.14*B*). Sedation is usually not necessary.
3. Examine the perianal and buttocks area for any lesions. Ask the patient to strain to see if there is any prolapse of the mucosa or internal hemorrhoids. After this, perform a rectal examination to ascertain any lesions before introducing the sigmoidoscope, to relax the sphincter before the procedure, and to ensure patency of the anal canal.
4. Insert the obturator into the sigmoidoscope and lubricate the tip.

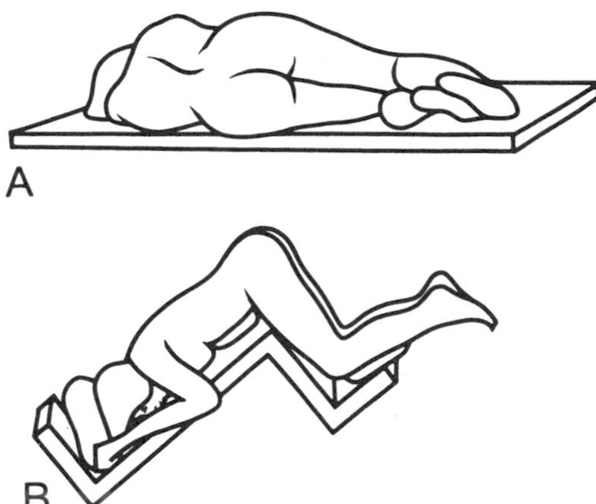

Figure 1.14. Two positions for performing sigmoidoscopy in the adult. *A:* The knee–chest position with the left knee and hip flexed and the right knee and hip slightly extended. This position is used on the examining table in the emergency center. When a sigmoidoscopy table is available, as shown in *B*, this is preferred.

Procedural Steps

1. Insert the sigmoidoscope into the rectum, aiming it anteriorly in the direction of the umbilicus (Fig. 1.15,*1*). Direct the sigmoidoscope in the midline and insert it into the anus with gentle and firm pressure.
2. Remove the obturator when the scope has been passed 4 cm into the canal (Fig. 1.16*A*). After removal of the obturator, visualize the anal mucosa, and suction fluid and fecal material (Fig. 1.16*B* and *C*).
3. Secure a glass covering over the end of the sigmoidoscope, and attach the insufflator and electric light source (Fig. 1.16*C*).
4. *Advance the sigmoidoscope into the bowel lumen only under direct vision* (Fig. 1.16*C*). The insufflation of air

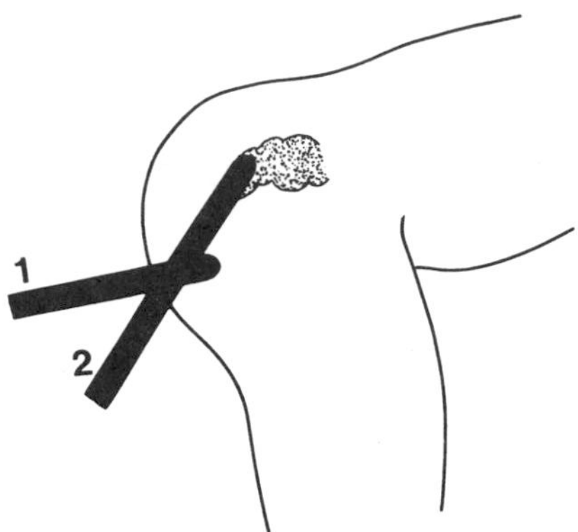

Figure 1.15. In passing the sigmoidoscope into the anus and anal canal, aim it first toward the umbilicus *(1)*. After the anal canal is passed, direct the sigmoidoscope posteriorly *(2)*. See text for details.

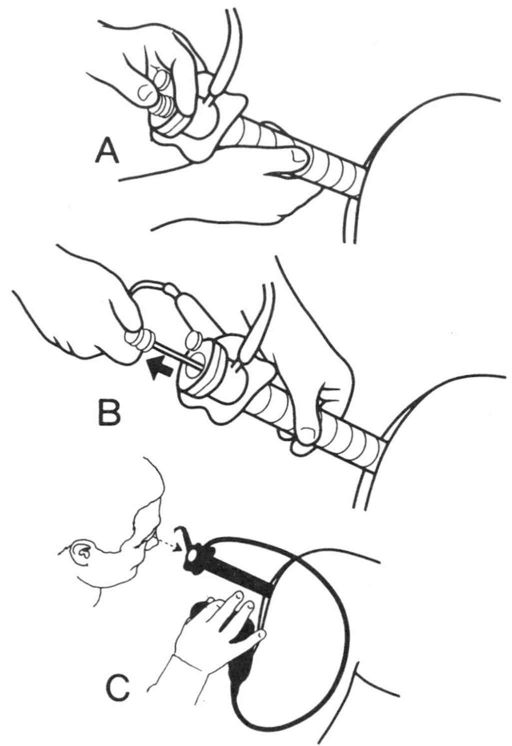

Figure 1.16. *A:* Remove the obturator so that direct visualization can be performed when passing the sigmoidoscope. *B:* Use a suction catheter to suction out secretions and fecal material during passage of the tube. *C:* Periodic insufflation of the rectum and sigmoid will permit direct visualization of the canal and aid in passage of the tube. See text for full discussion.

dilates the rectal lumen, facilitating identification of the mucosal structures, and aids in passing the scope. However, it also increases the risk of perforation.

5. After passing through the anal canal, direct the sigmoidoscope posteriorly (Fig. 1.15,*2*), keeping the sigmoidoscope in the midline toward the hollow of the sacrum. If resistance is met, withdraw slightly and visualize the lumen, and then pass the sigmoidoscope, instilling only small amounts of air to aid in visualizing the lumen. If the patient notes that the rectum has become uncomfortable, remove the glass shield, permitting air under pressure to be released.
6. At approximately 10 to 12 cm, the rectosigmoid junction is encountered, and the bowel angulates. At this point, direct the sigmoidoscope anteriorly and to the left side. One may encounter difficulty in passage of the instrument should acute angulation be present.

NOTE

In patients with diverticulitis, it is often impossible to advance the scope beyond 15 cm because of pain. In some patients, the angulation of the rectosigmoid juncture is so acute that one is unable to advance the scope beyond this point. Identify the sigmoid colon by its transverse folds, in contrast to the smooth mucosa of the rectum.

In patients with a sigmoid volvulus, the mucosa at the site of the obstruction may be sloughed or have ulcerations with dark blood noted. If this is not seen in a patient with a sigmoid volvulus and if obstruction is met at the site of the volvulus, then advance a soft rubber tube that is well lubricated through the obstructed segment, thus permitting decompression and rapid and often explosive passage of air and liquid. Caution must be exercised in doing so because the examiner may be sprayed with this material. Then remove the sigmoidoscope, and tape the rectal tube to the buttocks. Leave the rectal tube in place for several days until bowel function returns to normal.

---

7. When the sigmoidoscope has been inserted to its maximal extent, withdraw it, and perform careful inspection. This is best done with frequent insufflations of small amounts of air to separate the bowel walls and with aspiration of any fluid and feces or wiping the area with cotton swabs.

Because an inadequately processed fiberoptic endoscope leaves a significant bacterial load, it is important that certain aspects of the processing be mentioned: (a) cleaning, (b) disinfection, (c) rinsing, (d) drying, and (e) storage (59).

COMPLICATIONS

1. **Perforation.** Perforation may occur at the antimesenteric border. This occurs most frequently at the rectosigmoid junction at approximately 15 cm as a result of overzealous advancement of the sigmoidoscope. Perforation may be noted by a sudden "give" during sigmoidoscopy or by visualizing bowel serosa. Look for any evidence of peritonitis. Take an upright abdominal radiograph in all patients with suspected perforation after sigmoidoscopic examination to exclude this complication. Exercise extreme caution in performing sigmoidoscopic examination in the patient with colitis or inflammatory bowel disease, because perforation is most likely to occur in inflamed bowel.
2. **Trauma to the mucosa** after instrumentation.
3. **Bacteremia.** Bacteremia has been found to occur in 8% to 10% of all patients undergoing sigmoidoscopic examination.
4. **Bursting of a thin-walled sigmoid colon or rectum** as a result of excessive insufflation of air.

Rigid video-sigmoidoscopy has been compared with conventional sigmoidoscopy. It has been found that the examination is actually easier to do, particularly in women, and allows a visual record of the findings. It has been concluded that because the tube is thinner and longer, it allows a more effective means of looking at the proximal sigmoid colon, and despite being inserted farther, it causes less discomfort than conventional sigmoidoscopy (112).

ANOSCOPY

Anorectal symptoms are very common and are the primary reason for more than 1,000 physician visits per 100,000 patients (84). The rectum is approximately 15 cm long and extends approximately from the pectinate line to the sigmoid. The anal canal extends from the pectinate line distally and is approximately 3.5 cm long. An anoscope is a short instrument with an obturator that is used to examine the anal canal and distal aspect of the rectum. This procedure can be done without any bowel preparation or enema. The procedure is quite useful in examining the patient with suspected hemorrhoids, fistulas, and other lesions involving the anus.

TECHNIQUE

Always perform a digital rectal examination before anoscopy (see Sigmoidoscopy, earlier). Place the patient in the lateral decubitus position. Insert a well-lubricated anoscope gently into the anus. Direct the anoscope gently toward the midline anteriorly, following the direction of the anal canal. While the anoscope is being advanced, hold the obturator in place with thumb until the instrument is fully inserted. After the anoscope is fully inserted, remove the obturator. Rotate the anoscope through a 360-degree arc to inspect all the areas of the anus circumferentially as the instrument is withdrawn. Illumination is provided by an ordinary flashlight or a gooseneck lamp. Cotton swabs on a forceps may be necessary to clean the area. As the instrument is withdrawn, check for hemorrhoids, polyps, fistulas, or other lesions of the anal canal causing the patient's symptoms.

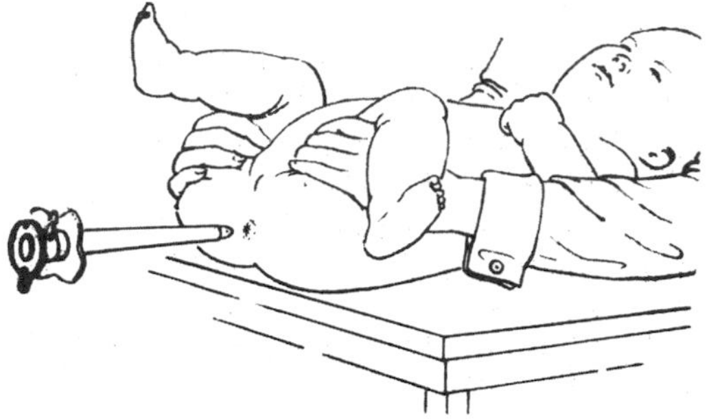

Figure 1.17. Position for proctoscopy for small infants. (From Hijmans J: Proctoscopy of the infant. Am J Dis Child 105:298, 1963, with permission.)

Proctoscopy in the Infant (33)

Proctoscopic examination is not commonly performed in the infant, but it can be quite useful in ascertaining the cause of symptoms referred to this area.

INDICATIONS

1. Prolonged or unexplained diarrhea.
2. Passage of bloody stools, pus, or mucus.
3. Abdominal pain of unknown etiology.
4. Perineal fistulas of abscesses.
5. Imperforate anus.

EQUIPMENT

The anoscope comes in various sizes, and one should have an anoscope with an outer diameter of approximately 1 cm and a length of 8 to 10 cm for the newborn and one with a diameter of 1.5 cm and a length of 12 to 25 cm for the older infant and child (54).

TECHNIQUE

1. Position the infant on the back (Fig. 1.17). A nurse puts his or her forearms alongside the child's body and grasps the thighs of the infant with his or her hands. He or she then abducts the thighs and flexes them so they touch the child's abdomen but do not compress the abdominal wall. Place the buttocks at the edge of the table so the instrument can be depressed easily during the procedure. Examine the child for fissures, hemorrhoids, or inflammatory changes before inserting of the instrument. Examine the rectum digitally to ascertain the size of the sphincter and the patency of the canal. Sedation is contraindicated for this procedure. Sedation may prevent a pain response that warns against an accident and, in addition, the sphincter relaxes during the inspiratory gasp after a prolonged cry, permitting the scope to slide more easily into the anal canal (30). Laxatives, suppositories, and enemas are not used because these may cause changes in the anal mucosa, leading to an erroneous diagnosis.
2. Grasp the instrument with the thumb held firmly over the obturator. Lubricate the tip and then press the instrument gently and evenly against the anal sphincter. Do not attempt to pass the instrument forcefully through; it will pass with gentle, even pressure when the sphincter relaxes. Wait patiently for this to happen. Once the tube is in the canal, remove the obturator, and advance the tube; the instrument is advanced only under direct vision. Cleanse the mucosa with a cotton swab or suction until the lumen is visualized and the mucosa examined. Do not use air to inflate in the infant and small child because this may

cause tears or pneumatic perforations (19). Examine for pitting edema, friability, inflammation, submucosal hemorrhagic ulcers, masses, or polyps. Take cultures when necessary. Do not pass the instrument beyond the angulation of the rectosigmoid junction. Instrumentation beyond this level should be performed only by an expert. One can easily tell when this junction is reached because the rectum passes backward and has longitudinal folds, whereas the sigmoid has transverse folds.

Video-endoscopic anoscopy is a time-efficient way to evaluate the anal canal (67). Insert a clear, plastic anoscope (Saniscope; Bard, Inc., Murray Hill, New Jersey) into the anal canal. Use a black, indelible marker to mark the innermost and outermost aspects of the anoscope so that the relative position in the anal canal can be determined. Withdraw the central plunger, and insert large cotton swabs through the anoscope to clear away any residual material. Then insert the video-sigmoidoscope into the channel of the anoscope. Maintain control of the anoscope and distal end of the sigmoidoscope by using the right hand, while the left hand is free to obtain endoscopic photographs. Start the examination with the anoscope at deep insertion in the anal canal, and continue it as the anoscope is slowly withdrawn. Duration of anoscopic examination is approximately 60 seconds (67).

EXTERNAL THROMBOSED HEMORRHOIDS

The arterial and venous supply of the rectum consists of, from top to bottom, the superior, middle, and inferior hemorrhoidal arteries and the superior, middle, and inferior hemorrhoidal veins. The middle hemorrhoidal vein anastomoses with the superior hemorrhoidal vein and also with the portal system. Therefore, in patients with portal hypertension, such as cirrhosis of the liver, high portal pressure is communicated to the middle hemorrhoidal vein and results in venous dilatation under a considerable amount of pressure.

Hemorrhoids represent a mass of dilated venules. If the hemorrhoids originate above the dentate line, they are called internal hemorrhoids. If they originate below the dentate line, they are termed external hemorrhoids. A prolapsed internal hemorrhoid is an internal hemorrhoid that extends lower than the dentate line. This type of hemorrhoid can prolapse outside the rectum.

Acute external thrombosed hemorrhoids are seen as a sudden, painful lump in the anus. On physical examination, a dark blue, tender nodule is noted at the anal verge. This nodule is covered with normal skin. The lesion is extremely painful, and treatment is directed to relieve this pain. If the patient has no pain, then only conservative treatment is necessary. If patients are seen in the first 48 hours, the entire lesion can be excised easily in an office procedure. If thrombosis occurs more than 48 hours before consultation, the best approach is to allow spontaneous resolution (84).

TECHNIQUE OF INCISION

Give the patient intravenous analgesics (meperidine; Demerol). We recommend intravenous analgesics in any operative procedure performed in the emergency center involving the anal region. After the patient is relaxed and in less pain, anesthetize the lesion by infiltrating 1% lidocaine with epinephrine (Fig. 1.18*A*) in the area under and around the thrombosed mass. Make an elliptical incision with a no. 11 blade over the thrombosed mass, and pick up the point of the ellipse with a hemostat or Allis forceps (Fig. 1.18*B* and *C*). Excise the underlying hemorrhoid along with the wedge of skin. Control bleeding with direct pressure, or, if unusually excessive, with locally applied

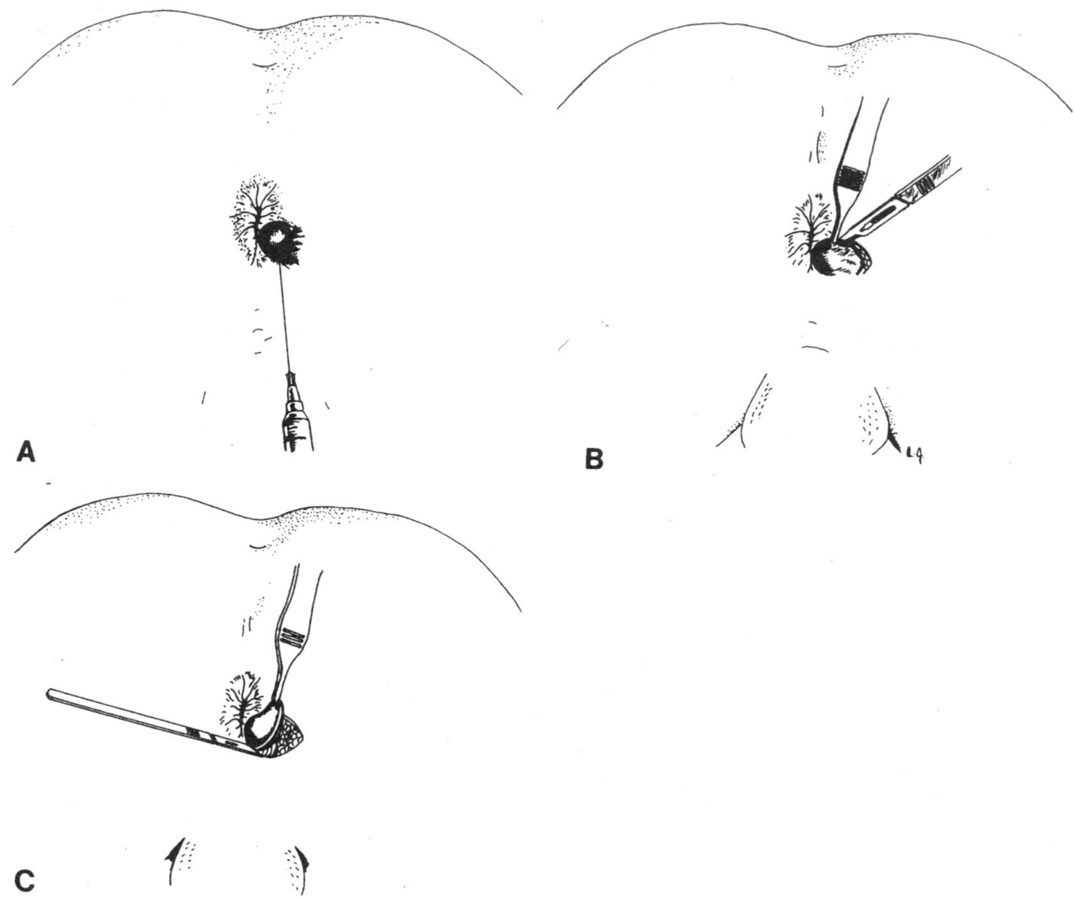

Figure 1.18. Anesthetize an external thrombosed hemorrhoid with 1% lidocaine with epinephrine *(A)* with a no. 15 or no. 11 blade. Excise the hemorrhoid in an elliptical fashion at its base *(B).* Be certain also to excise a wedge of skin and the subcutaneous tissue that contain additional clots, as shown above *(C).*

epinephrine. Apply a pressure dressing and keep it in place for a few hours.

There is almost always more than one clot, and it is important to express all of the clots to prevent recurrence. If all the clots are not expressed from the hemorrhoid, recurrence of thrombosis is likely. After removal of the clots, insert the tip of a gauze compress into the wound (Fig. 18*C*). No further dressing is necessary, but tape the buttocks together to create a pressure dressing. Leave this pad and pressure in place for approximately 8 hours, after which the patient removes the pack while in a sitz bath. In a recent study, application of topical nitroglycerin relieved pain for from 4 to 6 hours in all patients with thrombosed external hemorrhoids. All patients reported the need for few sitz baths when topical nitroglycerin was used for an average of 3 days (29, 43). Side effects were limited to transient headache in 40% of the patients (43).

Treatment of Gangrenous Prolapsed Hemorrhoids

These patients have severe pain and usually have a history of hemorrhoidal difficulty. Perform a perianal field block by using a solution of 0.5% bupivacaine (Marcaine) with epinephrine and, added to this,

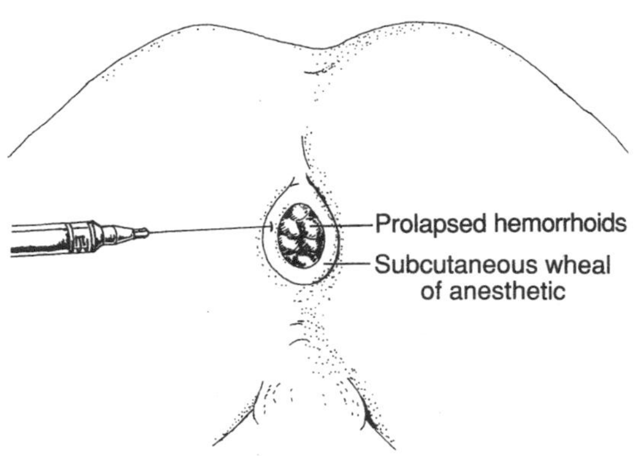

Figure 1.19. Deposit an anesthetic wheal subcutaneously around the prolapsed hemorrhoid. See text for discussion.

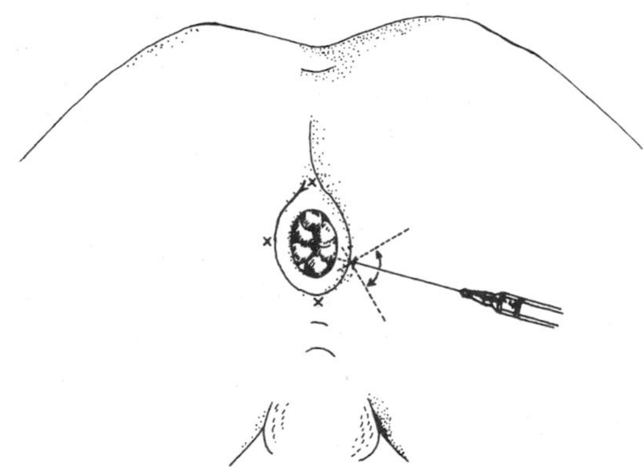

Figure 1.20. A four-quadrant infiltration of anesthetic solution will provide enough anesthesia to reduce prolapsed hemorrhoids. See text for discussion.

2 mL (two ampules) of hyaluronidase (300 units of Wydase). Then raise a subcutaneous circumanal wheal around the hemorrhoidal tissue (Fig. 1.19). After this, complete the field block by a four-quadrant deeper injection of lidocaine in the intersphincteric groove in each of the four quadrants (Fig. 1.20). This causes paralysis of the sphincter mechanism and creates total perianal anesthesia.

In doing this procedure, insert a finger in the rectum to guide the needle so that it does not penetrate the anal lumen. After a few minutes, apply pressure by direct massaging to reduce the hemorrhoidal mass. Apply a pressure dressing to the buttocks and tape it in place.

Severe Hemorrhoidal Bleeding

Use the usual therapy of intravenous fluids for the hypotensive patient or a massively bleeding patient. Hemorrhoidal bleeding usually occurs with a "squirting of blood" with defecation. To treat this with moderate or severe bleeding, ask the patient to bear down. If the bleeding site is visible, apply a hemostat to the bleeding site and tie a ligature around the hemostat. If the lesion is not visible, try to visualize the bleeding spot through the anoscope. When the bleeding point is visualized, apply a hemostat to the bleeding site and leave the hemostat in place for 5 minutes. After this period, cauterize the bleeding site with silver nitrate. If the hemorrhoidal bleeding is mild, the usual symptomatic therapy for hemorrhoids is recommended.

Posthemorrhoidectomy Bleeding

Within 10 to 14 days after a hemorrhoidectomy, the patient absorbs the sutures, and in 1.3% of cases, bleeding may ensue. Bleeding may be severe and require the insertion of a pack. Posthemorrhoidectomy bleeding packs are commercially available for this purpose. The packs should be inserted through the anoscope, and the strings pulled down to engage the pack against the bleeding site, causing tamponade (Fig. 1.21). Admit the patient to the hospital. When such a pack is not available, the emergency physician may insert a Foley catheter and inflate the balloon for temporary control of the bleeding. With either of these procedures, administer proper sedation because pressure from the pack or balloon causes significant discomfort to the patient. An alternative technique found to be effective in stopping active posthemorrhoidectomy bleeding is injecting the submucosal edge of the hemorrhoidectomy wound with 1 to 2 mL of 1:10,000 adrenalin with a 23-gauge

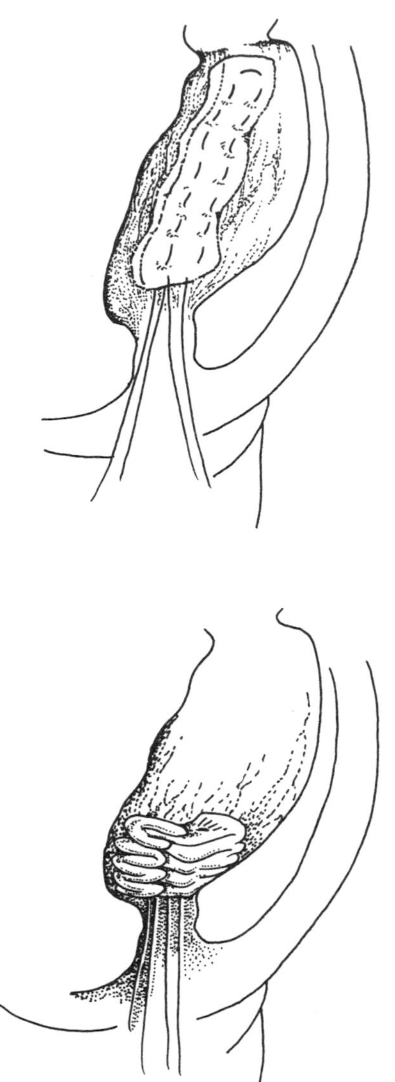

Figure 1.21. Insert a posthemorrhoidectomy accordion-like pack that contains two strings which are then pulled down to secure the pack in place in the anal canal; the pack tamponades bleeding.

needle. When bleeding is controlled, observe the patient in the hospital and allow the patient to return home after a normal bowel movement (91).

INTERNAL HEMORRHOIDS

Internal hemorrhoids may cause bleeding or prolapse but are rarely associated with severe pain, and this happens only when they become prolapsed, thrombosed, and/or strangulated. When it occurs, this is a surgical emergency (56). Internal hemorrhoids are graded by size:

- Grade I: Prominent hemorrhoidal vessels on endoscopy; no prolapse
- Grade II: Hemorrhoid prolapses but spontaneously reduces
- Grade III: Hemorrhoid prolapses and requires manual reduction
- Grade IV: Hemorrhoid prolapses and is not reducible

For persistent symptoms, several procedures are available. *Injection sclerotherapy* is easily learned and has a low complication rate. With a spinal needle inserted through an anoscope, instill a small volume of sclerosant in the submucosa of the internal hemorrhoid. This method is particularly useful for grade I and mild grade II hemorrhoids (88). *Rubber-band ligation* consists of a single sodium biphosphate enema taken approximately 1 hour before the procedure. Perform the procedure through an anoscope with a McGivney Rubber Band Ligator. This ligator consists of a drum on which the rubber ring is secured at a shaft that connects to a trigger handle. When that trigger is activated, the rubber ring slips off the drum (121). This procedure is beyond the scope of the emergency physician (88,121). In his study comparing emergency and elective hemorrhoidectomy, Eu (38) found that emergency hemorrhoidectomy appears to be as safe as the elective procedure. It offers several advantages, including definitive treatment of hemorrhoids at the time of admission, and may save the patient a subsequent admission for an elective operation. There are a number of acute and chronic complications of hemorrhoidectomy (12). In a study comparing hemorrhoidal treatments, it was found that patients who underwent hemorrhoidectomy had a better response to treatment than did those patients who had rubber-band ligation (75). Because the pain was better with rubber-band ligation, one can conclude that rubber-band ligation can be recommended as the initial modality of choice for grades I to III hemorrhoids. Although hemorrhoidectomy showed better responses, it is associated with more complications and pain and should be reserved for those hemorrhoids that fail to respond to rubber-band ligation (75).

Treatment of Anal Fissures

Anal fissures are usually successfully treated with stool softeners, high-fiber diet, and sitz baths. A sphincter-stretch procedure is used when conservative therapy fails, but is best done under general anesthesia. The stretch procedure can be done under the regional block described earlier for gangrenous prolapsed hemorrhoids. Insert the index finger gently into the anus and rectum (Fig. 1.22); after this, insert the index finger of the opposite hand (Fig. 1.23). Gentle lateral and circumferential retraction then ensues and continues for approximately 30 to 60 seconds. After this, insert a third finger (the long finger) and possibly a fourth finger into the anal canal. Perform careful stretching for 4 minutes. This procedure should not be performed by the novice because disruption of the sphincter muscles that support the anus can occur.

Internal fissure hypertonia appears to play a role in the etiology of the pain of anal fissure. Nitrous oxide has recently been identified as the "novel biologic messenger" that mediates the anorectal inhibitory reflex in humans. In one study, 500 to 1,000 mg of 0.5% nitroglycerin ointment was applied with the finger to the external anus and distal anal canal 4 or more times a day after bowel movements. All patients reported a dramatic relief of anal pain within 3 to 4 minutes of nitroglycerin ointment application, and 83% of those patients were healed within 2 weeks (43). Another study using glyceryl trinitrate (GTN) ointment showed a 68% healing rate after 8 weeks of treatment (61).

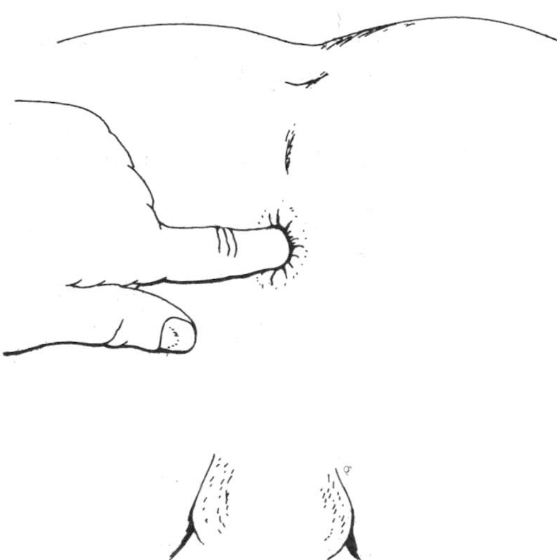

Figure 1.22. After adequate anesthesia, insert the index finger gently into the anus. See text for discussion.

Topical isosorbide dinitrate is an effective and safe treatment for chronic anal fissure. The optimal dose regimen is 2.5 mg, 3 times each day (73). Using nitric acid donor compounds has become an additional modality in the therapeutic endeavors required to heal and treat anal fissure (78).

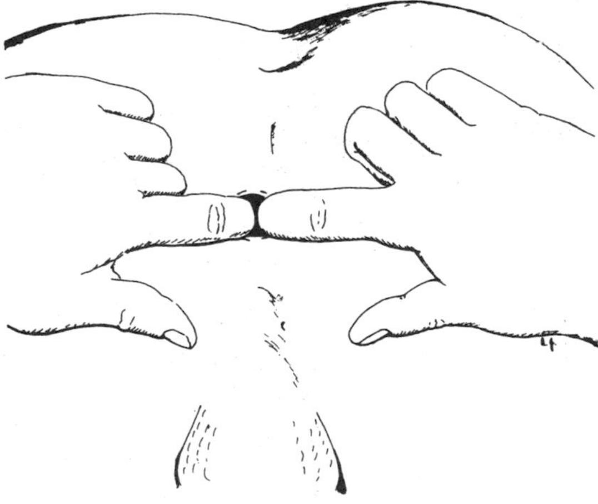

Figure 1.23. Gently insert the index fingers of both hands to separate the walls of the anus, as described in the text.

Anorectal Abscesses

The dentate or pectinate line represents a transverse series of openings or crypts in the anal mucosa. These crypts are the openings of the anal glands, which are in the connective tissue of the anus. The anal glands are mucus-secreting glands that drain via ducts into the anal crypts at the dentate line (Fig. 1.24). When a blockage occurs in the duct of the anal gland, inflammation and abscess formations are likely to occur. When an abscess occurs in an anal gland, one has a perianal abscess. The anal abscess may extend into several potential spaces (Fig. 1.24*A*). When the abscess extends to the skin surface, it is considered a perianal abscess. When extension occurs in the space between the sphincters in the posterior midline, it is called an intersphincteric abscess. Extension into the submucosal space of the ischiorectal fossa leads to an ischiorectal abscess (1). Two other rectal abscesses that are seen in the emergency center are submucosal and supralevator abscesses. Each of these abscesses is discussed separately later.

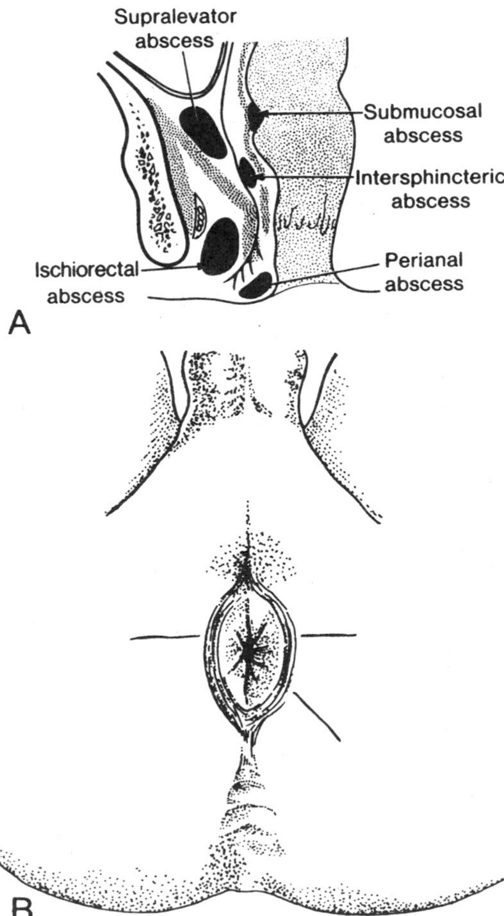

Figure 1.24. *A:* Various locations of rectal abscesses. *B:* Use a radial incision to drain a perianal abscess. The incision should be lateral to the sphincter muscle.

CLINICAL PRESENTATION

Perianal pain, local swelling, and sometimes fever are the cardinal symptoms of a perianal abscess. In the absence of an obvious, thrombosed external hemorrhoid or anal fissure, an abscess must be strongly suspected without the typical findings. For example, a higher abscess in the supralevator position may cause only gluteal pain or minimal or no external physical findings at all, other than mild lower abdominal pain. Similarly, there may be only vague erythema of the perianal skin, and the diagnosis of cellulitis is made. This diagnosis is usually incorrect, as this simply means that the abscess is more deep seated and potentially more dangerous. Failure to diagnose an abscess at this stage may on occasion lead to the development of life-threatening sepsis. Thus a diagnosis of "perianal cellulitis" means that an abscess is in need of drainage and should not be treated by a course of antibiotics. Delaying drainage in this setting only allows extension of the infection (58). The anal rectal region also may be a site of life-threatening necrotizing infections such as Fournier's necrotizing gangrene, which classically results from unrecognized or inadequately treated suppurative disease, particularly in a diabetic or other immunocompromised host (58).

Perianal Abscesses

Before draining any abscess around the anus, administer intramuscular analgesic and sedative 20 minutes before the procedure.

The patient should lie in the prone position. Separate the buttocks and tape them with 3-inch adhesive tape to the lateral aspect of the hip, thus exposing the anus (Fig. 1.25). Infiltrate the area around the abscess with 1% lidocaine with epinephrine, and infiltrate the roof of the abscess likewise. If adequate analgesia cannot be achieved, the patient needs general anesthesia. One of two techniques can be used to drain these abscesses. Either excise an elliptical wedge, by using a radial incision from the roof of the abscess (thus permitting wide drainage), or make a cruciate incision with edges excised to expose the abscessed cavity adequately (Fig. 1.26). Make an incision as close to the anal canal as possible so that any subsequent fistula tracks are as short as possible (58). Either method will permit adequate drainage of the abscess. Packing usually is very painful and may actually interfere with adequate drainage. In an alternative method, make a small stab wound, and then insert an appropriate-sized mushroom-type catheter. The catheter may be removed in 7 to 10 days. The use of the catheter provides continuous drainage while avoiding the traumatic dressing changes (58). Apply a gauze pad to the anal region, and release the buttocks around it. Advise the patient to take a sitz bath the following day and each day thereafter until healing is complete. Because of pain and complications, some institutions do not permit drainage of perianal abscesses in the emergency center.

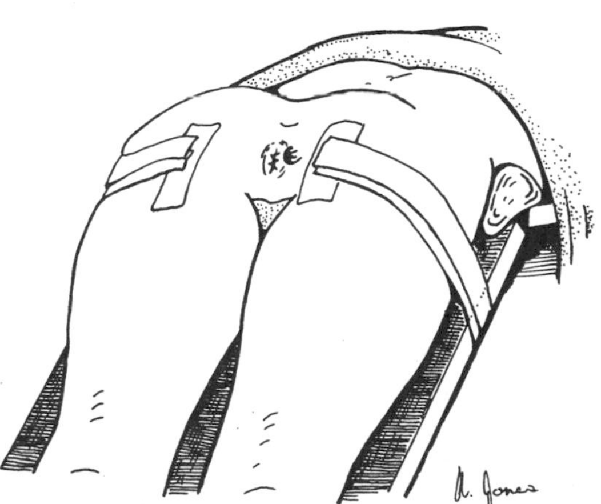

Figure 1.25. When excising a thrombosed external hemorrhoid or performing incision and drainage of an anal abscess, separate the buttocks by using 3-inch adhesive tape, as shown above, to provide optimal exposure.

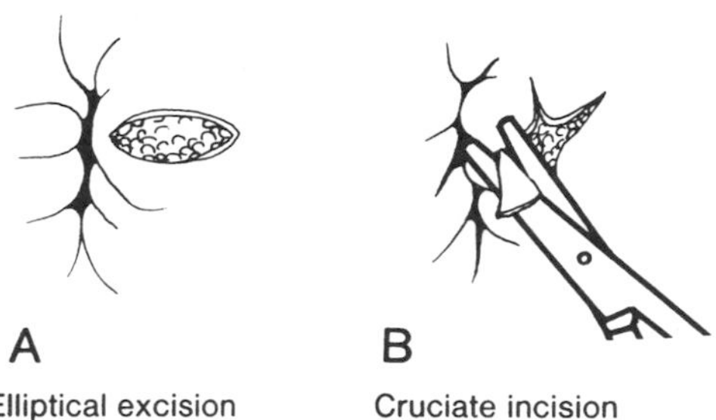

Figure 1.26. The most common type of rectal abscess drained in the emergency center is the perianal or perirectal abscess. To drain this abscess, use an elliptical excision to provide adequate opening for proper drainage to occur, as shown in *A*. Alternatively, use a cruciate incision when deeper abscesses are being drained, as shown in *B*.

Fistulas after drainage of acute anorectal abscesses can occur. In one study, it was found that in 37% of patients who had anorectal abscesses drained, a fistula had developed, and in 10%, a recurrent abscess developed (50). Perianal abscesses result in fewer persistent fistulas if drained properly and have no added risk of fecal incontinence (55).

Submucosal Abscess

Most submucosal abscesses may be drained in the emergency center. These patients have a deep, dull pain in the area of the rectum and usually have a history of diarrheal episodes or a mucous or purulent discharge from the rectum. Visualize these abscesses with a proctoscopic or sigmoidoscopic examination, and perform incision and drainage in the normal fashion.

Ischiorectal and Supralevator Abscesses

Because of their size and extension, drain ischiorectal and supralevator abscesses in the operating room.

Pilonidal Abscesses

A pilonidal abscess results from an infection in a pilonidal cyst. A pilonidal cyst develops when the posterior neuropore fails to close, resulting in a structure that becomes fluid filled. The cyst may develop tracts called pilonidal sinuses. When a cyst fails to drain, infection and abscess formation are likely to occur. The pilonidal sinus may become plugged with keratin, desquamated epithelial cells, or debris. Pilonidal cysts derive their name from the fact that many of the cysts have hair within the cavity. The abscesses that form may be treated in the usual manner; however, they almost always recur, and the patient should be referred after incision and drainage for definitive excision of the underlying lesion.

Drain the pilonidal abscess by using a midline vertical incision after adequate anesthesia by local infiltration. Open loculations and irrigate the abscess cavity with half-strength hydrogen peroxide. Then pack the cavity with iodoform gauze. Remove the gauze packing in 48 hours while the patient is in a sitz bath. Instruct the patient to continue sitz baths daily until healing is complete.

FOREIGN BODIES IN THE ANUS

Foreign bodies in the anus and rectum may present a formidable problem. The patient may or may not complain of pain in the rectal area. A thorough history and physical examination are necessary to ensure that the rectum has not been perforated. Plain radiographs are useful if the object is radiopaque to determine its size and location (42). Occasionally, foreign bodies may be removed in the emergency center; however, some patients may require a general anesthetic to remove the object. For removal, appropriate relaxation and sedation are usually necessary. Local anesthesia may be required to permit adequate relief of pain and relaxation of the anal sphincter (42). The foreign body must be stabilized before removal, because attempts to remove the object without stabilization may result in displacing it farther and farther away from one's grasp. A variety of unique ways to assist in the removal of foreign bodies of the rectum have been described, including using obstetric forceps. Use of a Foley catheter also has been described (42). Others have used a plaster of paris that has been placed in a hollow object with a string attached, allowing the plaster of paris to harden, thus facilitating removal of the hollow object (42). Insert a 24 French Foley catheter with a 50-mL balloon into the rectum through an anoscope and inserted past the foreign body. Then inflate the balloon proximal to the foreign body. Apply traction on the Foley catheter, thus stabilizing the foreign body in position (Fig. 1.27). If the object is small and round, use the inflated balloon to remove the object. In situations in which the object is either irregular or has sharp edges, use the inflated balloon of the Foley catheter to stabilize the object, and introduce a long forceps through the anoscope to grasp the foreign body and remove it. Use laparotomy only as a last resort for removal of a foreign body of the rectum (42).

COLOSTOMY PROBLEMS SEEN IN THE EMERGENCY CENTER

Sigmoid colostomy is the most commonly encountered surgical stoma and is usually permanent. The stoma is located on the left side and is usually fashioned to protrude as a spout above the surface of the lower abdominal wall (2). In sigmoid colostomies, formed stool is the output.

Descending colostomy is located slightly higher than the sigmoid colostomy, and slightly less formed stool occurs here.

Wet colostomy is a term applied when one or both ureters are implanted into the

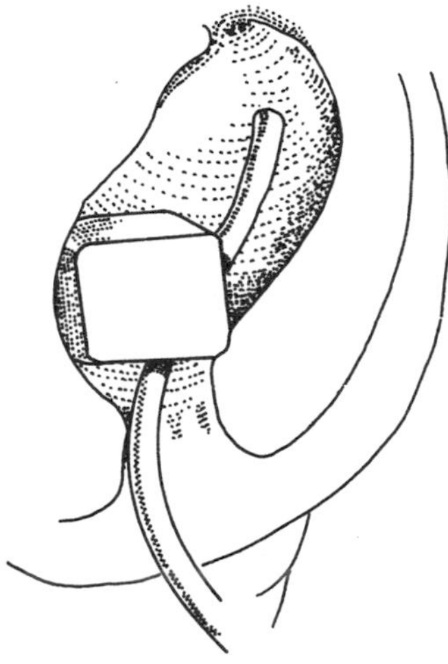

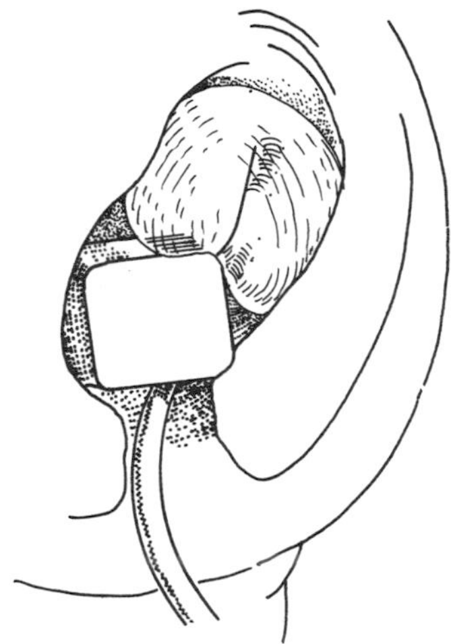

Figure 1.27. Use a size 24 French Foley catheter with a 50-mL balloon at its tip to stabilize a foreign body in the rectum while manipulating it for extraction.

colon. Problems that occur in management are leakage and odor.

A transverse colostomy or loop colostomy is usually temporary, and the output is often unformed stools.

Skin protection is the most difficult part of dealing with a colostomy and is largely dependent on fitting an effective appliance. Stoma adhesive, karaya gum, or a protective film such as a skin prep or skin gel is often useful.

Prolapse of a colostomy may be a problem requiring surgical correction. Parastomal herniation also may occur, and again, surgical revision may be necessary. Retraction or stenosis also is a commonly encountered problem that may require surgical intervention.

The most common problem seen in the emergency center, however, is the result of an ill-fitting appliance, whereby the patient has skin excoriation, allergies, and other problems related to the skin.

Ileostomy Problems Seen in the Emergency Center

Obstruction is one of the most common complications encountered (117). The obstruction causes the patient to have colic pain with abrupt stoppage of stool. Distention rarely occurs, but bowel sounds may be excessive or high pitched. Occasionally, the stoma may discharge extremely fluid contents immediately before complete cessation of efflux.

The obstruction is most frequently due to a bolus. A plain radiograph of the abdomen may confirm the presence of dilated air–fluid levels before the stoma. Stenosis occurs most often at the skin or fascial level and this itself may cause frequent bolus problems. A proper-size orifice may not have been created initially. The ileostomy orifice should fit two average-size fingers.

Abdominal wall stricturing may be a problem. Great care must be taken not to make the hole too large. Bolus obstruction may cause the stoma to swell. This is best dealt with by inserting a soft rubber catheter very gently, as far as it will go, withdrawing it slightly, and then instilling 100 mL of warm saline fairly rapidly while advancing the catheter. Allow the catheter to drain for a few moments before repeating the irrigation. This procedure may bring on an immediate relief of the symptoms.

Sometimes the bolus cannot be removed by conservative means, because an intraabdominal band may be the cause.

This type of obstruction may require operative intervention.

Recession is the most common cause of reoperation on a stoma, and this disorder occurs in about 10% to 15% of patients mostly because of the gap in the abdominal wall being too small.

Prolapse of an ileostomy is far less frequent. Typically, the ileostomy should protrude 1.5 to 2.5 cm. Prolapse beyond this length may cause the patient considerable difficulty; however, prolapse is seldom symptomatic.

Fistula formation may occur, usually because of recurrent disease, and more commonly from an ill-fitting or misapplied appliance in which the flange exerts pressure on the stoma and finally ulcerates through it. This condition will usually be seen as a leakage problem, but the cause is not often immediately apparent. Lift the stoma and carefully explore it for granulation tissue around a fistula.

Ulceration of the stoma may imply recurrent disease, such as Crohn disease. Granuloma formation may occur and suggests a fistula, probably because of persistent irritation. These granulomas usually do not respond to cauterization with silver nitrate, and they may recur.

Herniation of the stoma is rare if the stoma is correctly positioned through the rectus abdominis muscle. If it is lateral to this position, peristomal bulging is common because the intestine is inadequately supported as it passes through the abdominal wall.

REFERENCES

1. Abcarian H: Acute suppurations of the anorectum. Surg Annu 8:305, 1976.
2. Acworth LA: Part 2: Stoma care. Clin Gastroenterol 11:297, 1982.
3. Ahmad W, Polk HC: Blunt abdominal trauma. Arch Surg 111:489, 1976.
4. Aragon GE, Eiseman B: Abdominal stab wounds: Evaluation of sinography. J Trauma 16:792, 1976.
5. Arullani AJ, Cappello G: Diagnosis and current treatment of hemorrhoidal disease. Angiol J Vasc Dis 45:6/2, 1994.
6. Atkenson RJ, Nyhus LM: Gastric lavage for hemorrhage in the upper part of the gastrointestinal tract. Surg Gynecol Obstet 147:797, 1978.
7. Bain IM, Kirby RM, et al: Survey of abdominal ultrasound and diagnostic peritoneal lavage for suspected intra-abdominal injury following blunt trauma. Injury 29:65–71, 1998.
8. Balkan E, et al: Sigmoidoscopy in minor lower gastrointestinal bleeding. Arch Dis Child 78: 267–268, 1998.
9. Berggreen PJ, Harrison ME, et al: Techniques and complications of esophageal foreign body extraction in children and adults. Gastrointest Endosc 39:626–30, 1993.
10. Berry TK, Flynn TC, Miller PW, Fischer RP: Diagnostic peritoneal lavage in blunt trauma patients with coagulopathy. Ann Emerg Med 13: 879, 1984.
11. Blow O, Bassam D, et al: Speed and efficiency in the resuscitation of blunt trauma patients with multiple injuries: The advantage of diagnostic peritoneal lavage over abdominal computerized tomography. J Trauma 44:287, 1998.
12. Boccasanta P, Ventrui M, et al: Circular hemorrhoidectomy in advanced hemorrhoidal disease. Hepatogastroenterology 45:969–972,1998.
13. Boyle EM, Maier RV, et al: Diagnosis of injuries after stab wounds to the back and flank. J Trauma 42:260–5, 1997.
14. Breen PC, Rudolf LE: Potential sources of error in the use of peritoneal lavage as a diagnostic tool. J Am Coll Emerg Physicians 3:401, 1974.
15. Bull JC Jr, Mathewson C Jr: Exploratory laparotomy in patients with penetrating wounds of the abdomen. Am J Surg 116:223, 1961.
16. Burney RE: Peritoneal lavage and other diagnostic procedures in blunt abdominal trauma. Emerg Med Clin North Am 4:513, 1986.
17. Burns RK, Sariol HS, Ross SE: Penetrating posterior abdominal trauma. Trauma 25,429–431, 1994.
18. Burns SM, Martin M, et al: Comparison of nasogastric tube securing methods and tube types in medical intensive care patients. Am J Crit Care 4:198–203, 1995.
19. Byrne WD, Samson PC, Dugan DJ: Complications associated with the use of esophageal compression balloons. Am J Surg 104:250, 1962.
20. Caffee HH, Benfield JR: Is peritoneal lavage for the diagnosis of hemoperitoneum safe? Arch Surg 103:4, 1971.
21. Campbell DE: Complications of gastrointestinal intubation. Ann Surg 130:113, 1949.
22. Campbell JB, Quattromani FL, Foley LC: Foley catheter removal of blunt esophageal foreign bodies: experience with 100 consecutive children. Pediatr Radiol 13:116, 1983.
23. Cappell MS: Safety and clinical efficacy of flexible sigmoidoscopy and colonoscopy for gastrointestinal bleeding after myocardial infraction: A six year study of 18 consecutive lower endoscopies at two university teaching hospitals. Dig Dis Sci 39:473–480, 1994.
24. Caralps-Riera JM: Diagnostic value of Hypaque injection in the conservative management of upper abdominal stab wounds. Am J Surg 123: 612, 1972.
25. Carter JW, Sawyers JL: Pitfalls in diagnosis of abdominal stab wounds by contrast media injection. Am Surg 35:107, 1969.

26. Cohen DD: Nasogastric intubation in the anesthetized patient. Anesth Analg 42:578, 1963.
27. Conn HO: Sengstaken-Blakemore tube revisited [Editorial]. Gastroenterology 61:398, 1971.
28. Conn HO, Simpson JA: Excessive mortality associated with balloon tamponade of bleeding varices: a critical reappraisal. JAMA 202:135, 1967.
29. Cox SW, Senagore AJJ, et al: Outcome after incision and drainage with fistulotomy for ischiorectal abscess. Am Surg 63:686–689,1997.
30. Crohn BB: Trauma from sigmoid manipulation. Am J Dis Child 2:678, 1936.
31. Cue JI, Miller FB, et al: A prospective, randomized comparison between open and closed peritoneal lavage techniques. J Trauma 30:880–883, 1990.
32. Daly WM: Unusual complication of nasal intubation. Anesthesiology 14:96, 1953.
33. Davis JR, Morrison AL, et al: Ultrasound impact on diagnostic peritoneal lavage, abdominal computed tomography, and resident training. Am Surg 65:555–559, 1999
34. Dees G: Difficult nasogastric tube insertions. Emerg Med Clin North Am 7:177, 1989.
35. Dokler ML, Bradshaw J, et al: Selective management of pediatric esophageal foreign bodies. Am Surg 61:132–134, 1995.
36. Drew R, Perry JF, Fischer RP: The expediency of peritoneal lavage for blunt trauma in children. Surg Gynecol Obstet 145:885, 1977.
37. Engrav LH, Benjamin CI, Strate RG, et al: Diagnostic peritoneal lavage in blunt abdominal trauma. J Trauma 15:854, 1975.
38. Eu KW et al: Comparison of emergency and elective haemorrhoidectomy. Br J Surg 81: 308–310, 1994.
39. Fenig J, Richter RM, Levowitz BS: Gastric ulceration caused by Sengstaken-Blakemore balloon tamponade. N Y State J Med 76:404, 1976.
40. Fremstad JD, Martin SH: Lethal complication from insertion of nasogastric tube after severe basilar skull fracture. J Trauma 18:820, 1978.
41. Fry ENS: Positioning of nasogastric tubes [Letter]. Br Med J 1:110, 1978.
42. Fry RD: Anorectal trauma and foreign bodies. Surg Clin North Am 74:1491, 1994.
43. Gorfine SR: Treatment of benign anal disease with topical nitroglycerin. Dis Colon Rectum 38:453, 1995.
44. Greene JF Jr, Sawicki JE, Doyle WF: Gastric ulceration: A complication of double-lumen nasogastric tubes. JAMA 224:338, 1973.
45. Gregory JA, Turner PT, Reynolds AF: A complication of nasogastric intubation: Intracranial penetration. J Trauma 18:823, 1978.
46. Gremse DA: Effectiveness of nasogastric rehydration in hospitalized children with acute diarrhea. J Pediatr Gastroenterol Nutr 21: 145–148, 1995.
47. Gustavsson S, Albert J, Forsberg H, et al: The accidental introduction of a nasogastric tube into the brain. Acta Chir Scand 144:55, 1978.
48. Haddad GH, Pizzi WF, Fleischmann EP, et al: Abdominal signs and sinograms as dependable criteria for the selective management of stab wounds of the abdomen. Ann Surg 172:61, 1970.
49. Hafner CD, Wylie JH Jr, Brush BE: Complications of gastrointestinal intubation. Arch Surg 83:147, 1961.
50. Hamalainen KPJ, Sainio AP: Incidence of fistulas after drainage of acute anorectal abscesses. Dis Colon Rectum 41:1357–1362, 1998.
51. Hallfedt KK, Trupka AW, et al: Emergency laparoscopy for abdominal stab wounds. 12: 907–910, 1998.
52. Hanselman RC, Meyer RH: Complications of gastrointestinal intubation. Surg Gynecol Obstet Int Abstr Surg 114:207, 1962.
53. Hawkins DB: Removal of blunt foreign bodies from the esophagus. Ann Otol Rhinol Laryngol 99:935, 1990.
54. Hijams J: Proctoscopy of the infant. Am J Dis Child 105:297, 1963.
55. Ho YH, Tan M, et al: Randomized controlled trial of primary fistulotomy with drainage alone for perianal abscesses. Dis Colon Rectum 40: 1435–1438, 1997.
56. Hussain JN: Hemorrhoids. Prim Care 26:35, 1999.
57. Hyatt DF, Gordon LA: Abdominal stab wound sinogram. Arch Surg 104:340, 1972.
58. Hyman N: Anorectal abscess and fistula. Prim Care 26:69, 1999.
59. Jackson FW, Ball MD: Correction of deficiencies in flexible fiberoptic sigmoidoscope cleaning and disinfection technique in family practice and internal medicine offices. Arch Fam Med 6:578–582, 1997.
60. James RH: An unusual complication of passing a narrow bore nasogastric tube. Anesthesia 33: 716, 1978.
61. Kamm MA: Diagnostic, pharmacological, surgical and behavioral developments in benign anorectal disease. Eur J Surg Suppl 582: 119–123, 1998.
62. Kelemen JJ III, Martin RR, et al: Evaluation of diagnostic peritoneal lavage in stable patients with gunshot wounds to the abdomen. Arch Surg 132:909–913, 1997.
63. Koong Shiao SYP, et al: Nasogastric tube placement: effects on breathing and sucking in very-low-birth-weight infants. Nursing Res 44:82, 1996.
64. Kuo B, Castell DO: The effect of nasogastric intubation on gastroesophageal reflux: A comparison of different tube sizes. Am J Gastroenterol 90:10, 1995.
65. Lazarus HM, Nelson JA: A technique for peritoneal lavage without risk or complication. Surg Gynecol Obstet 149:889, 1979.
66. Lazarus HM, Nelson JA: Peritoneal lavage with low morbidity. JACEP 8:316, 1979.
67. Lazas J, Moses FM, Wong RKH: Videoendoscopy: A new technique for examining the anal canal. Gastrointest Endosc 42:4, 351, 1995.
68. Liebman R: New tube for the diagnosis and treatment of upper gastrointestinal hemorrhage. Am J Surg 127:171, 1974.
69. Liedberg G: Esophageal tamponade in the treatment of massive bleeding from esophageal varices, with special reference to volume and pressure in the balloons. Acta Chir Scand 134: 249, 1968.

70. Lind LJ, Wallace DH: Submucosal passage of a nasogastric tube complicating attempted intubation during anesthesia. Anesthesiology 49: 145, 1978.
71. Lucas CE: The role of peritoneal lavage for penetrating abdominal wounds [Editorial]. J Trauma 17:649, 1977.
72. Lyons MF, Tsuchida AM: Foreign bodies of the gastrointestinal tract. Gastrointest Emerg 77: 1101, 1993.
73. Lysy J, et al: Treatment of chronic anal fissure with isosorbide dinitrate: Long term results and dose determination. Dis Colon Rectum 41: 1406–1410, 1998.
74. Macpherson RI, Hill J, et al: Esophageal foreign bodies in children: diagnosis, treatment, and complications. AJR Am J Roentgenol 166: 919–924, 1996.
75. MacRae HM, McLeod RS: Comparison of hemorrhoidal treatments: a meta-analysis. Can J Surg 40:14–17, 1997.
76. Madureri V: Sonda de doble circulacion para lavado, gastrico. GEN 26:411, 1972.
77. Mahar J: An aid in the passage of gastrointestinal tubes. Am J Surg 135:866, 1978.
78. Manookian CM, Fleshner PH, et al: Topical nitroglycerin in the management of anal fissure: An explosive outcome! Am Surg 64:962–964, 1998.
79. Marcuard SP, Stegall KS, et al: Unclogging feeding tubes with pancreatic enzyme. JPEN 14: 198, 1989.
80. Markovchick VJ, Elerding SC, Moore EE, et al: Diagnostic peritoneal lavage. JACEP 8:326, 1979.
81. McDougal K: Modifications in the technique of gastric lavage. Ann Emerg Med 10:514, 1981.
82. McGahan JP, Rose J et al: Use of ultrasonography in the patient with acute abdominal trauma. J Ultrasound Med 16:653–662, 1997.
83. McGuirk TD, Coyle WJ: Upper gastrointestinal tract bleeding. Emerg Med Clin North Am 14: 3523, 1996
84. Mecalf A: Anorectal disorders: five common causes of pain, itching, and bleeding. Postgrad Med 98:81, 1995.
85. Mele TS, Stewart K, et al: Evaluation of a diagnostic protocol using screening diagnostic peritoneal lavage with selective use of abdominal computed tomography in blunt abdominal trauma. J Trauma 46:847, 1999.
86. Mendez C, et al: Diagnostic accuracy of peritoneal lavage in patients with pelvic fractures. Arch Surg 129:477–482, 1994.
87. Mundy DA: Another technique for insertion of nasogastric tubes. Anesthesiology 50:374, 1979.
88. Nagle D, Rolandelli RH: Primary care office management of perianal and anal disease. Prim Care 213:609, 1996.
89. Nickell MD, Schwitzer GA, Gremillion DE Jr: Overdistension of the gastric balloon: Complication with the Sengstaken-Blakemore tube. JAMA 240:1172, 1978.
90. Novishki N, et al: Does the size of nasogastric tubes affect gastroesophageal reflux in children? J Pediatr Gastroenterol Nutr 29:448–451, 1999.
91. Nyam DCNK, et al: Submucosal adrenaline injection for posthemorrhoidectomy hemorrhage. Dis Colon Rectum 38:776–777, 1995.
92. Ogawa H: A reliable technique for the insertion of a gastric tube during operation. Surg Gynecol Obstet 132:497, 1971.
93. Olsen WR, Hildreth DH: Abdominal paracentesis and peritoneal lavage in blunt abdominal trauma. J Trauma 11:824, 1971.
94. Olsen WR, Redman HC, Hildreth DH, et al: Quantitative peritoneal lavage in blunt abdominal trauma. Arch Surg 104:536, 1972.
95. Osgard E, Jackson JL, Strong J: A randomized trial comparing three methods of bowel preparation for flexible sigmoidoscopy. Am J Gastroenterol 93:1126, 1998.
96. Ozer S, Benumof JL: Oro- and nasogastric tube passage in patients: Fiberoptic description. Anesthesiology 91:137–143, 1999.
97. Parvin S, Smith DE, Asher WM, et al: Effectiveness of peritoneal lavage in blunt abdominal trauma. Ann Surg 181:255, 1975.
98. Pasquale MD, Cerra FB: Sengstaken-Blakemore tube placement: Use of tamponade to control bleeding varices. Crit Care Clin 8:743, 1992.
99. Perry JF Jr, Strate RG: Diagnostic peritoneal lavage in blunt abdominal trauma: Indications and results. Surgery 71:898, 1972.
100. Pitcher JL: Safety and effectiveness of the modified Sengstaken-Blakemore tube: A prospective study. Gastroenterology 61:291, 1971.
101. Robinson EP, Cox PM Jr: Feeding tube introduction an easier way. Crit Care Med 7:349, 1979.
102. Root HD, Hauser CW, McKinley CR, et al: Diagnostic peritoneal lavage. Surgery 57:633, 1965.
103. Rosemurgy AS II, Albrink MH, Olson SM, et al: Abdominal stab wound protocol: Prospective study documents applicability for widespread use. Am Surg 61:112–116, 1995.
104. Sader AA: New way to stabilize nasogastric tubes. Am J Surg 130:102, 1975.
105. Seebacher J, Nozik D, Mathieu A: Inadvertent intracranial introduction of a nasogastric tube: a complication of severe maxillofacial trauma. Anesthesiology 42:100, 1975.
106. Simon T, Fink AS: Current management of endoscopic feeding tube dysfunction: Case report. Surg Endosc 13:403–405, 1999.
107. Slavin S: A new technique for diagnostic peritoneal lavage. Surg Gynecol Obstet 146:446, 1978.
108. Sliwa JA, Marciniak C: A complication of nasogastric tube removal. Arch Phys Med Rehabil 70:702–704, 1989.
109. Spencer GT: Tracheostomy and endotracheal intubation in the intensive care unit. In: Gray TC, Nunn JF, eds. General Anaesthesia, 3rd ed. London: Butterworth, 1973, Vol 2, 566.
110. Stack LB, Munter DW: Foreign bodies in the gastrointestinal tract. Emerg Med Clin North Am 14:493, 1996.
111. Stenapien SJ, Dagradi AE: A double lumen tube for gastroesophageal lavage. Gastrointest Endosc 12:26, 1966.

112. Taffinder NJ, Gould SWT, et al: Rigid videosigmoidoscopy vs. conventional sigmoidoscopy: A randomized controlled study. Surg Endosc 13:814–816, 1999.
113. Tahis AH: A method of inserting a gastric tube during operation. Surg Gynecol Obstet 132: 497, 1971.
114. Tavilogu K, Gunay K, et al: Abdominal stab wounds: The role of selective management. Eur J Surg 164:17–21, 1998.
115. Thal ER: Evaluation of peritoneal lavage and local exploration in lower chest and abdominal stab wounds. J Trauma 17:642, 1977.
116. Thal ER, Shires GT: Peritoneal lavage in blunt abdominal trauma. Am J Surg 125:64, 1973.
117. Todd IP: Part 4: Mechanical complications of ileostomy. Clin Gastroenterol 11:268, 1982.
118. Trimble C: Stab wound sinography. Surg Clin North Am 49:1217, 1969.
119. Virtue RW: Simple and reliable method for inserting nasogastric tube during anesthesia. Br J Anaesth 45:234, 1973.
120. Webb WA: Management of foreign bodies of the upper gastrointestinal tract: Update. Gastrointest Endosc 51:39–51, 1995.
121. Wrobleski DE: Rubber band ligation of hemorrhoids. R I Med 78:172–173, 1995.
122. Wyler AR, Reynolds AF: An intracranial complication of nasogastric intubation. J Neurosurg 47:297, 1977.
123. Young RF: Cerebrospinal fluid rhinorrhea following nasogastric intubation. J Trauma 19: 789, 1979.
124. Zeid SS, Young PC, Reeves JT: Rupture of the esophagus after introduction of the Sengstaken-Blakemore tube. Gastroenterology 36:128, 1959.

SUGGESTED READINGS

Altemeier WA, Culbertson WR, Fullen WD, et al: Intra-abdominal abscesses. Am J Surg 125:70, 1973.

Bizzarri D, Giuffrida J, Latteri F, et al: Esophageal intubation for prevention of aspiration of gastric contents. Acta Anesth Scand Suppl 24:19, 1966.

Bizzarri D, Gremillion MDE Jr: Simple method for passage of small-bore nasogastric feeding catheter. Ann Intern Med 91:655, 1979.

Blades B: Ruptured diaphragm. Am J Surg 105:501, 1963.

Borja AR, Lansing AM: Immediate control of intermediate vascular bleeding. Surg Gynecol Obstet 132:494, 1971.

Bray PF, Herbst JJ, Johnson DG, et al: Childhood gastroesophageal reflux. JAMA 237:1342, 1977.

Burcharth F, Malmstrom J: Experiences with the Linton-Nachlas and the Sengstaken-Blakemore tubes for bleeding esophageal varices. Surg Gynecol Obstet 142:529, 1976.

Child CG, Braunstein PW: Gastroduodenal intussusception with massive hemorrhage. Surgery 34: 754, 1953.

Clarke JM: Culdocentesis in the evaluation of blunt abdominal trauma. Surg Gynecol Obstet 129:809, 1969.

Conway K: Letter to the editor. Anesth Analg 50: 1010, 1971.

Dennis C: The gastrointestinal sump tube. Surgery 66:309, 1969.

Durham MW, Holm JC: Simple perforated ulcer of the colon. Surgery 34:750, 1953.

Elerding SC, Aragon GE, Moore EE: Fatal hepatic hemorrhage after trauma. Am J Surg 138:883, 1979.

Galloway DC, Grudis J: Inadvertent intracranial placement of a nasogastric tube through a basal skull fracture. South Med J 72:240, 1979.

Grant GN, Elliott DW, Frederick PL: Postoperative decompression by temporary gastrostomy or nasogastric tube. Arch Surg 85:844, 1962.

Jahadi MR: Diagnostic peritoneal lavage. J Trauma 12:936, 1972.

Lawler NA, McCreath ND: Gastro-oesophageal regurgitation. Lancet 2:369, 1951.

Ledgerwood AM, Kazmers M, Lucas CE: The role of thoracic aortic occlusion for massive hemoperitoneum. J Trauma 16:601, 1976.

McCoy J, Wolma FJ: Abdominal tap: Indication, technic, and results. Am J Surg 122:693, 1971.

Moss CM, Levine R, Messenger N, et al: Sliding colonic Maydl's hernia: Report of a case. Dis Colon Rectum 19:636, 1976.

Nance FC: The early management of abdominal trauma. Curr Concepts Trauma Care 9:16, 1979.

Notaras MJ: A simple technique for continuous gastric aspiration. Lancet 2:476, 1966.

Orloff MJ, Snyder GB: Experimental ascites, I: production of ascites by gradual occlusion of the hepatic veins with an internal vena caval cannula. Surgery 50:789, 1961.

Palmer ED: The vigorous diagnostic approach to upper-gastrointestinal tract hemorrhage. JAMA 207:1477, 1969.

Palmer ED, Soderstrom CA, DuPriest RW, et al: Pitfalls of peritoneal lavage in blunt abdominal trauma. Surg Gynecol Obstet 151:513, 1980.

Palmer ED, Tucker A, Lewis J: Passing a nasogastric tube. Br Med J 281:1128, 1980.

Requarth W, Theis FV: Incarcerated and strangulated inguinal hernia. Arch Surg 57:267, 1948.

Richards JH: Bacteremia following irritation of foci of infection. JAMA 99:1496, 1932.

Sealy WC: Rupture of the esophagus. Am J Surg 105: 505, 1963.

Tobias S, DeClement FA, Cleveland JC: Management of abdominal stab wounds. Arch Surg 95:27, 1967.

Wavak P, Zook EG: A simple method of exsanguinating the finger prior to surgery. JACEP 7:125, 1978.

Wright RN, Arensman RM, Coughlin TR, et al: Hernia reduction en masse. Am Surg 43:627, 1977.

Yurko AA, Williams RD: Needle paracentesis in blunt abdominal trauma: A critical analysis. J Trauma 6:194, 1966.

2

Airway Procedures

ESSENTIAL ANATOMY OF THE AIRWAY

A thorough understanding of both the surface and structural anatomy of the airway, particularly that of the upper respiratory tract, is fundamental to the emergency physician. A detailed description and discussion of the upper respiratory tract anatomy is beyond the scope of this text.

The upper airway is best thought of as a "Y," with one arm of the "Y" being the oral passage, and the other, the nasal, and the two joining in the hypopharynx. The problems in either arm of the "Y" that the emergency physician deals with are primarily obstructive in nature. If either arm of the "Y" is obstructed, the patient will still be able to breath adequately; therefore, respiratory obstruction must have either both arms obstructed or an obstruction at the area where they join, the hypopharynx, or else an obstruction proximal to this site.

In the oral passage, obstruction is usually due to the tongue, which tends to fall posteriorly and cause obstruction when the patient is in the supine position. In the nasal passage, obstruction is usually due to swelling from nasal fractures and/or maxillofacial injuries and is less consequential than obstruction of the oral passage.

Four causes of respiratory inadequacy are seen in the emergency center:

1. Obstruction
2. Respiratory failure
   a. Parenchymal (emphysema, tension pneumothorax, tracheal tear)
   b. Neurogenic (drug induced, depression of the respiratory center due to metabolic causes)
3. Musculoskeletal disorders
   a. Chest wall trauma
   b. Diseases of muscles (myasthenia gravis)
4. Cardiorespiratory arrest

OBSTRUCTION

CRITICAL QUESTION

The physician must first ask, is the patient breathing normally, ventilating and moving air adequately, or is there evidence of obstruction?

Stages of Obstruction

The symptoms and signs of respiratory obstruction have been graded by Forbes (38) according to severity, and this system has been modified by Verrill (143).

Stage I. This stage is a mild form of upper airway obstruction characterized by hoarseness, cough, and stridulous respirations on moderate exertion. Generally, these patients have either oral or nasal obstruction alone and not both.

Stage II. These patients have stridor on slight exertion and have associated signs of increased work of breathing, rib retraction on inspiration, use of accessory muscles of respiration, alae nasi dilating on inspiration, and suprasternal retraction.

Stage III. Stridor occurs at rest; the patient is apprehensive and restless with sweating, pallor, and increased pulse rate and blood pressure. These patients have severe obstruction.

Stage IV. This stage represents very severe obstruction with slowing of respirations, hypotension, cyanosis, and impaired consciousness. If these patients are not treated immediately, death ensues shortly.

Those patients who are in stages III and IV are of most immediate concern to the emergency physician; accurate assessment of the cause and relief of symptoms is urgently needed.

Verrill (143) divided the common causes of airway obstruction into five groups: oral obstruction, nasal obstruction, pharyngeal obstruction, laryngeal obstruction, and tracheal obstruction. A modification of this system by grouping those disorders that should be considered in the patient in the emergency center according to site of obstruction is presented in Tables 2.1 through 2.4.

Common Traumatic Conditions

Maximal edema is reached in 24 to 48 hours after facial trauma (93). In patients with fractures of the mandibular arch, collapse may allow the base of the tongue to obstruct the entrance to the larynx and lead to signs of airway obstruction. When it is not possible to pass an oral or nasal airway easily in these patients, pass a large towel clip or suture through the anterior tongue to permit traction to be used to bring both the tongue and the mandibular arch forward (45).

Table 2.1
Causes of Oral Obstruction Seen in the Emergency Center

Neoplastic
Tumors of the palate and floor of the mouth, jaws, or tongue
Inflammatory
Oral infections
Osteomyelitis of the mandible
Dental infections with association trismus
Ludwig angina
Temporomandibular joint (TMJ) syndrome and TMJ arthritis
Caustic agents ingested
Traumatic
Fractures of the facial bones or mandible with swelling
Swelling associated with severe facial injuries
Neurologic
Tetanus
Allergies
Angioneurotic edema or severe allergic reactions

In obtunded patients with or without trauma, a common misconception is that "swallowing of the tongue" is prevented by placing the patient in a prone position. Studies have shown no difference in the incidence or the degree of pharyngeal obstruction with patients in either the

Table 2.2
Causes of Nasal Obstruction Seen in the Emergency Center

Congenital
Deviated septum
Postchoanal atresia in the neonate
Neoplastic
Polyps
Cysts
Carcinoma
Inflammatory
Coryza
Abscesses
Adenoids
Traumatic
Septal hematoma
Nasal fracture
Allergic
Allergic rhinitis
Foreign body
For example, buttons and beads (especially in children)

Table 2.3
Causes of Pharyngeal Obstruction Seen in the Emergency Center

Neoplastic
Carcinoma
Inflammatory
Hypertrophy of uvula
Hypertrophied tonsils
Peritonsillar abscess
Retropharyngeal abscess
Severe pharyngitis
Traumatic
Caustic burns with acids or alkali
Posteriorly displaced tongue in facial trauma
Blood and vomitus after facial and oral injuries
Neurologic
Bulbar palsy
Foreign bodies
Fish and chicken bones
Allergies
Angioneurotic edema
Stings

prone or supine position (113). Flexion of the neck was found to worsen obstruction significantly in both positions.

Some controversy is found in the literature regarding the management of patients with laryngotracheal trauma. Some authors preferred emergency tracheostomy (3, 18), and others believed that careful endotracheal intubation yields excellent results (71, 124). In our opinion, it would seem that careful endotracheal intubation via the orotracheal route yields good results and is advocated whenever possible.

Table 2.4
Causes of Laryngeal and Tracheal Obstruction Seen in the Emergency Center

Congenital
Stenosis
Cysts
Neoplastic
Carcinoma
Polyps
Inflammatory
Laryngitis
Diphtheria
Epiglottitis
Tracheitis
Croup Traumatic
Fracture of the larynx
Tracheal rupture
Allergic
Glottic edema
Angioneurotic edema
Neurologic
Laryngeal spasm
Laryngeal tetany
Foreign body
Laryngeal obstruction most common; tracheal obstruction is rare

Foreign Bodies

The sixth most common cause of accidental death in the United States is foreign-body obstruction of the airway (132). Most foreign bodies in the trachea that cause severe obstruction are located in the subglottic area (132). If the particle is distal to the cricoid cartilage, a bronchoscope is needed to remove it. In patients with airway obstruction so severe that they cannot speak, use the Heimlich maneuver. Otherwise, manipulate the patient as little as possible, and use emergency bronchoscopy. However, despite successful removal of foreign bodies, complications such as pulmonary complications followed by retropharyngel abscess and local infections may occur. An increased risk for the development of these complications is associated with delayed presentation, location of foreign body, and type of foreign body (104).

FOREIGN BODIES IN PEDIATRICS

It is well known that young children have a tendency to place objects in their mouths, frequently leading to aspiration of foreign bodies into the tracheal bronchial tree. Foreign-body aspiration is a leading cause of accidental death in children younger than 1 year and is the cause of death in 7% of children younger than 4 years. Food items, especially peanuts, are the most common items aspirated in infants and toddlers, whereas older children are more likely to aspirate nonfood items such as pen caps, pins, and paper clips. A high degree of suspicion is required to diagnose foreign-body aspiration. A history of a witness-choking episode is most important in early diagnosis. *An asymptomatic* period is common after aspiration and contributes to a delay in diagnosis of more than 1 week in 12% to 26% of patients. This delay in diagnosis causes morbidity from bronchial inflammation, obstruction, and pneumonia that is resistant to treatment. Prompt endoscopic removal of the foreign body with an open, rigid bronchoscope under general anesthesia is the mainstay of therapy.

Nasal foreign bodies, unlike foreign bodies inhaled into the lower airway, are not life threatening. The majority of patients with foreign bodies in the nose are aged 2 to 5 years (41). The most common nasal foreign bodies are beads (12%), rocks (10%), and plastic toys (10%) (65). Martes noted that 55% of patients with a nasal foreign body complained of pain or discomfort, and 36% had a foul odor or discharge noted (83).

Because of the many different types of nasal foreign bodies, the emergency physician should have several techniques at his or her disposal for removing nasal foreign bodies. The most commonly used techniques include forceps, Foley balloon catheter, positive pressure with an anesthesia bag, and a suction catheter tip. Kaish and Corneli (65) recommended that before any of these procedures, the patient should be placed in a supine position and premedicated with several drops of both 1% lidocaine without epinephrine and 0.5% phenylephrine instilled into the nostril to provide local anesthesia and decreased mucosal bleeding.

Other authors recommended the following method: examine children older than 5 years in a sitting position but restrain younger children in a lying position. Examine the nose with a bright light. The foreign body can usually be seen when the tip of the nose is lifted with the examiner's thumb. This makes it unnecessary to insert a speculum. If there is significant mucosal edema or bleeding because of the patient's attempts to remove the obstruction, gently insert a cotton wad soaked with local vasoconstrictor into the anterior part of the nasal cavity and leave it in place long enough for the vasoconstrictor to act (41).

Hooked Probe or Alligator Forceps

This approach usually works well if the foreign body is close to the anterior nares and can be easily grasped. Visualize the anterior of the nose with a nasal speculum and a headlight or a direct light source. Then use a hooked probe or alligator forceps, depending on the size and nature of the object, to remove the foreign body (65).

Balloon Catheter

Depending on the size of the patient, use a 5 French or 6 French Foley catheter to remove the foreign body. After checking that the balloon inflates properly, lubricate it with 2% lidocaine jelly and advance it past the object. Inflate the balloon with 2 to 3 mL of air, and withdraw the catheter, gently pulling out the foreign body. Varying the balloon's inflation may aid in removing various objects. Nandapalan and McIlwain (92a) reported removal of nasal foreign bodies with a Fogarty biliary balloon catheter. Henry and Chamberlain (54a) reported a removal with the use of an 8 French Foley catheter (65).

Positive Pressure

Positive pressure applied mouth to mouth or with an Ambu bag has been used to remove nasal foreign bodies. Occlude the contralateral nares with external pressure. Allow an anesthesia bag, connected to high-flow oxygen at 10 to 15 L/min with a mask that covers only the mouth, to expand with the thumbhole covered. If this pressure is not sufficient, compress the bag, expelling the foreign body. This technique usually works well for large objects occluding the entire nasal passage, which limit the ability to pass a Foley catheter or a hooked probe (65).

Suction Catheter

Use a Schunkt-Neck Suction Catheter. This is a metal suction catheter with a plastic umbrella at the tip. Place the plastic umbrella against the object, and turn on the suction to approximately 100 to 140 mm of mercury. The object is removed from the nose as the catheter is removed. This technique works well for round, smooth objects in the nares (65).

Although most fatal episodes of foreign-body injection in children involve asphyxia from airway obstruction, there are other causes. Asphyxia also may result from foreign bodies that lodge in the esophagus because of compression of the adjacent trachea. In infants, it has been reported that esophageal dysmobility may cause cardiorespiratory arrest secondary to the vasovagal reflex mechanism. Less commonly, death results from foreign-body migration. In some children, migration of foreign material has occurred from the pharynx and all levels of the esophagus, with death resulting from innominate artery erosion, carotid artery thrombosis, stroke, and sepsis (19).

BASIC AIRWAY MANEUVERS

The procedures listed and described in this section are divided into those useful when there is an adequate airway with no obstruction and those used when there is not an adequate airway with or without obstructive symptoms.

Breathing Adequately without Obstruction

If the patient is breathing adequately with no evidence of obstruction but needs supplemental oxygen, four modalities or modifications thereof are available for delivering oxygen.

NASAL CANNULA

This delivers an unpredictable amount of oxygen varying between 25% and 40%, with a flow rate of 6 L/min, depending on the ratio of mouth-to-nose breathing in a given patient.

Technique

1. Place the cannula into the patient's nostrils.
2. Lead the tubing around the patient's ears and tighten.

PLASTIC FACE MASK (SIMPLE MASK)

This supplies 50% to 60% oxygen at a flow rate of 10 L/min.

VENTURI MASK

The Venturi mask is used in the patient whose respiratory failure is secondary to chronic lung disease or who has hypercarbia, in whom it would be dangerous to administer an unpredictable volume of oxygen that may induce respiratory arrest by suppressing the respiratory center's "drive to breathe." These masks are available to deliver 24%, 28%, 35%, and 40% oxygen and require a flow rate of 4, 4, 8, and 8 L of oxygen per minute, respectively.

OXYGEN RESERVOIR MASK

This mask stores oxygen in a reservoir during expiration; when the patient inspires, this oxygen is inhaled from the reservoir. If a very tight seal is maintained, one can deliver an oxygen concentration of 90%. Fifty percent to 60% of the stored oxygen is the maximum delivered with the usual fit of a mask.

Breathing Spontaneously with Obstruction

With incomplete obstruction, the patient has labored breathing, excessive use of the accessory muscles, intercostal retraction, supraclavicular retraction, and a "crowing" sound on inspiration. The patient may

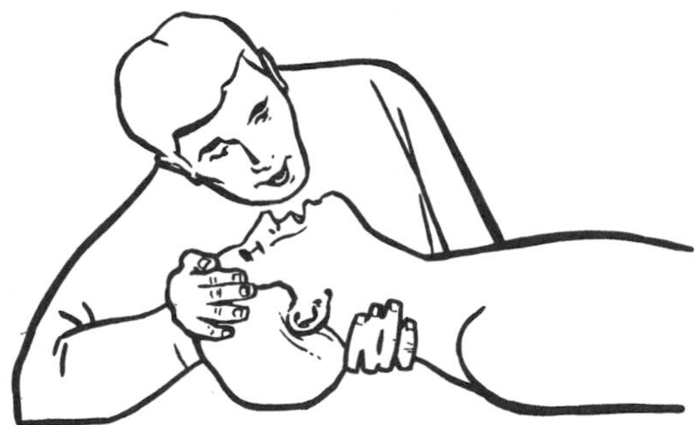

Figure 2.1. The head-tilt maneuver. See text for details. (From Guildner GW: Resuscitation: Opening the airway. JACEP 5:589, 1976, with permission.) We do not recommend this method.

be ashen gray or cyanotic, and there may be posterior displacement of the tongue. In the patient with signs of respiratory distress and signs of incomplete obstruction, consider the causes listed in Tables 2.1 and 2.4. Perform the following maneuvers, as indicated.

HEAD-TILT MANEUVER (FIG. 2.1)

CAUTION

The search for a foreign body obstructing the airway should be a very quick and superficial examination. One has no time to do a meticulous examination of the patient. Search for a bolus of food or foreign particle lodged in the posterior pharynx, dentures occluding the airway, or a large posteriorly displaced tongue. When one must provide an airway immediately, if the superficial search including jaw-thrust or chin-lift maneuvers discloses no obvious foreign-body obstruction that can be relieved immediately, then a cricothyroidotomy should be performed next.

Ruben et al. (112) evaluated three airway maneuvers and found the chin lift, jaw thrust, and head tilt useful techniques in the flaccid subject. For the chance rescuer, the head-tilt, chin-lift method is perhaps the easiest to master. When mouth-to-nose ventilation is used, the head tilt is the procedure of choice. With the exception of its use in the cardiac arrest victim, the traditional head-tilt maneuver is no longer advocated, however. Ruben et al. demonstrated the ineffectiveness of the procedure in relieving upper airway obstruction when compared with the chin lift or jaw thrust (112).

Procedural Steps

1. In the supine patient, place one hand behind the neck under the patient's occiput.
2. Place the heel of the other hand on the patient's forehead.
3. Displace the forehead back, and lift the occiput, thereby extending the head.

Contraindication

This maneuver should not be performed in cases of suspected cervical spine injury (79). This method has been deleted from the 1992 American Hospital Association (AHA) guidelines for cardiopulmonary resuscitation (CPR).

CHIN-LIFT MANEUVER (45, 79) (FIG. 2.2)

Procedure

1. Place the heel of the hand on the forehead.
2. Place the first two fingers of the other hand on the underside of the patient's chin.
3. Use traction on the chin and tilting motion on the forehead to extend the neck and open the airway. This method is the most adequate and consistent means of relieving airway obstruction (7).

In a recent study on the effects of this maneuver on upper airway dimensions during a routine magnetic resonance imaging (MRI) in pediatric patients sedated with propofol, it was concluded that

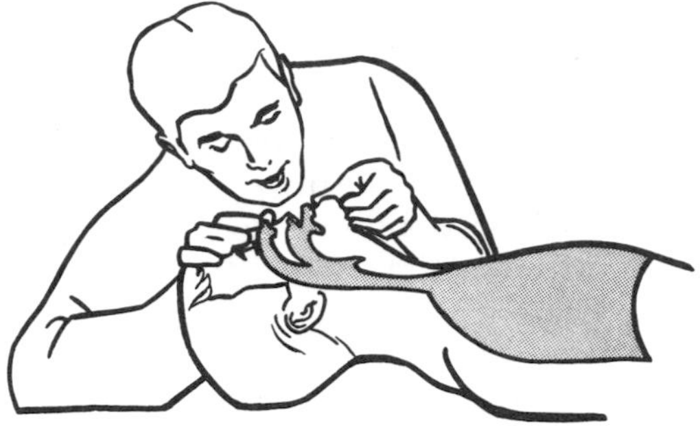

Figure 2.2. The chin-lift maneuver. See text for details. (From Guildner GW: Resuscitation: Opening the airway. JACEP 5:589, 1976, with permission.)

chin lifts cause a widening of the entire pharyngeal airway that is most pronounced between the tip of the epiglottis and the posterior pharyngeal wall (104). Thus it suggests that this maneuver is the treatment of choice because it is effective and more easily applied than other techniques in children (104).

Contraindication

This maneuver should not be performed in cases of cervical spine injury (71).

JAW-THRUST MANEUVER (TRIPLE-AIRWAY MANEUVER) (40, 71) (FIG. 2.3)

Procedure

1. While standing above the patient's head, place the fingers of each hand behind the angle of the mandible, lifting and displacing the jaw forward. While doing this, the patient's lower lip may be retracted to insert an oral airway.
2. Tilt the head backward, while the thumbs retract the lower lip and jaw.

In many instances, the airway is improved by these maneuvers. One should attempt these before resorting to any adjuncts. If they work, then place an oropharyngeal or nasopharyngeal airway as described later.

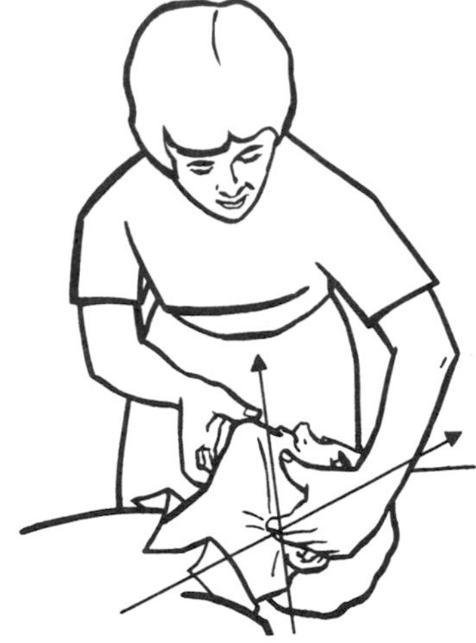

Figure 2.3. The jaw-thrust maneuver or triple-airway maneuver. See text for details. (From Guildner GW: Resuscitation: Opening the airway. JACEP 5:589, 1976, with permission.)

OROPHARYNGEAL AIRWAY (79)

The airway comes in various sizes from 000 for neonates to 4 for large adults. It is semicircular and curved to fit behind the tongue in the lower portion of the posterior pharynx. The airway is usually made of plastic but may be made of metal or rubber. The hard plastic form is the most commonly used. When in place, it extends from the lips to the posterior pharynx. The distal 2 cm includes a hard plastic guard to prevent the patient from biting and occluding the airway.

Contraindication

This procedure is contraindicated in a patient with an intact gag reflex.

Technique (Fig. 2.4)

1. Insert the airway between the patient's teeth with the convexity pointing toward the patient's feet (Fig. 2.4*A*).
2. As the airway passes the back of the tongue, it is rotated around to its resting position with the concavity pointing toward the feet. Then insert the airway to the hub (Fig. 2.4*B*).

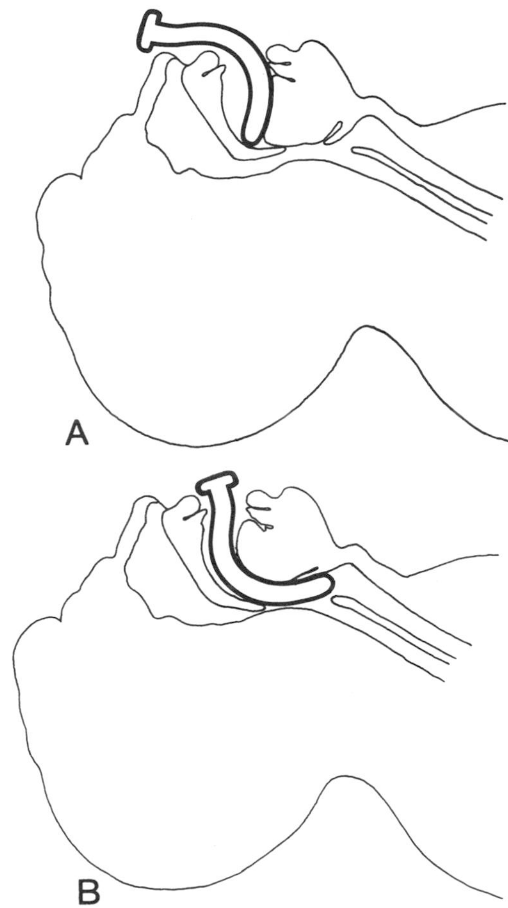

Figure 2.4. *A:* The oropharyngeal airway. Insert the airway between the patient's teeth with the convexity pointing toward the patient's feet. *B:* As the airway passes the back of the tongue, rotate it around into its resting position so the concavity points toward the feet.

Alternate Method

One also can insert the airway into its proper position by using a tongue depressor to depress the tongue inferiorly while passing the airway into the pharynx.

CAUTION

If the airway is not properly placed, it can increase the obstruction by pushing the tongue back into the pharynx.

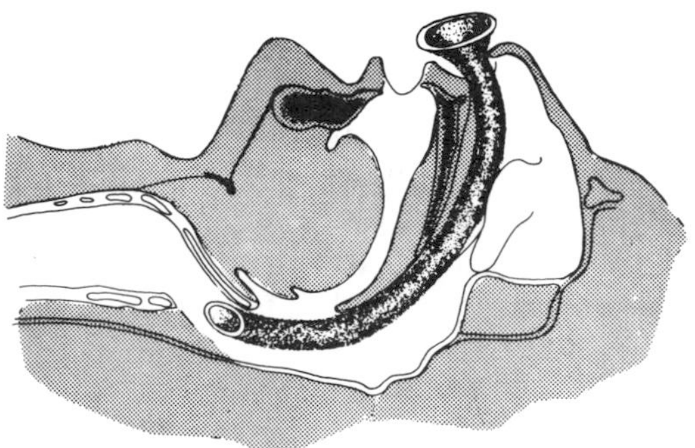

Figure 2.5. The position of the nasopharyngeal airway. (From Warner A: Nasopharyngeal airway: A facilitated access to the trachea. Ann Intern Med 75:594, 1971, with permission.)

Complications

Use of the oropharyngeal airway can cause retching and vomiting. To prevent this, do not use the airway in the conscious patient. To treat, remove the airway and suction the oropharynx.

NASOPHARYNGEAL AIRWAY (FIG. 2.5)

The nasopharyngeal airway is made of soft rubber and is approximately 6 inches in length. This airway is better tolerated in the conscious patient.

Contraindications

This airway should not be used in the presence of several nasal fractures that occlude the nasal passage.

Technique

1. Select the size of airway desired, judged by the largest size that will fit into the patient's nostril.
2. Look into both nostrils for septal deviation, polyps, and the like, and select the nostril that appears more open.
3. Lubricate the airway with an anesthetic lubricating solution [lidocaine (Xylocaine) ointment].
4. Pass the airway, with the bevel facing the nasal septum along the floor of the nose.

CAUTION

The floor of the nose lies parallel to the oral cavity. If one recalls this anatomic point in passing the tube, then the most common complication with this procedure (nasal bleeding) can be avoided.

5. Rotate the tube as it reaches the hypopharynx so that the tube sits as shown.

Some authors have described a modified nasopharyngeal tube to relieve high upper-airway obstruction in infants with craniofacial anomalies (Pierre–Robin syndrome, Down syndrome, idiopathic generalized hypotonia) that does not add airway dead space and resistance and is well tolerated. The device described allows simultaneous use of oxygen prongs. This potentially reduces the need for tracheostomy and other surgical interventions.

Preparation of the Tube

Estimate the required length of the tube (distance from lateral nostril to tragus of ipsilateral ear), and place a tracheal tube in the nasopharynx, adjust it, temporarily tape it, and assess its position radiologically. Record the tube length at the nostril when the correct position is established (the tube tip sits just superior to the epiglottis). Prepare a new tube (blue-line ivory tracheal tube; Portex, United Kingdom) by cutting at the measured length plus 5 cm. Then cut the tube down the midline of the under side of the tube to the measured length. Make two cuts to each side of the midline to create two thin strips 3 mm wide. These are used for anchoring the tube to the child's cheeks. Make a further cut, creating two additional strips on the top. Shorten one of these top strips to the measured length plus 2 cm and use it for anchoring the tube to the dorsum of the nose. Cut off the remaining top strip at the measured length. The wedge that is cut off depends on whether the nasopharyngeal tube is used for insertion into the right or left nasopharynx.

Securing the Tube

Before inserting the tube, apply a protective dressing (Duo Derm; Bristol-Myers, Montreal, Canada) approximately 4 ×2.5 cm to both cheeks to use as the base. Insert the prepared tube into the selected nostril, and anchor the side strips on the base tape with adhesive tape. Pass the smaller top strip across the ala and anchor on the dorsum of the lateral nasal aspect. In the initial period, the nasopharyngeal tube size and length may require minor adjustments. Change the nasopharyngeal tube every 2 to 4 days for the first 10 days and then every 5 to 7 days thereafter, and use alternate nostrils (83).

Complications

Nasal bleeding is the primary complication of use of the nasopharyngeal airway. Prevention involves careful passage of the airway (see step 4 under Technique). No treatment is usually indicated because the bleeding will subside spontaneously. If bleeding is significant, insert a nasal pack if necessary.

Apnea with Complete Airway Obstruction

If there is no spontaneous breathing and the airway is completely obstructed, the Heimlich maneuver is the procedure of choice.

HEIMLICH MANEUVER

The primary indication for use of the Heimlich maneuver is upper airway obstruction due to a bolus of food or any aspirated foreign material unrelieved by coughing and traditional means that now is causing complete airway obstruction and threatening asphyxiation.

Contraindications

Use of the Heimlich maneuver is contraindicated in the patient who has any chest injury such as fractured ribs or flail, cardiac contusion, or sternal fracture.

Technique

NOTE

Recent studies have shown that the traditional Heimlich maneuver causes more complications and is not so effective as the modified technique shown in this text.

---

1. Have the patient sit upright or stand. Place patients who are lying on the ground in the supine position.
2. In the patient who is sitting or standing, wrap both arms around the patient's chest with the right hand closed in a fist and placed over the midsternal region (between the nipples), while the left hand grasps the right "fist"' (Fig. 2.6). In the supine patient, place hands over the lower sternum with the right hand over the left and compress. Alternatively, place the right hand over the lower sternum just above the xiphoid process, as shown in Fig. 2.7. The technique remains the same except for positioning of the hand over the sternum. Both methods are equally acceptable.
3. With a rapid forceful thrust, compress the chest, and the bolus will be dislodged.

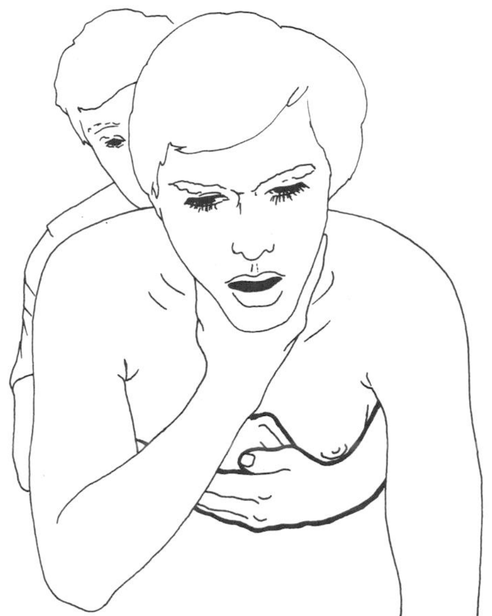

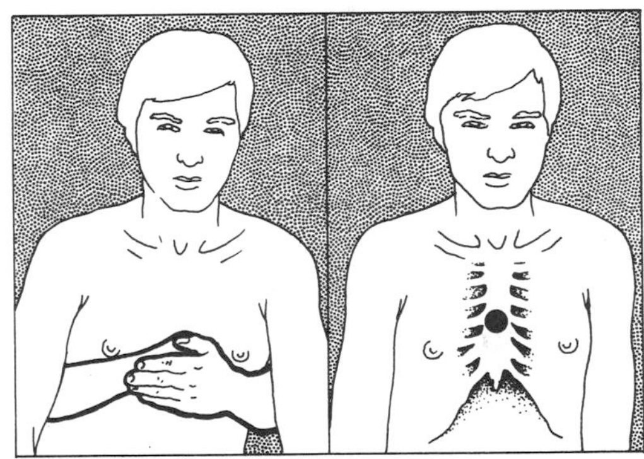

Figure 2.6. Heimlich maneuver. Wrap both arms around the patient's chest with the right hand closed in a fist and placed over the midsternal region, while the left hand grasps the right hand as shown in the *inset* in the lower left corner. Place the hand between the nipples, as shown in the lower left *inset*. Compression should be forceful and directed posteriorly.

NOTE

If repeated thrusts fail to dislodge the bolus and the patient is asphyxiating, immediately resort to a cricothyroidotomy or cricothyroid membrane puncture.

NOTE

A technique for dislodging a foreign body in a small child is shown in Fig. 2.8. Place the child upside down, held in the examiner's hand, as shown in the figure. Apply forceful compression with the right hand while the left hand is over the lower sternum. We have found this method to be quite successful in dislodging foreign bodies in smaller children. Its value compared with that of the Heimlich maneuver remains to be determined.

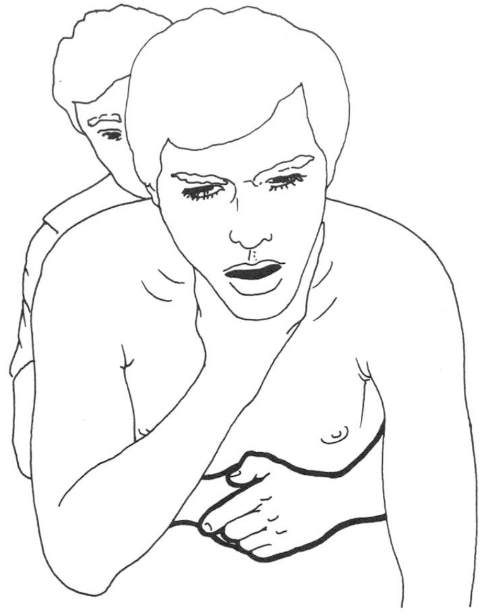

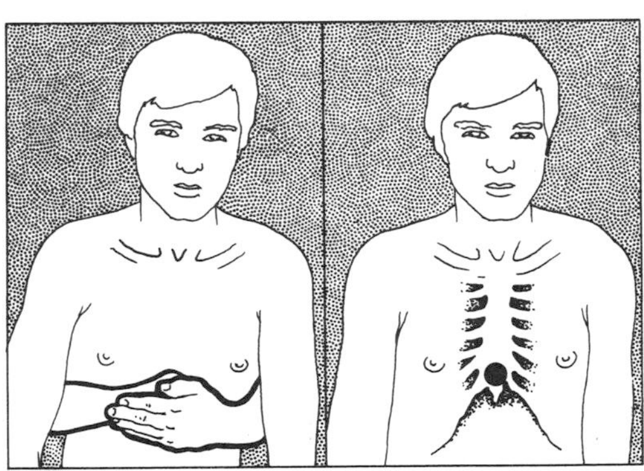

Figure 2.7. Heimlich maneuver: alternate technique. Place the right hand over the lower sternum, just above the xiphoid process. The technique remains the same, except for positioning of the hand over the sternum *(inset)*. See text for details.

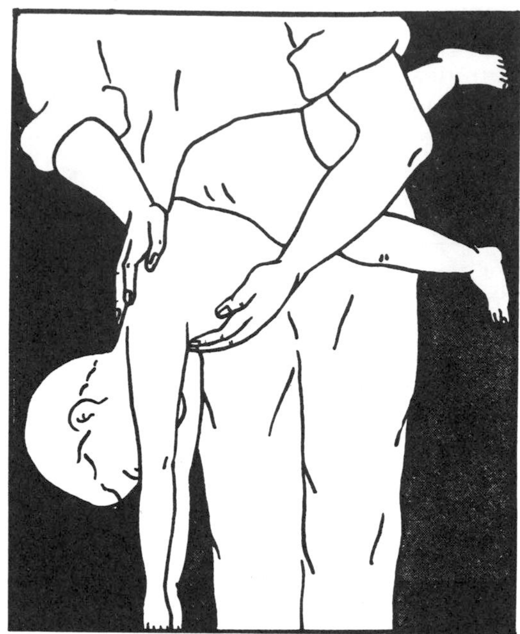

Figure 2.8. The technique for dislodging a foreign body in a small child. Invert the child and apply a sharp blow between the shoulder blades. (From JAMA 172:815, 1960, with permission.)

Complications

1. **Fractured ribs.** These are unavoidable, particularly in the elderly patient with a brittle rib cage. Treat as with any rib fracture.
2. **Rupture of the liver or spleen.** This is not associated with the procedure described earlier, but is a common complication of the traditional Heimlich maneuver.

Apnea without Airway Obstruction

If there is no spontaneous breathing and the possibility of complete airway obstruction is unlikely or has been eliminated by examination, proceed with the following techniques.

MOUTH-TO-MOUTH BREATHING

Exhaled air delivers 16% to 17% oxygen to the patient. Ideally this would have a Po_2 of 80 torr; however, because of the decreased cardiac output, ventilation–perfusion abnormalities, and physiologic shunting, the actual Po_2 is much less.

In the United States, debate continues about the necessity of ventilation during CPR. Three questions are being considered. First, is ventilation necessary for the treatment of cardiac arrest? Second, is mouth-to-mouth ventilation any better than no ventilation at all? Third, are other techniques of ventilation as effective or more effective than mouth-to-mouth ventilation during basic life support? Many studies have been performed, however, and taken together, the results provide some evidence that ventilation can be withheld when chest compression is initiated promptly after cardiac arrest, but this ventilation is important for survival when chest compression is delayed. In the Netherlands where CPR is given in the order "CAB"(chest compression, airway, breathing) with ventilation delayed and chest compression initiated as soon as possible, CPR survival rates are comparable to those reported in the United States.

Because exhaled gas contains so much CO_2 and less O_2 than air, it may have adverse affects during CPR and may be no better than no ventilation at all. Chest compression alone and spontaneous gasping each provides some pulmonary ventilation and gas exchange. Blood oxygenation can be improved with supplemental oxygen. Active compression–decompression (ACD) CPR in which force is applied during both the downstroke compression phase and the upstroke decompression phase may improve gas exchange compared with standard chest compression (59). The successful outcome of CPR is based on rapid identification and treatment of cardiac arrest.

The success of CPR is based on rapid identification and treatment of cardiac arrest. The first treatment goal is pulmonary ventilation and oxygenation, which require airway patency. Begin with the least invasive maneuvers (chin lift, jaw thrust, oral airways, and nasal airways) and progress down the options sequentially toward transtracheal ventilation.

Technique

1. Stand at the patient's right side and extend the head by placing the right hand under the chin. Apply upward pressure and lift the chin as a downward pressure is applied concomitantly over the head with the palm of the left hand (Fig. 2.9*A*).
2. With the thumb and index fingers of the left hand, pinch the nostrils shut so as not to permit the egress of air while using upward traction on the jaw or the patient's neck to open the mouth.
3. Take a deep breath, cover the patient's mouth with yours, and forcibly exhale air into the patient's oral cavity.

Alternate Technique: Mouth-to-Nose Breathing

An alternate technique that can be used effectively is that of providing mouth-to-nose artificial ventilation. In this procedure, stand at the patient's right side and extend the head as indicated earlier and as shown in Fig. 2.9*A*. Use the left hand to hyperextend the neck by placing it over the patient's forehead and applying downward and backward pressure, while the right hand is used to hyperextend the jaw and close the mouth (Fig. 2.9*B*). With the patient's mouth closed, the physician can then effectively give mouth-to-nose ventilation. For this technique to be effective there must be a patent nasal passage. It is particularly useful in those patients to whom one cannot give mouth-to-mouth ventilation because of vomitus, profuse bleeding from the mouth, or severe mandibular fractures. Then permit the mouth to open slightly to allow exhaling of air, as shown in Fig. 2.9*C*.

NOTE

In an infant or small child, exhale into both the oral and nasal passages by covering the infant's nose and mouth with that of the rescuer (Fig. 2.10). An alternate method of providing mouth-to-mouth ventilation in an infant is shown and discussed in Fig. 2.11.

For those patients who have vomited, it is extremely important that aspiration be prevented and that an airway be maintained. The technique of providing this is shown and discussed in Fig. 2.12.

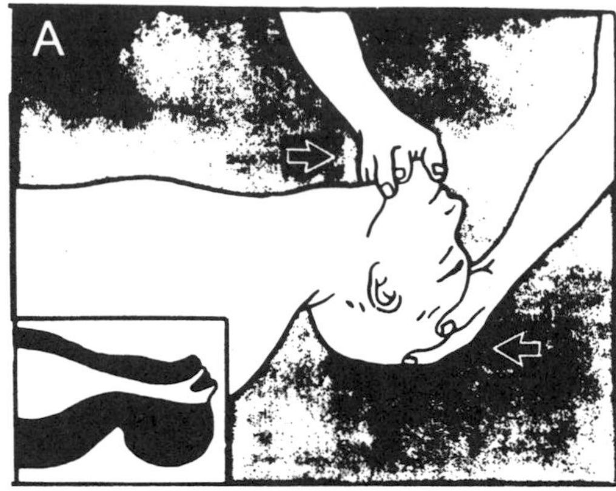

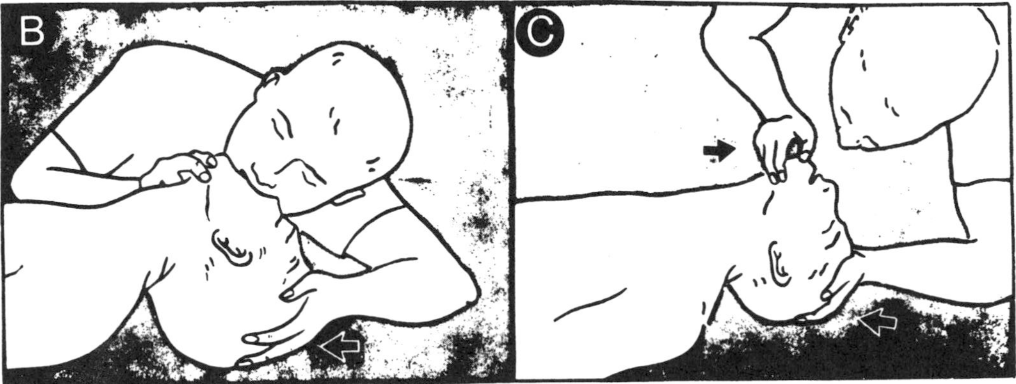

Figure 2.9. Technique for mouth-to-mouth breathing with the head-tilt oral method. *A:* Tilt the head back fully. *B:* Inflate the lungs via the nose or mouth. *C:* Patient exhales by him or herself, as necessary, through his or her mouth. (From JAMA 172:814, 1960, with permission.)

POCKET MASK

The pocket mask, which is particularly useful, has an inlet nipple for providing supplemental oxygen. With a 10-L flow rate, the mask will deliver an oxygen concentration of 50%. If the flow rate is increased to 30 L, the mask will supply oxygen at a concentration of 100%, and the rescuer can occlude the portal intermittently and provide adequate ventilation to the patient without any mouth-to-mask breathing.

Technique

Apply the mask to the patient's oral and nasal passages and hold it firmly by placing the thumbs on either side of the mask while the index, middle, and ring fingers grasp the mandible, pulling it upward, which opens the airway for ventilation.

Advantages of the Pocket Mask

1. Eliminates contact with the patient, especially because there is a fear of acquiring infection during mouth-to-mouth resuscitation.
2. Provides good ventilation.
3. Easier to use than the bag–valve–mask devices.
4. Contains an inlet for the provision of supplemental oxygen.

NOTE

The pocket mask should have a one-way valve to prevent contamination of the rescuer by regurgitation of the victim. This valve should remain a one-way valve despite biting of the mask by the victim. The mask should have been de-

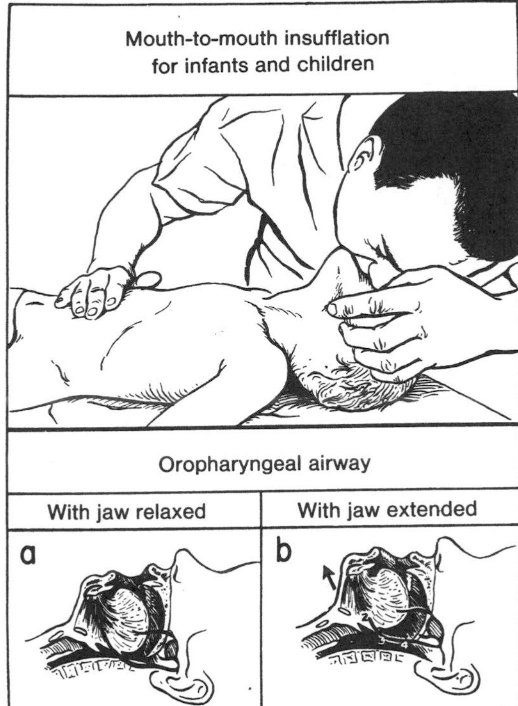

Figure 2.10. Technique for mouth-to-mouth resuscitation in an infant or small child. Place the infant in the supine position with the head in neutral position. Position the rescuer at the side of the head. Place the fingers of both hands beneath and behind the angles of the lower jaw and lift vertically upward, so that it juts out into a position shown above. This is the most important step in the entire procedure, because it effectively clears the oropharynx of obstruction by the tongue. In the unconscious patient, the jaw relaxes, and the tongue gravitates against the posterior pharyngeal wall to occlude the oropharynx *(A)*. When the mandible is extended by lifting it upward, the airway is opened *(B)*. (From JAMA 167:322, 1958, with permission.)

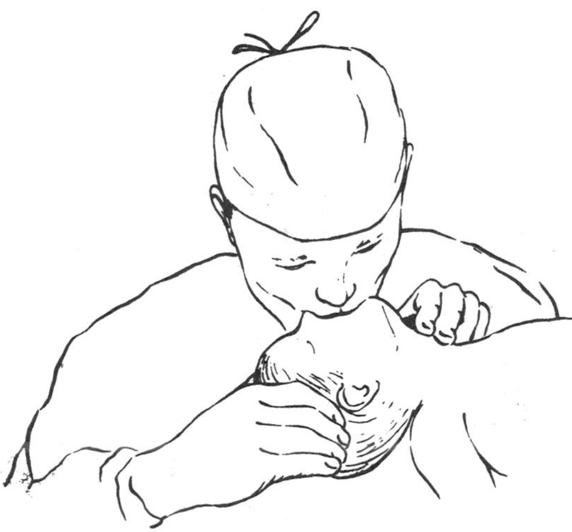

Figure 2.11. The application of gentle cricoid pressure during mouth-to-mouth resuscitation of a small infant. The use of cricoid pressure controls regurgitation of gastric contents. This also prevents inflation of the stomach during ventilation with a face mask or mouth-to-mouth. (From Anesthesiology 40:97, 1974, with permission.)

monstrated to pass no infections, even viral, from the victim to the rescuer or vice versa.

BAG–VALVE–MASK DEVICE (LAERDAL BAG)

This device is very familiar to all emergency personnel. It is found in every emergency center and ambulance. Although it is perhaps the most popular modality for providing artificial ventilation, it has numerous disadvantages when compared with the pocket mask and other adjuncts to ventilation that have not (until now) been adequately appreciated.

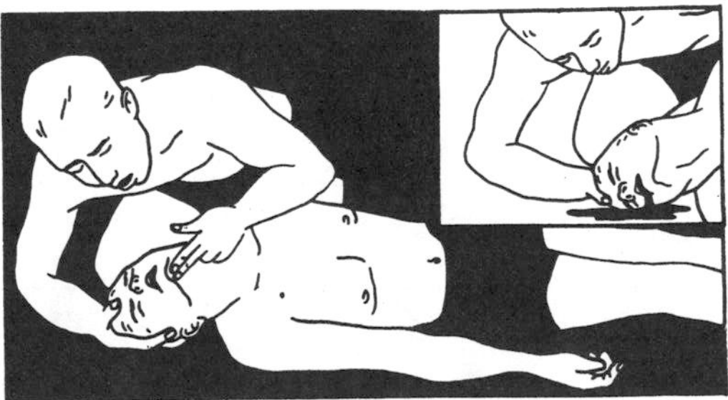

Figure 2.12. The semilateral position for gravity drainage of fluid from the patient's oropharynx. Pull up the patient's shoulders, and stabilize them with the knee. Apply gentle pressure over the epigastrium to facilitate emptying fluid from the stomach. (From JAMA 172:815, 1960, with permission.)

Features This Device Should Contain

1. The bag should be self-refilling and contain no sponge rubber on the inside lining. The sponge rubber can become friable and also is difficult to sterilize in cleaning the bag.
2. The bag must feature a non-jamming valve system. The purpose of this is that some valves may become jammed with vomitus and may function poorly or not at all. The newer bags contain a non-jam valve system that does not permit this to happen.
3. The mask should be made of transparent plastic to permit the examiner to see if there are any foreign particles or vomitus contained in the bag, which the black bags previously used do not allow.
4. Provisions for delivering supplemental oxygen.
5. A non–pop-off valve. The pop-off valve contained on some pediatric bags will pop off once a predetermined pressure is reached during the delivery of the air contained within the bag. Thus the patient does not receive the full volume of air contained within the bag when high pressures are necessary to deliver that volume.
6. The capability to be used with an oropharyngeal airway.

NOTE

The Ambu bag does not meet all of these requirements, and we recommend the Laerdal bag, which is available in several sizes for both pediatric and adult age groups.

NOTE

When attached to supplemental oxygen at 12 L/min, the bag–valve–mask device will deliver only 40% oxygen, provided there is a tight seal. If one attaches an oxygen reservoir and adapter, an oxygen concentration of 90% can be achieved.

Technique

1. Remove foreign material. Leave dentures in place unless they obstruct the airway. Dentures may render a good mouth–bag seal that is almost impossible to achieve in the edentulous patient.
2. Insert an oral airway.
3. Extend the neck and elevate the mandible to open the hypopharynx.
4. Apply the mask over the nose and mouth.

NOTE

Various size masks are available for children and adults. Select the mask that provides the tightest seal and conforms best to the patient's nose and mouth.

---

5. Squeeze the mask with the right hand and produce a tight seal, using the last two or three fingers to support the mandible while the thumb and first one or two fingers are placed over the mask on either side of the valve connection. Then use the left hand to squeeze the bag. When enough personnel are available, a better seal is provided with two operators, one to hold the mask in place and the mandible extended, while the other squeezes the bag.
6. Tilt the head and inflate the lungs.
7. Observe for chest movement.
8. For prolonged ventilation with this device, place a nasogastric tube to prevent gastric distention.

Advantages of the Bag–Valve–Mask Device

1. Provides an immediate means of ventilating the patient.
2. Supplies enriched oxygen if needed.
3. Permits the operator to assess the compliance of the lungs. This clinical determination is lost when oxygen-powered devices are used.

Disadvantages of Bag–Valve–Mask Device

1. A lower tidal volume is delivered than with the mouth-to-mouth technique or the pocket mask.
2. Difficult for even the skilled practitioner to provide a perfect seal.
3. Gastric distention is a very common sequela.

Contraindications

1. Oral bleeding or vomiting.
2. Upper airway obstruction or injury.
3. Severe maxillofacial fractures.

OXYGEN-POWERED MANUALLY TRIGGERED BREATHING DEVICE

In an arrest situation, one cannot use pressure-cycled respirators. When chest compression is performed, this triggers the device to shut off prematurely as a result of the increase in intrathoracic pressure associated with chest compressions. This abbreviated respiration causes the patient to receive an inadequate volume. Volume-cycled respirators cannot be used either, because one cannot properly synchronize compressions with ventilations.

With the oxygen-powered breathing devices, both these problems are overcome by the manual triggering of the device (timing) and the delivery of high-flow oxygen at 100 L/min. Do not use these devices for long periods, because they are associated with high incidence of gastric distention.

Two additional modalities should be mentioned, although not used. The S-tube is a device similar to the oropharyngeal airway in that it does assist in keeping the mouth open; however, it does not provide an adequate seal in the oropharynx and may induce emesis by irritating the oropharynx.

The accordion bag mask is totally unacceptable and should never be used. This device is no longer available in most facilities because it does not meet any of the requirements of a good bag–valve–mask device.

CAUTION

Remember to suction the patient's mouth and pharynx periodically while using any of the adjuncts described earlier in the patient who is not spontaneously breathing.

INTUBATION OF THE TRACHEA

ADVANTAGES OF ENDOTRACHEAL INTUBATION

1. Protects against aspiration and achieves complete control of airway.
2. Eliminates gastric distention associated with mouth-to-mouth, mouth-to-mask, bag–valve–mask, and oxygen-powered devices used for ventilation.
3. Suctioning of the trachea is possible.
4. Permits better elimination of CO_2.

INDICATIONS

1. Respiratory arrest or cardiorespiratory arrest.
2. Hypoventilation of hypoxia. Patients who have neuromuscular disturbances that impair respiratory function may require endotracheal intubation because of hypoventilation and hypoxia (17).
3. Inability to ventilate a patient who is unconscious by other conventional means.
4. Prolonged artificial ventilation.
5. Moderate to severe flail chest.
6. Isolation of the trachea to prevent aspiration.
7. Some believe that endotracheal intubation can be performed with little difficulty in acute epiglottitis (68).
8. Prevention of airway obstruction and aspiration of vomitus in central nervous system (CNS)-depressed patients (105).

NOTE

Endotracheal intubation is indicated if the lash reflex is absent, response to stimulation is not purposeful, or airway obstruction develops when the patient's neck is flexed (105).

A misconception exists about an empty stomach. The stomach is never completely empty no matter how long the depressed patient may have been without food. In the absence of recent food ingestion, the normal stomach will secrete at least 50 mL of gastric juice per hour (57). Patients are often thought of as having an empty stomach if intake has not occurred in the preceding 8 hours; however, in some situations, food ingested before this time may remain in the stomach (e.g., ulcers and obstructing lesions may delay gastric emptying). In addition, any acute abdominal process will delay gastric emptying. Sepsis, systemic diseases, and medications also may delay emptying.

Aspiration of blood, mucus, and saliva does not lead to serious complications in such patients (57). The acidic fluid is a severe respiratory irritant, causing large secretions and respiratory compromise.

CONTRAINDICATIONS

1. Severe injury to the larynx. Controversy exists regarding laryngotracheal trauma. Some authors (3) preferred emergency tracheotomy in these patients, whereas others (124) recommended careful endotracheal intubation. Careful endotracheal intubation has many advocates (71).
2. Severe maxillofacial trauma.
3. Fracture or possible fracture of the cervical spine.

EQUIPMENT

Laryngoscope with assorted sizes of blades

NOTE

Two types of blades are available, the MacIntosh and the straight blade (Fig. 2.13). Each is available in a variety of sizes for children and adults. The practitioner usually finds one or the other type more comfortable to use. Although the choice between the MacIntosh and the straight blade is primarily that of personal preference, in some distinct situations, one is preferred over the other. These are discussed in the appropriate area in the section on procedure.

Endotracheal tubes (ETTs) sizes 3 through 9.5.

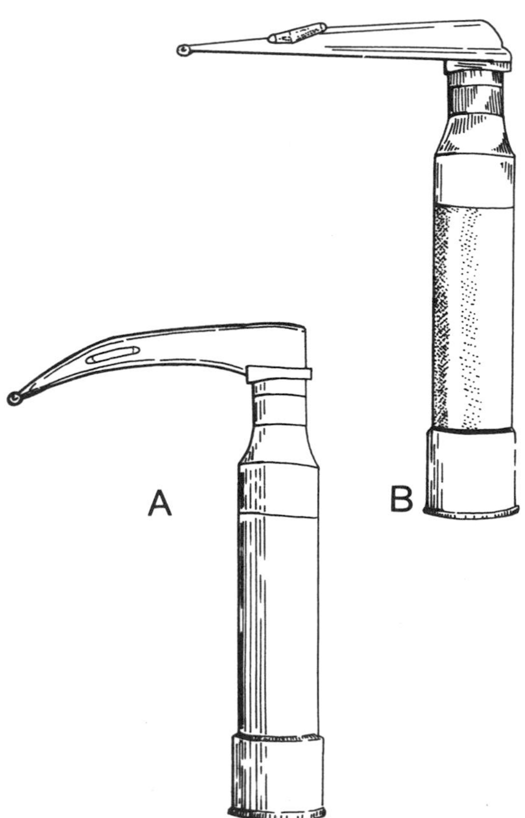

Figure 2.13. The MacIntosh *(A)* and straight *(B)* laryngoscope blades.

NOTE

All of these tubes have a standard 15-mm adapter to fit bag or ventilator. Tubes less than 7 mm do not have a cuff. Generally, patients younger than 8 years do not need a cuffed tube because the cartilaginous trachea is "soft" and a well-fitting ETT will sufficiently "seal" the airway.

Lubricating jelly
Stylet
Topical spray anesthetic
10-mL syringe
Suction catheters

NOTE

One should have both tracheal suction catheters to suction secretions from the tube and rigid (tonsil) suction for oral secretions and vomitus.

TECHNIQUE

Preparatory Steps

1. Select the proper tube. In urgent situations, remember that in the average adult, an 8-mm tube works well.

NOTE

The adult male patient generally takes an 8.5- to 9.5-mm tube. The average woman takes a 7.5- to 8.5-mm tube. In the child, the tube size should approximately equal the diameter of the patient's small finger.

In the patient with a narrow pharynx, a smaller tube than one would otherwise judge appropriate is indicated to facilitate visualization and placement (117). In determining whether a patient has a narrow pharynx, clinical judgment must be used. Those patients with a narrow, long neck and a small mouth and those with long faces can be assumed to have a narrow pharynx, and a smaller tube size would be used, such as a 7-mm tube in the average adult male.

2. Attach a syringe with 10 mL of air to the portal of the tube. A child between ages 8 and 12 years needs only 5 mL of air in the syringe. One must use clinical judgment here, because some 12-year-olds are large enough to be considered adults.
3. If time permits, check the cuff for air leaks.
4. If one is going to use a stylet, insert it into the tube at this time. The stylet must be recessed 1/2 inch from the end of the tube.

CAUTION

A stylet that sticks out of the end of the tube may cause tracheal perforation or injury to the vocal cords! This potential danger is the prime reason that many anesthesiologists do not permit stylets in their operating suites.

Note: Lighted stylets facilitate passage of ETTs into the trachea in a relatively noninvasive fashion. Lighted stylets are constructed of an energy source (battery), a shaft (which is often flexible), and a light bulb (106). Place an ETT on the shaft of the stylet in a position that allows the light bulb to approximate the tip of the tube. Illuminate the bulb before it is advanced blindly into the airway and around the base of the tongue. At that point, light is transilluminated through the anterior aspect of the neck. Then advance the stylet into the larynx. As the stylet enters the trachea, the transilluminated light remains bright and well circumscribed. Insert it into the esophagus. The light appears dim and diffuse. Reducing the ambient light, when possible, facilitates this distinction. If the tube is thought to be in the trachea, it is advanced of the stylet towards the carina. The stylet is then removed and the ETT is left in place (106).

5. Select a blade, either the MacIntosh or straight blade, of approximate size to negotiate the oropharynx.

NOTE

In patients with a short, thick neck, the MacIntosh blade may be somewhat easier to use in visualizing the glottic opening. These patients tend to have a more posteriorly placed tongue and epiglottis. In infants and small children, the straight blade is preferred, because of the large size of these patients' heads as compared with the rest of the torso. Although the curved blade can be used in these patients, because of the proximity and small size of the epiglottis in relation to the glottic opening, the curved blade may not provide sufficient visualization of the opening, as it does not displace the epiglottis as does the straight blade. Some individuals who have been well trained in the use of the curved blade, however, have not found this to be a problem.

---

6. Lubricate the tube.

Procedural Steps

Ideally, intubation should take no more than 20 to 30 seconds. If particular attention is paid to those steps that are in italics, the requisite skill will be attained. In a survey of difficult or unsuccessful intubations involving anesthetists, medical students, and physicians, one of these steps was either omitted or performed improperly, and this led to the difficulties encountered in the majority of cases (104).

CAUTION

Ventilate the patient well *before* attempting intubation, including between unsuccessful attempts! If this is not done, one may cause arrhythmias or sudden death (112). No attempt at endotracheal intubation should persist for more than 50 to 60 seconds without artificial ventilation.

---

1. **Align the axis** of the mouth, pharynx, and larynx in a straight line (58, 80). Accomplished this by extending the head at the atlantooccipital joint and flexing the neck (Fig. 2.14). (Note flex-

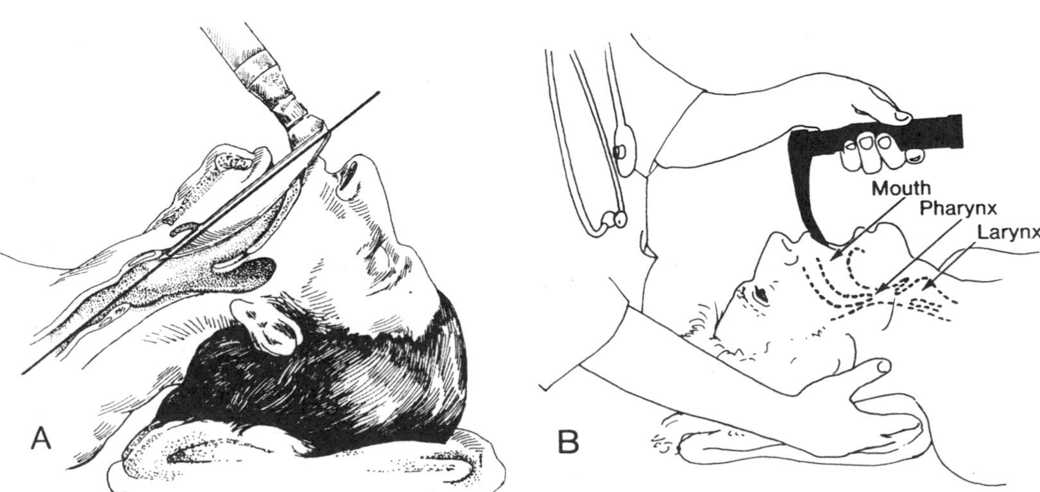

Figure 2.14. *A:* Aligning of the axis of the mouth, pharynx, and larynx. *B:* Extending the head at the atlantooccipital joint, and flex the neck. Note flexion of the neck by a small towel placed beneath the head for difficult cases.

ion of neck by small towel placed beneath the head). This maneuver of aligning the mouth with the posterior pharynx and the larynx converts their normal relationship to each other from that of a semicircular curve to more a gentle curve approximating a straight line. Facilitate this maneuver by first locating the tracheal axis and then proceeding to align the mouth and posterior pharynx with this axis. This places the patient in what is commonly referred to as the "sniffing" position.

NOTE

In the endotracheal intubation in which visualization of the glottis is difficult, two maneuvers may be of use. Place a *folded* towel under the occiput, which will flex the neck, aiding in aligning the axes of the larynx and the mouth (Fig. 2.14). Compression of the larynx often facilitates visualization of the glottis.

CAUTION

Do not permit the head to hang over the bed (extension of neck rather than flexion) during endotracheal intubation because this displaces the desired axes. At the very least, the head should be horizontal with the shoulders. Extension of the neck will cause anterior displacement of the larynx and make it difficult to visualize the glottis.

---

2. Use two fingers to open the mouth widely (thumb and index finger of left hand) and a third (middle finger) to displace the tongue to the left (117).

NOTE

A common error is not opening the patient's mouth wide enough for adequate visualization.

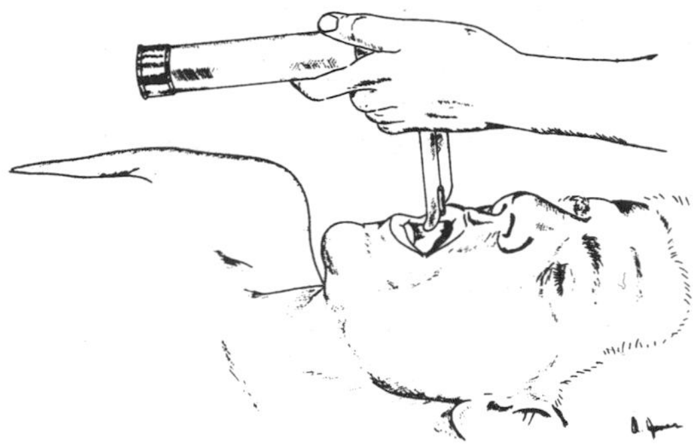

Figure 2.15. Always insert the laryngoscope blade along the right side of the patient's mouth (as shown above). Stand above the patient's head in doing so. After passing the laryngoscope blade along the right side of the patient's mouth, aim the tip of the blade toward the posterior midline of the tongue. Lift the tongue to visualize the glottic opening (as described in the text).

3. Remove dentures and foreign material with the right hand, and suction any secretions, blood, or vomitus from the oral cavity, using the tonsil suction. Keep dentures nearby. If the initial attempts at endotracheal intubation are unsuccessful, dentures may be needed for good seal with bag–mask ventilation.
4. With the laryngoscope held in the left hand, insert the blade from the right side of the patient's mouth on the right side of the tongue, aiming toward the posterior midline of the tongue (Fig. 2.15). Displace the tongue to the left with blade. "Walk down" the tongue (50).
5. Applying forceful leverage to the blade in an upward direction and not traction (the arrow in Fig. 2.16 shows the direction in which the traction is applied with the laryngoscope blade), advance the blade until the epiglottis is visualized. The eyes of the intubationist must be in line with the epiglottis for visualization of the glottis, which often requires the physician to crouch (Fig. 2.17).

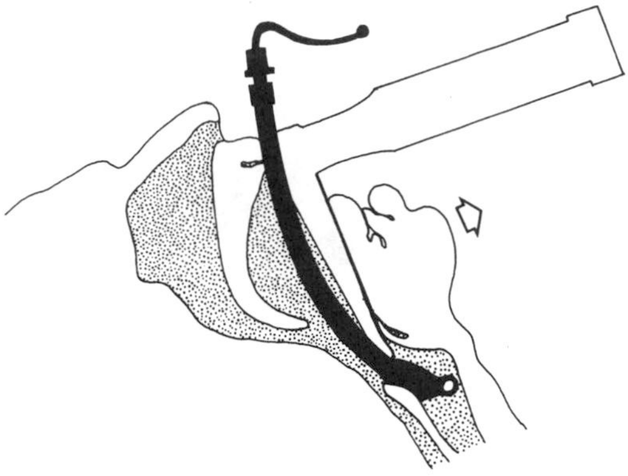

Figure 2.16. Apply forceful leverage to the blade in an upward direction *arrow*. Advance the blade until the epiglottis is visualized.

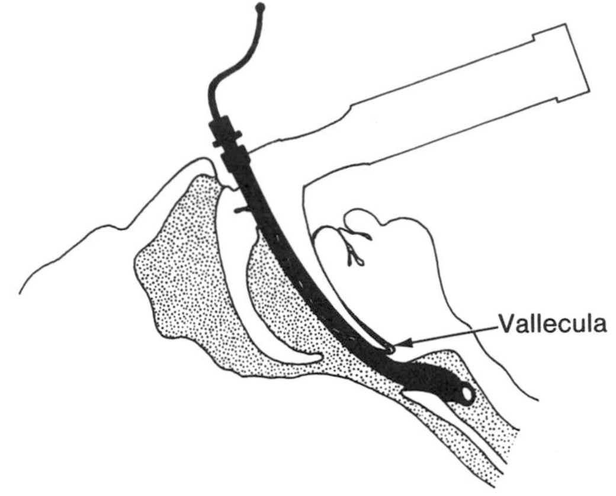

Figure 2.18. If the MacIntosh blade is used, position the tip of the blade into the vallecula.

CAUTION

Be careful not to use the laryngoscope as a lever against the upper incisors, because this process may fracture a tooth that can later be aspirated.

---

6. MacIntosh: If the MacIntosh is used, position the tip of the blade in the vallecula (Fig. 2.18). Straight blade:

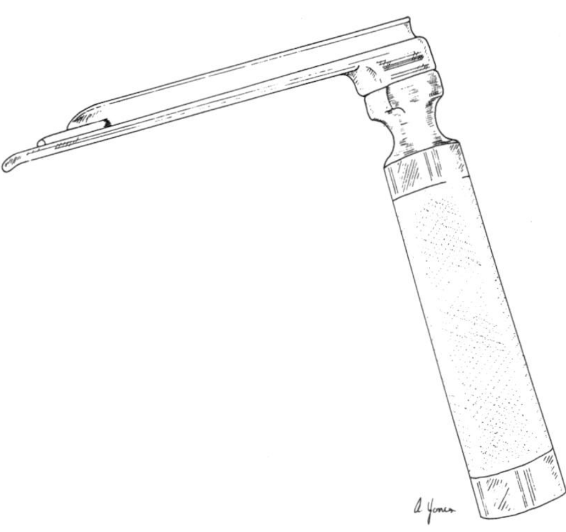

Figure 2.17. Please note that the hollow portion of the blade is the channel through which one visualizes the glottis; do not pass the tube through this portion of the blade, as visualization will be obstructed.

If the straight blade is used, uplift the epiglottis with the blade (Fig. 2.16).

7. MacIntosh: While applying upward leverage to the epiglottis with the blade positioned anterior to the epiglottis and in the vallecula, visualize the arytenoid cartilages or the glottic opening and advance the ETT into the trachea. Figure 2.19 shows the vocal cords and glottic opening as visualized through the laryngoscope. When using the curved blade (MacIntosh), one may see only the epiglottis and the arytenoid cartilages through the laryngoscope; however, the glottis lies between these two structures. All that is necessary to insert the ETT accurately into the trachea is visualization of the epiglottis and arytenoid cartilages through the curved blade.

Straight blade: Lift the epiglottis upward and visualize the vocal cords as you apply leverage. Pass the ETT into the trachea once the glottis is seen. With the straight blade the vocal cords are usually visualized making accurate placement more definitively assessable by the physician.

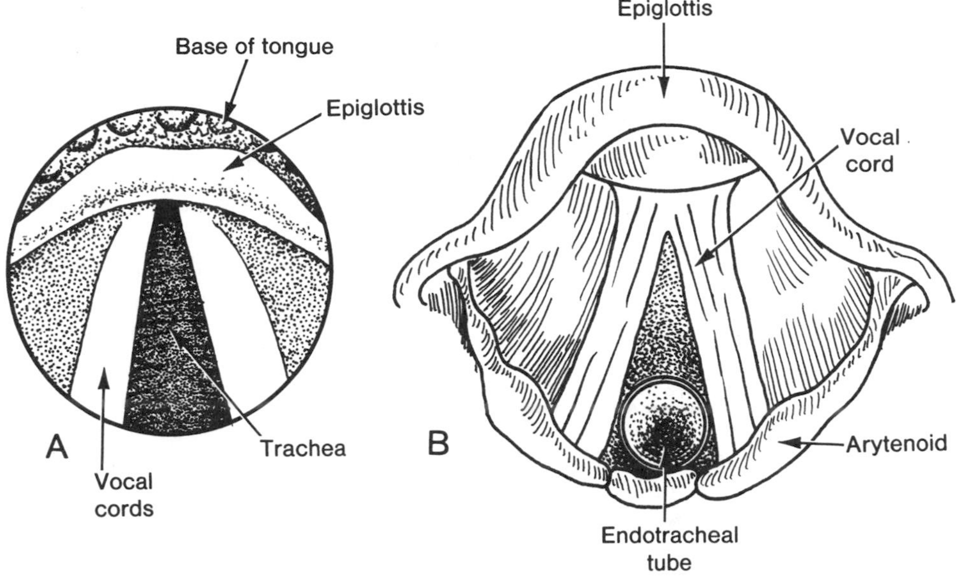

Figure 2.19. The glottic opening, as visualized through the laryngoscope. With the straight blade, lift the epiglottis to see the vocal cords and trachea through the channel of the laryngoscope. With the MacIntosh blade, one may see only the epiglottis and the arytenoid cartilages posterior to the vocal cord; pass the tube through the glottic opening.

NOTE

The tube should be passed only during inspiration in the patient who is spontaneously breathing. This technique will avoid damage to the vocal cords. External pressure on the larynx may bring an anteriorly placed larynx into view.

CAUTION

Laryngospasm is a frequent occurrence when attempting to pass the tube through the glottis. Should this occur, maintain gentle, but constant pressure against the cords with the tip of the tube, and the laryngospasm will usually reverse. Should this continue, insert lidocaine through the tube. Be certain that a stylet, if used, does not extend beyond the opening of the ETT.

8. In passing the tube, always insert it from the right side of the patient's mouth. Do not pass the tube down the channel of the blade because this obscures adequate visualization.
9. Inflate the cuff and auscultate both sides of the chest. If the right thorax is the only side on which breath sounds are heard, retract the tube 1 or 2 cm and recheck the breath sounds.

CAUTION

One may hear breath sounds on both sides even if the tube is in the esophagus or if the tube is located in one lung. Always auscultate in the anterior or midaxillary line inferiorly on both sides to avoid this problem.

NOTE

The left main stem bronchus comes off at a 45-degree angle to the trachea, whereas the right main stem bronchus is essentially continuous with the trachea. This anatomic difference causes one to pass the tube into the right main stem bronchus more commonly than into the left.

CAUTION

A tube in the esophagus may cause laryngospasm (67).

NOTE

Malposition of the tube is a hazard. If doubt exists about the location of the tip of the tube, advance the tube until breath sounds are lost, and then withdraw the tube 1 or 2 cm until *bilaterally equal* sounds are heard (144). In one study of 49 patients, the tube remained in the right main bronchus in 25 of the cases despite distinct breath sounds auscultated on both sides of the chest (53). Therefore, radiographs should be obtained to confirm the position of the tube (49, 144). Ideally the tube tip is 1 to 2 cm from the carina of the trachea with the head in the neutral position (49). To determine if the head was in the neutral position, on the anteroposterior film of the neck, the mandible should lie over C5 or C6. With the neck flexed, the mandible is at T1. The tube moves significantly with movement of the head. In one large study, the tube moved an average of 1.9 cm toward the carina with flexion from the neutral position and 1.9 cm away from the carina with extension. With lateral head rotation, the ETT moved 0.7 cm away from its neutral position (Fig. 2.20) (24). Thus it is best to place the tip of the

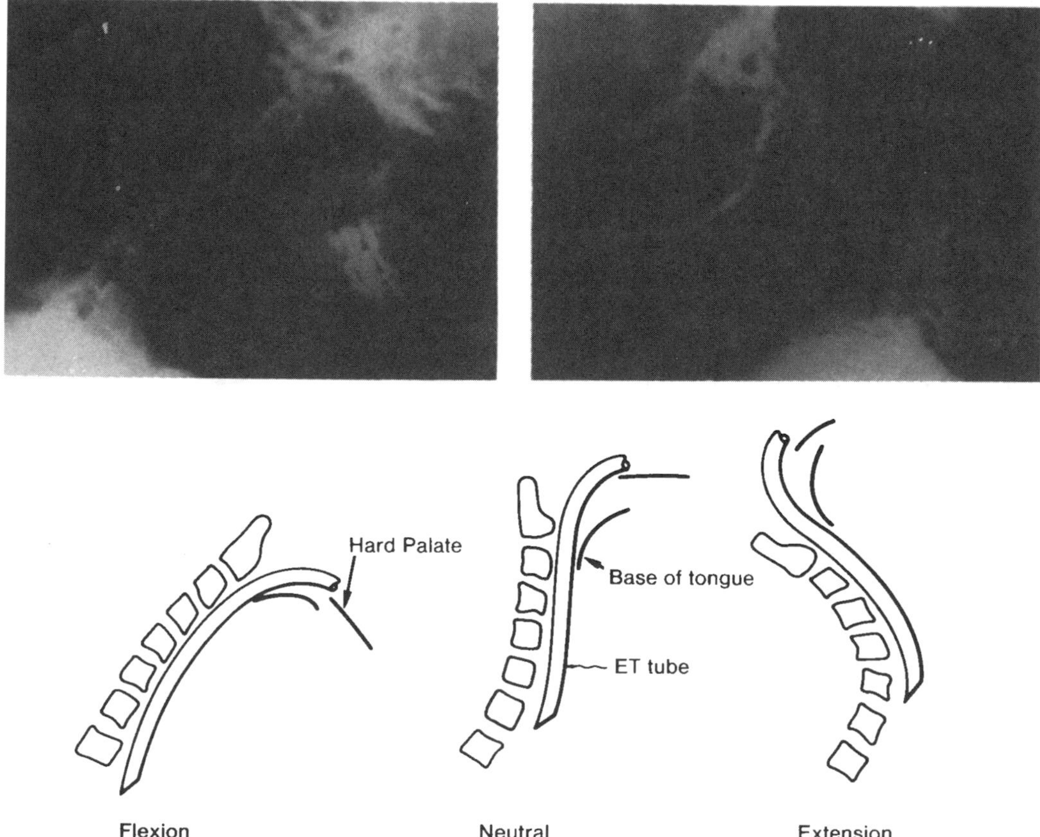

Figure 2.20. Endotracheal tube movement. The endotracheal tube is diagrammed so that the length is constant from the base of the hard palate to the tube tip. See text for details. (From Conrardy PA: Alteration of endotracheal tube position. Crit Care Med 4:10, 1976, with permission.)

tube in the middle third of the trachea with the neck in neutral, or 1 to 2 cm above the carina, rather than at the carina, in the average adult.

---

10. Insert an oral airway to prevent biting on the tube, and secure the tube in place. Always restrain the patient; it is part of securing the airway. There are a number of devices on the market for securing the ETT in place. The devices are made of synthetic plastics that encompass the ETT and serve as a bite block as well as safeguarding the tube in position. If one of these is not available, adhesive tape may be used to secure the tube in its proper position; however, this requires frequent rechecking of the patient because perspiration and motion often loosen the tape.

SPECIAL CONSIDERATIONS AND HELPFUL HINTS

Endotracheal intubation in the patient who has vomitus and secretions in the oral cavity can be a very challenging problem. Adequate suctioning is critical for visualization of the glottis to insert the ETT. However, suctioning is often followed by refilling of the oral cavity with secretions from the esophagus or stomach. In this situation it is not always easy to visualize the vocal cords. An important landmark is the esophageal surface of the larynx. The mucosal surface on the posterior (esophageal) surface of the larynx is unique and can usually be visualized with the laryngoscope that has been passed too far, as is often the case in such patients. The larynx is convex, and the mucosa is loosely attached, giving the appearance of transverse folds. This mucosal pattern is distinctive and is not present in the mucosal lining of the pharynx or the esophagus, in which the mucosa is smooth. If this distinctive surface is seen in passing the blade, then the blade is in the midline and is in too far. Withdraw the blade slightly, and the glottis will fall into place, making endotracheal intubation possible.

Exchanging a Damaged Endotracheal Tube (Cuff Ruptured)

A flexible stylet 4 mm in diameter and twice the length of the ETT may be passed through the damaged ETT; remove the old tube over the stylet, and place a new tube over the stylet (35, 38, 63, 99, 110).

Dealing with the Obstructed Endotracheal Tube (52)

CAUTION

Be prepared to bag ventilate the patient.

---

1. First turn and hyperextend the head.
2. If obstruction persists, deflate the cuff because it may herniate around the ETT orifice.
3. If obstruction persists, insert a catheter into the ETT and, if it can be passed only part way, place a finger in the mouth to see if the ETT is kinked.

NOTE

Using a large ETT diminishes the risk of kinking.

---

4. If obstruction persists, withdraw the tube a short distance; if there is still obstruction, withdraw the tube entirely.

Suctioning an Endotracheal Tube

Handle suction catheters as aseptically as possible, and suction should be applied only on withdrawal of the catheter after it has been inserted through the ETT into the trachea and bronchi. Suction for 15 seconds and avoid high intratracheal pressures (greater than 50 cm of water) (39). Turning the patient's head to the right does not promote catheter inserting into the left main stem bronchus, as has been the popular belief (39, 51). By bending the tip of the plastic catheter or using a catheter with an angled tip, catheterization into the left main stem bronchus may be achieved (39, 51, 68). Always use an aseptic technique. Use sterile gloves and a sterile catheter during suctioning of the ETT. Forty seconds of suctioning resulted in a decrease in Po_2 more than twice as large as the decrease in Po_2 from only 20 seconds of suctioning (13). Therefore bag–mask ventilate with oxygen 3 times before suctioning to prevent arrhythmias (125).

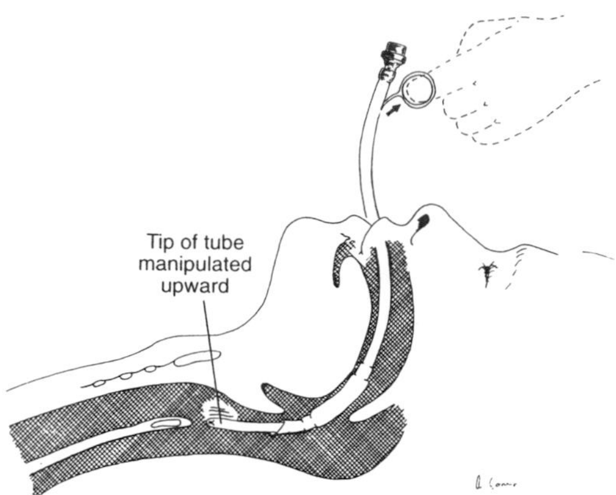

Figure 2.21. The use of the fiberoptic laryngoscope in assisting endotracheal intubation. See text for discussion.

GUIDELINES FOR THE DIFFICULT ENDOTRACHEAL INTUBATION

If, after following standard technique, one either does not see the glottis or cannot pass the tube, what should be done? Five common situations, in addition to those already indicated, are discussed separately, and some helpful hints are given to aid difficult intubation.

Normal Anatomy

In the patient with normal anatomy in whom the physician cannot pass the tube, check the following common causes for inability to pass a tube:

1. The patient's neck should be flexed rather than extended. One may have to place a folded towel or a small pillow under the patient's head to facilitate this position (sniffing position) so that the larynx is aligned with the posterior pharynx and the mouth to facilitate visualization of the glottis (Fig. 2.14).
2. An assistant can supply pressure over the laryngeal notch or cricoid cartilage to displace the glottis posteriorly and facilitate visualization. A tube that has been recently introduced can be used in patients with an anteriorly placed glottis difficult to visualize. This tube has a trigger at the end that allows manipulation of the tube tip anteriorly to facilitate intubation (Fig. 2.21).
3. Check the size of the laryngoscope blade and be certain that it is not too narrow (the tongue will "fold" around the blade, obstructing visualization) or too short. The laryngoscope blade should be approximately half the width of the tongue to displace it properly.
4. A smaller tube may have to be placed if the size routinely used causes obstruction of visualization of the glottis because of a narrow oral cavity or pharynx.

Large Tongue

When a large tongue causes difficulty with visualization of the glottis or epiglottis, a wider blade than routinely used is suggested. In our experience, a MacIntosh blade facilitates endotracheal intubation of these patients more readily than does a straight blade.

A Patient with a Short, Squat Neck

These patients are perhaps the hardest to intubate endotracheally. Check to be certain that the axes of the larynx, pharynx, and mouth are accurately aligned. One of us (R.S.) routinely places a folded towel beneath the head of such patients before endotracheal intubation because accurate alignment of the structure seems most difficult in these patients. A MacIntosh blade permits more adequate visualization of the glottic opening than does the straight blade, which requires more displacement anteriorly of the epiglottis and tongue. A smaller size ETT is suggested in these patients to facilitate visualization and accurate placement. When all else fails and endotracheal intubation is mandatory, we suggest nasotracheal intubation, retrograde intubation, or cricothyroidotomy as a last resort.

Glottic Edema

When glottic edema after an allergic reaction is a problem, use either a small ETT tube or a nasotracheal intubation with a small nasotracheal tube.

Abnormal Anatomy

1. **Epiglottitis.** As is indicated in the section on Nasotracheal Intubation later, a number of studies have shown that patients with epiglottitis can be intubated using the nasotracheal route without difficulty. We recommend using the same philosophical approach as when examining a third-trimester bleed, that is, have a cricothyroidotomy set ready and open, resuscitative drugs (including succinylcholine) nearby, an intravenous route established, and a catheter for retrograde intubation, should this become necessary. The decision whether to perform nasotracheal intubation or cricothyroidotomy in these patients must be individualized, based on the physician's experience, skill, and preference. Retrograde intubation as described earlier is not suggested in these patients, because the swollen epiglottis may be displaced over the glottis by the passing ETT and may obstruct passage of that tube.
2. **Congenital anomaly.** In the patient with a congenital anomaly, endotracheal intubation may be difficult depending on what the anomaly involves. Obviously one must individualize each situation. In the patient in whom the anomaly causes a narrow pharynx and oral cavity, use a smaller tube. When the anomaly makes it difficult to visualize adequately the structures necessary to intubate a patient, and intubation is necessary, a cricothyroidotomy may have to be performed.
3. **Cancer.** A number of patients who have received radiotherapy to the head and neck have stiffening of those structures, and one is unable to extend the head or flex the neck in these patients to perform endotracheal intubation. In such patients, nasotracheal intubation is the preferred route; when this is not possible, go directly to a cricothyroidotomy.
4. **Maxillofacial trauma.** In patients with maxillofacial trauma causing an abnormal anatomy, we recommend either a cricothyroidotomy or nasotracheal intubation when possible.

When a patient in the emergency center is difficult to intubate endotracheally for any of the reasons listed and either has an esophageal obturator airway in place or is unconscious and an esophageal obturator airway can be inserted, this should be done. After insertion of the esophageal obturator airway and ventilation through it, perform endotracheal intubation over the esophageal obturator airway. The technique is the same as for endotracheal intubation except that a smaller ETT is usually used, particularly in the patient with a small mouth and oropharynx. Leave the esophageal obturator airway in place during endotracheal intubation and remove it only after the patient has been successfully intubated and the cuff inflated. Removal of the esophageal obturator airway often is accompanied by vomiting, and if an ETT is not in place to protect the trachea, aspiration may result. After endotracheal intubation, deflate the esophageal obturator airway cuff, and remove the tube.

The roles of nasotracheal intubation, cricothyroidotomy, and retrograde intubation have either been discussed in this section or are discussed in their respective sections.

COMPLICATIONS

1. **Perforation of the trachea with the stylet.** For prevention, see step 4 in Preparatory Steps (p. 59).
2. **Esophageal intubation.**
   a. Adequate visualization of either the glottis or the vocal cords will prevent passage into the esophagus.
   b. Auscultate both sides of the chest after endotracheal intubation. If no breath sounds are heard, remove the tube and re-intubate or check tube for proper placement. When vomiting occurs, leave the tube in place because this acts as a conduit for the vomitus, and endotracheally intubate around the ETT in the esophagus.
3. **Injury to the vocal cords.** To prevent, use a lubricated tube and if the patient is breathing, pass the tube only during inspiration when the vocal cords are retracted and the glottic opening is widest.
4. **Injury to the teeth.** For prevention, see step 5 in Procedural Steps (p. 59).
5. **Intubation of the right main stem bronchus (45).** In a recent series, this complication occurred 11% of the time and, interestingly enough, often was not detected by chest radiography. If the left bronchus is not totally occluded, the air that comes from the right main stem bronchus may successfully partially ventilate the left lung. On all occasions, listen and make sure that both lungs are being equally ventilated and confirm the position of the tube by careful inspection of the chest radiograph.
6. **Dislodged tube.** This complication occurs in up to 2.5% to 3.0% of the reported cases. Secure the tube properly with either tape or, preferably, with one of the commercially available devices for holding the ETT in place, and restrain the patient.
7. **Obstruction of the tube.** Thick secretions or particulate foreign matter (125) aspirated into the lungs may obstruct the ETT. Should ventilation become ineffective, expect this obvious complication, and either suction to relieve the obstruction or replace the tube (see Dealing with the Obstructed Endotracheal Tube, earlier) (45).
8. **Aspiration of stomach contents.** In a recently published series (48), this complication occurred in 14% of endotracheal intubations involving drug overdoses. The incidence of aspiration during endotracheal intubation is increased when the patient is hypotensive or difficult to intubate. Aspiration is associated with a definite increase in pneumonia and mortality rates. A new design of tracheal tube cuff to prevent leakage of fluid into the lungs was evaluated by Young et al. (147). The new design offers the protection against leakage provided by the low-volume high-pressure (LVHP) cuffs, and the protection against excessive tracheal wall pressures that is provided by the high-volume low-pressure (HVLP) cuffs. It is made of latex with inflation characteristics that allow the tracheal wall pressure to remain constant.
9. **Pneumothorax (45).** Pneumothorax occurs in patients with decreased pulmonary compliance who, therefore, require high ventilatory pressures or in those with endotracheal intubation of the right main stem bronchus. Frequent chest auscultation and appropriate chest radiographs would alert the physician to the development of a pneumothorax.

10. **Atelectasis.** This may occur with intubation into the right main stem bronchus, in which the left side of the lung is not ventilated, and atelectasis will result (149).
11. **Cuff damage.** Cuff damage may occur with repeated attempts at endotracheal intubation or with a defective cuff. Gastric distention may result from an air leak. After three or four attempts at intubation, switch the ETT or check the cuff again for air leak (125).
12. **Arrhythmias.** Hypoxia may result from poor ventilation between attempts at endotracheal intubation or from prolonged attempts at intubating a patient. Hypoxia may result in the development of arrhythmias. Do not prolong an attempt at intubation beyond 40 seconds. If unsuccessful, immediately ventilate the patient with a bag–mask device. Arrhythmias also may result secondary to vagal stimulation during intubation. Bradycardia is the most common arrhythmia noted in patients who have increased sensitivity of the vagus during attempts at endotracheal intubation (136).
13. **Laryngospasm.** Laryngospasm has been reported after attempts at endotracheal intubation, particularly in the patient with inflammation around the glottis, which would predispose to laryngospasm or polyps in this region (125).

Tactile Oral Tracheal Intubation

A method used on a patient who is deeply comatose, who has aspirated, and who is difficult to intubate by direct visualization of the glottis was described by Stewart (133). The technique consists of the introduction of an intratracheal tube by palpation of the epiglottis. The advantage of this technique is that it can be performed despite secretions or blood in the upper airway.

1. Select the appropriate intratracheal tube and place a stylet carefully so that the distal end is at the level of the side hole of the ETT.
2. Gently curve the tip of the ETT to form a "hook" in the shape of the letter "J." Apply lubricant.
3. Stand or kneel facing the patient's right shoulder, holding the ETT in the right hand.
4. Then place the index and middle finger of the left hand into the patient's mouth on the right side and, while depressing the tongue and opening the mouth, slide the fingers along the tongue until the epiglottis is palpated in the midline (see Fig. 2.22).
5. Slide the ETT along the side of the open mouth by using the medial aspect of the middle finger and the palmar surface of the index finger to guide the tube toward the palpated epiglottis. Then place the tube against the epiglottis anteriorly with the middle and index fingers posteriorly directed.
6. The fingers then provide firm anteriorly directed pressure to guide the tube through the glottic opening. Do not pass the tube too far into the larynx because the tip may irritate the anterior walls of the trachea. Once the tube is beyond the vocal cords, withdraw the stylet, and the usual procedure for passing the tube is completed (Fig. 2.22).

Retrograde Intubation

In difficult endotracheal intubations, pass a 14-gauge, 12-inch Intracath, as shown in Fig. 2.23, through the cricothyroid membrane and into the oral cavity. Then thread the ETT over this catheter (117, 145). Retrograde intubation is indicated when the patient requires endotracheal intubation, and an esophageal obturator airway cannot be used (e.g., awake patient), and when several attempts at endotracheal intubation have been unsuccessful because of either abnormal

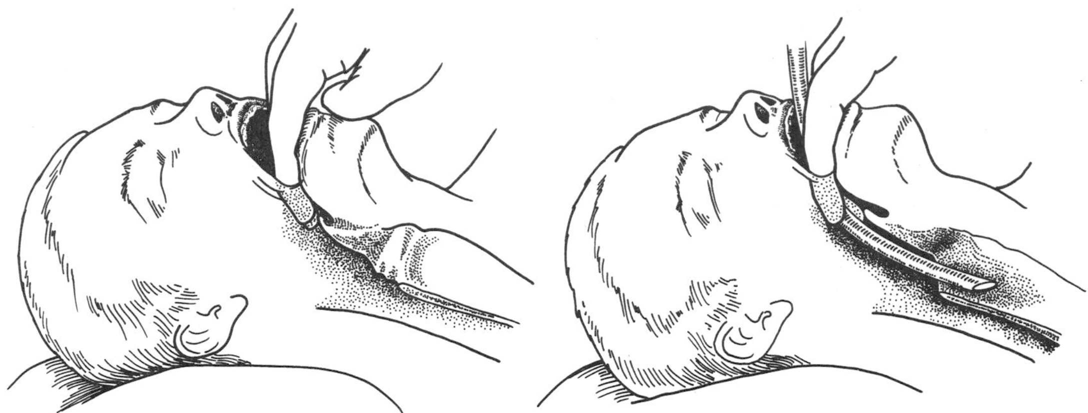

Figure 2.22. *A:* While the long finger holds the epiglottis, the index finger serves as a guide for the endotracheal tube into the glottic opening. Remember that the endotracheal tube must be curved upward in the shape of a "J." This is best done by inserting a stylet which should be removed once the tube is through the glottic opening. *B:* After removing the stylet from the endotracheal tube, push the tube through the vocal cords and into the trachea.

anatomy or the patient's condition (e.g., multiple facial injuries resulting from an automobile accident). Also use retrograde intubation in medical situations such as patients with acute respiratory distress from asthma, emphysema, or a neck tumor in whom nasotracheal intubation is either unsuccessful or cannot be performed.

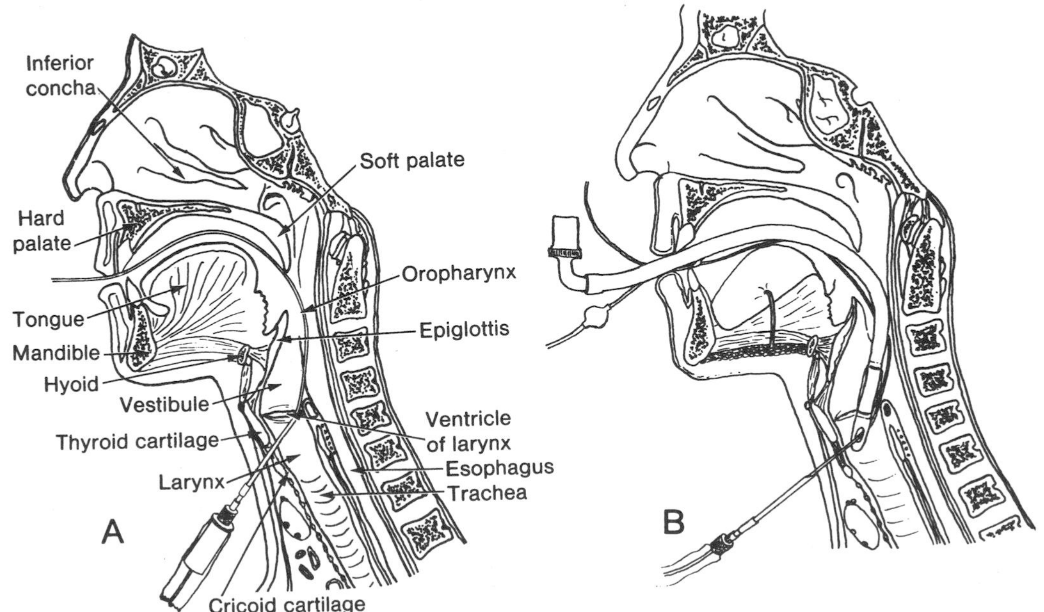

Figure 2.23. With difficult endotracheal intubations, pass a 14-gauge, 12-inch Intracath as shown above. *(A)* Position of Intracath after percutaneous insertion through the cricothyroid membrane for oral intubation. Then thread the endotracheal tube over the catheter as shown *(B)*. The position of the Intracath before cutting and withdrawing the catheter is shown *(B)*. (From Powell WF, Ozdil T: A translaryngeal guide for tracheal intubation. Anesth Analg 46:232–233, 1967, with permission.)

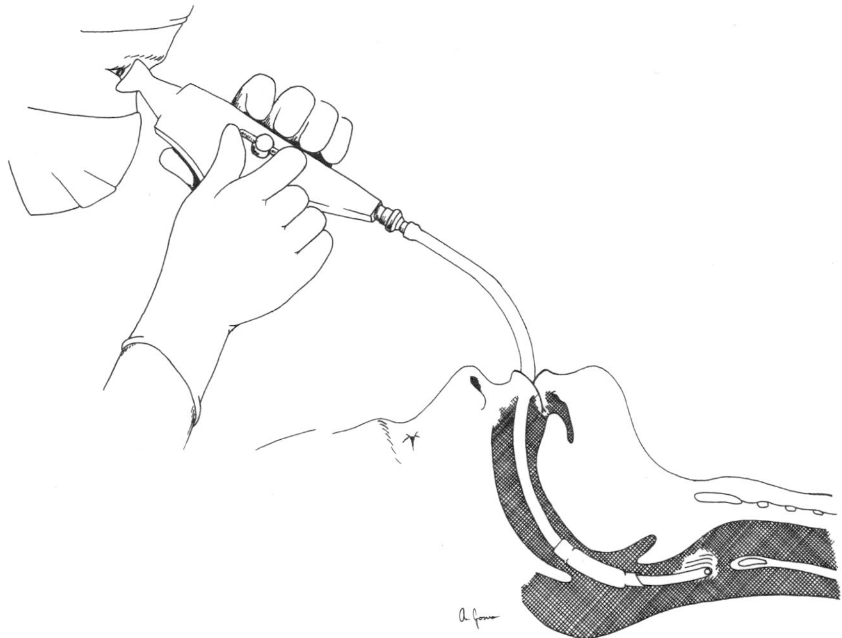

Figure 2.24. A special lever at the proximal end of the tube allows the physician to manipulate the tip when inserting the tube into the glottic opening. This is useful in a patient with an anteriorly placed glottis.

When performing endotracheal intubation over the catheter, hold the catheter tightly at both ends to provide a "rigid" channel over which the ETT may pass.

Fiberoptic Endoscopes

Fiberoptic endoscopes were thought to be the answer to difficult endotracheal intubations, but they have significant shortcomings, making their usefulness in the emergency center limited. Secretions accumulate over the scope and make visualization difficult, and it is often harder to identify structures with the endoscope than with conventional laryngoscopy (117). Endoscopes are very useful in the patient who does not have a problem with secretions, vomitus, or blood.

Endotracheal tube insertion with the fiberoptic endoscope is a procedure that requires much practice, time to learn, and the manual dexterity to use in the emergency setting. Unless the physician has experience with this technique, we do not recommend it (Fig. 2.24). In this procedure, a bilateral superior laryngeal nerve block as well as transtracheal blocks, combined with good topical oral and nasal anesthesia, are helpful (90).

Nasotracheal Intubation

There are many advantages to nasotracheal intubation, especially in patients with oral injury or in preoperative patients. Some believe it is better than tracheostomy when oral intubation is not possible (81, 96). Many authors believe nasotracheal intubation is the preferred procedure when endotracheal intubation is necessary (21, 73) because the tube is more easily secured to the face, cannot be bitten, and does not increase salivation (73). This route also appears to be better tolerated by the patient, with fewer patients attempting self-extubation. Some think that even with a swollen epiglottis, nasotracheal intubation is not difficult to do. Schuller and Birch (87) showed that 85% of patients with epiglottitis were intubated without difficulty, and nasotracheal intubation was possible in all patients with epiglottitis in their series. Others also have supported this contention (9, 139). Nasotracheal intubation is the only procedure by which endotracheal intubation can be performed in the patient who is sitting upright.

INDICATIONS

1. The primary indication for nasotracheal intubation occurs in the traumatized patient with cervical spine injuries (18, 28, 38, 72).
2. Decreased patency of the oral airway due to neoplasm, inflammatory disease, or neurogenic disturbances.
3. Inability to open the mouth, markedly retruded mandible, and previous head and neck surgery, all of which make oral intubation difficult with a laryngoscope (7, 28, 117).
4. Mandibular fractures and extensive maxillofacial deformities.
5. Alert and conscious patient who requires endotracheal intubation, as for example, a patient who is asthmatic or has chronic obstructive pulmonary disease (COPD) with exacerbation.
6. Possible or actual cervical spine injury, possible or actual herniated disk, poor mobility of the cervical spine (7, 117), or chronic atlantoaxial dislocation (e.g., rheumatoid arthritis).
7. Postradiation fibrosis of the neck (76).
8. Patient who requires endotracheal intubation but who cannot lie supine (severe asthma with respiratory distress).

CONTRAINDICATIONS

Nasotracheal intubation is contraindicated in patients with severe nasal or maxillofacial fractures, basilar skull fractures, or if an upper airway foreign body is a possibility (16, 25, 39).

EQUIPMENT

Equipment for endotracheal intubation
Magill forceps
Topical anesthetic spray
4% cocaine
2% lidocaine (Xylocaine) with adrenaline (1:100,000)
Cotton balls or gauze strips
Lubricant
Lidocaine jelly

TECHNIQUE

NOTE

There are essentially three requirements to a successful blind nasotracheal intubation.

1. A well-lubricated tube (47, 75, 148).
2. Topical anesthesia to the nose, pharynx, and larynx (46, 117, 143).
3. Spontaneously breathing patient (117, 148).

Preparatory Steps

1. Select a tube that will fit well, but not loosely, into the nose. In the adult man, a size 7.5 or 8.0 may be passed, and in women, a size 7 is generally selected (148).
2. Lubricate the tube with lidocaine jelly.
3. Anesthetize the nose, pharynx, and larynx.
   a. In the awake, spontaneously breathing patient, Pedersen (71) uses the following method. Anesthetize the nose with a spray of 4% cocaine, followed by cotton plugs impregnated with cocaine and instilled into the nostril with a bayonet forceps. Leave these in place for a few minutes. Cocaine reduces the risk of bleeding as well as shrinking the nasal membranes. Induce nasopharyngeal analgesia by spraying the back of the throat. This can be done

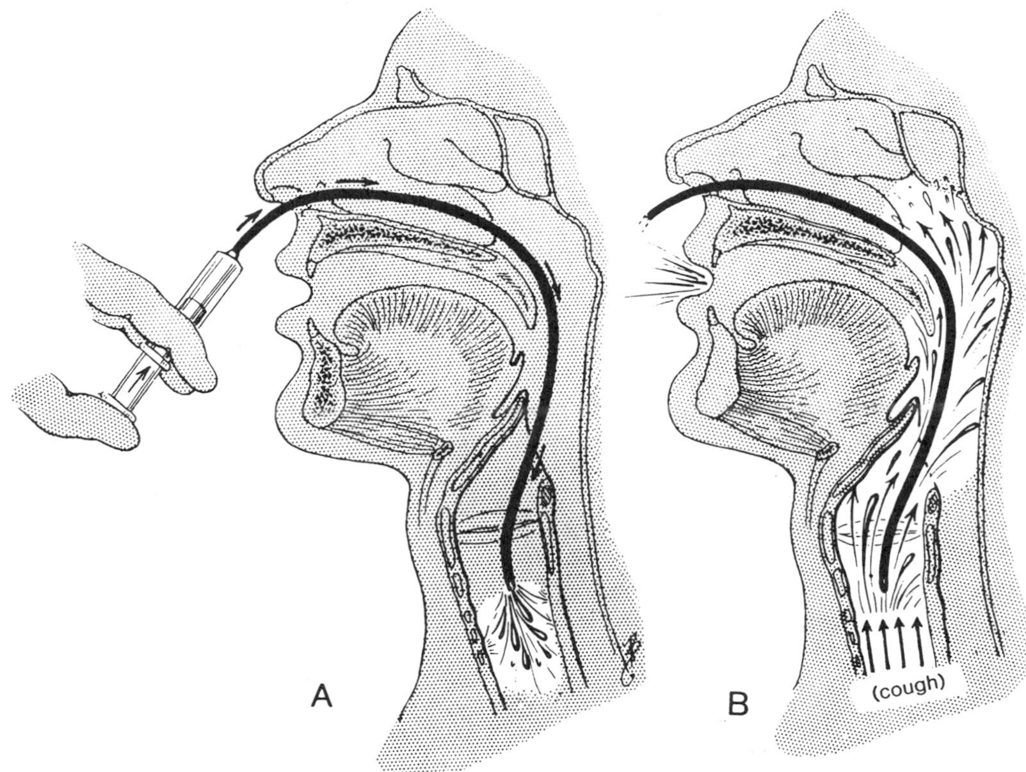

Figure 2.25. Method for anesthetizing the posterior pharynx and glottis. When good breath sounds are heard, ask the patient to take a deep breath and simultaneously compress the spray containing the cocaine solution. *A:* Nasotracheal instillation of cocaine. Notice the firm control of the syringe barrel to prevent expulsion during coughing. *B:* Dissemination of cocaine by coughing, with resultant oropharyngeal anesthesia. (From Starzi TE: A simple method for the induction of topical laryngo-tracheo-bronchial anesthesia. J Thorac Surg 37:652, 1959, with permission.)

using 10% lidocaine spray or cocaine, if available. Pass the nasotracheal tube, and listen for good breath sounds through the tube. When good breath sounds are heard, ask the patient to take some deep breaths and compress the spray simultaneously, anesthetizing the larynx (Fig. 2.25). As the patient coughs, the anesthetic is dispersed over the nasopharynx.

b. An alternate method in awake, spontaneously breathing patients is advocated by several authors (46, 76, 148). Spray the nasal passage with 4% cocaine. Then block the internal branch of the superior laryngeal nerve (Fig. 2.26). Perform a bilateral superior laryngeal nerve block with a total of 6 mL of 2% lidocaine. In addition, instill 4 mL of lidocaine into the trachea via puncture of the cricothyroid membrane. The superior laryngeal nerve innervates the base of the tongue, the epiglottis, and the laryngeal mucosa as far inferiorly as the vocal cords. With the patient lying supine and the head maximally extended, draw 2% lidocaine into a syringe and attach to a 21- or 22-gauge needle. Direct the needle parallel to the floor, at a right angle to the skin, through the

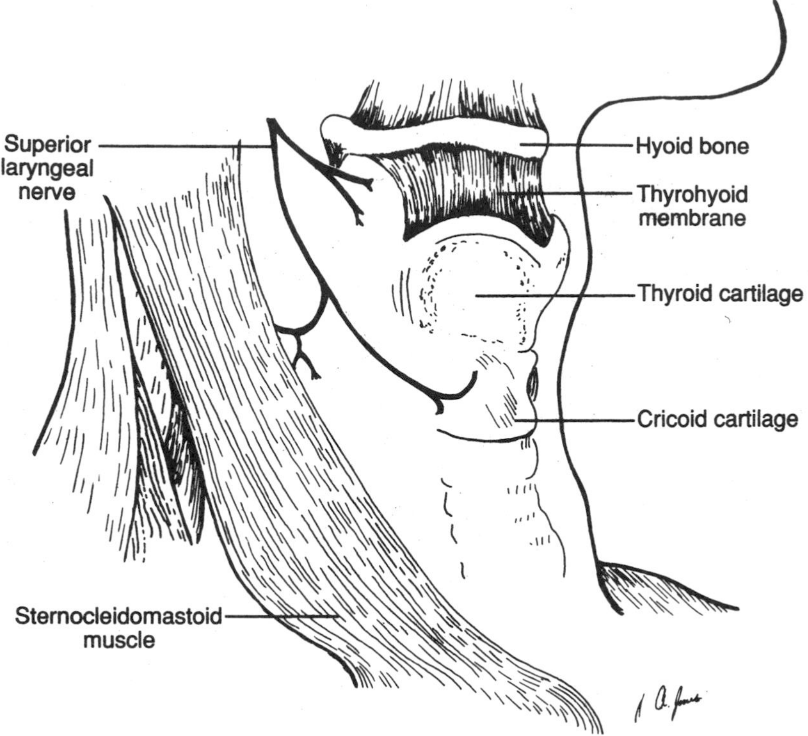

Figure 2.26. The superior laryngeal nerve block. See text for details.

skin, and onto the hyoid bone. After contact is made, direct the needle caudad until it just slips off the bone (see Fig. 2.27). Remember that the nerve is located just beneath the cornu of the hyoid bone on both sides. It may be possible to feel the resistance of the thyrohyoid membrane as it is penetrated. After passing through the membrane, the tip of the needle will be in a space bounded medially by the laryngeal mucosa and laterally by the thyrohyoid membrane. This space contains the ramifications of the nerve. When this space cannot be found, and one cannot feel the needle penetrate the thyrohyoid membrane, the needle should go all the way through until air is aspirated; then inject the lidocaine while withdrawing the needle (49). Perform the same procedure on the opposite side. Finally, anesthetize the tracheal mucosa and into the trachea with 2 mL lidocaine.

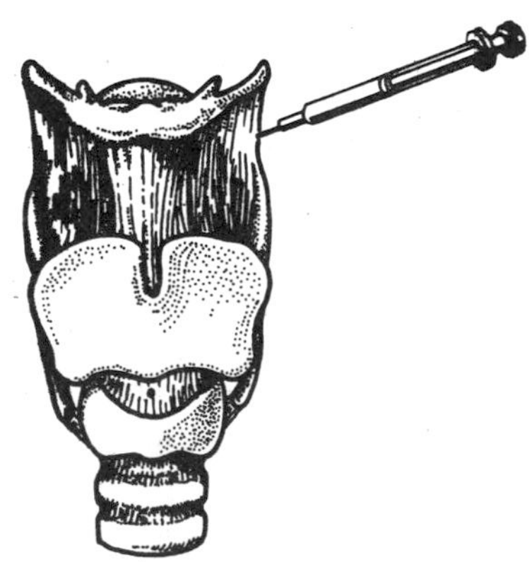

Figure 2.27. The superior laryngeal nerve can be found at the posterior aspect of the hyoid bone, just over the thyrohyoid membrane. At this point, the thyrohyoid membrane is pierced, and the superior laryngeal nerve is blocked as the needle is removed.

c. In the unconscious, spontaneously breathing patient, spray the nostril and the posterior pharynx with a 4% cocaine spray. This reduces epistaxis and shrinks the mucosa (143). The maximal dose is 3 mg/kg.

4. Position the patient's head, and select the nostril to enter. Nasotracheal intubation can be done in the recumbent or sitting position (e.g., in an asthmatic in respiratory distress) (148), whichever is more comfortable. Often endotracheal intubation by this route is easier with the patient sitting because the head can be manipulated more easily (74). Inspect the nose and select the side with the freer airway without nasal obstruction from septal deviation or congested membranes (117). The optimal position of the head for nasotracheal intubation is the sniffing position (81, 117); excessive extension of the neck causes the tube to enter the anterior commissure, and excessive flexion causes it to enter the esophagus. With the patient lying down, support the head with a small pillow or folded towel to achieve this optimal position (75, 80, 101, 148).

Procedural Steps

1. Insert the tube through the nose with the bevel facing the nasal septum so as not to irritate the turbinates, and introduce the tube along the floor of the nose into the hypopharynx (104). When the pharynx is reached, rotate the tube into its normal position.

When a patient is taking anticoagulants or may develop a problem with nasal bleeding from other causes, Fry (42) advocated the following after shrinking the nasal membranes with cocaine. Cut the digit off a size 8 glove. Then excise the tip, and place a slit longitudinally. After lubricating both the inside and outside of the "digit," introduce it along the floor of the nostril with a bayonet forceps, leaving part of the glove protruding so that it can be held with a hemostat. When introducing the nasotracheal tube, pass it through the inside of the "digit." This prevents the tip of the tube from striking against and irritating the nasal membranes as the tube passes.

2. Advance the tube into the hypopharynx and trachea.

NOTE

It is often helpful in passing the tube to tilt the patient's head laterally a small amount to the side of the nasal cavity that is being used (76, 101).

Advance the tube into the hypopharynx and listen for breath sounds over the portal (Fig. 2.28). Locate that point at which the breath sounds are heard maximally over the portal. From here onward, movement of the tube must be bold and rapid because a slow-moving tube is easily deflected from its course (75, 101). The tube should be in the hypopharynx in a position where breath sounds are maximally audible. When the tube is in its proper position, the patient is usually comfortable. With the tube held in the right hand and the left hand palpating the larynx (to stabilize it and "feel" the tube entering), quickly pass the tube during the terminal instances of exhalation or the onset of inhalation. If the tube goes into the esophagus, then withdraw the tube and apply pressure over the larynx shown in Fig. 2.28*B*. This will displace the larynx posteriorly and permit entry into it. When the trachea is entered, the patient often coughs briskly (148).

NOTE

Often one may think one is hearing breathing sounds over the portal, when the tube is in fact in the esophagus, because of respirations around the tube from the contralateral nostril. If this is a

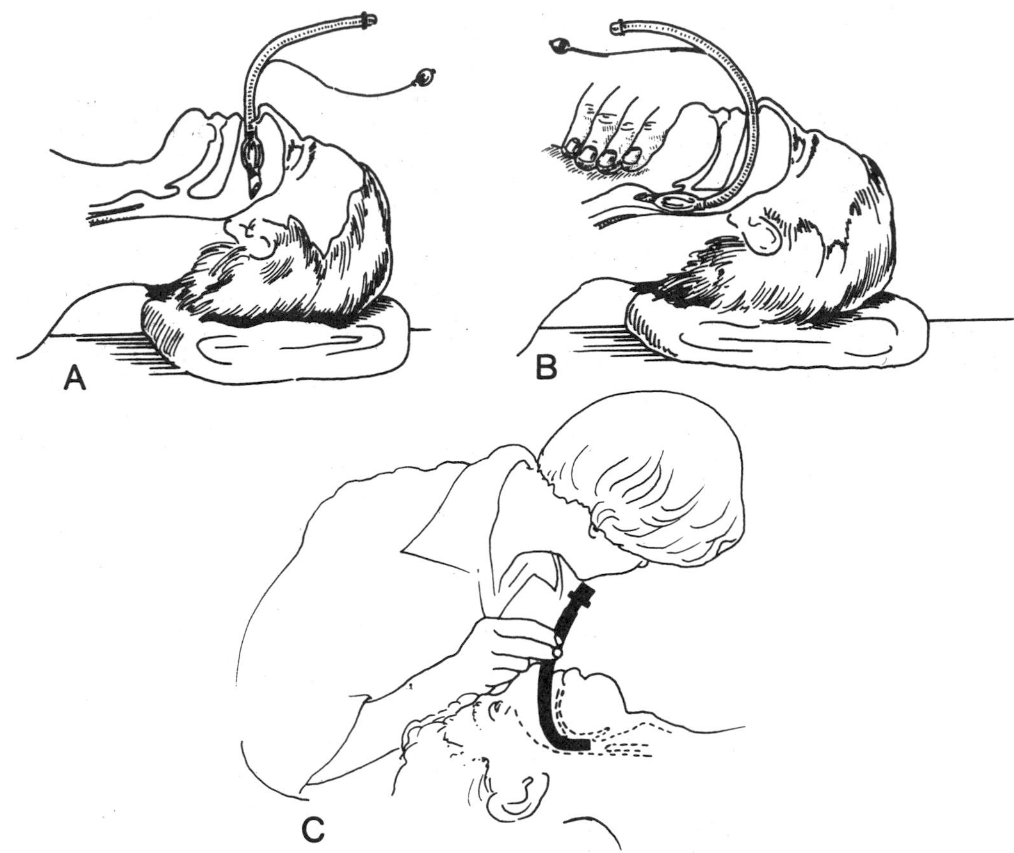

Figure 2.28. In the supine patient, flex the neck *(A).* Insert the tube into the nares, and advance it past the nasopharynx. As it passes the nasopharynx and into the oropharynx, a "give" will be felt. Gently displace the larynx posteriorly with one hand *(B).* Advance the tube until maximal breath sounds are audible through it. Listen over the orifice of the tube for this point *(C).* Pass the tube rapidly during the very beginning of inspiration or terminal instance of exhalation.

problem, close this nostril (55) and assess respiration.

NOTE

If airflow stops during the advancement of the tube, it may be easily passed into the esophagus without meeting any obstruction. In this case, withdraw the tube until airflow is again audible and then rotate the tube slightly to the right or left and advance it again with the neck rotated slightly to the right or left and with the neck slightly extended. In a patient with a deviated septum, it may be impossible to align the tube tip with the epiglottis, and blind nasotracheal intubation may be unsuccessful (45). Esophageal intubation can be differentiated from the tube entering the vallecula or pyriform sinuses because when the vallecula or pyriform sinuses are entered, the breath sounds cease, and one is unable to advance the tube farther. If one enters the vallecula or pyriform, flex the neck until the tube passes the epiglottis, and then place the neck in neutral position and advance the tube (148). The ETT can be deflected laterally or in an anteroposterior direction. Lateral deflection can be ascertained by looking into the pharynx through the oral cavity after the tube has been passed into the pharynx. Anterior

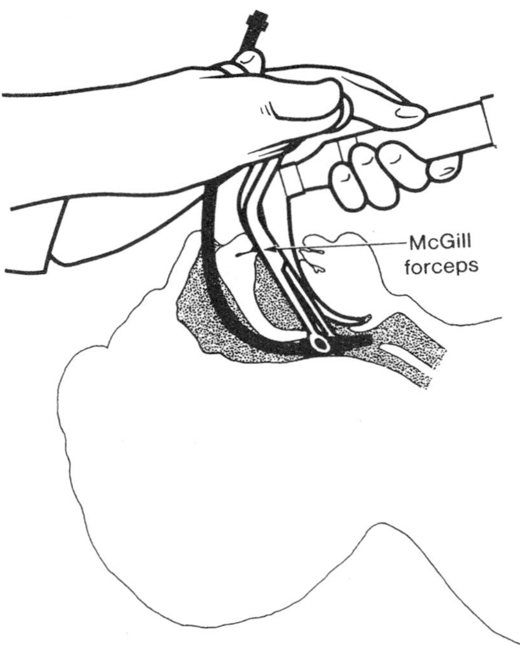

Figure 2.29. The use of the McGill forceps to aid in passing a nasotracheal tube into the trachea.

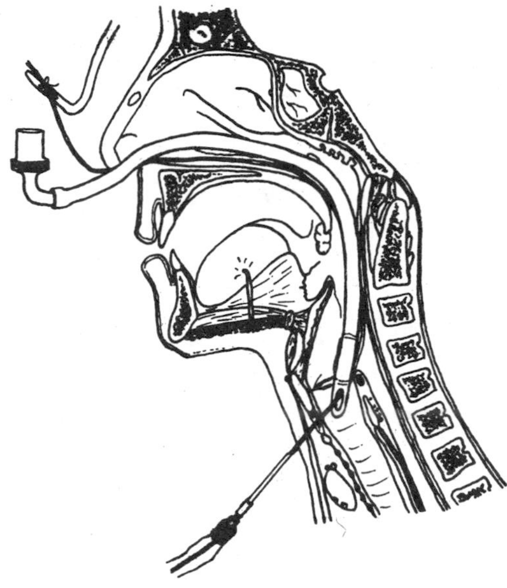

Figure 2.30. The use of a 14-gauge Intracath inserted through the cricothyroid membrane to aid in passage of a nasotracheal tube in difficult patients. The drawing shows the position of the Intracath after urethral catheter has been passed to pull the catheter through the nose. Keep the catheter taut, so the nasotracheal tube can be threaded as shown into the trachea. (From Powell WF, Ozdil T: A translaryngeal guide for tracheal intubation. Anesth Analg 46:234, 1967, with permission.)

and posterior deflection can be similarly ascertained. To correct lateral deflection, rotate the tube until breath sounds are at their loudest, and the tube is passed successfully. When, because of septal deviation or other anatomic aberrations, the tube cannot be rotated from its lateral course, three alternatives are available:

A. A Magill forceps, a specially shaped forceps, can be used once the nasotracheal tube is at the level of the oropharynx (Fig. 2.29). In this situation, use the laryngoscope to visualize the epiglottis and the glottic opening (when possible) and guide the tube with the Magill forceps during inspiration while an assistant pushes the distal end of the tube (75). Alternatively, pass the tube with the Magill forceps; however, this is more difficult.

B. When one cannot deviate the tube, another alternative is to pass the ETT over a nasotracheal suction catheter that has been previously passed. Use the nasotracheal suction catheter to direct the tip of the ETT while it is passed (101, 135). Alternatively, pass a long, 14-gauge Intracath through the cricothyroid membrane, as shown in Fig. 2.30, and pass the nasotracheal tube using the catheter as a guide.

C. A technique that is especially useful in children is to use a copper wire bent to form a hook, which is then used as a guide to help pass the tube. The dimensions of the hook are a 6- to 8-inch long handle with the bottom bent into a hook about 1/2 to 1 inch long (Fig. 2.31). This forms a rectangular hook. After intubating the nose and exposing the larynx, visualize the tip of the nasotracheal tube in the oropharynx. Then insert the copper wire into the mouth, with the hook portion placed gently against the posterior pharyngeal wall. An assistant then advances the nasotracheal tube until the tip over-

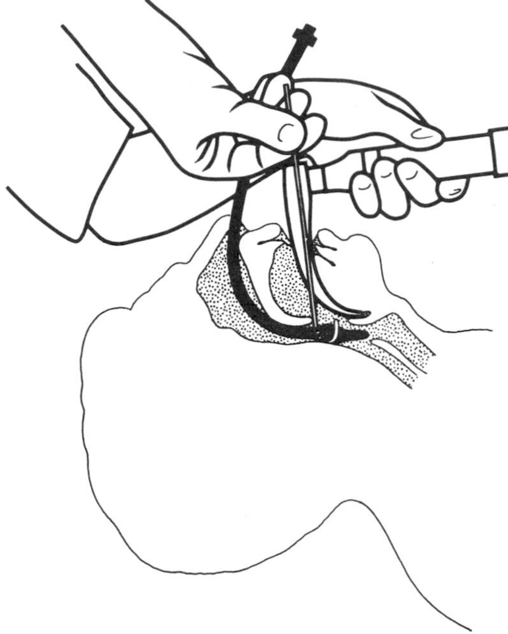

Figure 2.31. Use a hook to aid in the passage of a nasotracheal tube. See text for details.

rides the hook. By lifting the wire while the assistant advances the nasotracheal tube, it can be directed into the larynx with the aid of a laryngoscope. This method is especially useful when a Magill cannot be introduced easily without obstructing vision (e.g., in a child).

NOTE

Pressing down on the larynx with the left hand will displace the glottic opening posteriorly and permit passage of the tube through the glottis when recurrent esophageal intubation occurs. Slight extension of the neck from the neutral position also will assist in avoiding recurrent esophageal intubation.

CAUTION

Touching the cords without advancing the tube will result in laryngospasm, coughing, or breath-holding. Should this occur, hold the tube against the vocal cords, and they will usually open spontaneously, or inject 2% lidocaine down the ETT.

---

3. The "fogging" of the ETT itself is the ideal method to determine the proper placement of the tube. Breath sounds sometimes may be heard even if the tube is in the esophagus.
4. Inflate the endotracheal cuff and secure the tube.
5. Auscultate bilaterally to ensure that the ETT has not entered the right main stem bronchus.

ALTERNATE TECHNIQUE

Another maneuver that has been described as an aid to blind nasotracheal intubation in patients with cervical spine injury and that has been compared with intubation using fiberoptic bronchoscopy, is the use of an inflated ETT. Inflate the ETT cuff in the oropharynx using 15 mL of air, and then advance it gently until a slight resistance is felt. At this time, because the breath sounds can still be heard, the inflated cuff makes contact with the vocal chords. Deflate the cuff, and advance the ETT into the trachea. After satisfactory insertion, withdraw the ETT, and intubate the trachea by using the second procedure. When ETT cuff inflation was used, intubation was successful in 95% of patients. The first attempt at intubation was successful in 70%. Intubation was successful in 95% of patients with fiberoptic bronchoscopy instead of this procedure. Mean times to intubate were less when the ETT cuff was inflated in the oropharynx than when using fiberoptic bronchoscopy.

In the presence of normal pharyngeal anatomy, inflation of the ETT cuff in the pharynx is likely to center the tip of the tube and to direct it anteriorly toward the larynx. As a result, misplacement of the ETT into the esophagus or pyriform fossa may be avoided. In conclusion, the ETT cuff inflation method is easy to perform and does not require a skilled operator or additional equipment.

COMPLICATIONS

1. **Nasal bleeding.** Always look into the nostrils with a nasal speculum and determine which nostril is more dilated. The nares must be free of polyps and should not have a deviated septum; introduce the tube through the more dilated side. Nasal bleeding is the most common complication of this procedure. Fry's method (42) (described earlier) is probably the best preventive measure for the patient who is predisposed to this condition. Usually the bleeding will stop, and no treatment is indicated; however, in some cases in which continuous bleeding is a problem and tamponade by the tube does not occur, the tube may have to be removed and an alternate site selected for nasal intubation. Some cases may have minor bleeding, but this bleeding may compromise the airway in a patient with severe respiratory distress; therefore Fry's method is strongly recommended.
2. **Laryngeal spasm.** This is an uncommon complication. If it cannot be relieved, attempted passage of the ETT may cause injury to the vocal cords, and cricothyroidotomy should be selected (21).
3. **Esophageal intubation.** The aforementioned techniques should aid in reducing this problem. If, after attempting all modifications to avoid esophageal intubation, there is still difficulty, then select alternate routes for endotracheal intubation.
4. **Retropharyngeal insertion.** Retropharyngeal insertion has been described as a complication occurring from nasotracheal intubation (136).

INTUBATING LARYNGEAL MASK

The recently introduced intubating laryngeal mask (ILM; Fastrach, Intravert, United Kingdom) is a new device that may be useful in cases of failed or difficult intubation. Patients with cervical spine disease and injury are at increased risk of difficult intubation, particularly if there is involvement of atlantooccipital joints.

Technique

Insert the proper size intubating laryngeal mask, and inflate the cuff with 30 mL of air; then pass a reinforced, straight, cuffed, silicone tracheal tube (SMIS Portex, United Kingdom) blindly through the mask into the trachea. Remove the mask over the tracheal tube, and then secure it. Blind trachea intubation through the ILM has many potential advantages. The ILM can be placed with the head in the neutral position. Only sufficient mouth opening is needed to accommodate the ILM. There is no need to visualize the larynx; consequently, negligible cervical spine movement is needed during placement. The ILM allows ventilation to continue during attempts at intubation, and the additional equipment required is minimal. The operator does not need to be at the head of the patient. In conclusion, the ILM may prove to be a useful adjunct to facilitate tracheal intubation in cases of difficult or failed intubation and allows both fiberoptic and blind tracheal intubation (98).

The retropharyngeal space is a potential space lying between the middle (buccopharyngeal or alar fascia) and the deep (prevertebral) layers of the deep cervical fascia. It extends from the base of the skull to the level of the T4, where the two layers fuse. Thus blood entering the space can cause airway obstruction at different levels. Retropharyngeal hematomas are associated with a range of conditions including cervical trauma, anticoagulation, bleeding diathesis, after arteriography, carotid sinus massage, and internal jugular vein cannulation (122). Although the latter is uncommon, when it happens, suspect inadvertent arterial puncture. The incidence of carotid artery puncture during internal jugular vein cannulation is 2% to 4% (70). The diagnosis can be difficult. The symptoms may include neck pain, dysphagia, dyspnea, and a hoarse voice. The signs include those of superior mediastinal obstruction and bruising on the neck appearing within 48 hours and spreading to the chest wall. The diagnosis is aided by a lateral radiograph of the neck, which will show a widening of the prevertebral space. The normal width of the larynx is less than the width of the adjacent cervical vertebrae (122). The external appearance of the neck swelling may underestimate the degree of pharyngeal edema, which is more likely to be the mechanism of the airway obstruction secondary to venous and lymphatic obstruction by the hematoma (70). In this situation, the Combitube, which can be inserted blindly without the use of a laryngoscope, is useful.

LARYNGEAL MASK AIRWAY

The laryngeal mask airway (LMA) is effective for maintaining airway patency during anesthesia. Application to CPR has been encouraging, but vast experience in CPR is lacking (106). The LMA is a mask that fits over the larynx, similar to the way a face mask fits over the face. The mask is oval with an inflatable balloon surrounding its periphery and a tube that serves as a conduit for the mask to the gas source. It has "ribs" that prevent the epiglottis from falling into and occluding the airway. It is reusable after autoclaving at 120°C to 134°C for 3 minutes. Preparing the LMA for insertion involves the following steps: insert the balloon completely and inspect the cuff for leaks; bend the LMA and search for kinking of the shaft; and deflate the LMA with its concave (anterior) face pressed against a firm, flat surface. The object of deflation is to produce a smooth, pointed, wedge-shaped mask that can be easily inserted into the airway. The convex (posterior) side is lubricated. During placement of a LMA, gag reflexes must be suppressed. Place the patient's head in the sniffing position. The mouth must be wide open.

Techniques

Grasp the LMA with the dominant hand and insert it into the mouth; push the convex (posterior) surface up against the hard pallet. The index finger supplies the forward driving force to advance the LMA around the base of the tongue. Before inserting one's fingers into a patient's mouth that may involuntarily close because of pharyngeal stimulation, test the airway with a tongue depressor or other instrument. Alternatively, insert the device into the patient's mouth and advance it by holding the 15-mL airway adapter rather than inserting fingers between the patient's teeth. After resistance to passage is overcome, the tip of the LMA should abut the upper esophageal sphincter, which is at the bifurcation of the airway and gastrointestinal tracts. Allow the device to remain in the airway without support while the balloon is inflated. During cuff inflation, a correctly seated LMA often moves slightly out of the airway. The black strip should be at the posterior aspect of the upper lip.

The relative contraindications are not so important as is immediately securing the airway for oxygenation and ventilation during CPR. Inability to achieve the sniffing position may increase the difficulty of insertion but does not contraindicate use of the LMA. The LMA can be correctly inserted with the patient's head in the neutral position. Patients who have an increased risk of aspiration pneumonitis are not ideal candidates for LMA insertion. Examples of such situations include morbidly obese patients or patients with a hiatal hernia. LMAs offer many advantages in the cardiac arrest situation. They are easy to insert, and inexperienced personnel have placed them successfully without the use of a laryngoscope. After brief training sessions, medical personnel achieved an 80% to 94% success rate on first attempt. When initial insertions fail, subsequent attempts are successful in 98% of adult cases and 95% of pediatric cases. Finally, a well-positioned LMA also can facilitate endotracheal intubation under direct vision (106).

The Combitube (Sheridon Catheter Corporation, Argyle, NY, U.S.A.) is a new double-lumen airway. One lumen serves as a tracheal channel comparable to a conventional tracheal airway with a distal open end. The second lumen, the esophageal channel, acts as an esophageal obturator with a blocked distal and perforation at the level of the pharynx. At the proximal end, both lumens continue as short tubes with connectors at the ends. At the distal end, the airway is surrounded by an inflatable cuff. The inflated cuff obturates either the trachea or the esophagus. At the oropharyngeal section, there is a long, elastic balloon. This oropharyngeal balloon, when inflated, is pressed against the base of the tongue and closes the soft palate, thereby sealing the hypopharynx against the oral and nasal cavities. The airway is correctly positioned when the ventral side of the oropharyngeal balloon reaches the posterior part of the hard palate, thus ensuring a strong anchoring. In conclusion, this study (82) indicates that in selected intensive care unit (ICU) patients, the Combitube can be an alternative technique for airway control, providing a clear unobstructed trachea. Patients unsuitable for this method include those with a history of esophageal disease, with markedly noncompliant lungs, edema of the upper airway, and those who require very frequent suction (82).

Inflate the large pharyngeal balloon with 100 mL of air. As inflation proceeds, the esophageal tracheal Combitube (ETC) often retracts out of the mouth a short distance. This movement is part of the "seating" process, and it does not need to be returned to its original position. The small cuff is then inflated with 10 to 15 mL of air. The ETC has been successfully used to provide airway patency during CPR, in the ICU, and during general anesthesia. Airway patency has been achieved with the ETC in patients in whom intubation was not technically possible with standard, rigid laryngoscopic techniques. In critically ill patients, arterial blood gas analysis demonstrates comparable results with the ETC and ETTs. No complications have been reported with the ETC other than frequent difficulty during placement. Although reminiscent of the esophageal opturnal airway, the ETC has not been linked with esophageal rupture airway obstruction, if positioned in the trachea, or aspiration pneumonitis after removal (106).

INFANT AND CHILD ENDOTRACHEAL INTUBATION

Prominence of the maxilla is usual until the fifth postnatal month, and mandibular retrusion also may exist. Either anatomic variation (posterior displacement or mandibular retrusion) may lead to poor support of the tongue of the infant by the muscles attached; obstruction of the airway occurs more easily in the child than in the adult (29). The cranium dominates the small body of the infant, and excess adenoidal tissue also may be present. The larynx of the infant is more anterior and cephalad, and so the angle between the laryngeal opening and the pharynx is even more acute; thus, even though the large heads of infants are given some degree of flexion, usually there must be additional flexion which is aided by a pillow placed under the head. The laryngoscope blade with a curve (MacIntosh) will increase the anterior displacement of the glottis; therefore a straight blade should be used in the manner recommended, with the tip of the blade lifting the epiglottis. In the child, it is difficult to lift the epiglottis, and slight posterior pressure exerted by a hand placed on the skin anterior to the larynx will give full view of the glottic opening. Because of the softness of the neck structures and cartilage, the larynx is easily displaced.

During endotracheal intubation, it is important to be extremely gentle in the infant. When the vocal cords are tightly apposed, a 1.5-cm depression of the sternum for 1 second by an assistant with the tips of the fingers will open the glottis during a forced expiration, at which time a tube can be safely passed (89).

A formula that may be used for calculating tube sizes in infants and children is the following (102):

Younger than 6.5 years, tube size (mm) = (age in years/3) + 3.5
Older than 6.5 years, tube size (mm) = (age in years/4) + 4.5

In most cases, the preferred route from endotracheal intubation is oral (137). Although cuffed ETTs are not recommended for patients younger than 6 to 8 years, it should be remembered that it is the pressure from the cuff inflation and not the cuff that causes the damage. If a cuffed ETT is used, a half-size smaller tube should be chosen, and the cuff inflated with the least amount of air necessary to prevent an excessive air leak (137).

Pediatric Oral Tracheal Intubation

A number of anatomic features differ between infants and adults. In the infant, the larynx is located at the C3–C4 level, whereas in the adult, it descends to the C5–C6 level. In the infant, the larynx is funnel shaped, whereas in the adult, it is cylindrical. The epiglottis is floppy and is "V"-shaped in the infant, whereas in the adult, it is flat and close to the tongue and parallel to the trachea. In the infant, the epiglottis is at a 45-degree angle to the anterior pharyngeal wall, with the narrowest portion of the airway occurring at the cricoid cartilage. Because of the larger size of the head in relation to the body in the infant, endotracheal intubation of the infant should be performed with the head in the neutral position. In the older child, however, the sniffing position should be used, similar to that in the adult, as described earlier.

Table 2.5
Recommended Endotracheal Tube Size for Infants and Children

Age	Diameter (mm)
Newborn	3.0
6–12 mo	3.5–4.0
12 mo–3 yr	4.0–4.5
3–6 yr	4.5–5.0
6–8 yr	5.5–6.0
10–12 yr	6.0–6.5

The technique for inserting ETTs in infants is similar to that used with the adults. Difficulties with visualization occur with a curved blade in a child. Rotate the laryngoscope handle toward the maxillary teeth and thus push the larynx forward, obscuring visualization.

The appropriate size of the ETT is important, and the recommended sizes are listed in Table 2.5.

The use of stylets remains controversial. There is always the potential for trauma; however, a stylet should be available for use when anatomic abnormalities make it difficult to intubate endotracheally.

DRUGS USED IN INFANT INTUBATION

Succinylcholine, a depolarizing neuromuscular blocking agent, depresses neuromuscular transmission, and in infants, a larger dose is required on a weight basis than in older children and adults. The action of succinylcholine is prolonged when a child has liver disease, hypothermia, or elevated potassium or alkaloid levels (95). The action is shorter when the patient has acidosis, decreased cardiac output, or decreased potassium (95). The recommended dosage of succinylcholine is 2 mg/kg intravenously for infants and 1 mg/kg for older children and adults (92).

In infants and children, intragastric pressure does not become markedly increased after the use of succinylcholine

(25). Serum potassium increases within 30 seconds after administration of this drug and peaks by 5 minutes, with a return to a more normal level in 15 minutes (25).

The advantages of succinylcholine include a rapid onset of action (30 to 45 seconds) and a short duration of action (4 to 5 minutes). The latter may be particularly important in patients with head trauma or suspected cervical spine injury, so that immediate reassessment of their clinical status is possible. Contraindications to the use of succinylcholine are the following (137):

1. Burns
2. Severe metabolic acidosis
3. Hyperkalemia
4. Degenerative CNS diseases (137)

Nondepolarizing muscle relaxants are used in situations or underlying conditions that contraindicate succinylcholine. Several different nondepolarizing agents are available (137):

1. Pancuronium
2. Vecuronium
3. Rocuronium

The primary differences include onset and duration of action, metabolic fate, and cardiovascular effects. Significant histamine release can occur with several of the agents, including curare, atracurium, and mivacurium, thereby limiting their use in the emergency setting. Pancuronium (0.15 mg/kg) will provide acceptable conditions for intubation in 90 to 120 seconds, with paralysis lasting from 45 to 90 minutes. Mild histamine release and an increase in heart rate related to its vagolytic effects may be seen. Pancuronium (70% to 80%) is dependent on renal excretion, with a significantly prolonged effect in patients with renal insufficiency or failure. A more rapid onset of paralysis can be achieved with either vecuronium or rocuronium. As vecuronium is devoid of cardiovascular effects, increased doses can be used to speed the onset of neuromuscular blockage. Doses of 0.3 mg/kg will provide acceptable conditions for endotracheal intubation in 60 to 90 seconds, with a duration of blockade of 60 to 90 minutes.

Priming also may be used to speed the onset of vecuronium. To do this, administer 0.01 mg/kg followed in 2 to 3 minutes by the remainder of the intubating dose of 0.15 mg/kg. In the emergency setting, a priming dose generally is not recommended because it may induce significant amounts of neuromuscular blockade.

One can reverse the effects of neuromuscular blocking agents with anticholinesterase drugs. In addition, an anticholinergic drug is usually given to block the muscarinic effects of the anticholinesterase drug used. Atropine at a dose of 0.02 mg/kg or neostigmine at a dosage of 0.06 mg/kg is used for this purpose. The maximal dose of atropine given at one time should never exceed 1 mg. The maximal dose of neostigmine should never exceed 2.5 mg.

The suggested sequence of events in the infant and child depends on whether the patient is awake or obtunded. In the obtunded or apneic patient, administer oxygen by bag–mask ventilation in the apneic patient, followed by endotracheal intubation and hyperventilation with 100% oxygen. In the obtunded patient who requires sedation and paralysis before laryngoscopy and endotracheal intubation (23), use the agents described earlier.

In the awake patient who can be sedated safely, sedation with a rapidly acting agent such as thiopental, diazepam, or ketamine provides loss of consciousness and amnesia. Use oxygenation through bag–mask ventilation, followed by muscle relaxants to obtain paralysis and then endotracheal intubation. Administer thiopental at a dosage of 2 to 4 mg/kg, i.v. Use ketamine at 0.5 to 2 mg/kg, i.v. Use diazepam in the infant in the dosage of 0.1 to 0.2 mg/kg, i.v. (Table 2.2) (137).

Unlike patients with endotracheal intubation performed for elective surgery, patients with acute medical emergencies frequently do not have an empty stomach. Trauma, pain, and anxiety all delay gastric emptying; therefore, regardless of when the patient last ate, he or she is still considered to have a full stomach. Therefore use techniques to minimize the risk of regurgitation of stomach contents. Cricoid pressure is a technique that prevents the passive regurgitation of stomach acid. Compress the upper esophagus against the cervical vertebral column by applying anteroposterior pressure on the cricoid cartilage, which is the only complete ring of the trachea and can be used to compress the esophagus without interfering with the ability to pass an ETT. Maintain cricoid pressure from the time consciousness is lost until proper placement of the ETT is confirmed or until the patient awakens, if intubation is unsuccessful (137).

RAPID-SEQUENCE INTUBATION

In children who require endotracheal intubation and have a full stomach, consider rapid-sequence intubation. When doing crash induction for endotracheal intubation, do not use positive pressure ventilation to avoid gastric distention. Preoxygenate the patient with 100% oxygen, and position the head properly, with suction readily available.

Give thiopental or ketamine, in the doses previously described, followed by pancuronium plus succinylcholine in rapid sequence intravenously. Apply external pressure to the cricoid cartilage to compress the esophagus (92).

An alternative to using succinylcholine is rapid infusion of a full dose of the nondepolarizing agent pancuronium and maintenance of external cricoid pressure until full relaxation is achieved. Succinylcholine causes muscle fasciculations and an increase in intragastric pressure. Thus a de-fasciculating dose of nondepolarizing muscle relaxant must be given before the administration of succinylcholine.

INTUBATION WHEN AN INFANT MUST BE KEPT AWAKE

When a patient has a possible upper airway obstruction, acute epiglottitis, a history compatible with cervical spine fracture or temporomandibular joint disease, or any other anatomic abnormalities, endotracheal intubation may have to be performed while the infant is awake. In the cooperative patient with a suspected difficult airway, awake intubation may be easier with the combination of small doses of intravenous sedation (midazolam, 0.03 to 0.5 mg/kg) and topical anesthesia of the airway with a local anesthetic solution. Aerosolize a local anesthetic, apply topically the local anesthetic to the mucosa of the oral pharynx, or perform a direct blockade of the innervation of the airway.

The superior laryngeal branch of the vagus nerve supplies sensory innovation to the larynx, epiglottis, and vocal cords. The nerve block is described elsewhere in this chapter (60).

Achieve transtracheal block of the trachea, below the cords, by injecting lidocaine through the cricothyroid membrane (88).

Basically, this technique is useful in the cooperative patient in whom visualization of the larynx is difficult or impossible. In addition to direct laryngoscopy with oral endotracheal intubation, other options exist for oral endotracheal intubation in the awake patient, including the Bullard laryngoscope, the light wand, and fiberoptic-guided endotracheal intubation. The majority of experience with any of these techniques has been in the adult population, and their use in the awake state requires an alert, cooperative patient. The Bullard laryngoscope is an anatomically shaped laryngoscope that uses fiberoptic technology to view the larynx. The blade is in the shape of a curved L. Once a blade has been rotated around the base of the tongue, apply force superiorly to visualize the larynx. Whereas visualization of the larynx is usually excellent, passage of the ETT into the glottis may be difficult. The current design has an intubating stylet that is incorporated into the laryngoscope and lies along the right posterolateral aspect of the blade in an attempt to align correctly the ETT and the airway. As there is limited movement of the cervical spine with both placement and subsequent use, it has been recommended as a useful tool for managing the airway in patients with suspected or confirmed cervical spine injury.

The light wand is a malleable, illuminated stylet that can be used for blind, oral intubation. The illuminating stylets can be inserted into an ETT greater than or equal to 5 mm. The technique is limited to patients who are at least 5 to 6 years old. Bend the distal end of the stylet and ETT 90 degrees to facilitate entry into the trachea. Instruct the patient to protrude the tongue, and insert the stylet with the ETT blindly into the oropharynx. As the device passes around the posterior aspect of the tongue and into the larynx, the light can be visualized in the anterior aspect of the neck at the level of the thyroid cartilage. The light can be followed into the suprasternal notch if entry into the trachea occurs, whereas the light disappears if the tube passes into the esophagus. Because the neck movement is not required for successful placement, it can be used in patients with cervical spine injuries and also has been suggested as a backup or alternative means of intubating the trachea when direct laryngoscopy fails, as described earlier (137). Fiberoptic-guided endotracheal intubation may be used via the oral or nasal route to aid in endotracheal intubation of difficult airways (137).

Cricothyroidotomy in the Infant

The complication rate associated with oral tracheal intubation is 10%. Complication rates associated with tracheostomy are 26% (69). However, when creating a surgical airway is indicated, cricothyroidotomy is faster and requires less skill and instrumentation than does formal tracheostomy.

In the infant, locate the cricothyroid membrane with a technique similar to that described for adults. The cricoid cartilage is smaller in the infant, and the cricothyroid membrane is more difficult to identify. To ventilate through the cricothyroid membrane, insert an intravenous cannula (over the needle, such as an Angiocath) into the membrane, and use a 3.0 endotracheal adapter to connect the cannula to an oxygen source. The cannula should come from a 16-gauge needle setup, and a flow of 50 psi will result in 500 mL/s ventilation (114).

Complications in the infant include difficulty in palpating the landmarks, bleeding, formation of false passages, and injury to the structures in the neck (69, 114).

NEONATAL RESUSCITATION

Neonatal resuscitation is perhaps the most mentally taxing situation that confronts the emergency physician. An approach must be devised that will permit the rapid assessment and judicious care of the neonate. The approach advocated later can be modified according to the individual needs of the neonate (138). The emphasis here is on the newborn, because this is the most common situation for neonatal resuscitation by an emergency physician.

Congenital Causes of an Obstructed Airway in the Newborn

Intrinsic obstructing lesions of the larynx and trachea are rare. When they occur, they cause almost immediate asphyxiation after birth. They are manifested by stridor or crowing and usually require endoscopy to confirm the diagnosis (108).

Choanal Atresia

All infants are obligate nasal breathers until age 9 months. Infants with choanal atresia will develop respiratory distress, especially during feeding. Catheter probing of the nose demonstrates a block bilaterally. If this patient is seen in the first month of life in the emergency center with a compatible history, the treatment consists of an oral airway, tube feeding, and admission for operative perforation of the posterior membrane (108).

Macroglossia

These infants usually have a lymphangioma. The treatment consists of placing the neonate in the prone position for mild obstruction; tracheostomy or percutaneous transtracheal ventilation (PTV) in the emergency center may be necessary in severe cases.

Micrognathia

This condition often is seen in association with cleft palate. In severe cases, sternal retraction, cyanosis, and sudden asphyxia may be noted. For mild cases, the treatment consists of placing the infant in the prone position and performing a temporary anterior glossopexy with a suture placed through the mid or posterior tongue and tied in the anterior sublingual region to displace the tongue forward.

Other Causes

Other causes include tumors (e.g., cystic hygroma) of the mouth, pharynx, or neck, which may require emergency treatment when the patient has airway obstruction. A congenital goiter may obstruct the airway of the child of a mother who is taking goitrogenic drugs, especially iodides. Usually respiratory difficulty subsides with appropriate treatment after delivery.

ASPHYXIA AND THE AIRWAY

In studies on puppies and monkeys (31) that were asphyxiated at birth, the first stage observed was very rapid dyspneic breathing. After 1.5 to 2.5 minutes of asphyxia, apnea ensued. This stage is called primary apnea and lasts for approximately 2 minutes. If the asphyxia continues, then the animal begins gasping, which continues for 3 minutes. After 8 minutes of total asphyxia, the last gasp occurs, and secondary apnea ensues. This period of apnea continues until death. If asphyxia is relieved after primary apnea, the animal will recover and begin gasping. If secondary apnea has occurred, recovery will not be spontaneous. The duration of secondary apnea will determine the time needed for assisted ventilation before breathing occurs on its own. As a rough rule, for every minute of secondary apnea before the onset of ventilation, 2 minutes of ventilation will be required before breathing begins on its own, and 4 minutes before spontaneous regular ventilation occurs. Thus for 5 minutes of secondary apnea, a total of 20 minutes of ventilation will be needed before breathing occurs on its own.

The newborn is sensitive to hypoxia. Eight to 10 minutes of total anoxia will result in permanent brain damage (31). Bradycardia in the newborn usually means hypoxia (108). To clear the airway, the nares and anterior oral cavity should be aspirated with a bulb syringe. Suction should precede bagging. If the newborn is meconium stained, bag–mask ventilation is contraindicated before the cords are exposed by a laryngoscope and direct suctioning is performed; otherwise meconium aspiration and severe pneumonitis are likely (2). Any child can be adequately ventilated by bag–mask ventilation without endotracheal intubation unless unusual circumstances exist. If bag–mask ventilation does not suffice and an airway is needed, orotracheal intubation should be performed in the infant with agonal or no spontaneous breathing. If the child has spontaneous respirations, some authors prefer nasotracheal intubation with a small Magill forceps (2) because of the more stable fixation of the tube. A nasotracheal tube of size similar to that of the orotracheal tube may be used. No cuff is needed because the subglottic tracheal diameter is narrow, which ensures a good tracheal seal. With orotracheal intubation, do not hyperextend the head; instead, slightly elevate the head with the neck flexed in a sniffing position.

If time permits, insert a gastric tube before endotracheal intubation and suction the stomach. Remove this tube (suctioning while removing it) when the infant is to be endotracheally intubated.

CARDIAC COMPRESSION AND DEFIBRILLATION IN THE NEONATE

Two acceptable methods are advocated for cardiac compression in the neonate (2, 10, 31, 37). Wrap both hands around the infant's chest, encircling the chest, and with both thumbs at the midpoint of the sternum, compress the sternum approximately 1.5 to 2 cm at a rate of 100 to 120 per minute. Alternatively, place one hand beneath the infant and the other over the sternum with the index and middle fingers touching the midsternum, and compress in a similar fashion. When these two methods were compared, and the pressures generated were quantitated via a femoral catheter, the two-handed method encircling the infant's chest was found to be superior (136).

The energy dose needed for defibrillating a neonate is 2 W/s/kg or about 1 W/s/lb. This energy is adequate for defibrillating children weighing less than 50 kg. If the first attempt does not work, then double the energy dose and repeat (50).

GUIDELINES FOR NEONATAL RESUSCITATION

On the basis of the foregoing considerations, the following guidelines are suggested for treating infants who have depressed respirations after delivery (10, 31, 37).

1. Gently aspirate the mouth and nares of the newborn with a bulb syringe as soon as the head is delivered. Hold the newborn in the head-down position to permit gravity to aid in the drainage of secretions. After delivery, continue this position and perform further suctioning with the bulb syringe or a DeLee suction trap. The DeLee suction trap has a catheter connected to a small container, which permits suctioning of copious secretions and analysis of secretions retained within the trap.

CAUTION

Over vigorous suctioning of the posterior pharynx will result in vagally induced bradycardia and laryngospasm.

---

2. Place neonate on warm resuscitation table in head-down position with heat source overhead.

CAUTION

The newborn is unable to shiver to produce heat and generates heat through the oxidation of its brown fat, which consumes oxygen. This oxidation induces further hypoxia and acidosis, so the infant must be placed on a warm resuscitation table with a radiant heater over it.

---

3. Quickly check for congenital causes of airway obstruction. This check includes probing the nose with a small catheter to demonstrate a block bilaterally (choanal atresia). Examine the mouth to check for macroglossia, micrognathia, cleft palate, a goiter in the neck, or "tumors" in the mouth, the pharynx, or the neck. A detailed discussion of these is given in the earlier section, Congenital Causes of Airway Obstruction in the Newborn.
4. If the infant does not respond to these measures, moderate depression exists. Clear the airway before ventilating with a bag and mask.

NOTE

Neonates born through particulate meconium are prone to develop aspiration pneumonitis. When this occurs, deliver the infant and pass it to the resuscitation table with minimal stimulation. Stimulation of the infant who has meconium staining may cause aspiration of the meconium as the infant takes a breath. Clear the trachea by passing an ETT under direct vision with a laryngoscope and putting suction on this tube as it is withdrawn from the infant's trachea. This will remove the plugs of meconium that are too large to be aspirated by a suction catheter. Repeat this procedure until the aspirate is clear. Remember that oxygenation of the infant is necessary after each endotracheal intubation and suction. Provide this oxygenation by gently bagging the patient, using supplemental O_2, after suctioning through the ETT. Meconium may not be present in the pharynx in these infants and may still be present in the trachea, so this procedure should be followed in all meconium-bathed infants.

---

5. Ventilate the infant by mouth-to-mouth resuscitation if a bag and mask are not available. Remember that in the newborn, it is necessary to cover the baby's nose and mouth for effective ventilation. In those infants who have spontaneous respirations in whom mouth-to-mouth or bag–mask ventilation is not necessary, supply supplemental O_2 with a small O_2mask held over the patient's mouth and nose. In this early stage, retrolental fibroplasia, although a concern, should not prevent the physician from giving high concentrations of oxygen in the immediate efforts to resuscitate the infant.

   If these initial resuscitative measures have produced no response by 1.5 minutes after delivery, the progressing asphyxia may lead to decreased muscular tone and a decrease in heart rate.
6. Insert a small plastic oropharyngeal airway into the mouth, and ventilate the infant with a bag–mask device with supplemental oxygen applied (ideally under a pressure of 16 to 20 cm of water) for 1 to 2 seconds. It is difficult to estimate this pressure unless previous experience shows what this amount of pressure feels like.

NOTE

The newborn generates negative intrathoracic pressures of 80 cm of water spontaneously on its first breath. The bag-and-mask oxygen will not produce these kinds of pressure; however, oxygen will be forced down to the level of the terminal bronchioles where some gas exchange does take place. The increase in intrabronchial pressure stimulates the pulmonary stretch receptors and will initiate a gasp in about 85% of infants (37).

---

7. If there is no respiratory effort and the heart rate continues to decrease, visualize the larynx with a laryngoscope; if foreign material obstructs the larynx, administer quick brief suction. When the glottis is visualized, insert a curved ETT. Blow brief puffs of air through the tube with enough force to cause the lower chest to rise to initiate spontaneous respiration. With the first or second application of positive pressure, the infant usually makes an effort to breathe, and the ETT may be withdrawn after the infant has taken five or six breaths (37). A severely depressed infant may need 6 to 8 minutes of artificial ventilation before spontaneous gasping ensues (37).

NOTE

In infants born to heroin-addicted mothers administer naloxone. The dose is 10 μg/kg in one to three parts. Because the narcotically depressed infant has normal circulation, the drug is effective intramuscularly (31).

---

8. If, despite adequate ventilation and external massage for 2 to 3 minutes, there is no improvement in the color, muscle tone, or heart rate, then insert an umbilical catheter (see Chapter 12: Vascular Procedures) and administer sodium bicarbonate.
   a. Dilute 5 mL of bicarbonate with 5 mL of 5% dextrose and water. This 10-mL solution then contains 5 mEq of sodium bicarbonate and can be administered to the neonate who weighs 3 kg at a dose of 1.5 mEq/kg. If no response is elicited, then administer an additional 0.75 mEq/kg.
   b. Obtain blood for pH, Po_2, Pco_2, and bicarbonate as soon as possible.
9. Administer 1 to 2 mL/kg of 50% glucose if there is no response to these steps.
10. If no marked improvement is elicited after the preceding steps, dilute 1 mL (1 mg) of a 1:1,000 epinephrine solution in 10 mL of isotonic saline, and give 0.5 to 2.0 mL of this solution until the heart rate is increased to more than 70 beats/min.
11. Continue ventilation and cardiac massage throughout this period, as indicated by the infant's status. Remember to minimize heat loss and oxygen consumption.
12. Place the infant in a bassinet after resuscitation, and transfer to the nursery.

TRACHEOTOMY

Percutaneous Tracheostomy

The complication rate of emergency tracheostomy is 2 to 5 times greater than that of the elective procedure (60, 92). A technique has been described for percutaneous tracheostomy in the literature (67, 103). We, along with some of our colleagues, do not favor the technique (84) because the complication rate is higher than that for simple cricothyroidotomy. In 94 cases studied, approximately 14% had complications (140). A severe complication is that the device can be inserted into the peritracheal area rather than the intratracheal area. This complication is due to the mobility of the larynx. The problem is that this procedure does not stabilize the airway, before insertion, because there is no tracheal incision, and thus no tracheal hook is inserted to hold the trachea in place.

Other complications described are pretracheal hematoma, subcutaneous emphysema, pretracheal cellulitis, bilateral pneumothorax, or injury to the great vessels (140). The most common of these complications is pretracheal hematoma (88).

TECHNIQUE

1. Place a needle in the trachea, and aspirate air through it to ascertain positioning in the tracheal lumen.
2. Through the needle, pass a dilator with an airway on it through the trachea by using a wire-reinforced polyethylene guide. In an adult, make a small incision in the skin of the neck to reduce tissue tension during insertion of the dilator.
3. Insert the dilator with the tracheal tube into the airway as a unit.
4. Then remove the dilator, leaving the tracheal tube in place.

The procedure of percutaneous dilatational tracheostomy (PDT) requires readjustment of the position of the existing tracheal tube, so there is a risk of potential loss of the airway. A number of methods have been adopted for safer airway management. A study (145) that evaluated the adequacy of ventilation via the Combitube during performance of PDT showed that the potential advantages, compared with those of the standard technique with the tracheal tube, are: no need for laryngeal readjustment of the existing tracheal tube; trachea is free and unobstructed; blood flow to the trachea is not impeded by the tracheal tube; and the reduced possibility of loss of the airway. Computerized tomographic scans at C7/T1 performed with a Combitube in situ in a patient before tracheostomy demonstrated slight displacement of the trachea anteriorly toward the right side. A tracheostomy may be needed if there is upper airway obstruction. In the case of lower cervical mediastinal hematomas, tracheal intubation and ventilation may be needed. In these cases, a tracheostomy does not solve the problem because the obstruction is below the level of the tracheostomy stoma (142).

NOTE

We do not recommend this procedure in that, although this procedure seems simple to perform, the complication rate due to mobility of the airway is greater than that for simply cricothyroidotomy.

Cricothyroidotomy

The cricothyroid membrane is recommended as an ideal area for performing an emergency laryngotomy by many authors (14, 16, 20, 48, 93, 94, 97). It is our opinion that the cricothyroid membrane puncture is the safest and simplest method for establishing a satisfactory airway under adverse conditions. Even the most skilled surgeon would be unwise to attempt emergency tracheostomy when cricothyroid membrane puncture would admirably control the crisis (94). Brantigan and Grow (16), in 1975, conducted the largest study on cricothyroidotomies. They performed 655 cricothyroidotomies, both electively and in emergency situations, and found an extremely low incidence of complications, much lower than that reported with tracheostomy.

When critical airway obstruction is seen in the emergency center, an orderly plan of action is essential; otherwise, irreversible brain damage or death may ensue shortly. The four basic steps are (a) recognition of the obstruction; (b) maneuvers to relieve obstruction (e.g., Heimlich maneuver); (c) artificial ventilation (mouth-to-mouth, bag, mask, etc.) to relieve obstruction; and (d) diagnosis of persistent obstruction and treatment by the establishment of an emergency surgical airway by cricothyroidotomy (94).

INDICATIONS

1. Any situation in which a standard endotracheal or nasotracheal intubation cannot be performed.
   a. Excessive oropharyngeal or nasopharyngeal hemorrhage.
   b. Massive regurgitation.
   c. Massive congenital or traumatic deformities of oropharynx or nasopharynx.
   d. Complete airway obstruction such that endotracheal intubation is impossible (e.g., foreign body), and maneuvers that should open the airway are unsuccessful.
2. Suspected or proven cervical spine fracture in a patient who needs an airway but in whom nasotracheal intubation is unsuccessful or contraindicated.
3. Unsuccessful attempts at endotracheal intubation in a patient in whom inordinate delay would result in cerebral anoxic damage.

CONTRAINDICATIONS

Cricothyroidotomy is contraindicated in patients with fracture or serious injury to the larynx or cricoid cartilage, in which case a tracheostomy should be performed.

EQUIPMENT

No. 11 blade
Scalpel
Trousseau dilator
Plastic tracheostomy tube (Silex or Portex tracheostomy tubes). Standard ETT can be used. The size of the ETT is dependent on the age of the patient and size of the trachea. In general, one can insert a

size 6, 7, or 8 tube in the adult. The tube is cut to the proper size once in place.
Small curved hemostats
Prep solution
1 dozen 4 × 4-inch gauze pads
Scissors
10-mL syringe
Tracheal suction catheter
Tracheal hook

TECHNIQUE

NOTE

There are currently devices on the market that can be inserted percutaneously through the cricothyroid membrane. Although they are reported to be easy to use, we have found them too dangerous to recommend when compared with the standard procedure described here. These devices do not allow the user to stabilize the larynx and result in similar complications to those described in the section on percutaneous tracheostomy.

1. Place the patient in the recumbent or semirecumbent position.
2. Locate the cricothyroid membrane by standing on the patient's right side and, with the palm of the left hand placed against the chin, use the thumb and middle finger to palpate the hyoid bone (Fig. 2.32). With the index finger, palpate the *thyrohyoid membrane* and then the larynx. Then remove the middle finger and thumb to a position on either side of the larynx to stabilize this structure while the index finger "walks down" the thyroid notch toward the cricoid cartilage until an indentation is felt between the cricoid and thyroid cartilages (Fig. 2.33). This indentation is the cricothyroid membrane (Figs. 2.34 and 2.35). Go past the cricoid cartilage and palpate the tracheal rings and then return with the index finger to redefine the cricothyroid membrane. This process establishes with absolute certainty that the cricothyroid membrane is defined.

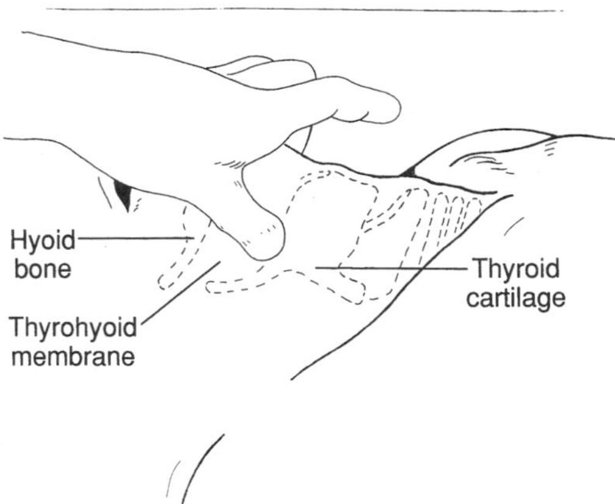

Figure 2.32. Grasp the thyroid cartilage with the thumb and long finger, and use the index finger to walk down the midline, locating the cricothyroid membrane. See text for discussion.

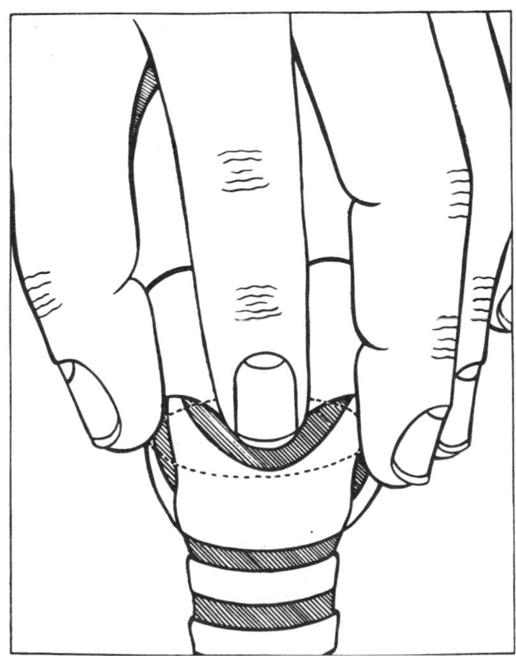

Figure 2.33. The larynx stabilized between the left thumb and middle finger. Insert the tip of the index finger over the cricothyroid membrane. To puncture the membrane, direct a no. 11 scalpel and blade along the nail of the index finger and through the membrane in one step.

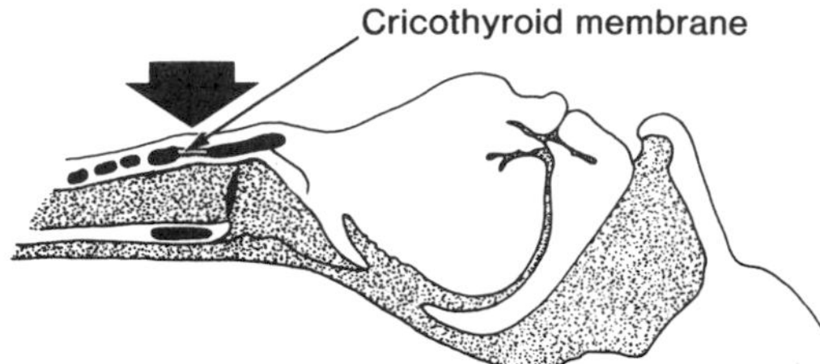

Figure 2.34. The indentation of the cricothyroid membrane.

CAUTION

One of the most common complications in this procedure is not identifying properly the cricothyroid membrane and performing a "cricothyroidotomy" erroneously on the thyrohyoid membrane. This complication can be avoided by using the technique described.

3. If time permits and the patient is awake, infiltrate the skin and subcutaneous tissue with 1% lidocaine with epinephrine.
4. While holding the larynx between the thumb and middle finger and, with the fingertip of the index finger against the cricothyroid membrane, make a stab incision (using an 11 blade) through the cricothyroid membrane (Fig. 2.36).
5. Make a transverse incision through the membrane with a single motion (Fig. 2.37) (16, 97), first in one direction, and then, rotating the blade 180 degrees, carry the incision in the opposite direction (Fig. 2.38).

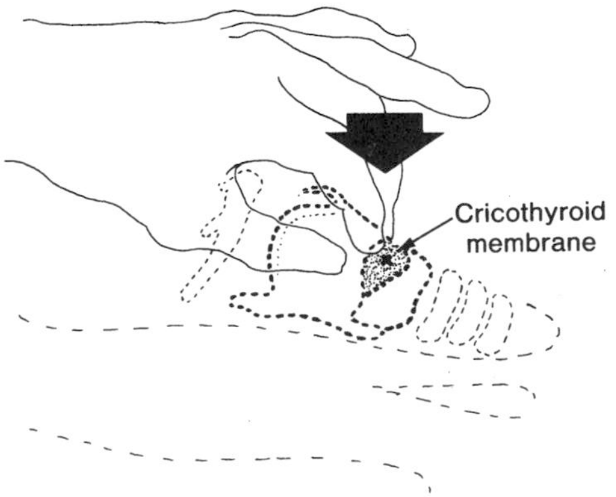

Figure 2.35. Hold the larynx as shown in Fig. 2.35, with the index finger placed over the cricothyroid membrane.

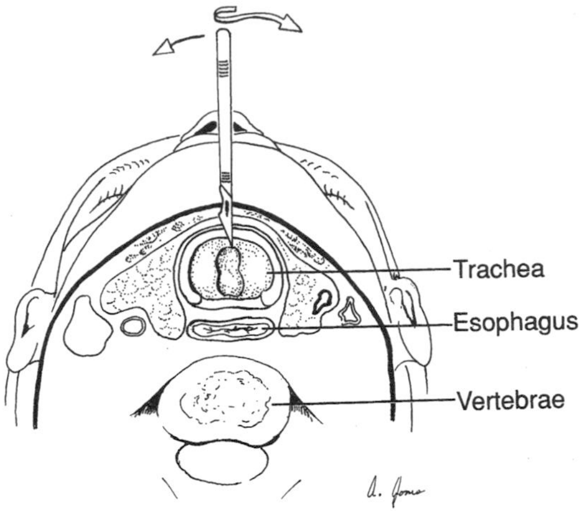

Figure 2.36. Note the depth at which the no. 11 blade is inserted. Be careful to avoid the esophagus, which is directly behind the trachea.

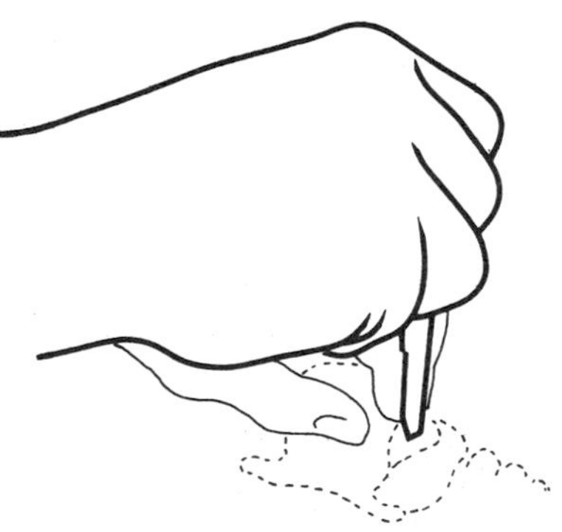

Figure 2.37. Make a transverse incision after puncture through the membrane with a single step. Hold the scalpel between the thumb and index finger in such a manner that only the tip of the blade can enter the trachea to the depth desired. This prevents penetration too deeply into and perforation of the esophagus during the initial stab incision (not shown above). After this, place the hand in the position shown above for extending the incision transversely across the membrane.

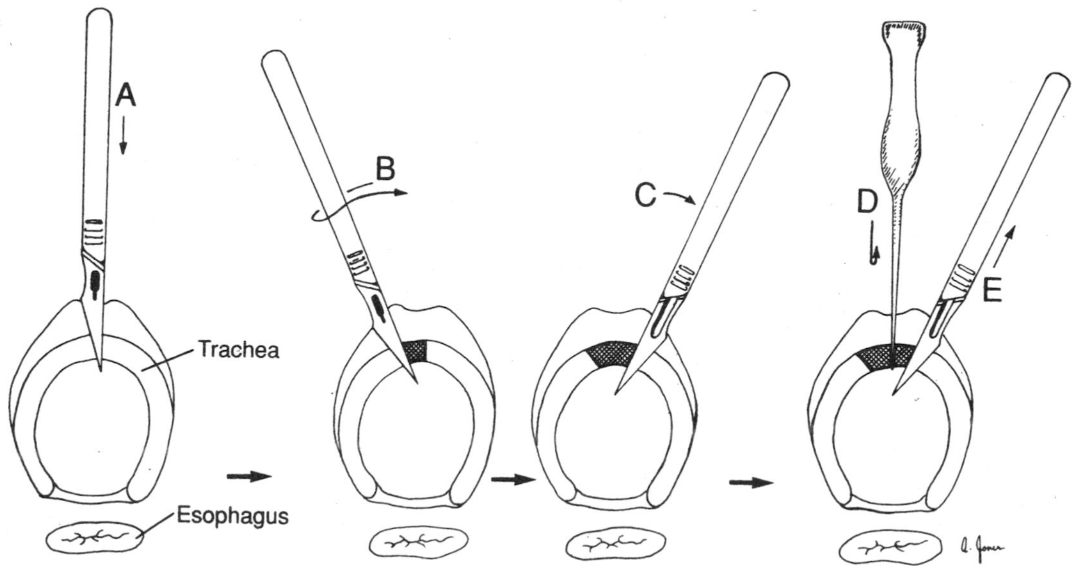

Figure 2.38. After inserting the blade *(A)*, carry the incision laterally *(B)*, and then rotate the blade 180 degrees with the sharp edge interiorly, and then continue the incision in the opposite direction *(C)*. Do not remove the no. 11 blade until a tracheal hook has been inserted through the incision to grasp the thyroid cartilage *(D)*. This is a critical point, in that if the no. 11 blade is removed before this, one may lose the tract created into the trachea and a false passage may be found when attempting to put in the tracheal hook.

NOTE

Hold the scalpel between the thumb and index finger in such a way that only the tip of the blade can enter the trachea during the initial stab incision.

CAUTION

The esophagus is located behind the cricoid cartilage. If the blade is not held in a manner that will keep one from going too deeply, then the esophagus may be perforated. It is for this reason that we advocate this somewhat unorthodox method of holding the scalpel when making the initial incision.

6. Once the trachea is entered, if the patient is breathing, a spurt of air will come through the incision. It is critical to leave the no. 11 blade in place, insert a tracheal hook into the hole, and retract the larynx upward; only then remove the no. 11 blade (Fig. 2.39). If this is not done, the tract from the skin to the trachea may be lost because of mobility of the trachea.
7. Placc a curved hemostat or a Trousseau dilator through the incision and open the membrane perpendicular to the incision (Fig. 2.40).

NOTE

Vessels have been identified that course through the cricothyroid membrane. In a recent cadaver study, 79% of 34 cadavers had vascular structures identified in this area (77). Sixty-two percent had vertically oriented arteries or veins that would be at risk of being severed during cricothyroidotomy. Hemorrhage has been reported; however, this is not a major problem in

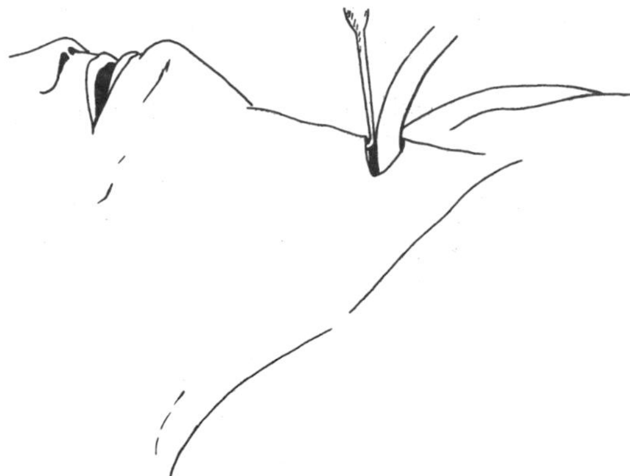

Figure 2.39. The tracheal hook stabilizes the airway and prevents mobility while the tracheostomy tube is being inserted. See text for discussion.

most cases (13, 73), because these vessels are quite small and easily controlled (5, 16, 20, 22, 91, 114, 130).

NOTE

In some patients, on insertion of the Trousseau dilator or hemostat, the larynx displaces posteriorly on attempting to insert the tracheostomy or ETT, making insertion difficult. When this occurs, a skin hook should be inserted through the cricothyroidotomy incision and the larynx uplifted to aid in stabilizing the larynx in position while passing the tracheostomy tube.

---

8. The ETT will of course be too long; it should be cut to an appropriate length and the adapter attached to the cut end. Inflate the cuff of the tube.
9. Ventilate lungs and auscultate to ensure proper tube placement.

COMPLICATIONS

1. **Esophageal perforation.** For prevention and treatment, see step 5 in Technique.
2. **Subcutaneous emphysema.** To prevent, do not carry the incision beyond that needed to pass the tracheostomy or ETT. A laterally placed incision that requires suturing around the tube is prone to subcutaneous emphysema. No treatment is indicated.
3. **Hemorrhage.** This complication will not be encountered if the incision is not too wide. Occasionally a small vessel crossing the cricothyroid membrane causes significant bleeding, and this may require ligation. Treat this complication with simple pressure unless a major vessel is bleeding, in which case ligation is indicated.

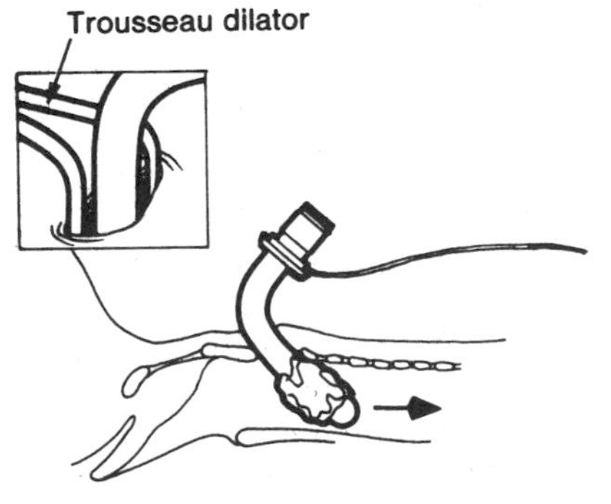

Figure 2.40. Use the Trousseau dilator or curved hemostat to open the cricothyroid membrane vertically *(inset)*. Then insert the Pyrex tube as shown above.

Cricothyroidotomy in the Pediatric Age Group

In the pediatric age group, cricothyroidotomy becomes progressively more difficult as the patient becomes smaller. Sufficient literature documenting the complication rate of this procedure is not yet available. We have been involved in approximately 10 cases of pediatric cricothyroidotomy. We found it efficacious and life saving. Thus this procedure merits further study (145). Some authors recommended needle cricothyroidotomy if an emergency airway is required. Emergency tracheostomy is preferable under controlled conditions.

Tracheostomy

When airway obstruction is secondary to acute injuries to the larynx or trachea, tracheostomy may be indicated (39, 52, 58, 73, 120, 126, 141); however, overall, this procedure has been replaced by cricothyroidotomy.

INDICATIONS

1. Acute injuries to the larynx and trachea.
2. Similar to those of cricothyroidotomy.

CONTRAINDICATIONS

In our opinion, tracheostomy is no longer regarded as the procedure of choice in emergency airway management in which the traditional "emergency tracheostomy" is indicated. Cricothyroidotomy is currently regarded as the procedure of first choice in emergency medicine. Although it is beyond the scope of this text to discuss the controversies relating to the use of one technique over another, it is our belief that this vital topic deserves some discussion. The emergency tracheostomy, even in the most skilled hands, can be a time-consuming and difficult procedure because of the very nature of the situation that makes it an emergency rather than an elective procedure. Brantigan and Grow (16) settled this issue during a large study in which they performed more than 600 cricothyroidotomies and showed that the complications often thought to be associated with this technique do not occur. The reader is urged to read this classic study. The burden of proof lies distinctly on any individual who believes that tracheostomy is as simple to perform as, and possesses distinct advantages over, cricothyroidotomy.

EQUIPMENT

No. 10 blade and scalpel
No. 11 blade and scalpel
Preparation cut and iodinated solution
10-mL syringe
18- and 25-gauge needles
Eight small curved hemostats (5.5 inch)
Tracheostomy tube with inflatable cuff (plastic tube preferable); size of the tube should be 6, 7, or 8 for the average adult
Seven towels and towel clips
Two dozen 4 × 4-inch gauze pads
3-0 catgut and 4-0 silk
Two Allis forceps
Mastoid retractor
Two small rakes
Two skin forceps
Two tissue forceps without teeth
Suture scissors and curved scissors
Needle holder
Kocher forceps
One medium tracheal dilator
Frazier suction tip and suction tubing
2-0 and 3-0 catgut
3-0 nylon suture

TECHNIQUE (54, 73, 93, 115)

Preparatory Steps

1. Place the patient in the recumbent or semirecumbent position.
2. Hyperextend the neck with a folded sheet placed behind the scapula. This hyperextension is obviously not done when one suspects a fracture of the cervical spine.
3. Prepare and drape the patient to expose the area bordered by the manubrium, root of the neck, supraclavicular space, and chin.

Procedural Steps

1. Choose the incision. This choice is dependent on the degree of urgency. In the emergency situation, the vertical incision is usually preferred over the transverse incision; however, a description is given of both methods.
   Vertical incision:
   a. Requires minimal dissection.
   b. Is associated with less bleeding.

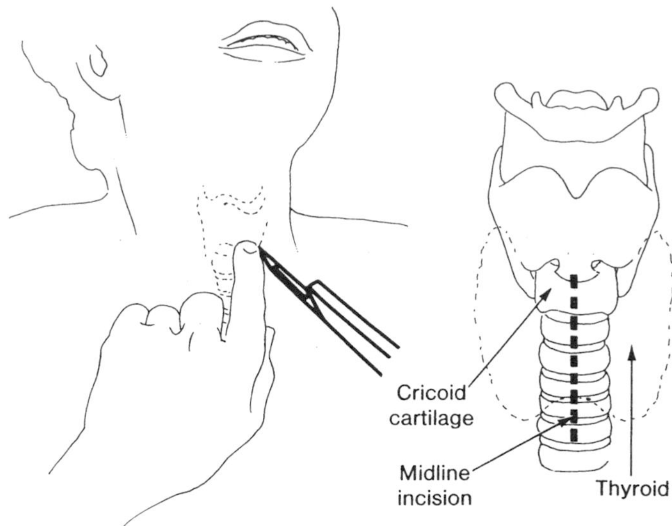

Figure 2.41. Make a midline incision vertically with a no. 10 blade, extending from the cricoid cartilage to the suprasternal notch. See text for details.

c. Affords more rapid access to the trachea.
d. Avoids the superficial veins.
e. Is easier to perform in the patient with a short neck.
f. Heals cosmetically worse than the transverse incision.

Transverse incision:

a. Heals better cosmetically.
b. Takes more time.
c. Is associated with more bleeding.
d. Requires more dissection.

2. *Vertical incision:* Make a midline incision using the no. 10 blade and carry the incision from the cricoid cartilage to the suprasternal notch (Fig. 2.41).

   Transverse incisions: Carry the incision from the point approximately one finger breadth below the cricoid cartilage, making an incision approximately 6 cm long. The incision should extend through the skin, subcutaneous tissue, and platysma.
3. *Vertical incision:* Continue through the medial raphe and dissect between the anterior strap muscles until the pretracheal fascia is reached.

CAUTION

Hemorrhage is a major complication occurring in this step. Stay in the midline to avoid this potentially lethal complication.

   Transverse incision: Separate the platysma from the anterior strap muscles until 4 to 5 cm of the medial raphe is exposed, and incise the raphe transversely.
4. Retract the wound edges with the mastoid retractor or small rakes (Fig. 2.42*A*).
5. Palpate the tracheal and cricoid cartilages. Locate the thyroid isthmus, and retract the isthmus upward. We find it easier to retract the thyroid inferiorly and hook the cricoid superiorly. Use blunt dissection with small curved hemostat to separate the thyroid isthmus from the trachea.
6. Place two small clamps on the isthmus, one on each side, and divide the isthmus. Later one can suture these divided edges with silk (Fig. 2.42*B*).

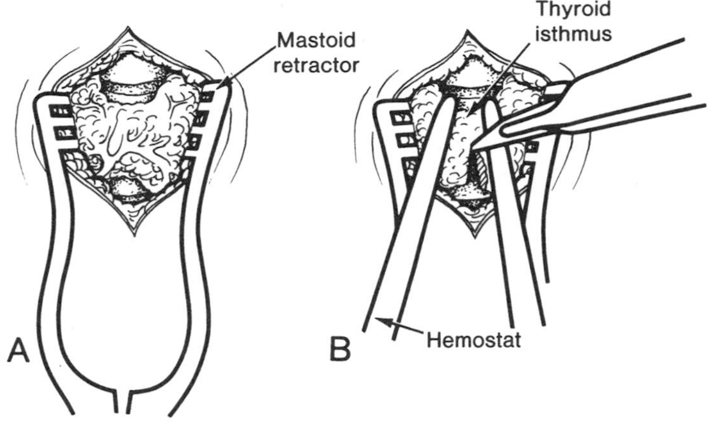

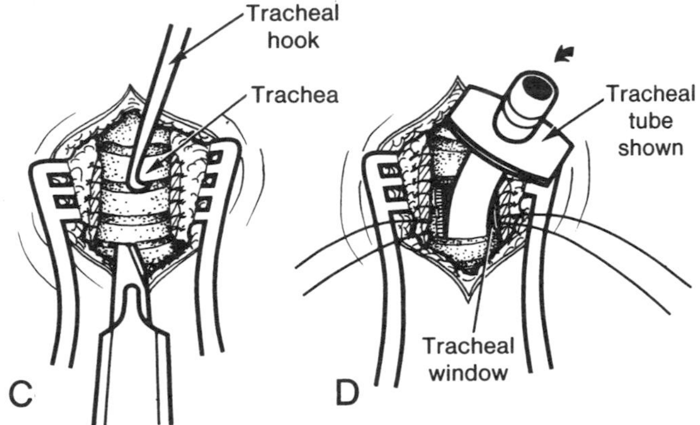

Figure 2.42. Performance of an emergency tracheostomy. See text for discussion.

7. Locate the second through the fourth rings (Fig. 2.42*C*).

CAUTION

Avoid the first ring because incision of this area causes subglottic stenosis.

---

8. Make a vertical incision through the third and fourth rings.

NOTE

One can make a window in the trachea through the third and fourth rings as shown (Fig. 2.42*D*). Although this is perfectly acceptable, it again is more time consuming in the emergency situation.

---

9. Suction the tracheal secretions.
10. Insert the tracheal tube and obturator, sizes 6, 7, or 8 in the adult, smaller in the child (Fig. 2.42*D*).
11. Remove the obturator and inflate the cuff.

CAUTION

The tube should fit comfortably in the trachea and not obstruct the carina.

AFTERCARE

1. Tie tube in place with umbilical tape around the neck.
2. Approximate the muscles with chromic catgut. To avoid subcutaneous emphysema, do not close the subcutaneous tissue.
3. Close the skin loosely. Dress the wound with 4 × 4-inch gauze.

COMPLICATIONS

1. **Mediastinal emphysema.**
2. **Outer tube coughed out,** causing severe mediastinal and subcutaneous emphysema. To prevent this complication:
   a. Secure the tube in place.
   b. Keep patient under observation.
3. **Hemorrhage.** Stay within the midline to avoid vessels that lie laterally.
4. **Subglottic stenosis.** This can be prevented by using the second through fourth tracheal rings.
5. **Obstruction of the carina.**
6. **Erosion into major vessels or the trachea.** Erosion into major vessels of the neck or through the trachea is a late complication. It can be avoided by the use of low pressure within the ETT cuff and periodic deflation when prolonged intubation is necessary. Periodic deflation will avoid pressure necrosis of the mucosa lining the trachea. This complication, because of its late occurrence, is not a problem in the emergency center. However, the emergency physician may see such a patient when called in the middle of the night to the ICU to deal with major bleeding around a tracheostomy tube previously placed.

Tracheostomy in the Patient with Massive Neck Swelling

A modified technique for emergency tracheostomy in the patient with massive neck swelling has recently been introduced (126). The patient who has massive neck swelling secondary to hematoma, subcutaneous emphysema, or hemorrhage may have nonpalpable landmarks (4). The hematoma may deviate the trachea and make it difficult to establish the midline. Such patients often require emergency tracheostomy within a matter of minutes. Using traditional methods of establishing an airway through a tracheostomy or cricothyroidotomy in such patients often is fraught with considerable hemorrhage and loss of time trying to identify structures in the distended neck.

The hyoid bone serves to anchor the trachea and larynx superiorly to the mandible, tongue, and base of the skull. The structure is rarely injured during massive neck trauma. It provides an ideal point on which to place traction to stabilize the trachea and larynx for a tracheostomy. Because the body of the hyoid is a midline structure, by attaching an instrument to it and retracting superiorly and anteriorly, one can pull the trachea and larynx forward as well as stabilize them so that no motion occurs during an emergency tracheostomy. To perform this procedure:

1. Measure the distance from the angle of the mandible to the point of the chin, as shown in Fig. 2.43 (*line A*). Measure half the distance of this line down the anterior aspect of the neck from the midpoint of the chin inferiorly (*line B,* Fig. 2.43*A*). The ratio of line *A* to line *B* is 2:1. The point at which a no. 11 blade should be inserted is at the end of line *B* (*point C*).
2. Direct the no. 11 blade posteriorly, remaining in the midline and angling the tip as if going toward the angle of the mandible (Figs. 2.43*A* and 2.44). The hyoid bone will be reached at various depths, depending on the amount of swelling and fat deposition in the anterior neck.
3. Insert a skin hook alongside the track established by the no. 11 blade and grasp the hyoid by hooking the skin hook underneath, as shown in Fig. 2.45.

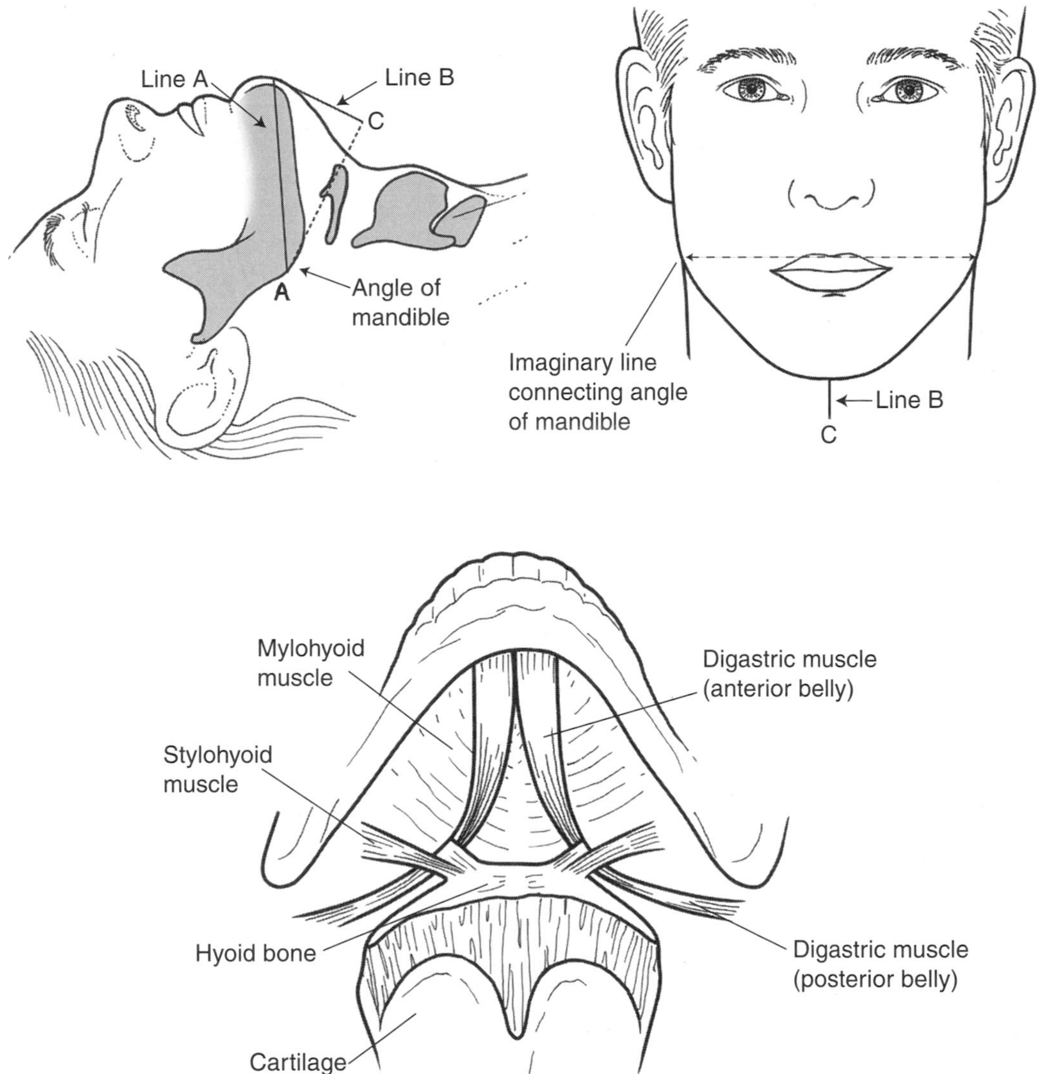

Figure 2.43. Measure the distance from the angle of the mandible to the tip of the chin (point *A* to *B*) and measure down from the tip to the chin inferiorly (point *B* to point *C*), half of the distance from the angle of the mandible to the chin. See text for details.

Retract the hyoid superiorly and anteriorly as shown by the arrow. Because the hyoid will have been grasped in the midline, retracting it superiorly will pull forward the larynx and the trachea.

4. Make an incision inferiorly from the point of the skin hook through the puncture site of the no. 11 blade, remaining in the midline, as shown in Fig. 2.46. Because the skin hook is grasping the body of the hyoid in its midpoint, an incision can be easily planned that will remain in the midline even though the patient may have a hematoma, which distorts the perception of the midline.
5. Identify the cricothyroid membrane and make a transverse incision through that membrane (Fig. 2.46).

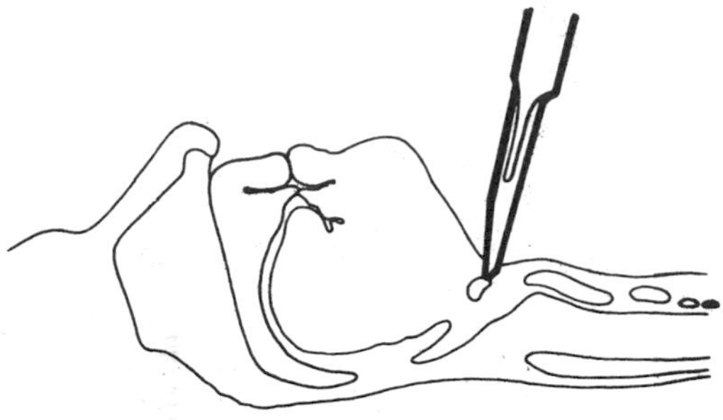

Figure 2.44. Insert a scalpel blade at the point identified (point *C*) at the end of line *B* (see Fig. 2.43*A*), and aim the tip of the blade toward the imaginary line connecting the angles of the mandible. The hyoid bone will be reached.

6. Insert a standard Pyrex tracheostomy tube through the cricothyroid membrane as one would routinely do for performing a cricothyroidotomy (Fig. 2.47).
7. Finally, close the incision, and connect the patient to a bag–valve–mask device.

ANCILLARY PROCEDURES

Percutaneous Transtracheal Catheter Ventilation

Percutaneous transtracheal catheter ventilation is a useful procedure in treating a patient who needs ventilation and oxygenation and in whom one cannot easily place an ETT for various reasons. The advantages of this technique are the rapid access through the cricothyroid membrane, and that it requires very little skill to perform. The procedure achieves good ventilation of the lungs within seconds with adequate oxygenation. Some studies in the past demonstrated a tendency toward CO_2 retention and poor CO_2 washout, but recent studies demonstrated that it is a useful procedure in patients who are hypoxic and hypercarbic (12, 107, 129). The use of 100% oxygen and appropriate ventilation volumes produces positive pressure ventilation with exhalation of carbon dioxide during recoil of the diaphragm and chest wall (129). One is able to achieve a Po_2 of 300 mm Hg and a Pco_2 of 40 mm Hg by using this technique. Without this recoil, despite continuous insufflation of oxygen under pressure up to 50 psi, hypercarbia will result (129); thus it is critical that at least 50-psi bursts of oxygen be used intermittently to avoid retention of CO_2.

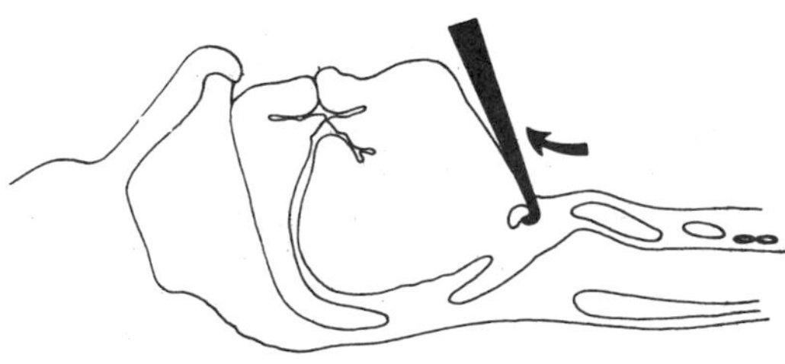

Figure 2.45. Insert a skin hook alongside the scalpel in the puncture site and track made by the no. 11 blade, and grasp the hyoid, lifting it upward and superior as shown above.

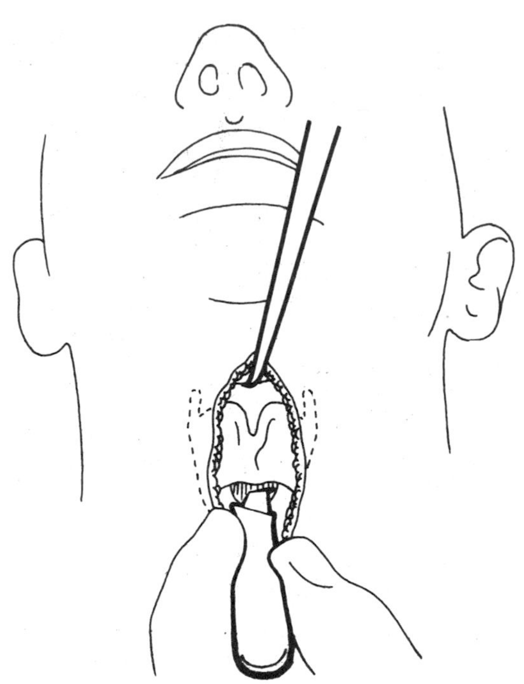

Figure 2.46. Make an incision from the skin hook downward to just above the suprasternal notch. Enter the cricothyroid membrane with a no. 11 blade. See text for details.

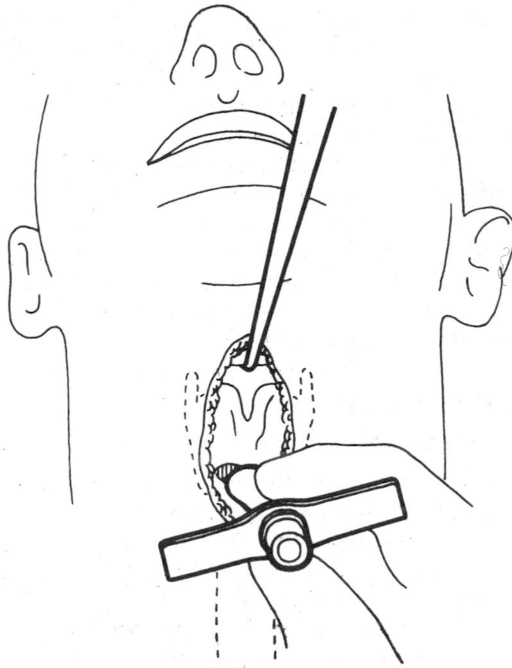

Figure 2.47. Insert the tracheostomy tube through the cricothyroid membrane. See text for details.

The disadvantage of this technique is that it does not safeguard against aspiration. The catheter does not allow complete control of the patient's airway. In addition, one is unable to suction through the catheter.

INDICATIONS

Percutaneous transtracheal ventilation should be used in patients with possible cervical spine injuries in which there is difficulty visualizing the airway, and in whom it is difficult to perform endotracheal intubation (23).

EQUIPMENT

Ordinary flow meter
Oxygen providing 50 psi from ordinary wall oxygen source
Standard oxygen tubing
14-gauge Angiocath
Three-way plastic stopcock

A manual in-line valve to interrupt the flow of oxygen is preferable. This may be a pushbutton device or a "T" piece inserted into the oxygen line. The 50 psi is available by means of a connector that can be attached directly through the piped oxygen line of any hospital. A cannula with side holes is available through Actronics Corporation (Zurich, Switzerland). Hold the cannula firmly in position and begin ventilation.

Some authors have indicated that the hand-operated release valve is not necessary, but this is useful when available (34, 42, 62, 128). Levinson et al. (74) modified the device described so that it could be assembled from parts found at any hospital emergency center.

TECHNIQUE

Preparatory Steps

To assemble the device, cut a side hole near the distal end of a length of standard oxygen tubing. Attach a standard three-way plastic stopcock made for intravenous tubing to the oxygen tubing. Set the flow meter attached to the wall oxygen source at the wide-open (flush) position, which provides a high flow rate necessary for PTV.

Procedural Steps

1. Identify the cricothyroid membrane.
2. Place the patient in a recumbent or semirecumbent position.
3. Prepare the patient with the neck slightly extended.

NOTE

Although extension of the neck is desirable, it is not essential to performance of this procedure.

---

4. Stabilize the larynx with the thumb and middle finger, and place the index finger over the cricothyroid membrane.

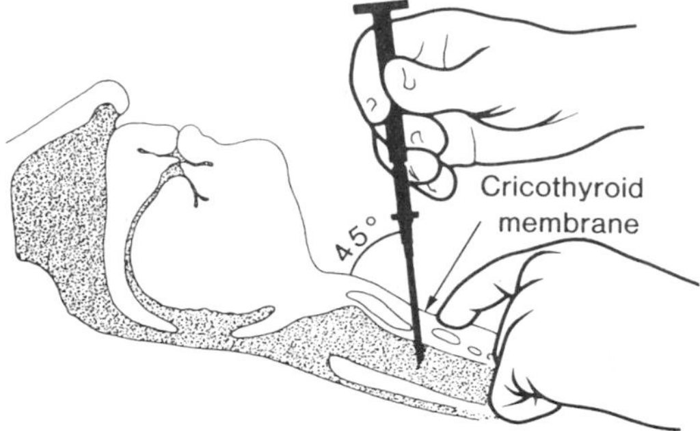

Figure 2.48. Percutaneous transtracheal catheter ventilation. Insert the needle into the cricothyroid membrane at a 45-degree angle, directed inferiorly. See text for discussion.

5. Pass the needle at a 45-degree angle, and cannulate the trachea through the cricothyroid membrane (Fig. 2.48).

CAUTION

The posterior wall of the trachea is membranous below the cricoid cartilage, and the esophagus lies posterior to it. Stop passing the needle the moment air is aspirated into the syringe, to avoid perforation of the esophagus.

---

6. Attach the catheter to the oxygen tubing.
7. **Turn on the oxygen to flush position if not already done**.
8. With the thumb placed over the side hole cut in the oxygen tubing, deliver a jet of pressurized air. Removal of the thumb permits oxygen to escape through the side hole and allows exhalation passively. There should be 20 bursts per minute. The inspiratory phase should last 1 second. Exhalation should last for 2 seconds (56, 134).

NOTE

An oxygen flow rate of approximately 50 psi is provided with a flow meter attached to a wall oxygen source set at the flush position (wide open). One can achieve a gas flow rate of 800 mL/s with the standard oxygen tubing connected to a 14-gauge Angiocath. All ventilations will be with 100% oxygen. Direct this oxygen flow intermittently into the trachea with the thumb over the portal of the three-way valve inserted between the oxygen tubing and the 14-gauge Angiocath. A 1-second jet of oxygen followed by 4 seconds of an expiratory phase in which the oxygen is permitted to escape achieves good ventilation (21).

COMPLICATIONS

1. **Subcutaneous emphysema** (34, 45, 128). This may be caused by incorrect catheter placement and is a very common problem. The oxygen escapes into the subcutaneous tissue.
2. **Mediastinal emphysema** (45, 128).
3. **Coughing.** This may occur with each ventilation jet in a conscious patient (34).
4. **Hemorrhage** at site of needle puncture (34, 45).
5. **Esophageal or mediastinal puncture** if the needle is passed too far (34, 45).
6. **Tracheal mucosal damage** (34). This is due to the high-pressure jets of oxygen and is not usually a problem. It becomes a problem when high-pressure oxygen is permitted to continue striking the mucosa too many times.
7. **Kinking of catheter** (34). This may occur as the catheter enters the neck. If this is a problem, a large catheter may have to be used.
8. **Pneumatocyst** (34). A pneumatocyst is a collection of air that occurs around the trachea, usually within a fascial plane, that is secondary to the high pressures of oxygen being delivered through the catheter. This is particularly prone to occur with improper use of the catheter and displacement. The pneumatocyst can be drained by simple needle aspiration.
9. **Arterial perforation** (106).

Bronchoscopy

There are situations in the emergency center in which rigid bronchoscopy is necessary. The procedure is easy to perform and may be lifesaving.

INDICATIONS

1. Massive hemoptysis. Bronchoscopy permits identification of the site of bleeding (85). Massive hemoptysis has a high mortality rate (27). Eighty-seven per cent of patients with massive hemoptysis have a history of pulmonary bleeding, and more than half die without surgical intervention (27). In patients who have more than 600 mL of bleeding in 16 hours, the mortality related to the rate of bleeding exceeds 75%. As is noted later, one may tamponade massive bleeding by instilling a temporary pack through the bronchoscope. Massive hemoptysis is a definite indication for rigid bronchoscopy, because flexible fiberoptic instruments become cloudy when in contact with blood (72). The airway also is better controlled, and packing can be placed, which cannot be performed through the fiberoptic bronchoscope (85).
2. Foreign-body retrieval. Although the flexible instrument is more useful here (72, 146), one can use the rigid bronchoscope in an acute emergency.
3. Massive aspiration. The bronchoscope can be used to remove large particulate matter to permit adequate ventilation.

EQUIPMENT

The following list is for emergency center bronchoscopy.

Rigid bronchoscope with light source
Adrenaline (1:1,000)
Medicine cup
Small sterile gauze ball sponges
Sterile saline
Jackson bronchoscopic sponge carrier
Suction
Oxygen source
Fogarty balloon catheter
4% cocaine solution
2% lidocaine with epinephrine

TECHNIQUE (FOR MASSIVE HEMOPTYSIS)

1. Place the patient in the Trendelenburg position with the head in the sniffing position by placing a folded towel under the head.
2. Induce light sedation.
3. Apply topical anesthesia with 4% cocaine spray to the pharynx and instill 2% lidocaine through the cricothyroid membrane. If needed, perform a block of the internal branch of the superior laryngeal nerve as indicated in preparatory step 3b for nasotracheal intubation (p. 70).
4. Insert the bronchoscope after hyperextending the head at the atlantooccipital joint (Fig. 2.49).
5. Remove blood and maintain the airway.
6. Once a site of bleeding has been identified, the topical application of epinephrine with pressure is used to control bleeding temporarily.
7. If bleeding continues, use one of two methods for control (55, 85, 121, 146). Under extreme circumstances, passage of a gauze pack through the

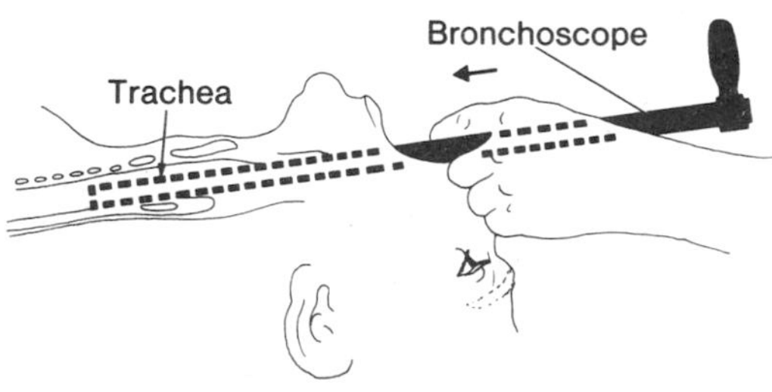

Figure 2.49. Insert the bronchoscope after hyperextending the head at the atlantooccipital joint. See text for details.

bronchoscope into the involved bronchus may be necessary for temporary control of bleeding. Apply the sponge with Jackson forceps and soaked with adrenaline. Irrigate that bronchus with 10-mL aliquots of sterile saline.

Alternatively, place the scope into the uninvolved main stem bronchus to maintain and isolate the airway. In one study with massive hemoptysis involving 10 patients who refused surgery, a balloon-tipped catheter was placed and left for 24 hours and then deflated, and this worked quite well (120). A Fogarty balloon catheter can be passed through the bronchoscope and the balloon inflated to obstruct bleeding from a secondary bronchus.

NOTE

Not all patients will tolerate isolation of one lung.

Transtracheal Aspiration

Transtracheal aspiration of tracheobronchopulmonary secretions in patients with lower respiratory tract disease is superior to expectorated sputum specimens for both Gram staining and culture of specimens (66, 100, 109). Transtracheal aspiration is a simple bedside procedure that should be used in cases of uncomplicated disease of the lower respiratory tract in which sputum has not been produced or in which examination of expectorated sputum has been uninformative (66). A comparison of cultures obtained with the bronchoscope and with transtracheal aspiration indicated that the latter is more reliable (100). In one large study involving 154 patients (109), the diagnosis of bronchopulmonary infection caused by anaerobic bacteria could not have been made without transtracheal aspiration. Gram stain of transtracheal aspirates provided prompt and accurate bacteriologic diagnosis in more than 90% of cases, whereas Gram stains of expectorated sputum were nonspecific (109).

TECHNIQUE

1. Place the patient in a supine position with the neck hyperextended by a pillow placed beneath the shoulders.
2. Cleanse the anterior aspect of the neck over the cricothyroid membrane with isopropyl alcohol.
3. Raise an intradermal wheal over the cricothyroid membrane with 1% lidocaine injected through a 23-gauge needle.
4. Pass a 14-gauge intracatheter needle through this membrane, directed at a 45-degree angle in a caudad direction with the bevel up.
5. Thread an 8-inch polyethylene catheter into the trachea. Quickly withdraw the 14-gauge needle.
6. Inject 2 to 5 mL of sterile 0.9% saline and then aspirate. Invariably a paroxysm of coughing is evoked. At this instant, apply suction through a 10-mL syringe attached to the catheter.
7. Remove the catheter and apply pressure for 3 to 5 minutes to assure hemostasis.

COMPLICATIONS

When this procedure is performed properly, reported complications are uncommon but include subcutaneous and mediastinal emphysema that may be extensive in some patients (66, 109).

Pulmonary Aspiration and Nasotracheal Suctioning

A number of misconceptions exist about nasotracheal suctioning, proper methods of maintaining an airway, and immediate treatment of aspiration.

Drainage of foreign matter from the lungs in the prone position is as unlikely as in the supine position because the trachea remains horizontal in both positions. The optimal position in which an unconscious person who is not in need of resuscitation should be placed in bed is in the lateral position, maintained with pillows behind (8, 113). Raise the foot of the bed 6 to 9 inches (8) for optimal drainage. When aspiration does occur, perform suction to remove the fluid aspirate, and optimally oxygenate the patient. Perform diagnostic and therapeutic bronchoscopy with a flexible fiberoptic scope. If one sees material that cannot be removed through the fiberoptic scope because of its size, insert a rigid bronchoscope and remove the material. With the aid of the fiberoptic scope, determine the location of foreign particles better. When aspiration occurs, roll the patient to the right side so the material remains in the dependent lung (116). Clear the mouth and pharynx and suction the patient. Bronchial lavage with normal saline solution after endotracheal intubation has been advocated by some (116). This lavage has been shown to decrease the risk of pulmonary edema after aspiration (66). Five to 10 mL of sterile saline solution is injected by syringe into the ETT, followed by immediate suction and oxygenation, and this is repeated until aspirated fluid is clear (86, 116). Lavage using large volumes of fluid increases the spread of acid and the extent of lung damage and is ineffective in neutralizing the acid reaction in pulmonary aspiration. A volume of saline equal to the volume of acid secretions will increase the hydrochloric acid pH from 1.6 to only 1.8 (86). This also increases the airway resistance and causes a decrease in the lung compliance and Po_2; thus lavage with large volumes of fluid is contraindicated.

Data available show that using a straight catheter and varying the head position do not help guide the catheter into the desired bronchus (51, 68). The catheter enters the right side in most patients regardless of the head position (51, 68). The best method to increase the likelihood of left main stem catheterization is to use a curved-tip catheter (6, 51, 68).

REFERENCES

1. Ablaza VJ: Positioning the nasal oxygen cannula. Am Plast Surg 41:97–98, 1998.
2. Akinyemi OO: Complications of guided blind endotracheal intubation. Anaesthesia 34:590, 1979.
3. Alonso WA, Caruso VG, Roncace EA: Minibikes: A new factor in laryngotracheal trauma. Ann Otol Rhinol Laryngol 82:800, 1973.
4. Alonso WA, Pratt LL, Zollinger WK, et al: Complications of laryngotracheal disruption. Laryngoscope 84:1276, 1974.
5. Anderson JE: Grant's Atlas of Anatomy, 8th ed. Baltimore: Williams & Wilkins, 1983, Fig. 9-28.
6. Anthony JS, Sieniewicz DJ: Suctioning of the left bronchial tree in critically ill patients. Crit Care Med 5:161, 1977.
7. Aro L, Takki S, Aromaa U: Technique for difficult intubation. Br J Anaesth 43:1081, 1977.
8. Atkinson WJ: Posture of the unconscious patient. Lancet 1:854, 1969.
9. Battaglia JD, Lockhart CH: Management of acute epiglottis by nasotracheal intubation. Am J Dis Child 129:334, 1975.
10. Behrman RE, James LS, et al: Treatment of the asphyxiated newborn infant. J Pediatr 74:981, 1969.
11. Bennett EJ, Ramamurthy S, Dall FY, et al: Pan and the neonate. Br J Anaesth 47:75, 1975.
12. Bougas TP, Cook CD: Pressure-flow characteristics of needles suggested for transtracheal resuscitation. N Engl J Med 262:511–513, 1960.
13. Boutros AR: Arterial blood oxygenation during and after endotracheal suctioning in the apneic patient. Anesthesiology 32:114, 1970.
14. Boyd AD, Colan AA: Emergency cricothyroidotomy: Is its use justified? Surg Rounds 2:19–23, 1979.
15. Boyd AD, Romita MC, Conlan AA, et al: A clinical evaluation of cricothyroidotomy. Surg Gynecol Obstet 149:365, 1979.
16. Brantigan CO, Grow JB: Cricothyroidotomy: Elective use of respiratory problems requiring tracheotomy. J Thorac Cardiovasc Surg 72:80, 1976.
17. Browne DRG: A guide to tracheal tubes. Anaesthesia 24:620, 1969.
18. Butler RM, Moser FH: The padded dash syndrome: Blunt trauma to the larynx and trachea. Laryngoscope 78:1172, 1968.
19. Byard RW: Mechanism of unexpected death in infants and young children following foreign body ingestion. J Forensic Sci 41:438–441, 1996.
20. Caparosa RJ, Zavatsky AR: Practical aspects of the cricothyroid space. Laryngoscope 67: 577–591, 1957.
21. Chandra P: Blind intubation. Br J Anaesth 38: 207, 1966.
22. Clemente CD: Anatomy: A Regional Atlas of the Human Body, 2nd ed. Baltimore, Urban & Schwarzenberg, 1981, Fig. 669.

23. Cole WI, Stoelting VK: Blood gases during intubation following two types of oxygenation. Anesth Analg 50:68, 1971.
24. Conrady PA: Alteration of endotracheal tube position. Crit Care Med 4:8, 1976.
25. Cook DR: Muscle relaxants in infants and children. Anesth Analg 60:335, 1981.
26. Coorey A, Brimacombe J, Keller C: Saline as an alternative to air filling the laryngeal mask airway cuff. Br J Anasth 819:398–400, 1998.
27. Crocco JA, Rooney JJ, Fankushen DS, et al: Massive hemoptysis. Arch Intern Med 121:495, 1968.
28. Dauphinee K: Nasotracheal intubation. Emerg Med Clin North Am 6:715–723, 1988.
29. Davenport HT, Rosales JK: Endotracheal intubation of infants and children. Can Anaesth Soc J 6:65, 1959.
30. Denlinger JK, Ellison N, Ominsky AJ: Effects of intratracheal lidocaine or circulatory responses to tracheal intubation. Anesthesiology 41:409, 1974.
31. DeVore JS: Resuscitation of the newborn. Clin Obstet Gynecol 19:607, 1976.
32. Donlon JV: Anesthetic management of patients with compromised airways. Anesth Rev 7:22, 1980.
33. Doolan LA, O'Brien JF: Safe intubation in cervical spine injury. Anaesth Intens Care 13:3, 319, 1985.
34. Dunlap LB: A modified simple device for the emergency administration of percutaneous transtracheal ventilation. JACEP 7:42, 1978.
35. Edens ET, Sia RL, et al: Flexible fiberoptic endoscopy in difficult intubations. Ann Otol 90: 307–309, 1981.
36. Fell T, Cheney FW: Prevention of hypoxia during endotracheal suction. Ann Surg 174:24, 1971.
37. Finster M: Resuscitation of the newborn. Acta Anaesth Scand Suppl 37:86, 1970.
38. Finucane BT, Kupshik HL: A flexible stylet for replacing damaged tracheal tubes. Can Anaesth Soc J 25:153, 1978.
39. Fitchett VH, Pomerantz M, Butsch DW, et al: Penetrating wounds of the neck. Arch Surg 99: 307, 1969.
40. Forbes JA: Croup and its management. Br Med J 1:389, 1961.
41. Francois M, Hamrioui R, Narcy P: Nasal foreign bodies in children. Eur Arch Otorhinol 255: 132–134, 1998.
42. Fry ENS: Letter to the editor. Can Anaesth Soc J 24:144, 1977.
43. Furgurson JE, Meislin HW: Airway problems in the trauma victim. Top Emerg Med 1:9, 1979.
44. Gandhi BS, Sahni JK, Gajaj Y: Two unusual cases of foreign body in larynx. Ind J Chest Dis Allied Sci 40:135–139, 1998.
45. Gaskill JR: Nasotracheal intubation in head and neck surgery. Arch Otolaryngol 86:115, 1967.
46. Gold MI, Buechel DR: A method of blind nasal intubation for the conscious patient. Anesth Analg 39:257, 1969.
47. Gonzalez S: A new instrument for uncomplicated emergency cricothyroidotomy. South Med J 69:309, 1976.
48. Goodman LR, Conrady PA, Laing F, et al: Radiographic evaluation of endotracheal tube position. AJR Am J Roentgenol 127:433, 1976.
49. Gotta AW, Sullivan CA: Superior laryngeal nerve block: An aid to intubating the patient with fractured mandible. J Trauma 24:83, 1984.
50. Gutgesell HP, Tacker WA: Energy dose for defibrillation of children. Pediatrics 58:898, 1976.
51. Haberman PB, Green JP, Archibald C, et al: Determinants of successful selective tracheobronchial suctioning. N Engl J Med 289:1060, 1973.
52. Harris HH, Tobin HA: Acute injuries of the larynx and trachea in 49 patients. Laryngoscope 80:1376, 1970.
53. Heinonen J, Takki S, Tammisto T: Effect of the Trendelenburg tilt and other procedures on the position of endotracheal tubes. Lancet 1:850, 1969.
54. Hemenway WG: The management of severe obstruction of the upper air passages. Surg Clin North Am 41:201, 1961.
54a. Henry LN, Chamberliain JW: Removal of foreign bodies from esophagus and nose with the use of a Foley catheter. Surgery 71:18–921, 1972.
55. Hiebert CA: Balloon catheter control of life-threatening hemoptysis. Chest 66:308, 1974.
56. Hoffman LA, Johnson JT, Wesmiller SW, et al: Transtracheal delivery of oxygen: Efficacy and safety for long-term continuous therapy. Ann Otol Rhinol Laryngol 100:108–115, 1991.
57. Hogg CE: Airway emergencies. Int Anesthesiol Clin 10:13, 1972.
58. Holinger PH, Schild JA: Pharyngeal, laryngeal and tracheal injuries in the pediatric age-group. Ann Otol 81:538, 1972.
59. Idris AH: Reassessing the need for ventilation during CPR. Ann Emerg Med 27:569–575, 1996.
60. Iserson KV, Sanders AB, Kaback K, et al: Difficult intubations: Aids and alternatives. Am Family Physician 31:3, 99–112, 1985.
61. Jacobs HB: Emergency percutaneous transtracheal catheter and ventilator. J Trauma 12:50, 1972.
62. Jacoby JJ, Hamelberg W, Ziegler CH, et al: Transtracheal resuscitation. JAMA 162:625, 1956.
63. Johnson C, Roberts JT, et al: Clinical competence in the performance of fiberoptic laryngoscopy and endotracheal intubation: A study of resident instruction. J Clin Anesth 1:5, 344–349, 1989.
64. Johnson RM, Owen JR, Hart DL, et al: Cervical orthoses: A guide to their selection and use. Clin Orthop 154:34, 1981.
65. Kaish HA, Corneli HM: Removal of nasal foreign bodies in the pediatric population. Am J Emerg Med 15:54–56, 1997.
66. Kalinske RW, Parker RH, Brandt D, et al: Diagnostic usefulness and safety of transtracheal aspiration. N Engl J Med 276:604, 1967.
67. Kato I, Uesugi K, Kikuchihara M, et al: Tracheostomy: The horizontal tracheal incision. J Laryngol Otol 104:322–325, 1989.

68. Kirimli B, King JE, Pfaeffle HH: Evaluation of tracheobronchial suction techniques. J Thorac Cardiovasc Surg 59:340, 1970.
69. Kress TD, Balasubramaniam S: Cricothyroidotomy. Ann Emerg Med 11:197, 1982.
70. Kua JS, Tan IK: Airway obstruction following internal jugular vein cannulation. Anaesthesia 52:776–778, 1997.
71. Lambert GE, McMurry GT: Laryngotracheal trauma: Recognition and management. JACEP 5:883, 1976.
72. Landa JF: Indications for bronchoscopy. Chest 73:160, 1978.
73. Lazoritz S, Saunders BS, Bason WM: Management of acute epiglottis. Crit Care Med 7:285, 1979.
74. Levinson MM, Scuderi PE, Gibson RL, et al: Emergency percutaneous transtracheal ventilation (PTV). JACEP 8:396, 1979.
75. Lewis I: Endotracheal anaesthesia. Br Med J 2: 630, 1937.
76. Liew RPC: A technique for naso-tracheal intubation with the soft Portex tube. Anesthesiology 28:567, 1973.
77. Linscott MS, Horton WC: Management of upper airway obstruction. Otolaryngol Clin North Am 12:2, 351, 1979.
78. Little CM, Parker MG, Tarnopolsky R, et al: The incidence of vasculature at risk during cricothyroidotomy. Ann Emerg Med 15:7, 63–65, 1986.
79. Lumpkin JR: Airway obstruction. Top Emerg Med 2:15, 1980.
80. Magill IW: Endotracheal anesthesia. Am J Surg 34:450, 1936.
81. Magill IW, Macintosh RR, Hewer CL: Lest we forget. Anaesthesia 30:476, 1975.
82. Mallick A, Quinn AC, et al: Use of the Combitube for airway maintenance during percutaneous dilatational tracheostomy. Anaesthesia 53:349–355, 1998.
83. Masters IB, Chang AB, et al: Modified nasopharyngeal tube for upper airway obstruction. Arch Dis Child 80:186–187, 1999.
84. Mathisen DJ: Percutaneous tracheostomy: A cautionary note. Chest Editorials 98:5, 1049, 1990.
85. McCollum WB, Mattox KL, Guinn GA, et al: Immediate operative treatment for massive hemoptysis. Chest 67:152, 1975.
86. McCormick PW: Immediate care after aspiration of vomit. Anaesthesia 30:658, 1975.
87. McGill J, Clinton JE, Ruiz E: Cricothyroidotomy in the emergency department. Ann Emerg Med 11:361–364, 1982.
88. McLaughlin J, Iserson KV, et al: Emergency pediatric tracheostomy: A usable technique and model for instruction. Ann Emerg Med 15:4, 17–129, 1986.
89. Milstein JM, Goetzman BW: The Heimlich maneuver as an aid in endotracheal intubation of neonates. Pediatrics 60:749, 1977.
90. Mishkel L, Wang JF, Gutierrez F, et al: Nasotracheal intubation by fiberoptic laryngoscope. South Med J 74:11, 1407–1409, 1981.
91. Morain WD: Cricothyroidotomy in head and neck surgery. Plast Reconstr Surg 65:424–428, 1980.
92. Morris IR: Pharmacologic aids to intubation and the rapid sequence induction. Emerg Med Clin North Am 6:4, 754–768, 1988.
92a. Nandapalan V, McIlwain JC: Removal of nasal foreign bodies with a Fogarty biliary balloon catheter. J Laryngol Otol 108:758–760, 1994.
93. Nahum AM: Immediate care of acute blunt laryngeal trauma. J Trauma 9:112, 1969.
94. Nicholas TH, Rumer GF: Emergency airway: A plan of action. JAMA 174:98, 1960.
95. Nugent SK, Laravuso R, Rogers MC: Pharmacology and use of muscle relaxants in infants and children. J Pediatr 94:481, 1979.
96. Oh TH, Motoyama EK: Comparison of nasotracheal intubation and tracheostomy in management of acute epiglottis. Anesthesiology 46: 214, 1977.
97. Oppenheimer RP: Airway–instantly. JAMA 230:76, 1974.
98. Parr MJ, Gregory M, Baskett PJ: The intubating laryngeal mask: Use in failed and difficult intubation 53:343–348, 1998.
99. Patil V, Stehling LC, Zauder HL, et al: Mechanical aids for fiberoptic endoscopy. Anesthesiology 57:69–70, 1982.
100. Pecora DV: A comparison of transtracheal aspiration with other methods of determining the bacterial flora of the lower respiratory tract. N Engl J Med 269:664, 1963.
101. Pedersen B: Blind nasotracheal intubation. Acta Anaesth Scand 15:107, 1971.
102. Penlington GN: Endotracheal tube sizes for children. Anaesthesia 29:494, 1974.
103. Piotrowski JJ, Moore EE, et al: Emergency department tracheostomy. Emerg Med Clin North Am 6:4, 737–744, 1988.
104. Reber A, Wetzel SG, et al: Effect of combined mouth closure and chin lift on upper airway dimensions during routine magnetic resonance imaging in pediatric patients sedated with propofol. Anesthesiology 90:1617–1623, 1999.
105. Redding JS, Tabeling BB, Parham AM: Airway management in patients with central nervous system depression. JACEP 7:401, 1978.
106. Reed AP: Current concepts in airway management for cardiopulmonary resuscitation. Mayo Clin Proc 90:1172–1184, 1995.
107. Reed JP, Kemph JP, Hamelberg W, et al: Studies with transtracheal artifical respiration. Anesthesiology 15:28–41, 1954.
108. Richardson WR: Thoracic emergencies in the newborn infant. Am J Surg 105:524, 1963.
109. Ries K, Levison ME, Kaye D: Transtracheal aspiration in pulmonary infection. Arch Intern Med 133:453, 1974.
110. Rogers S, Benumof JL, et al: New and easy techniques for fiberoptic endoscopy-aided tracheal intubation. Am Soc Anesth 59:569–572, 1983.
111. Rowbotham ES: Intratracheal anaesthesia by the nasal route for operations on the mouth and lips. Br Med J 2:590, 1920.
112. Ruben HM, Elam JO, Ruben AM, et al: Investigation of upper airway problems in resuscitation, I: Studies of pharyngeal x-rays and

performance by laymen. Anesthesiology 22:271, 1961.
113. Safar P, Escarraga LA, Chang F: Upper airway obstruction in the unconscious patient. J Appl Physiol 14:760, 1959.
114. Safer P, Penninckx J: Cricothyroid membrane puncture with special cannula. Anesthesiology 28:943–948, 1967.
115. Salem JE: Intubation of conscious patients with combat wounds of upper respiratory passageway in Vietnam. Oral Surg 24:701, 1967.
116. Salem MR: Anesthetic management of patients with "a full stomach": A critical review. Anesth Analg 49:97, 1970.
117. Salem MR, Mathrubhutham M, Bennett EJ: Difficult intubation. N Engl J Med 295:879, 1976.
118. Schachner A, Ovil J, Sidi J, et al: Rapid percutaneous tracheostomy. Chest Editorials 98:5, 1266–1270, 1990.
119. Schuller DE, Birch HG: The safety of intubation in croup and epiglottis. Laryngoscope 84:33, 1975.
120. Seed RF: Traumatic injury to the larynx and trachea. Anaesthesia 26:55, 1971.
121. Selecky PA: Evaluation of hemoptysis through with bronchoscope. Chest 73:741, 1978.
122. Senthuran S, Lim S, Gunning KE: Life threatening airway obstruction caused by a retropharyngeal hematoma. Anesthesia 5497:674–678, 1999.
123. Shapiro SL: Emergency airway for acute laryngeal obstruction. Eye Ear Nose Throat Mon 49: 35, 1970.
124. Sheeley CH II, Mattox KL, Beall AC Jr: Management of acute cervical tracheal trauma. Am J Surg 128:805, 1974.
125. Shim C, Fine N, Fernandez R, et al: Cardiac arrhythmias resulting from tracheal suctioning. Ann Intern Med 71:1149, 1969.
126. Shumrick DA: Trauma of the larynx. Arch Otolaryngol 86:109, 1967.
127. Simon RR, Brenner BE: Emergency tracheostomy in the patient with massive neck swelling. Crit Care Med 11:119, 1983.
128. Smith RB: Transtracheal ventilation during anesthesia. Anesth Analg 53:225, 1974.
129. Smith RB, Babinski M, Klain M, et al: Percutaneous transtracheal ventilation. JACEP 5: 765–770, 1976.
130. Snell RS: Atlas of Clinical Anatomy. Boston: Little, Brown, 1978, 390.
131. Spoerel WE, Narayanan PS, Singh NP: Transtracheal ventilation. Br J Anaesth 43:932, 1971.
132. Stark DCC, Biller HF: Aspiration of foreign bodies: Diagnosis and management. Int Anesthesiol Clin 15:117, 1977.
133. Stewart RD: Manual translaryngeal jet ventilation. Emerg Med Clin North Am 7:1, 155–164, 1989.
134. Stewart RD: Tactile orotracheal intubation. Ann Emerg Med 13:175, 1984.
135. Tahir AH: A simple manoeuvre to aid the passage of a nasotracheal tube into the oropharynx. Br J Anaesth 42:631, 1970.
136. Tintinalli JE: Complications of nasotracheal intubation. Ann Emerg Med 10:142, 1981.
137. Tobias JD: Airway management for pediatric emergencies. Pediatr Ann 25:317–320, 323–328, 1996.
138. Todres ID, Rogers MC: Methods of external cardiac massage in the newborn infant. J Pediatr 86:781, 1975.
139. Tos M: Nasotracheal intubation in acute epiglottis. Arch Otolaryngol 97:373, 1973.
140. Toye FJ, Weinstein JD, et al: Clinical experience with percutaneous tracheostomy and cricothyroidotomy in 100 patients. J Trauma 26:11, 1034–1040, 1986.
141. Urschel HC, Razzuk MA: Management of acute traumatic injuries of tracheobronchial tree. Surg Gynecol Obstet 136:113, 1973.
142. Van Elstraete AC, Mami JC, Mehdaoui H: Nasotracheal intubation in patients with immobilized cervical spine: A comparison of tracheal tube cuff inflation and fiberoptic bronchoscopy. Anesth Analg 87:400–402, 1998.
143. Verrill PJ: Anaesthesia in upper respiratory obstruction. Br J Anaesth 35:237, 1963.
144. Wallace CT, Cooke JE: A new method for positioning endotracheal tubes. Anesthesiology 44: 272, 1976.
145. Walls RM: Cricothyroidotomy. Emerg Med Clin North Am 6:4, 725–736, 1988.
146. Wilson HE: Control of massive hemorrhage during bronchoscopy. Dis Chest 56:412, 1969.
147. Young PJ, Ridley SA, Downward G: Evaluation of a new design of tracheal tube cuff to prevent leakage of fluid to the lungs. Br J Anaesth 80: 796–799, 1998.
148. Zuck D: A technique for tracheobronchial toilet in the conscious patient. Anaesthesia 6:226, 1951.
149. Zwillich CW, Pierson DJ, Creagh CE, et al: Complications of assisted ventilation: A prospective study of 354 consecutive episodes. Am J Med 57:161, 1974.

SUGGESTED READINGS

Agosti L: Modification of Magill's intubating forceps [Letter]. Anaesthesia 31:574, 1976.

Ashworth C, Williams LF, Byrne JJ: Penetrating wounds of the neck: Reemphasis of the need for prompt exploration. Am J Surg 121:387, 1971.

Atkins JP: Current utilization of tracheotomy as a therapeutic measure: A review of the literature and an analysis of 526 cases. Laryngoscope 70: 1672–1690, 1960.

Barkin RM: Pediatric airway management. Emerg Med Clin North Am 6:4, 687–692, 1988.

Bearman AJ: Device for nasotracheal intubation. Anesthesiology 23:130, 1962.

Beatrous WP: Tracheotomy (tracheostomy): Its expanded indications and present status. Laryngoscope 78:3–5, 1986.

Bergen RP: Lost or broken teeth. JAMA 221:119, 1972.

Berman RA: A method for blind oral intubation of the trachea or esophagus. Anesth Analg 56:866, 1977.

Black AE, Hatch DJ, Nauth-Misir N, et al: Complications of nasotracheal intubation in neonates, infants and children: A review of 4 years' experience in a children's hospital. Br J Anaesth 65:461, 467, 1990.

Boyles JH: Lacerations of the larynx. Arch Otolaryngol 87:114, 1968.

Coghlan CJ: Blind intubation in the conscious patient. Anesth Analg 45:290, 1966.

Coldiron JS: Estimation of nasotracheal tube length in neonates. Pediatrics 41:823, 1968.

Curtin JW, Holinger PH, Greeley PW: Blunt trauma to the larynx and upper trachea. J Trauma 6:493, 1966.

Danzl DF, Thomas DM: Nasotracheal intubation in the emergency department. Crit Care Med 8:11, 677, 1980.

Dauphinee K: Orotracheal intubation. Emerg Med Clin North Am 6:4, 699–713, 1988.

Ducrow M: Throwing light on blind intubation. Anaesthesia 33:827, 1978.

Echols DH: The management of acute head injuries. N Orleans Med Surg J 102:97–101, 1949.

Egol A, Culpepper JA, Snyder JV, et al: Barotrauma and hypotension resulting from jet ventilation in critically ill patients. Chest 88:1, 98–102.

Eross B: Nonslipping, nonkinking airway connections for respiratory care. Anesthesiology 34:571, 1971.

Evans JA: Fundamentals of infant resuscitation. Int Anesth Clin 11:141, 1973.

Feinberg SE, Peterson LJ, et al: Use of cricothyroidotomy in oral and maxillofacial surgery. J Oral Maxillofac Surg 45:873–878, 1987.

Foster CA: An aid to blind nasal intubation in children [Letter]. Anaesthesia 32:1038, 1977.

Galloway TC: Tracheotomy in bulbar poliomyelitis. JAMA 128:1096–1097, 1943.

Gaskill JR, Gillies DR: Local anesthesia for per-oral endoscopy. Arch Otolaryngol 84:94, 1966.

Gold MI, Buechal DR: Translaryngeal anesthesia: A review. Anesthesiology 20:181–185, 1959.

Harris HH, Ainsworth JZ: Immediate management of laryngeal and tracheal injuries. Laryngoscope 75: 1103, 1965.

Head JM: Tracheostomy in the management of respiratory problems. N Engl J Med 264:587–591, 1961.

Hey VMF: Relaxants for endotracheal intubation: A comparison of depolarizing and non-depolarizing neuromuscular blocking agents. Anesthesia 28:32, 1973.

Holinger PH, Johnston KC: Factors responsible for laryngeal obstruction in infants. JAMA 143:1229, 1950.

Jackson C: The drowning of a patient in his own secretion. Laryngoscope 21:1183–1185, 1911.

Jacobs HB: Needle-catheter brings oxygen to the trachea. JAMA 222:1231, 1972.

Jacobson S: Upper air obstruction. Emerg Med Clin North Am 7:2, 205–217, 1989.

Jorden RC: Airway management. Emerg Med Clin North Am 6:4, 671–686, 1988.

Jorden RC: Percutaneous transtracheal ventilation. Emerg Med Clin North Am 6:4, 745–752, 1988.

Kerr M: Pre-lubrication before nasal intubation. Br J Anaesth 40:632, 1968.

LeMay SR: Penetrating wounds of the larynx and cervical trachea. Arch Otolaryngol 94:558, 1971.

Linder N, Aranda JV, Tsur M, et al: Need for endotracheal intubation and suction in meconium-stained neonates. J Pediatr 112:4, 613–615, 1988.

Lynn HB, van Heerden JA: Tracheostomy in infants. Surg Clin North Am 53:945, 1973.

Lyons GD, Garrett ME, Fourier DG: Complications of percutaneous transtracheal procedures. Am J Otolaryngol 86:633–640, 1977.

Mattila MAK, Heikel P-E, Suutarinen T, et al: Estimation of a suitable nasotracheal tube length for infants and children. Acta Anaesthesiol Scand 15:239, 1971.

McMillan DD, Rademaker AW, Buchan KA, et al: Benefits of orotracheal and nasotracheal intubation in neonates requiring ventilatory assistance. Pediatrics 77:1, 39–43, 1986.

Meltzer SJ, Auer J: Continuous respiration without respiratory movements. J Exp Med 11:622, 1909.

Morch ET, Saxton GA, Gish G: Artificial respiration via the uncuffed tracheostomy tube. JAMA 160: 864, 1956.

Munnell ER: Fracture of major airways. Am J Surg 105:511, 1963.

Nakayama DK, Gardner MJ, Rowe MI, et al: Emergency endotracheal intubation in pediatric trauma. Ann Surg 211:2, 218–223, 1990.

Nilsson RK, Brendstrup A: Fixation of nasotracheal tubes. Lancet 2:260, 1973.

Olson NR, Miles WK: Treatment of acute blunt laryngeal injuries. Ann Otol Rhinol Laryngol 80:704, 1971.

Ovassapian A: Failure to withdraw flexible fiberoptic laryngoscope after nasotracheal intubation. Anesthesiology 63:124–125, 1985.

Pearson FG, Goldberg M, DaSilva A: A prospective study of tracheal injury complicating tracheostomy with cuffed tube. Ann Otol 77:868, 1968.

Pecora DV, Brook R: A method of securing uncontaminated tracheal secretions for bacterial examination. J Thorac Med Surg 37:653, 1959.

Pennington CL: External trauma of the larynx and trachea. Ann Otol Rhinol Laryngol 81:546, 1972.

Pittinger C, Adamson R: Antibiotic blockage of neuromuscular function. Annu Rev Pharm 12: 1969, 1972.

Pons PT: Esophageal obturator airway. Emerg Med Clin North Am 6:4, 693–698, 1988.

Powell WF, Ozdil T: A translaryngeal guide for tracheal intubation. Anesth Analg 46:231, 1967.

Ripoll I, Lindholm C-E, Carroll R, et al: Spontaneous dislocation of endotracheal tubes. Anesthesiology 49:50, 1978.

Rosen M, Hillard EK: The use of suction in clinical medicine. Br J Anaesth 32:486, 1960.

Safar P: Recognition and management of airway obstruction. JAMA 208:1008, 1969.

Safar P, Penninckx J: Cricothyroid membrane puncture with special cannula. Anesthesiology 28: 943, 1967.

Saha AK: The estimation of the correct length of oral endotracheal tubes in adults [Letter]. Anaesthesia 32:919, 1977.

Salem MR, Wong AY: Efficacy of cricoid pressure in preventing aspiration of gastric contents in pediatric patients. Br J Anesth 44:401, 1972.

Schellinger RR: The length of the airway to the bifurcation of the trachea. Anesthesiology 25:169, 1964.

Schwab JM, Hartman MM: The management of the airway and ventilation in trauma. Med Clin North Am 48:1577, 1964.

Sellick BA: Cricoid pressure to control regurgitation of stomach contents during induction of anaesthesia. Lancet 2:260, 1973.

Sercer A: Tracheotomy through 2000 years of history. CIBA Symp 10:78–86, 1962.

Simon RR: Emergency tracheotomy in patients with massive neck swelling. Emerg Med Clin North Am 7:1, 95–101, 1989.

Smith RM: The critically ill child: Respiratory arrest and its sequelae. Pediatrics 46:108, 1970.

Sophocles AM, Atkins JP: The widening scope of tracheotomy: An analysis of 400 cases. J Med Soc N J 57:23–25, 1960.

Szold PD, Glicklich M: Children with epiglottitis can be bagged. Clin Pediatr 15:792, 1976.

Timmis HH: Tracheostomy: An overview of implications, management and morbidity. Adv Surg 7:199–233, 1973.

Vollmer TP, Stewart RD, Paris PM, et al: Use of a lighted stylet for guided orotracheal intubation in the pre-hospital setting. Ann Emerg Med 14:4, 81–85, 1985.

Waldron J, Padgham ND, Hurley SE, et al: Complications of emergency and elective tracheostomy: A retrospective study of 150 consecutive cases. Ann R Coll Surg Engl 72:218–220, 1990.

Wang KP, Wise RA, Terry PB, et al: A new controllable suction catheter for blind cannulation of the main stem bronchi. Crit Care Med 6:347, 1978.

Yealy DM, Paris PM, et al: Recent advances in airway management. Emerg Med Clin North Am 7:1, 83–93, 1989.

Yoshikawa TT, Chow AW, Montgomerie JZ, et al: Paratracheal abscess: An unusual complication of transtracheal aspiration. Anesthesiology 32:1268, 1970.

3

Anesthesia and Regional Blocks

THE CLINICAL PHARMACOLOGY OF LOCAL ANESTHETICS

Two general types of local anesthetics currently exist: ester compounds (procaine, cocaine, and tetracaine) and amide compounds (mepivacaine, bupivacaine, lidocaine). Ester anesthetics are hydrolyzed by pseudocholinesterase in the serum, whereas amide-type compounds are metabolized in the liver. The only local anesthetic agent excreted unchanged in the urine is cocaine (12). The mechanism of action of local anesthetics is a decrease in the rate of increase of depolarization of the action potential such that after excitation of the cell, depolarization does not reach threshold for firing; thus a propagated action potential fails to occur (12).

All local anesthetic agents are vasodilators because of the relaxant effect on smooth muscles. Only cocaine produces immediate vasoconstriction preceded by a brief period of vasodilation. This vasoconstriction is due to inhibition of uptake of catecholamines by cocaine (12). Vasoconstrictors are often added to local anesthetics (e.g., lidocaine) to diminish bleeding in a wound. Vasoconstrictors are less effective subcutaneously than intradermally because the blood supply is more abundant intradermally (4). Thus local anesthetics containing epinephrine should be injected intradermally. Effective vasoconstriction is obtained by using a dilution of 1:100,000 of epinephrine.

In using local anesthetics, aspiration is essential before all injections because some of the nerves being blocked course with the major vessels. In most regional nerve blocks, it is desirable to elicit paresthesias before infiltration of an anesthetic solution; however, when resistance to injection is encountered combined with a paresthesia, it is likely that one is depositing the anesthetic solution intraneurally. Thus when paresthesia is elicited, withdraw the needle 1 or 2 mm before the deposition of the agent to avoid injection into the nerve fiber itself. The clinical uses, concentrations, onset and duration of action, and maximal single doses of common local anesthetics are listed in Table 3.1.

The most commonly used anesthetic is 2% lidocaine with 1:100,000 epinephrine. Other anesthetics may provide a longer period of anesthesia, such as 0.5% bupivacaine with 1:200,000 epinephrine. Some of the agents contain no vasoconstrictor at all, such as 3% mepivacaine. The choice of anesthetic and whether a vasoconstrictor will be used depends on the procedure and the patient's medical history (18, 19). The pain of a local anesthetic injection and the

Table 3.1
Local Anesthetic Agents: Concentrations and Clinical Uses

Agent	Concentration and clinical use	Onset and duration of action	Maximal single dose (mg)	Comments
		AMIDES		
Lidocaine (Xylocaine)	0.5%–1.0% for infiltration or i.v. 1.0%–1.5% for peripheral nerve 4.0% for topical	Rapid onset; short to intermediate duration (60–120 min)	300 plain 500 adrenaline	Excellent spreading ability. Wide range of applications
Prilocaine	0.5%–1.0% for infiltration or i.v. block 1.0% for peripheral nerve	Slower onset; short to intermediate duration (60–120 min)	400 plain 600 adrenaline	0.5% is choice for intravenous block. Most rapidly metabolized and safest of all amide-type agents. Doses in excess of 600 mg produce significant amounts of methemoglobin. Therefore, avoid doses >600 mg and repeated doses. Good choice in outpatient block. Not suitable for obstetrics
Mepivacaine (Carbocaine)	1.0% for infiltration 1.0%–1.5% for peripheral nerve	Slower onset; intermediate to longer duration (90–180 min)	300 plain 500 adrenaline	Duration slightly longer than equal dose of lidocaine, and blood levels not so sensitive to inclusion of adrenaline as lidocaine; thus may be useful if adrenaline not desirable
Etidocaine	0.5% for infiltration 0.5%–1.0% for peripheral nerve	Rapid onset; long duration (4–8 h)	200 plain 300 adrenaline	Capable of producing profound motor block. Useful in postoperative pain management by peripheral blocks
Bupivacaine (Marcaine)	0.25%–0.5% for infiltration 0.25%–0.5% for peripheral nerve	Slow onset; long duration (4–8 h)	175 plain 250 adrenaline	Favored for obstetric nerve blocks because of minimal fetal effects. Excellent for postoperative analgesia because of minimal motor block

ESTERS				
Procaine (Novocaine)	1.0% for infiltration	Slow onset; short duration (30–45 min)	500 plain 600 adrenaline	Indicated with history of malignant hyperpyrexia (MH). Ideal for skin infiltration. Very rapidly metabolized
Chlorprocaine	1.0%–2.0% as for procaine	Rapid onset; short duration	600 plain 750 adrenaline	Drug of choice for obstetric and outpatient neural blockade. Metabolized four times more rapidly than procaine
Amethocaine (Tetracaine)	0.5%–1.0% for topical 0.1%–0.2% for infiltration and peripheral nerve	Slow onset; long duration	100 approx.	May be useful alternative if amides contraindicated (e.g., MH). Metabolized four times more slowly than procaine
Cocaine	4.0%–10.0% for topical	Slow onset; medium duration	150 approx. (1.5 mL of 10% or 4 mL of 4%)	Topical use only. Addictive. Indirect adrenoceptor stimulation. No evidence that 10% solution more effective than 4%. Patients sensitive to exogenous catecholamines should receive topical lidocaine rather than cocaine
Benzocaine	0.4%–5.0% for topical only. Usually dispensed in admixture with other therapeutic ingredients related to site of application	Rapid onset; short duration	No information	Occasionally dispensed in urethane solution. Urethane is a suspected carcinogen and should not be used

area of anesthesia one obtains can be influenced by the following factors:

1. Temperature of the solution. At body temperature, the solutions hurt less than cool injectibles.
2. pH of the anesthetic solution. Sodium bicarbonate addition to a solution attenuates the pain of injection.
3. Number of injections (i.e., using direct approaches for anatomic block instead of multiple regional infiltrative injections).
4. Composition of solution. Addition of hyaluronidase expedites the speed of the anesthetic.
5. Rapidity of injection. Rapid infiltration hurts more (14).

Lidocaine toxicity involves an initial excitement, apprehension, disorientation, nausea, and vomiting, which are often prodromal signs of convulsions. Frequently this prodrome is overlooked or the symptoms are termed hysteria by physicians who are unaware of the hazards of local anesthesia. The severity and duration of the convulsions vary with the nature of the drugs used, the quantity and rapidity of absorption, and the susceptibility of the patient. Large quantities of lidocaine rapidly infused intravenously may cause fleeting convulsive manifestations that may quickly be followed by severe central nervous system collapse. This reaction is characterized by coma, areflexia, apnea, and circulatory collapse. The cardiovascular responses of lidocaine toxicity involve myocardial depression as well as vasodilation. Local anesthetics also may slow conduction in the myocardium. For more extensive discussion, see Chapter 10: Plastic Surgery Principles and Techniques. Tachycardia is a common complication caused by the vasoconstrictor. If the patient experiences a rapid pulse, he or she should be watched closely for the next 15 minutes. The amount of vasoconstrictor used is minimal, and the tachycardia is generally short in duration. The reflex mechanism in response to a rapid pulse and elevated blood pressure may produce vasovagal syncope (18, 34).

ALLERGIC REACTIONS TO ANESTHETIC AGENTS

There is a high incidence of allergic reactions with ester-type local anesthetics. The incidence of allergic reactions to lidocaine is extremely low. Procaine, an ester type local anesthetic, is hydrolyzed by pseudocholinesterase in the serum. This reaction results in the formation of *p*-aminobenzoic acid and diethylaminoalcohol. *p*-Aminobenzoic acid will competitively inhibit sulfonamide antibiotics (12). In patients who are allergic to lidocaine, an amide compound (e.g., procaine) can be safely used for local anesthesia.

LONG-ACTING LOCAL ANESTHETICS

Bupivacaine is a long-acting anesthetic in common use today. In a review of 2,077 cases by Moore et al. (30), the onset of action of this drug was within 4 to 10 minutes, and the maximal analgesic effect was achieved within 15 to 30 minutes. When the drug was used for peripheral nerve blocks, 0.25% and 0.5% were satisfactory in most cases. An inadvertent intravenous injection of 100 mL of bupivacaine occurred twice in their series without any untoward sequelae (30). Although bupivacaine is often listed as the "moderate" onset-of-action category drug compared with lidocaine, which is classified as having "fast" onset, many emergency physicians have noted equal rapidity of onset of anesthesia for bupivacaine and lidocaine. In one study (11), it was concluded that bupivacaine 0.25% digital block induces anesthesia in the same period and with equivalent pain of injection as a 1:1 lidocaine 1%/bupivacaine 0.25% combination and that it is not necessary to use lidocaine and bupivacaine in an attempt to achieve faster onset of local anesthesia (11).

Types of Local Anesthesia

Local infiltration is the production of analgesia by direct infiltration of the wound. This type of local anesthesia is probably the most commonly used in the emergency center. Its disadvantages are that it distorts the wound margins and is more painful at the site of injury than peripheral nerve block or other types of anesthesia.

Field block anesthesia is the production of regional anesthesia by creating a wall of anesthetic around the operative field by local infiltration around the wound site.

Regional nerve block is regional anesthesia produced by directly injecting around the nerve or nerves supplying the area with sensation. This type of anesthesia is the type on which this chapter concentrates. The following factors make regional nerve block anesthesia the procedure of choice (6) for a number of procedures performed in the emergency center: (a) it does not increase or cause tissue anoxia, (b) the complications of general anesthesia are avoided, (c) it does not disturb the wound edges, and (d) it does not propagate infection in contaminated wounds (13). Regional nerve block anesthesia is commonly used for repair of extensive lacerations because it avoids multiple injections and the use of large volumes of local anesthetics (35). It is particularly useful in situations in which local infiltration produces much pain, such as abscesses and arthrocentesis for acute arthritis.

There is little evidence that topical anesthetics are of any value on unbroken skin (12). They are of value on broken skin and on mucous membranes, as is discussed in Chapter 10.

To avoid intravascular injection, one must be certain to aspirate before the deposition of any anesthetic agent (8). We prefer injection during advancement rather than withdrawal of the needle, because this produces less pain for the patient as one advances the needle. This facilitates deposition in the correct line and plane. All blocks used in this chapter are those with easily recognized landmarks. We have purposely omitted those blocks that are more difficult to perform and are of little value in the emergency center.

EQUIPMENT

The equipment needed for regional nerve block anesthesia is not discussed separately and includes the following:

1% lidocaine without epinephrine
1% lidocaine with epinephrine
2% lidocaine with epinephrine
0.25% bupivacaine (when a long-acting anesthetic agent is desired)
4% and 10% cocaine solution
Assortment of needles (23-, 25-, and 18-gauge) for drawing up the anesthetic solution. The lengths should be 1.5 to 3 inches
Syringes: 10, 20, and 30 mL
Iodinated prep solution
4 × 4-inch gauze pads (1 dozen)
Sterile towels
Sterile gloves

HEAD AND NECK BLOCKS

Mental Nerve Block

The mental nerve is a branch of the inferior alveolar nerve, which in turn is a branch of the mandibular division of the fifth cranial nerve. It exits from the mental foramen, which is directly below the level of the second premolar and inside the lower lip at its junction with the lower gingiva (called the inferior sulcus) (Fig. 3.1). This nerve supplies sensation to the skin and mucous membranes of the lower lip (Fig. 3.2).

INDICATIONS

Repair of lacerations of the lower lip.

TECHNIQUE

Although the extraoral route has been described, we prefer the intraoral route

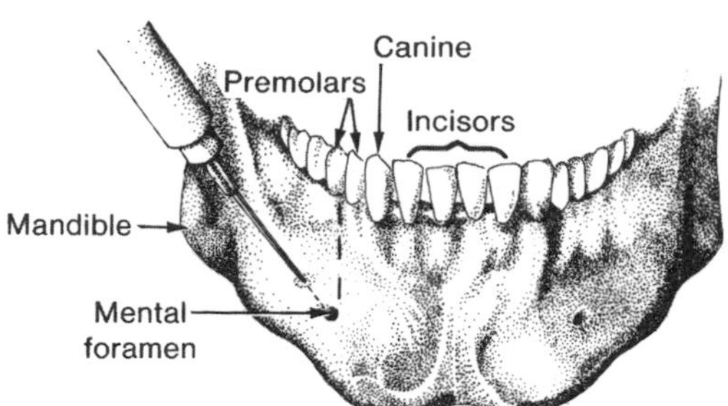

Figure 3.1. The mental foramen through which the mental nerve exits lies directly below the level of the second premolar.

for anesthetizing this nerve because it is less painful to the patient and easier to perform. Block the nerve as it exits from the mental foramen (19). Use the left index finger to palpate the point where the nerve exits from the mandible. Insert the needle at the inferior sulcus of the mouth and direct it toward the foramen. Although the site of insertion of the needle has been described to be between the apices of the bicuspid (19), in our experience, it has been easier to retract the lower lip with the thumb of the left hand and insert the needle at the level of the canine, directing it to the mental foramen (Fig. 3.3). Direct the needle point at the foramen, and inject 2 mL of lidocaine with 1:100,000 aqueous epinephrine. Perform the same on the opposite side to achieve complete block of the lower lip (Fig. 3.4). As the solution is injected, vigorous shaking of the lower lip will decrease the pain of injection. This procedure gives excellent anesthesia, and block is usually complete. When the foramen cannot be palpated, then inject about 0.5 cm below the second premolar, and massage the area to achieve good distribution.

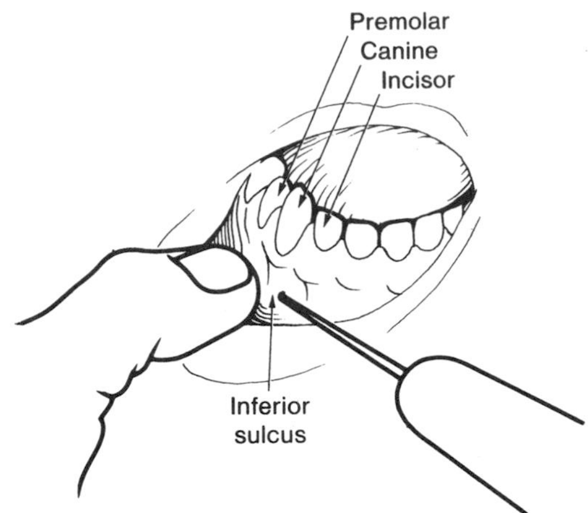

Figure 3.3. Retract the lower lip with the thumb of the left hand, and insert the needle at the level of the canine, directing it under the mental foramen.

At other times, the nerve to the mylohyoid supplies some sensation to the chin and/or lateral to it. The nerve to the mylohyoid that branches from the inferior

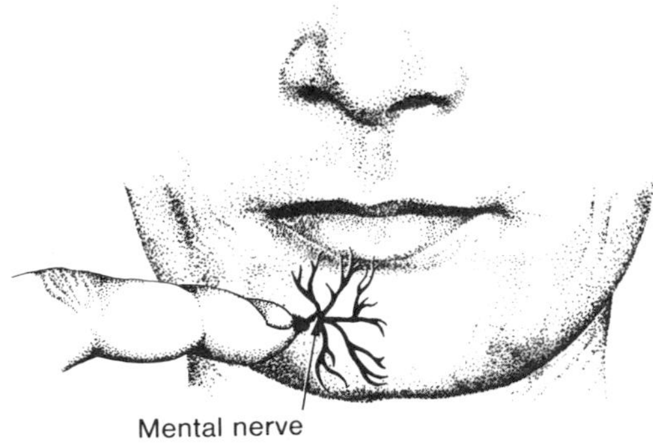

Figure 3.2. The mental nerve supplies sensation to the skin and mucous membranes of the lower lip.

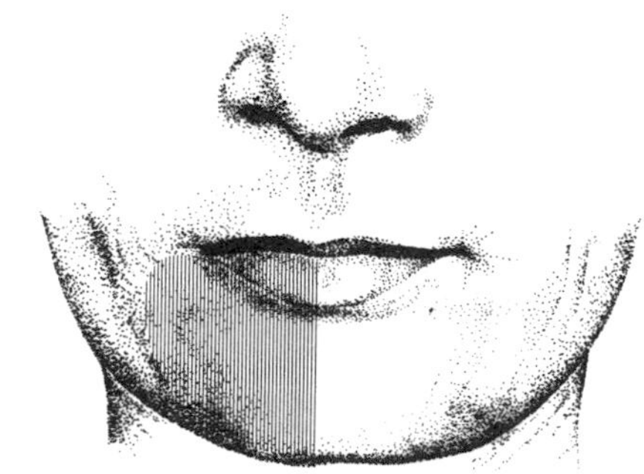

Figure 3.4. Infiltration provides anesthesia for half of the lower lip. Bilateral infiltration of the mental nerve will provide good anesthesia for the entire lower lip.

alveolar nerve just proximal to entering the lingula of the mandibular medial ramus can be blocked at the medial mandibular ramus. The terminal branches, the lowest mental nerve branch, or the sensory mylohyoid nerve supplying the chin, can be blocked just before reaching the chin by using the *mental plus block 2.*

Technique

This block can be done immediately after the mental block by an anterior premandibular injection anterior to the vestibule in front of the anterior teeth. Change your position to behind the patient, turn the syringe more vertically, and inject in the *supraperiosteal plane* with at least a 1.5-inch needle. Inject anterior to and beyond the lower border of the mandible (actually out of the lip) but not quite out of the skin. Only the mental plus block obviates the need for the inferior alveolar block (14).

Mandibular Nerve Block

The mandibular nerve contains both sensory and motor fibers. The sensory branches include the auriculotemporal nerve, which courses anterior to the external auditory meatus and innervates the skin of the temple as well as that of the external auditory canal and a portion of the pinna. The lingual nerve runs between the ramus of the mandible and the medial pterygoid bone and supplies sensation to the anterior two thirds of the tongue. The inferior alveolar nerve courses through the mandibular foramen and traverses the mandibular canal, supplying sensation to the teeth, gums, and lower jaw. This third division of the mandibular nerve branches to form the mental nerve, which innervates the lower lip.

INDICATIONS

1. Repair of gingival and oral lacerations along the mandible.
2. Reduction of displaced or avulsed teeth of the lower jaw.

TECHNIQUE

Achieve complete block of sensory distribution of the mandibular nerve by injecting the anesthetic solution proximal to the division of the nerve into its sensory branches. The site of injection is the mandibular sulcus on the inner surface of the ramus. This blocks the inferior alveolar and lingual nerves. Palpate the retromolar trigone with the patient's mouth partly opened (Fig. 3.5). Insert a needle at the apex of the pterygomandibular raphe and advance it to the ramus of the mandible and the muscles over the internal surface of the ramus. A point of resistance will be felt against the posterior wall of the ramus and will halt further advancement of the needle. At this point,

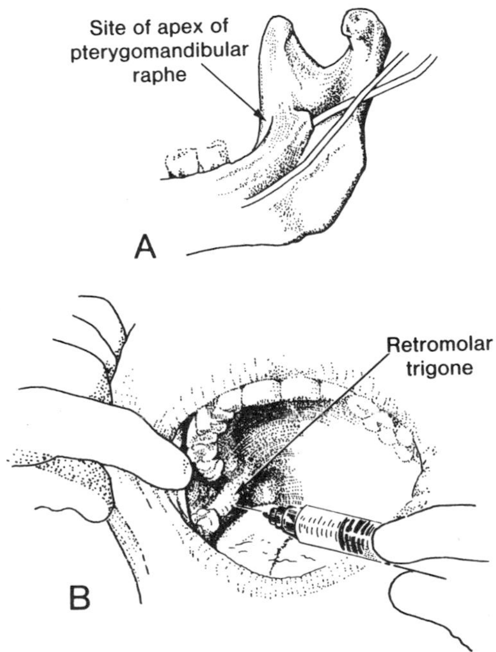

Figure 3.5. *A:* The site of injection for mandibular nerve block on the inner surface of the ramus of the mandible. This can be found by locating the retromolar trigone, which lies behind the third molar. Insert the needle at the apex of the pterygomandibular raphe or apex of the trigone. *B:* Advance the needle to the ramus of the mandible on the inner surface, and inject 2 mL of anesthetic solution.

deposit 2 mL of anesthetic solution (lidocaine with epinephrine) here, and deposit another 2 mL as the needle is withdrawn.

Maxillary Nerve Block: Greater Palatine and Nasopalatine Block

The maxillary nerve is entirely sensory. It exits through the foramen rotundum and enters the pterygopalatine fossa, where it divides. The sensory nerves that are of importance to the emergency physician are the posterior nasal branches, which supply the mucous membrane lining the posterior inferior portion of the nasal cavity. One of these branches, the nasopalatine nerve, courses forward and downward along the nasal septum to exit through the incisive foramen and supplies sensation to the anterior part of the hard palate and the adjacent gums. The greater palatine nerve is another important branch of this nerve that supplies sensation to the posterior two thirds of the palate. The infraorbital nerve, a branch of the maxillary nerve, supplies sensation to the malar region and side of the nose and upper lip.

INDICATIONS

1. Repair of injuries involving the face over the sensory distribution of the nerve.
2. Reductions of displaced or avulsed superior incisors.
3. Repair of lacerations involving the palate.

TECHNIQUE

Individual branches of this nerve are anesthetized, rather than the entire nerve. There is no indication for block of the maxillary nerve in the emergency center. Those individual divisions that are blocked are discussed later.

Block the **nasopalatine nerve** by injecting 1 mL of 1% lidocaine with epinephrine at the point where the nerve exits from the anterior midline of the hard palate, behind and between the upper incisors. This provides anesthesia to the anterior third of the palate and the adjacent gingiva.

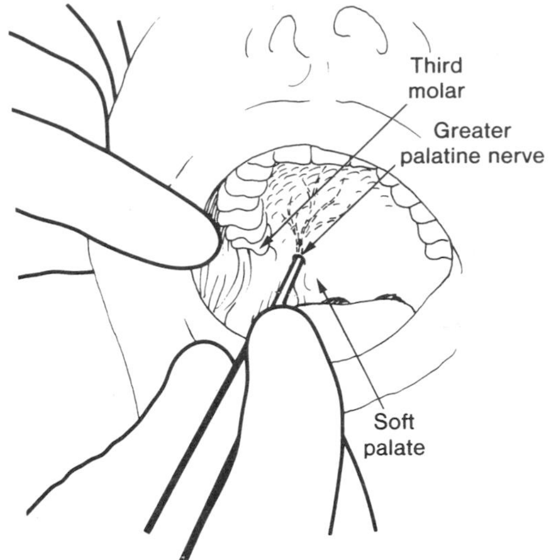

Figure 3.6. Block of the greater palatine nerve. See text for discussion.

Block the **greater palatine nerve** by injecting 1 mL of 1% lidocaine with epinephrine at the site where the nerve exits from the greater palatine foramen. This is just medial to the third molar, anterior to the junction of the soft and hard palate. This anesthetizes the posterior two thirds of the palate and gingiva (Fig. 3.6).

Supraorbital and Supratrochlear Nerve Block

The supraorbital and supratrochlear nerves emerge through notches or depressions at the upper border of the orbital ridge about 2.5 cm from the midline, after which they are distributed to the forehead and the scalp (Figs. 3.7 and 3.8). The depression of the supraorbital notch as it exits from the upper border of the orbit is easily palpated.

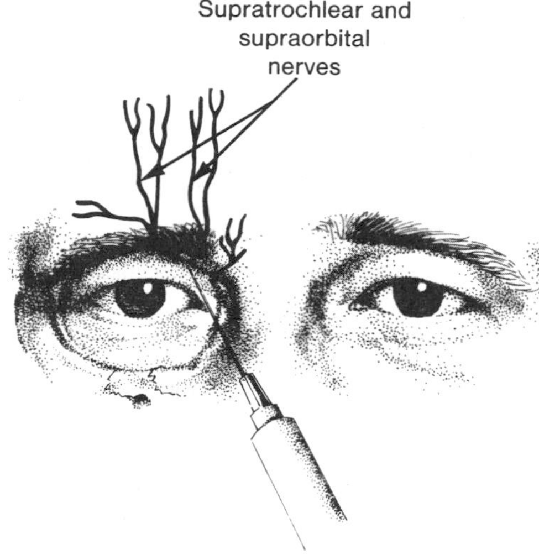

Figure 3.7. The supraorbital and supratrochlear nerves emerging through the notches at the upper border of the orbital ridge.

INDICATIONS

1. Extensive lacerations of the forehead.
2. Debriding abrasions of the forehead and removal of particles of dirt or glass.

TECHNIQUE

These nerves are easily located by palpating the supraorbital ridge with the index finger of the right hand until the notch is palpated just medial to the midpoint of the eyebrow (Fig. 3.9). This marks the point where the supraorbital nerve exits. The supratrochlear nerve exits just medial to this point. Block the nerves by one of two methods. Insert a 23-gauge, 1.5-inch needle attached to a 3-mL syringe filled with 1% lidocaine with epinephrine and direct it by the index finger of the left hand toward the notch palpated earlier (Fig. 3.9). This is the site of injection. Paresthesias do not have to be elicited. Infiltrate a site approximately 0.5 to 1 cm medial to this point to anesthetize the supratrochlear nerve.

In some cases, the lateral branches of the supraorbital nerve exit a foramen above the rim. If these lateral branches are missed with the orbital rim block, deposit local anesthetic 1 cm above the rim. This subfrontalis injection starts 1 cm above the rim at the zygomaticofrontal suture and proceeds toward the medial eyebrow (14).

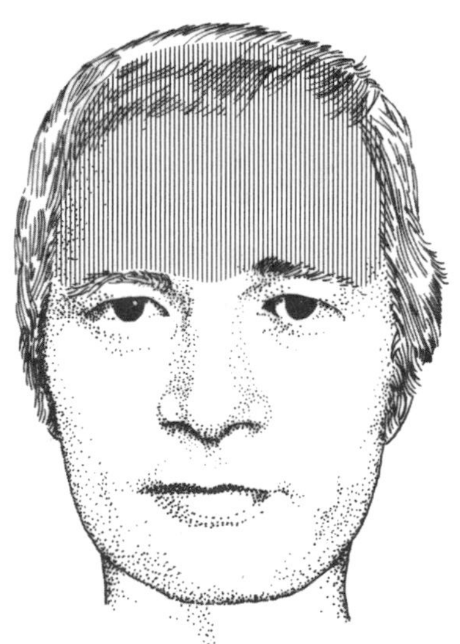

Figure 3.8. The supraorbital and supratrochlear nerves supply sensation to the forehead and scalp as far back as the coronal suture.

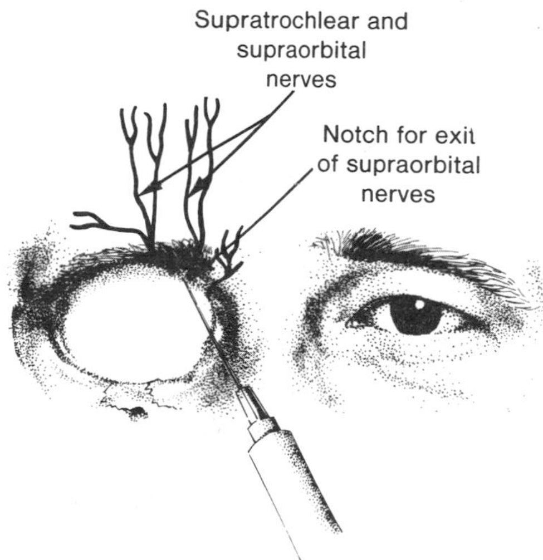

Figure 3.9. Block the supraorbital and supratrochlear nerves by inserting the needle just beneath the supraorbital ridge and directing it to the notch where the supraorbital and supratrochlear nerves emerge.

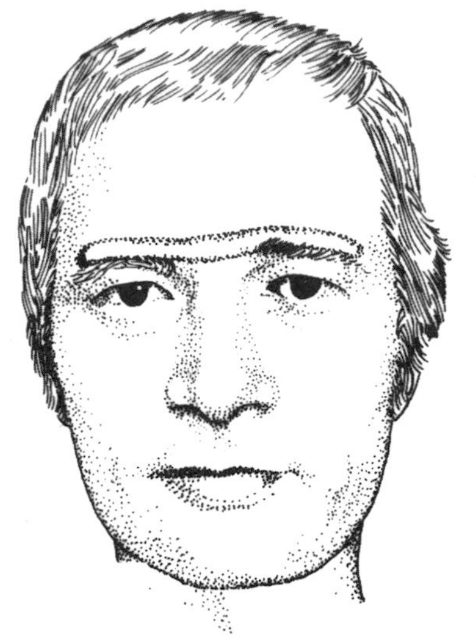

Figure 3.10. Deposit a line of anesthetic solution horizontally to block all the branches of the supraorbital and supratrochlear nerves.

ALTERNATE TECHNIQUE

An alternate method assures infiltration of all the branches of the nerves. Deposit a line of anesthetic solution horizontally extending across both supraorbital ridges (Fig. 3.10).

Infraorbital Nerve Block

The infraorbital nerve exits along the infraorbital ridge at a point directly below the exit of the supraorbital nerve superiorly. The site of exit can be palpated as a depression or foramen just inferior to the infraorbital ridge (Fig. 3.11). This nerve supplies sensation to the infraorbital region of the cheek and the lateral aspect of the nose and upper lip (Fig. 3.12).

INDICATIONS

1. Extensive lacerations of the malar area of the upper lip.
2. Drainage of facial abscess in the cheek.
3. Debridement of abrasions of the cheek.

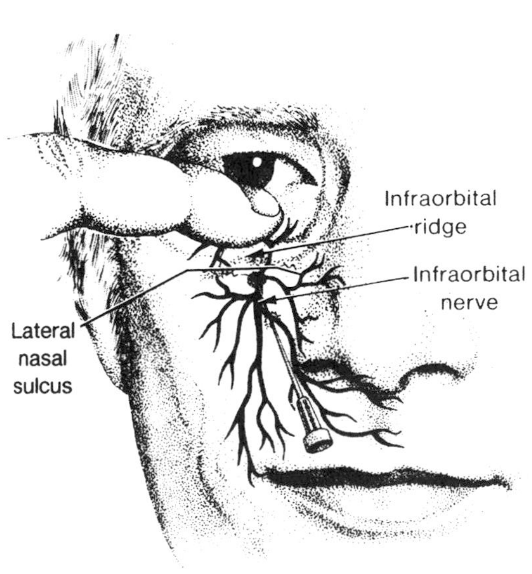

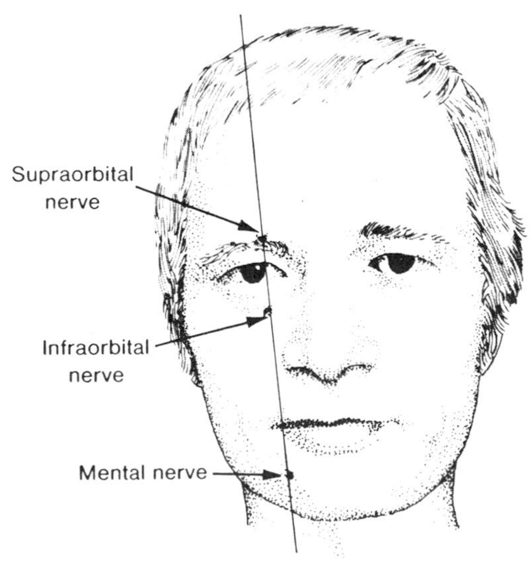

Figure 3.11. *A:* The infraorbital nerve courses through a foramen that lies inferior to the infraorbital ridge. *B:* In many patients in whom an infraorbital nerve block is desirable but in whom the malar area is markedly swollen, one cannot palpate or find the infraorbital foramen. In such cases, extend a line from the supraorbital notch to the mental foramen, and this will traverse the infraorbital foramen.

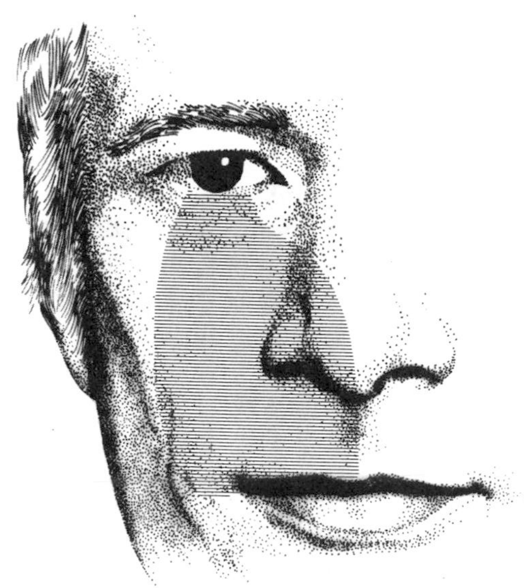

Figure 3.12. The sensory distribution of the infraorbital nerve.

TECHNIQUE

Although two methods are described in the literature, one intraoral and the other extraoral, we prefer the intraoral route because it is less painful and easier to perform (24). Attach an 18-gauge, 1.5-inch needle to a 5-mL syringe filled with 1% lidocaine with epinephrine. Infiltrate the site of injection of the mucous membrane with a 25-gauge needle and lidocaine, or swab the mucosa with a topical anesthetic on a cotton-tipped applicator and wipe clean with gauze after about 1 minute (18). This site is at the buccogingival fold just medial to the canine tooth of the maxilla on the side to be blocked. Insert the needle at this point and advance it to the infraorbital foramen, guided by the index finger of the left hand externally. Infiltrate 1 to 2 mL of anesthetic solution at this point, and anesthesia usually is complete within 5 minutes. Vigorous shaking of the upper lip will decrease the pain of injection. With a bilateral block, good anesthesia can be obtained for the entire upper lip. The injection with this method does not have to be exactly at the foramen.

ALTERNATE TECHNIQUE

An alternate extraoral method has been described (12). The lateral nasal sulcus 1 cm from the ala of the nose is the site of injection (Fig. 3.11). Insert the needle here, and advance it upward and laterally, guided by the index finger of the left hand palpating the depression of the infraorbital ridge. At 0.5 cm below the infraorbital ridge, inject 1 to 2 mL of anesthetic solution.

Anesthesia to the Nose

The sensory innervation of the nose is provided by branches of the first and second divisions of the fifth cranial nerve. The anterior ethmoidal arises from the first (ophthalmic) division within the orbit and reenters the skull by passing through the anterior ethmoidal foramen on the medial wall of the orbit. It then courses down through the cribriform plate and innervates the anterior third of the nasal septum and the lateral walls in the upper nasal cavity. The posterior two thirds of the septum and the lateral walls inferiorly and posteriorly receive their supply from the sphenopalatine nerve arising from the sphenopalatine ganglion of the maxillary division of the fifth cranial nerve.

INDICATIONS

1. Nasal lacerations.
2. Nasal fracture reduction.
3. Epistaxis.
4. Drainage of a septal hematoma or abscess.

TECHNIQUE

Two techniques have been described for anesthetizing the nose. When anesthesia is required for reduction of nasal fractures, further steps are needed to provide adequate anesthesia than when intranasal mucosal anesthesia is indicated. These are discussed separately.

Modified Sluder's Technique (9, 29)

Dip a nasal tampon into a solution of 1:1,000 epinephrine, and remove the excess fluid by squeezing the tampon between the fingers. Then dip the tampon into 10% cocaine, and again remove the excess. Place this tampon between the turbinates and the septum, and leave it in place for 5 minutes. Remove this tampon from the nose; the membranes are now maximally shrunken. Now wind a small amount of cotton onto the end of a metal applicator and moisten with 1:1,000 epinephrine, press this dry, and dip into cocaine flakes. Then pass the applicator into the nose at the angle between the middle and posterior thirds of the middle turbinate and septum until it reaches the face of the sphenoid sinus (Fig. 3.13). Place a second applicator in the cleft of the nose at a point between the anterior end of the middle turbinate and the septum until it comes to rest on the inferior surface of the cribriform plate. The first applicator provides anesthesia to the sphenopalatine ganglion, and the second, to the anterior ethmoid nerve.

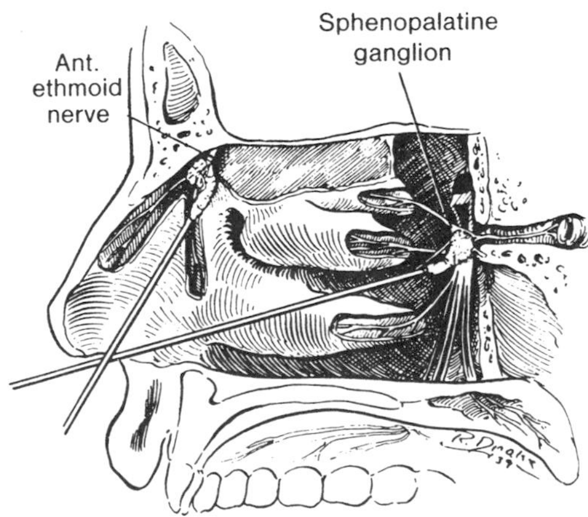

Figure 3.13. Cotton-tipped applicators in position to anesthetize the anterior ethmoid nerve and the nasal branches of the sphenopalatine ganglion. (From Mousel LH: Anesthesia for operations about the head and neck. Anesthesiology 2:61–73, 1941, with permission.)

Leave these applicators in place for at least 10 minutes. This technique provides excellent anesthesia for all intranasal procedures.

Moffett's Technique (15)

This is not our preferred procedure. It is indicated when one is dealing with an uncooperative patient or a child who will not permit placement of applicators into the proper position. The technique requires no applicators and so is less traumatic. Lying supine and with the head tilted as far back as possible, the patient is in the optimal position for blocking these nerves to the nose. Deposit 2 mL of anesthetic solution into the nostril with a dropper so that it reaches the site of the anterior ethmoid nerve. To anesthetize the sphenopalatine nerve, tilt the patient's head slightly forward. The solution used is 4% or 10% cocaine, and permit this to remain in the nose for 10 minutes. Both nostrils are anesthetized at the same time.

Additional Anesthesia for Reduction of Nasal Fractures

In addition to the intranasal blocks indicated earlier, the following nerves should be blocked for nasal fracture reduction:

1. The infraorbital nerve (technique described earlier) (Fig. 3.14).
2. Infratrochlear nerve. This nerve courses just above the inner canthus of the eye (Fig. 3.14). It is blocked with a 1.5-inch needle passed just lateral to the bridge of the nose and superior to the inner canthus. Instill 1 to 2 mL of 1% lidocaine with epinephrine at this site.
3. Anesthetize the external nasal nerves by inserting a needle on the outside of the nose at the point where the superior rim of the lateral cartilage joins the nasal bone (Fig. 3.14). The external nasal nerve courses at the junction of the lateral cartilage and the nasal bone; apply the anesthetic solution

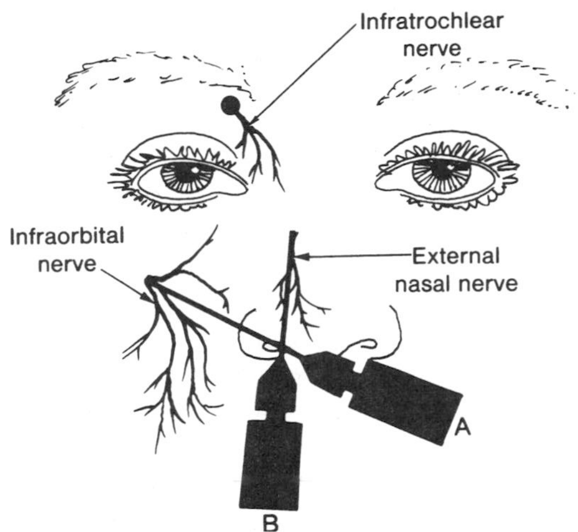

Figure 3.14. For reduction of nasal fractures and for complex nasal repairs, anesthetize the infratrochlear, infraorbital *(A)*, and external nasal *(B)* nerves as shown and described in the text.

there bilaterally. This provides anesthesia for the distal part of the nose, including the tip of the nose. Anesthetize the infraorbital nerve by the intraoral approach described earlier in this chapter.

NOTE

The nasociliary nerve is a branch of the ophthalmic nerve, giving off several important groups of branches while in the orbital cavity. The ethmoidal branches and the nasal branches supply the mucous membrane of the anterior part of the septum, the lateral wall of the nasal cavity, and the skin of the ala, and apex of the nose by the internal and external branches, respectively. To block the nasociliary nerve or its branches, insert a 3-cm, 25-gauge needle 1 cm above the inner canthus and direct it posterolaterally, keeping contact with bone. At a depth of 1.5 cm, the needle should be at the anterior ethmoidal foramen; inject 2 mL of anesthetic solution. Advance the needle slowly 1 cm farther to reach the postero ethmoidal foramen; inject 1.5 mL of solution to block the antero ethmoidal nerve that supplies the posterior sinuses. The two injections also are likely to block another branch of the nasociliary nerve, the infratrochlear nerve, which supplies the roof of the nose. The nasociliary blocks are produced without adrenaline to eliminate any risk of retinal artery spasm (28).

Scalp Block

Almost the entire nerve supply to the scalp is superficial (Figs. 3.15 and 3.16). Anteriorly the supraorbital and supratrochlear nerves, which are terminal branches of the first division of the fifth cranial nerve, reach the forehead through a depression in the superior bony ridge of the orbit. They supply the scalp as far as the crown of the head, supplying innervations to both the forehead and the front of the scalp. Laterally, the auriculotemporal nerve, a branch of the mandibular division of the fifth cranial nerve, passes beneath the parotid gland to reach the temporal fossa posterior to the superficial temporal artery, where it supplies innervation to

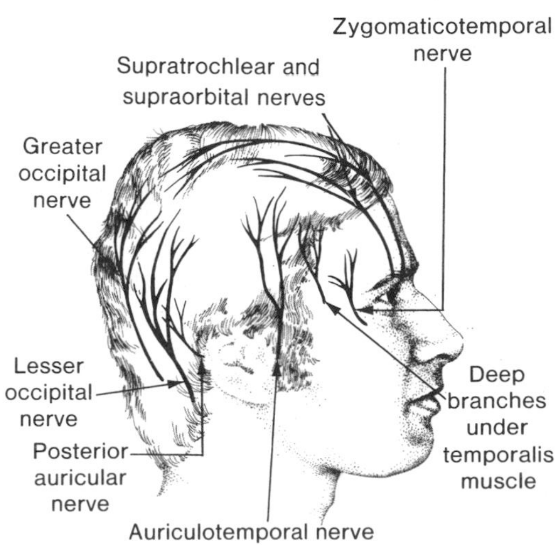

Figure 3.15. Nerve supply to the scalp. See text for discussion.

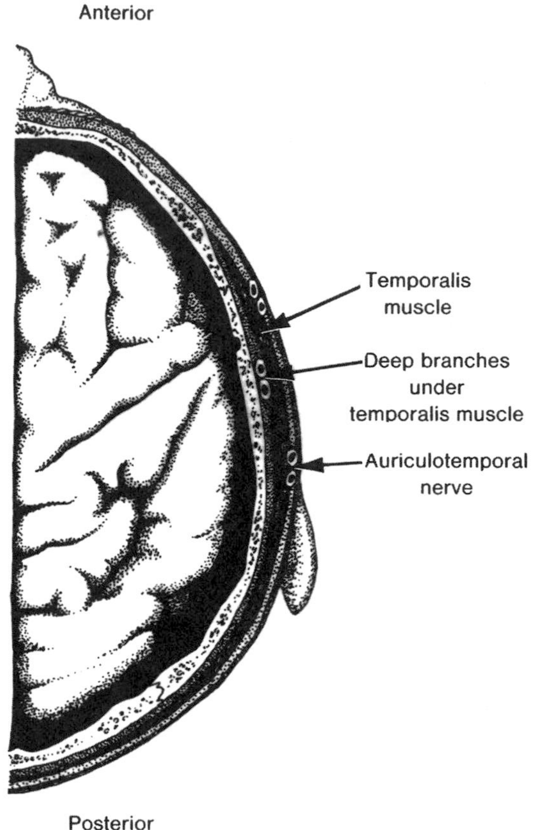

Figure 3.16. Portions of the sensory nerve supply to the scalp over the temporal region lie deep to the temporalis muscle. See text for discussion.

the temporal aspect of the scalp. A small area between these two nerves is innervated by the zygomaticotemporal nerve, a branch of the maxillary nerve. The posterior scalp is supplied by the greater and lesser occipital nerves, which are branches of the first through the third cervical roots after they pierce the erector spinae muscle and become superficial as they cross the occipital ridge. These nerves supply the posterior scalp as far anteriorly as the vertex and laterally to the mastoids (6, 9).

INDICATIONS

This block is useful when repairing extensive lacerations of the scalp.

TECHNIQUE

With a 3-inch, 22-gauge needle, infiltrate intradermally and subcutaneously with 0.5% to 1.0% lidocaine with epinephrine circumferentially around the scalp. The temporal regions may require extra anesthetic to be deposited deep to the temporalis muscle because of the depth of the nerves in this area. A "cap" of analgesia is produced over the head above the line of infiltration (Fig. 3.17).

When only a portion of the scalp must be anesthetized (anterior or posterior portion), specific nerves may be blocked. The supraorbital and supratrochlear nerve blocks providing anesthesia for the anterior portion of the scalp and forehead were discussed earlier in this chapter. When a posterior nerve block is indicated, anesthetize the greater occipital nerve as it courses through its hiatus along the superior aspect of the trapezius muscle where that muscle attaches to the base of the occiput (Fig. 3.18*A*). In performing this block, elicit paresthesias. Alternatively, deposit a line of anesthesia subcutaneously at the base of the occiput, at the level of the external occipital protuberance, which can be palpated along the occipital bone (Fig. 3.18*B*). This block will

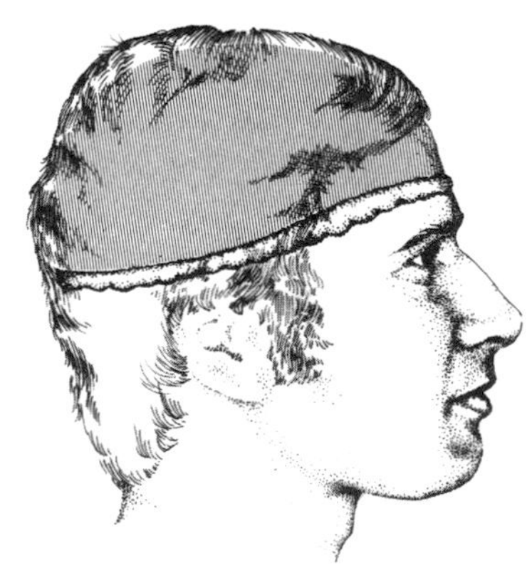

Figure 3.17. Deposit a cap of anesthesia circumferentially around the scalp for complex lacerations of the scalp. In addition, anesthetize the deep branches that lie beneath the temporalis muscle, as shown in Fig. 3.16.

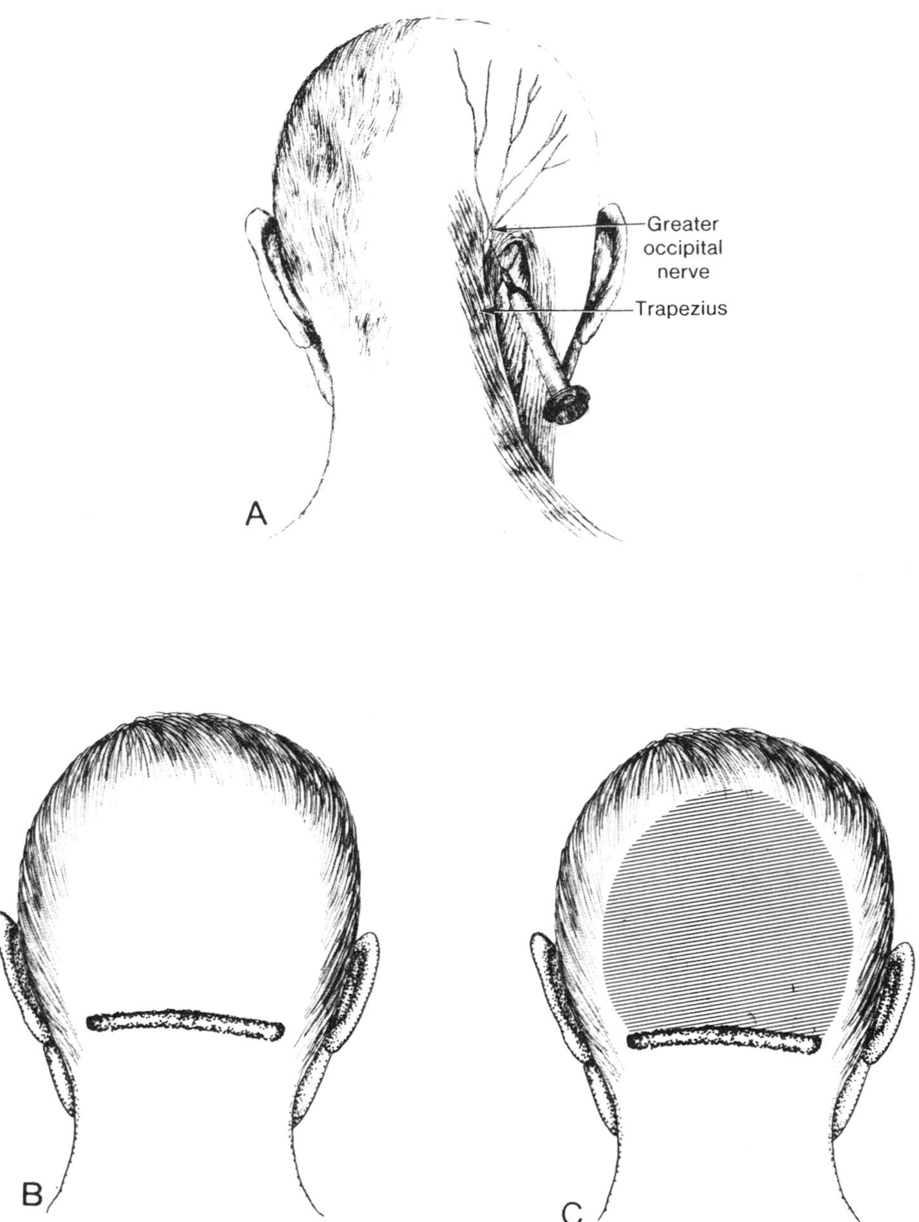

Figure 3.18. *A:* Block of the greater occipital nerve. *B:* Alternatively, deposit a line of anesthetic subcutaneously at the base of the occiput, at the level of the external occipital protuberance. *C:* The area of anesthesia provided by this block. See text for discussion.

provide anesthesia to the greater occipital nerve, lesser occipital nerve branches, and the third occipital nerve (Fig. 3.18*C*). The amount of anesthetic solution required is approximately 10 mL of 1% lidocaine and epinephrine.

Anesthesia of the Ear

Four nerves are of importance in considering anesthesia to the ear (Fig. 3.19). The innervation of the auricle is mainly via the *greater auricular nerve*, which is a branch of the cervical plexus (10). It be-

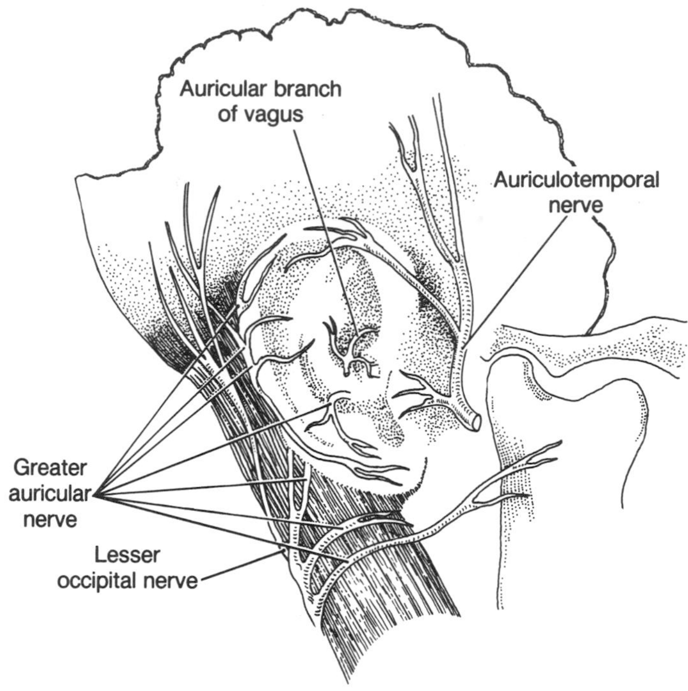

Figure 3.19. The nerves supplying the ear.

comes subcutaneous posterior to the midpoint of the sternocleidomastoid muscle, from which it runs directly toward the ear. This nerve supplies the medial portion of the auricle and the lower and peripheral portion of the lateral aspect of the ear by the anterior branch. The auriculotemporal nerve, a branch of the mandibular nerve, supplies the anterosuperior portion of the lateral surface of the auricle. This nerve comes immediately in front of the external auditory canal. The *auricular branch of the vagus* nerve supplies innervation to the concha (Fig. 3.20) as it emerges through the tympanomastoid fissure just anterior to the mastoid process and behind the external meatus.

The external auditory meatus is innervated by two of the previously discussed nerves: the auriculotemporal nerve and the auricular branches of the vagus nerve. The auriculotemporal nerve gives off a branch to the canal and supplies the skin of the superior, anterior, and inferior boundaries of the canal as well as the tympanic membrane. The auricular branch of the vagus innervates the skin of the inferior or posterior walls of the auditory canal. Another nerve supplying sensation to the ear is the tympanic nerve, which is a branch of the glossopharyngeal nerve and innervates the middle ear.

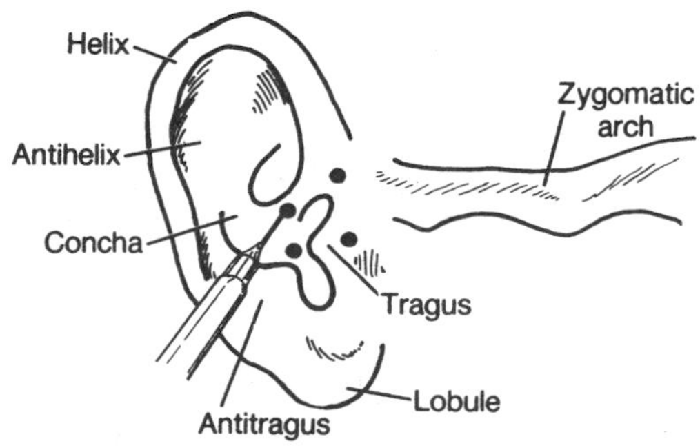

Figure 3.20. The four-quadrant block for anesthetizing the auditory canal. See text for discussion.

INDICATIONS

1. Lacerations of the ear. In patients with extensive lacerations of the ear, it is difficult to provide anesthesia by local infiltration of the wound edges because of the close apposition of the skin to the cartilaginous surface. Block of the greater auricular nerve and auriculotemporal nerve provides adequate anesthesia to repair the wound in the majority of cases. In lacerations extending posterior to the ear, one may find it necessary to block the lesser occipital nerve, which supplies innervation to the skin behind the ear. This is discussed later.
2. Irrigation of the ear and removal of impacted cerumen. In patients with otitis externa and in patients who have cerumen impacted close to the tympanic membrane, block of the ear canal may be necessary to cleanse the canal of debris for topical antibacterials to work adequately or to dislodge a particle of cerumen without discomfort.
3. Myringotomy. Myringotomy requires anesthesia of the canal and tympanic membrane. This anesthesia may be difficult to accomplish; the techniques described later relate the procedures specifically.
4. Foreign-body removal. Removal of foreign bodies, particularly in children, may be difficult without adequate anesthesia of the external auditory canal.

TECHNIQUE FOR BLOCK OF THE AURICLE

Deposit a line of anesthetic solution subcutaneously in the sulcus behind the auricle and immediately anterior to the mastoid (Fig. 3.21), extending semicircularly from the inferior to the superior pole (Fig. 3.22). This blocks the greater auricular nerve and the lesser occipital nerve supplying much of the external ear. Then block the auriculotemporal nerve by deposition of 1 to 2 mL of solution just ante-

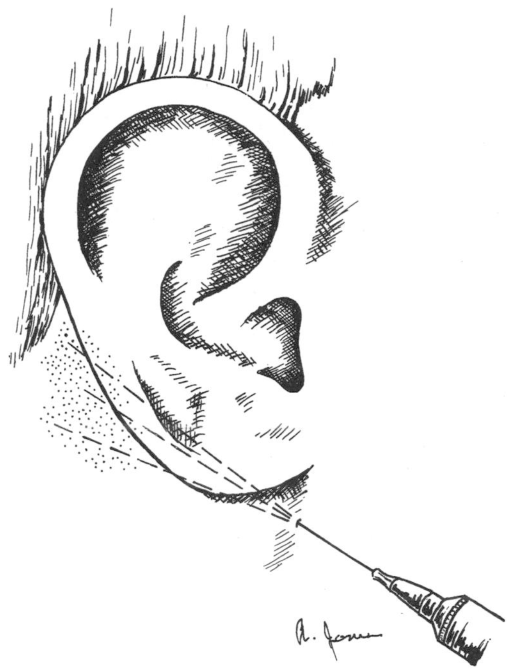

Figure 3.21. Deposit anesthetic solution in the sulcus behind the auricle. Raise a wheal under the skin that lies over the mastoid process.

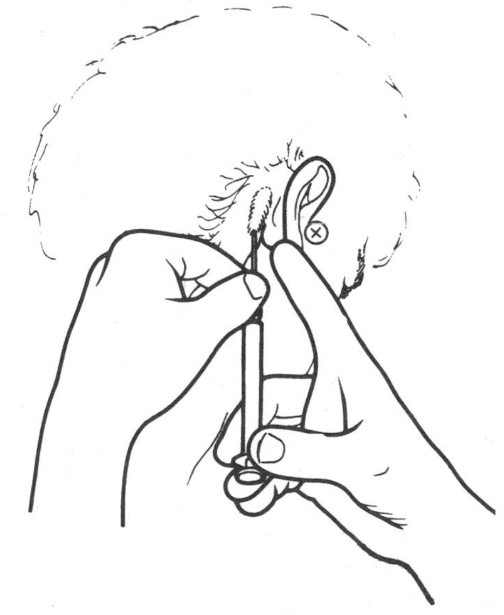

Figure 3.22. Accompany subcutaneous infiltration in a semicircle behind the ear by a block of the auriculotemporal nerve anteriorly (see text for discussion) to provide anesthesia for the auricle.

rior to the tragus, at the point where the zygomatic arch meets the tragus. This is easily palpable with the index finger. The success rate of this block is approximately 60% to 70% in our experience.

TECHNIQUE FOR BLOCK OF THE AUDITORY CANAL

Inject 1 mL of 2% lidocaine with epinephrine at the points indicated in Fig. 3.20. This *four-quadrant block* is used to anesthetize the ear canal. This generally provides adequate anesthesia of the ear canal and tympanic membrane for foreign-body removal and irrigation. For myringotomy, one may have to spray or instill several drops of anesthetic into the ear canal and leave it in place for 5 to 10 minutes. This block is usually incomplete in its effectiveness when compared with other blocks. With large foreign bodies entrapped near the tympanic membrane, the patient may need general anesthesia or iontophoresis.

UPPER EXTREMITY BLOCKS

Brachial Plexus Block

This is one of the most widely used nerve blocks. It produces anesthesia of the arm and forearm and hand for virtually any procedure necessary in this region. Two approaches are described in the literature, the supraclavicular approach and the axillary approach (3, 8, 41, 42). The axillary approach is the procedure of choice in the emergency center (1, 3, 7, 16, 20, 27). The supraclavicular approach is fraught with hazards, especially pneumothorax and trauma to the great vessels (3, 9). The advantage of the supraclavicular approach is that anesthesia is achieved in 10 to 15 minutes, whereas by the axillary route, a good block is not achieved for 30 minutes. In addition, the musculocutaneous or axillary nerve may not be adequately blocked with this approach (3, 25).

The brachial plexus is formed by the anterior primary rami of the lower four cervical nerves and the greater portion of the first thoracic nerve. The plexus emerges from the lateral border of the anterior and middle scalene muscles. As it emerges from this region, it carries with it an investing fascial sheath from the paravertebral fascia that completely encircles the plexus. This investing sheath is called the axillary sheath. This sheath is composed of tough fibrous connective tissue extending laterally to a little beyond the pectoralis minor. Regardless of the level (interscalene, supraclavicular, or axillary) at which this sheath is encountered, an effective block of the brachial plexus is possible because the anesthesia will remain within the sheath.

INDICATIONS

1. Repair of extensive lacerations of the forearm, arm, or hand.
2. Reduction of fractures of the forearm, elbow, and hand.
3. Debridement of extensive abrasions to the upper extremity, with embedded dirt, resulting from a motorcycle accident.
4. Reduction of fracture dislocations of the elbow and wrist.

TECHNIQUE

Preparatory Steps

1. Position the patient supine, with the arm on the side to be injected held at 90 degrees of abduction and externally rotated.
2. Rotate the head to the opposite direction.
3. Stand at the side that is to be injected.
4. Prepare and drape the axilla.
5. Locate landmarks.
   a. Palpate the humeral insertions of the latissimus dorsi posteriorly and the pectoralis major anteriorly (Fig. 3.23). Draw a vertical line between these two points. Bisect the line and mark the point. This point lies directly over the brachial artery,

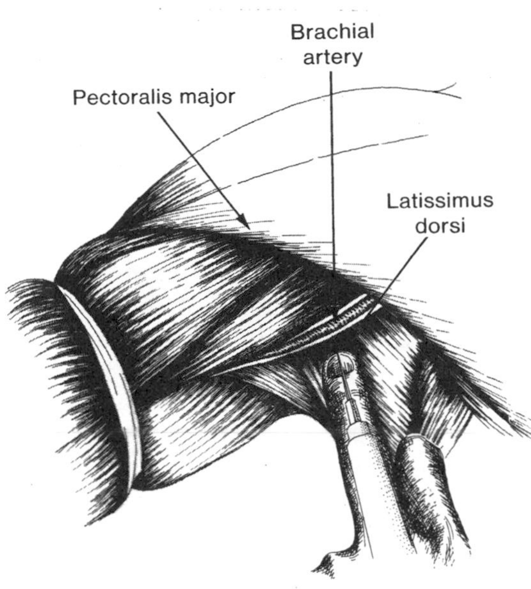

Figure 3.23. Brachial plexus block. See text for discussion.

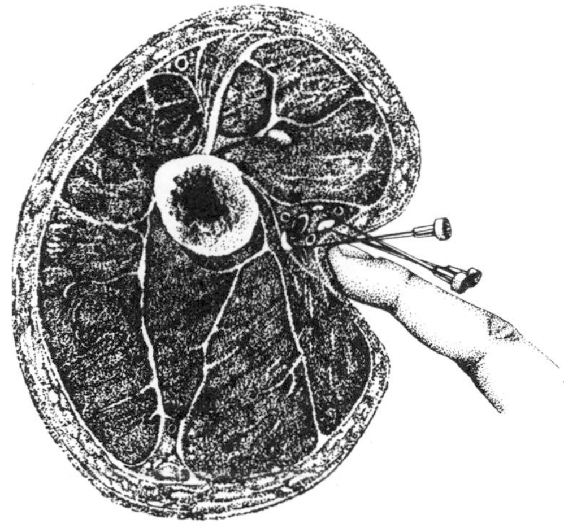

Figure 3.24. Insert the needle at a right angle to the skin alongside the palpating finger, which is placed over the point of maximal pulsation of the axillary artery. When the needle is within the sheath that encloses the axillary and brachial plexus, the needle will "pulsate." At this point, aspirate and inject the anesthetic solution within the sheath.

which can be palpated in all but the very obese (1, 3).

b. When the axillary artery is easily palpable, this procedure is not necessary. The point of maximal pulsation of the axillary artery is the only landmark.

6. Calculate amount of anesthetic necessary for adequate block. All of the solutions should be 1% lidocaine with 1:200,000 epinephrine at approximately 0.33 mL/kg.

80-kg man, 25 to 30 mL
70-kg, 20 to 25 mL
40 to 60 kg, 15 to 20 mL
25 to 30 kg, 14 to 20 mL

Use a 25-gauge, 5-cm needle attached to a 20- to 30-mL syringe.

Procedural Steps

1. Palpate the axillary artery with the index finger of the left hand.
2. Insert the needle at a right angle to the skin alongside the palpating finger, which is placed at the point of maximal pulsation or the region indicated in step 5 earlier (Fig. 3.24).
3. When the needle is properly placed, the pulsation of the artery is transmitted to the needle, and one may feel a give as the axillary sheath is entered.
4. Inject the anesthetic solution directly into the sheath after aspiration to be certain one is not in the lumen of the artery.

NOTE

Sometimes the musculocutaneous nerve is not reached, and patchy anesthesia is achieved on the radial side of the forearm. Place a tourniquet high on the arm or the blood pressure cuff inflated to between systolic and diastolic pressures at about the level of insertion of the deltoid (Fig. 3.23). This effectively limits the spread of the solution, causing distention of the sheath and permitting an effective block (8).

COMPLICATIONS

Intraarterial puncture and a small hematoma in the sheath are the only complications of significance. This produces little difficulty if aspiration is performed and a small-gauge needle is used.

NOTE

A new fluoroscopically guided approach for brachial plexus block was found to be a reliable and easy technique associated with a low complication rate. Advance the needle near the first rib and posterior to the subclavian artery, which is identified by the groove where the first rib starts to curve posteriorly. In a recent study, more than 1,000 blocks were performed with this technique, and it was found that the solution spread into the interscalene space, despite neither hearing the "click" nor eliciting paresthesias simply by placing the tip of the needle at some part of the first rib. This new approach for brachial plexus block was termed the *supracostal* approach (33). The technique requires fluoroscopic control and thus is of little use in emergency medicine.

Median Nerve Block at the Elbow (32)

The median nerve courses in the arm medially and is included in the large neurovascular sheath that contains the brachial artery. In the antecubital fossa, the nerve courses laterally to the brachial artery and is covered by the aponeurosis of the biceps muscle.

INDICATIONS

1. Repair of lacerations over the sensory distribution of the nerve in the hand and forearm.
2. Debridement of abrasions in the distribution of the nerve to the forearm and hand.

TECHNIQUE

The landmark for blocking this nerve is the brachial artery, and the nerve is best blocked on the ulnar side of this artery. The medial condyle of the humerus and the tendon of the biceps form two additional landmarks for locating the nerve. Place the patient in the supine position, with the arm abducted and the forearm extended. Moisten an applicator with iodine, and place it in the antecubital fossa. Next ask the patient to flex the arm to an angle of 90 degrees. A transverse line results that is at the same level as a line drawn between the two epicondyles. The nerve lies superficially here and can be palpated in some thin individuals. One can feel the tendon of the biceps by flexing and extending the forearm with the hand in supination. The brachial artery is medial to the tendon, and the nerve is medial to the artery and superficial at the level of the line drawn (Fig. 3.25). Raise an intradermal wheal medial to the artery, and introduce a needle through the skin and fascia to achieve paresthesia. Inject 5 mL of 1% lidocaine at this site in a fan-wise fashion (6).

Ulnar Nerve Block at the Elbow

The ulnar nerve courses along the medial aspect of the arm and, in the distal

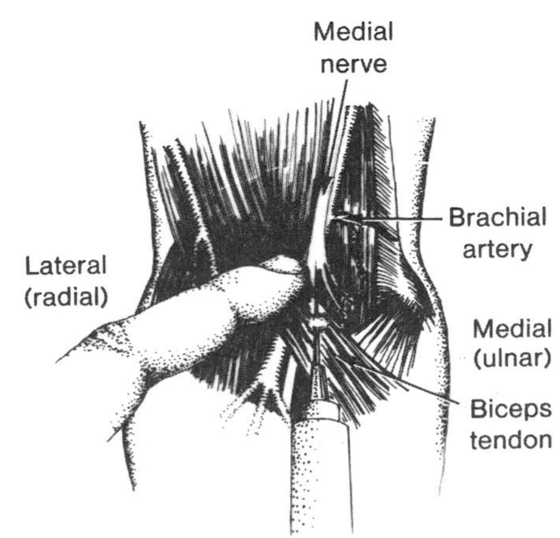

Figure 3.25. The median nerve block at the elbow. See text for discussion.

one third, perforates the medial intermuscular septum to enter the extensor compartment of the forearm. In doing so, it passes behind the posterior aspect of the medial epicondyle of the humerus. The nerve can be easily palpated in this area, usually without difficulty. Almost everyone has at some time or another struck the "funny bone"; the paresthesias elicited are those from the ulnar nerve.

INDICATIONS

1. To repair injuries over the sensory distribution of the nerve.
2. To augment an inadequate brachial plexus block. The fibers of C8 and T1 are often difficult to block.

TECHNIQUE

Place the patient in the lateral prone position on the side opposite the one to be injected. The elbow should be flexed at 90 degrees. The landmarks are the groove between the medial condyle of the humerus and the olecranon process, particularly in the obese patient in whom palpation of the nerve behind the medial epicondyle may be difficult (Fig. 3.26). Palpate the nerve and grasp the skin and subcutaneous tissue above this groove with the thumb and index finger of the left hand. After raising an intradermal wheal in the skin grasped, introduce a 25-gauge, 1.5-inch needle in the direction of the nerve (Fig. 3.26). The injection should ideally be 1 to 2 cm above the position of the nerve in the groove behind the epicondyle. This avoids the possibility of neuritis, which may result from injection at the epicondyle. Paresthesias should be elicited, and 3 to 5 mL of 1% lidocaine introduced at this site (35).

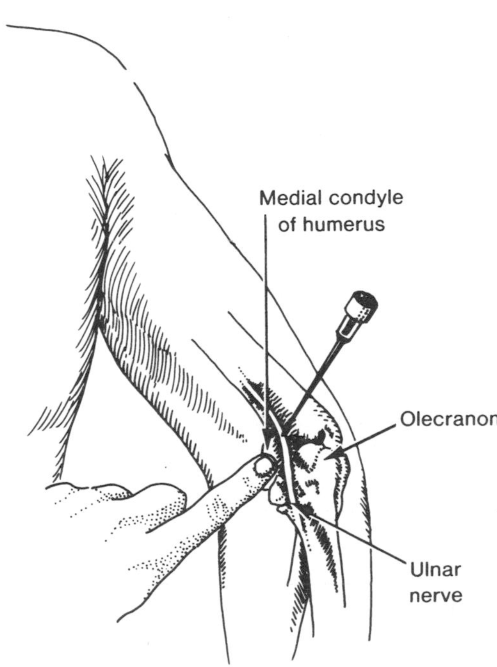

Figure 3.26. The ulnar nerve block at the elbow. See text for discussion.

Median Nerve Block at the Wrist (3, 8, 35)

The median nerve courses between the superficial and deep flexor tendons supplying the digits. At the level of the proximal wrist crease, the nerve courses superficially to lie immediately radial to the tendon of the palmaris longus (Fig. 3.27). In patients who do not have a palmaris longus, the median nerve courses between the flexor carpi radialis and the flexor superficialis tendons. The landmarks for performing a median nerve block at the wrist are the tendons of the palmaris longus and the flexor carpi radialis. The nerve lies deep to the tendon of the palmaris longus on its radial side; however, whereas the tendon of the palmaris longus is superficial, all other flexor tendons and the nerve itself lie deep to the flexor retinaculum.

INDICATIONS

1. Lacerations of the hand over areas supplied by the median nerve.
2. Removal of foreign bodies in the hand.

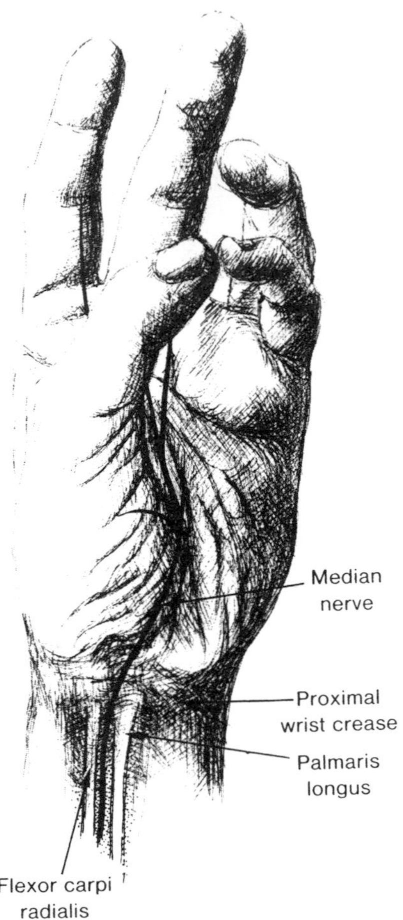

Figure 3.27. The median nerve block at the wrist. At the level of proximal wrist crease, the nerve courses superficially and lies immediately radial to the tendon of the palmaris longus. See text for discussion.

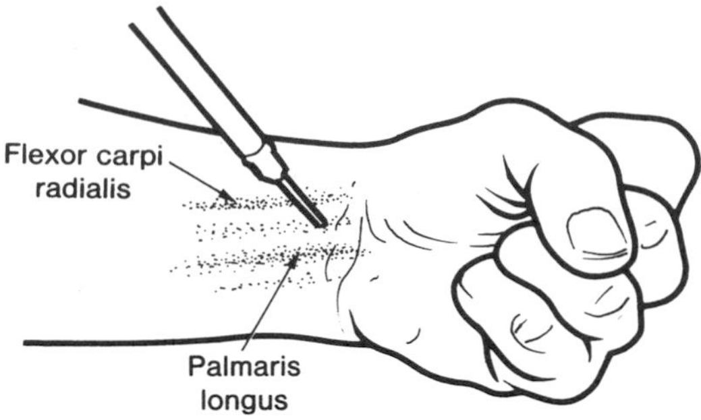

Figure 3.28. Locate the flexor carpi radialis by having the patient make a fist and flex the wrist against resistance. The point of injection is immediately radial to the palmaris longus tendon at the level of the proximal skin crease of the wrist. See text for discussion.

TECHNIQUE

To perform the block, locate the palmaris longus and the flexor carpi radialis tendons by asking the patient to oppose the thumb and small finger while flexing the wrist against resistance as shown in Fig. 3.27. In patients who are missing the palmaris longus, locate the flexor carpi radialis and the flexor digitorum superficialis tendons by having the patient make a fist and flex the wrist against resistance (Fig. 3.28). Mark the palmaris longus and the flexor carpi radialis tendons. The point of injection is immediately radial to the palmaris longus tendon at the level of the proximal skin crease of the wrist (Fig. 3.28). Insert a 23-gauge, 1.5-inch needle through the skin at right angles to the tendon. One may feel the resistance of the flexor retinaculum. The nerve lies deep to the retinaculum and, unless the nerve is palpated, it is difficult to appreciate the depth for infiltration. Insert the needle approximately 0.5 cm beyond the retinaculum and attempt to obtain paresthesias in the hand, which indicate that the nerve has been touched by the needle point. At this point, inject 2 mL of 1% lidocaine. If paresthesias are not elicited, inject approximately 5 mL of 1% lidocaine in an in-and-out fashion to spread the anesthetic throughout the area.

Ulnar Nerve Block at the Wrist

The ulnar nerve divides into a palmar and dorsal branch approximately 5 cm proximal to the wrist (8, 35). The ulnar artery accompanies the palmar branch of the nerve (Fig. 3.29). The dorsal branch is entirely sensory and courses beneath the tendon of the flexor carpi ulnaris to reach the dorsal aspect of the wrist and supplies sensation to the ulnar side of the dorsum of the hand. The palmar branch is a mixed nerve and continues along the tendon

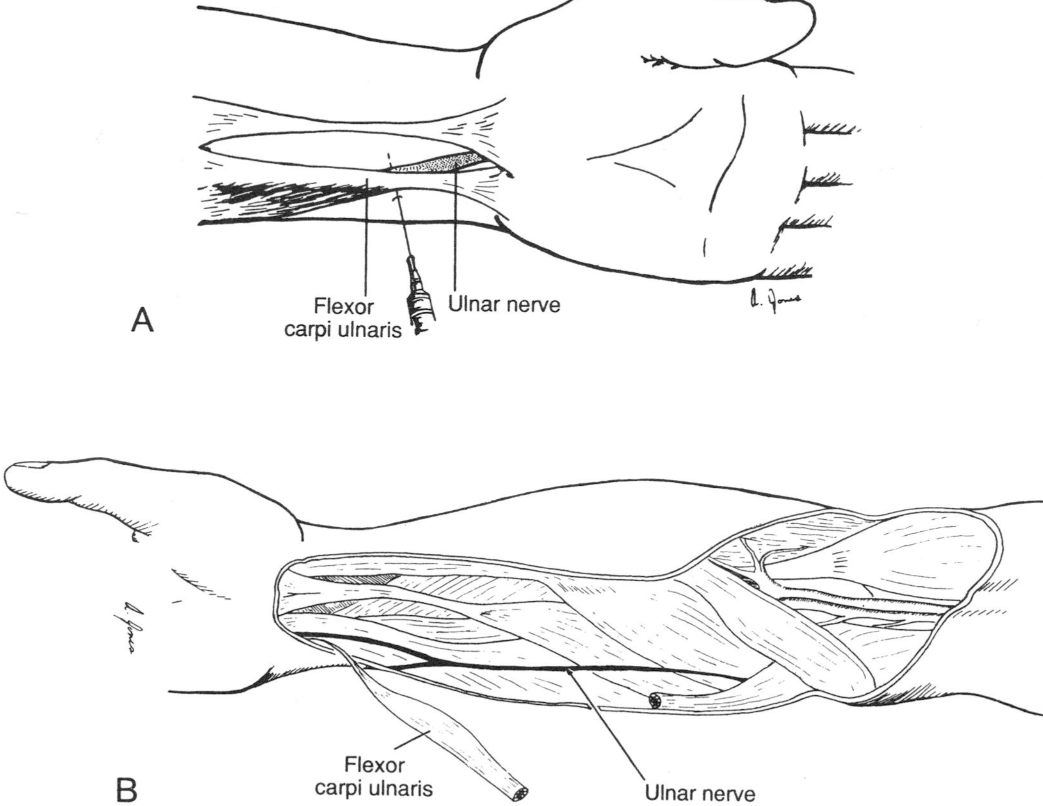

Figure 3.29. The ulnar nerve courses directly under the flexor carpi ulnaris. To anesthetize the ulnar nerve, inject several centimeters proximal to the wrist/crease. See text for discussion.

flexor carpi ulnaris to divide on the radial side of the pisiform bone into a superficial and a deep branch. The superficial branch is entirely sensory and supplies sensation of the ulnar side of the palmar portion of the hand and to the fourth and fifth fingers.

INDICATIONS

1. Lacerations of the hand over areas supplied by the ulnar nerve.
2. Removal of foreign bodies in the hand.

TECHNIQUE

Palpate the tendon of the flexor carpi ulnaris at the level of the styloid process of the ulna (Fig. 3.29*A*). The flexor carpi ulnaris can be easily identified at its attachment to the pisiform bone by palpating the pisiform and asking the patient to flex the wrist against resistance, which makes the tendon stand out. Insert a 23-gauge, 1.5-inch needle perpendicular to the skin on the radial side of the flexor carpi ulnaris tendon at the level of the proximal skin crease (3, 8). The palmar branch lies superficial to the flexor retinaculum, and the injection should be beneath the flexor ulnaris tendon. Then inject 2 mL of 1% lidocaine. To anesthetize the dorsal cutaneous branch of the ulnar nerve, one must understand its anatomy (Fig. 3.29*B*). The dorsal cutaneous branch of this nerve separates from the main trunk of the ulnar nerve approximately 5 to 7 cm proximal to the ulnar styloid. To anesthetize this branch of the ulnar nerve, deposit 2 to 3 mL of anesthetic solution at this level, immediately beneath the flexor carpi ulnaris tendon. This method should provide good anesthesia for both the dorsal and the palmar branches of the ulnar nerve (3, 8, 35).

Radial Nerve Block of the Wrist

The radial nerve accompanies the artery alongside the brachioradialis muscle in the forearm. Approximately 7 cm proximal to the wrist joint, the superficial branch passes laterally beneath the tendon of the muscle and goes to the dorsal aspect of the wrist. At this point, the nerve breaks up into superficial rami to supply the radial side of the dorsum of the hand with sensation. At the level of the skin crease of the wrist, all the sensory branches of the radial nerve are superficial (8).

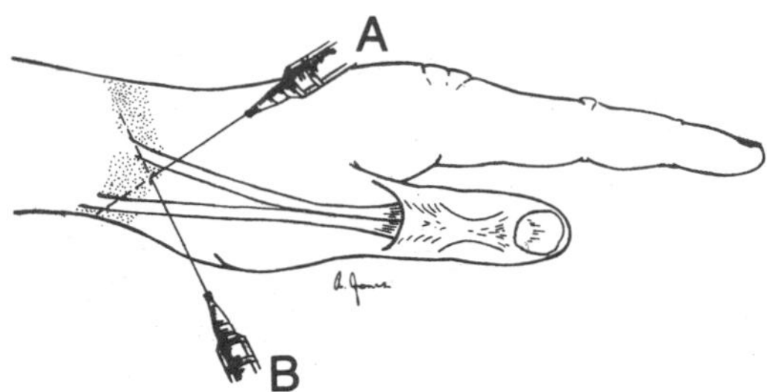

Figure 3.30. Radial nerve block at the wrist. Deposit anesthetic at radial styloid, volar aspect *(A)*, and continue to dorsal aspect of wrist *(B)*.

INDICATIONS

1. Extensive lacerations involving the hand. It is unusual to do a radial nerve block as an isolated procedure, and usually this block accompanies the ulnar and median nerve blocks to provide complete anesthesia of the hand in dealing with extensive lacerations.
2. Removal of foreign bodies from areas of the hand supplied by the radial nerve.

TECHNIQUE

Inject approximately 10 mL of anesthetic solution (1% lidocaine) subcutaneously in a band along the radial side of the wrist at the level of the proximal skin crease. Begin the injection at a point along the volar aspect of the radial styloid (Fig. 3.30) and deposit the anesthetic subcutaneously in a half-moon shape, proceeding to the dorsal aspect of the wrist (Fig. 3.31) (23, 24).

Digital Nerve Blocks

The digital nerves lie in pairs on either side of the phalanges, two on the ulnar and two on the radial aspect. The nerves of the digits are easily blocked at the base of the involved digit.

INDICATIONS

1. Lacerations involving isolated fingers.
2. Applying a skin graft or rotating a flap in a patient with an amputation of a fingertip.
3. Procedures requiring removal of a nail or repair of a nailbed of an isolated finger.
4. Reduction of an interphalangeal joint dislocation or a fracture of the phalanx.
5. Complex repairs involving the individual digits.

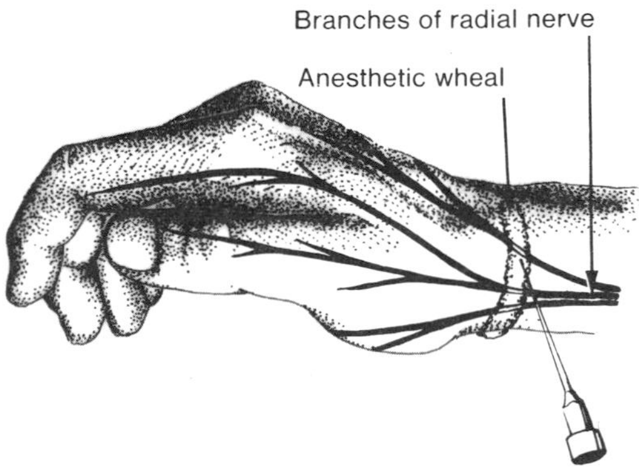

Figure 3.31. Deposit a subcutaneous wheal of anesthesia in a semicircular fashion to block all branches of the radial nerve.

TECHNIQUE

It is difficult to reach the nerves on both sides of the bone by a single injection at the midpoint; thus two separate needle insertions are made on either side of the digit (Fig. 3.32) (2, 8). No attempt is made to elicit paresthesias. Infiltrate superficially with 1 mL of 1% lidocaine and deeply, almost to the bone, on both sides of the proximal phalanx on the involved finger at the base so that a half-ring block is made.

In the early part of the century, when adrenaline first became widely available, it was used in an uncontrolled manner in cases of ischemic necrosis, which led to its falling into disfavor for hand surgery. It is widely thought that it will cause irreversible digital artery vasospasm. In a prospective study on 100 patients who underwent digital blocks with 2% lidocaine with 1:80,000 adrenaline, it was observed that adrenaline-containing digital blocks produced intense local vasoconstriction at the site of injection. This is no doubt due to the local vasoconstriction of arterioles and capillaries; however, perfusion of the fingers persisted in every case, as confirmed by the clinical impression, digital blood pressure, and fingertip temperature readings. Thus contrary to traditional teaching and conventional expectations, none of the patients in the study had irreversible digital artery vasospasm or digital ischemic necrosis (40).

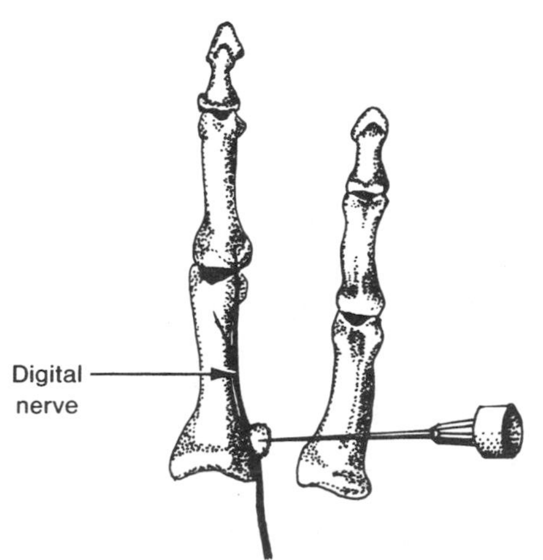

Figure 3.32. Digital nerve block. See text for details.

Metacarpal Nerve Block

Pressure from the anesthetic solution in the small space containing the digital nerve may obstruct flow into the digit, and for this reason, we prefer a metacarpal block. The digital nerves are the terminal branches of the ulnar and median nerves. One must understand the anatomy of the digital nerves to anesthetize them adequately. The common digital nerve passes volar to the lumbrical canal (Fig. 3.33) between the metacarpals and bifurcates into the proper digital nerves that supply the

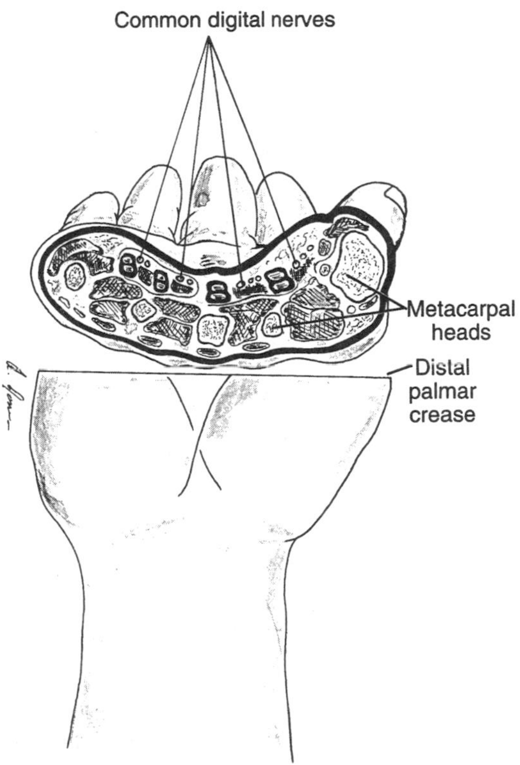

Figure 3.33. Metacarpal nerves. Cross-section of the hand showing the volar placement of the neurovascular bundle.

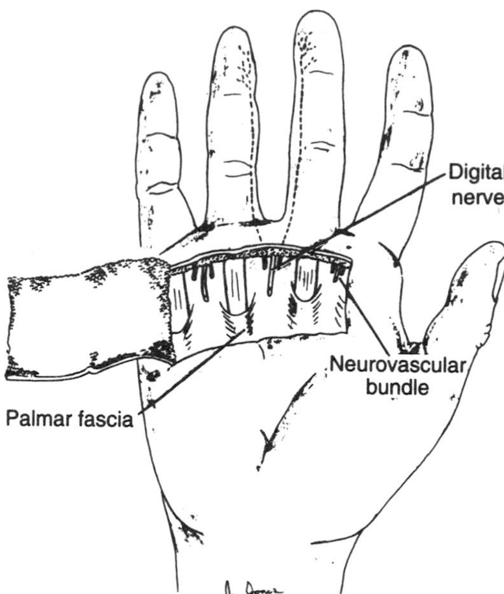

Figure 3.34. The metacarpal nerve block, also called the common digital nerve block, requires knowledge of the depth and location of the nerve. Note that this nerve and the arteries course adjacent to the flexor tendons, along the volar side of the palm. The interosseous muscles are dorsal to the nerve. Thus with the hand pronated and the fingers flexed, anesthetize the metacarpal nerve by inserting a needle in the dorsal web space between the metacarpal heads and directing the tip volarly, so that one can palpate swelling along the volar side of the web space, as the anesthetic is deposited.

adjacent fingers. This bifurcation occurs just proximal to the intermetacarpal ligament, at about the level of the distal palmar crease. The digital nerves lie very close to the palmar fascia and pass into individual digits just volar to the midlateral line and adjacent to the phalanges. Thus the digital nerves are 1 to 2 mm volar to the mid-axial line (Fig. 3.34).

The mid-axial line joins the loose dorsal skin and the tight volar skin. In performing this procedure, flex the metacarpophalangeal (M-P) joints to 30 degrees, and hold a finger in the web space where the anesthetic will be deposited. With a finger placed on the volar aspect of the web space, one should feel a sense of fullness as the lidocaine bolus is injected into the area (Fig. 3.35). If this fullness is not palpable, the needle is probably dorsal to the intermetacarpal fascia, and thus above the nerve.

Block the radial side of the index finger and the ulnar side of the little finger at the level of the distal palmar crease. Introduce the needle laterally just volar to the midaxial line, and inject 1 to 2 mL of 2% lidocaine solution (Fig. 3.36).

TECHNIQUE FOR BLOCKING A THUMB

The proper digital nerves to the thumb can be blocked at the level of the most proximal thumb flexor crease. These nerves are superficial and lie immediately adjacent to the readily palpable flexor pollicis longus tendon (Fig. 3.37). Introduce the needle at a depth of 2 to 3 mm in a slightly distal direction, along either side of the thumb flexor tendon. Inject 1 to 2 mL of 2% lidocaine, and palpate the subcutaneous fullness.

NERVE BLOCKS OF THE FOOT

Nerve blocks of the foot are commonly used in the emergency center when dealing with extensive lacerations involving the foot, particularly the sole, and when a deep exploratory procedure is needed for the removal of a foreign body (23). A number of nerves supply the foot, and these are discussed separately (Fig. 3.38).

Posterior Tibial Nerve Block

The posterior tibial nerve is located along the medial aspect of the ankle, coursing between the medial malleolus and the Achilles tendon (Fig 3.39) (3, 6, 23). The nerve accompanies the posterior tibial artery, lying just posterior and slightly deep to the artery. The nerve courses between the tendons of the flexor digitorum longus and the flexor hallucis longus muscles and is covered by the laciniate ligament. The nerve divides into medial and

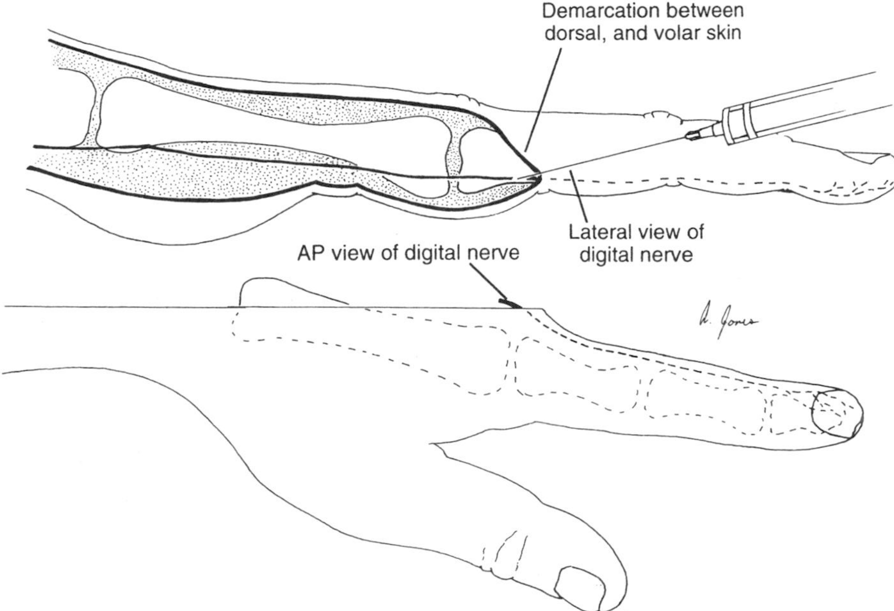

Figure 3.35. Note again that the common digital nerves are anesthetized by directing the needle as shown (Fig. 3.34). Hold a fingertip along the volar surface of the web space while injecting the anesthetic. Swelling should be palpated as the anesthetic is deposited. If swelling is not palpated, the anesthetic has probably gone dorsal to the ligaments and will not adequately anesthetize this nerve.

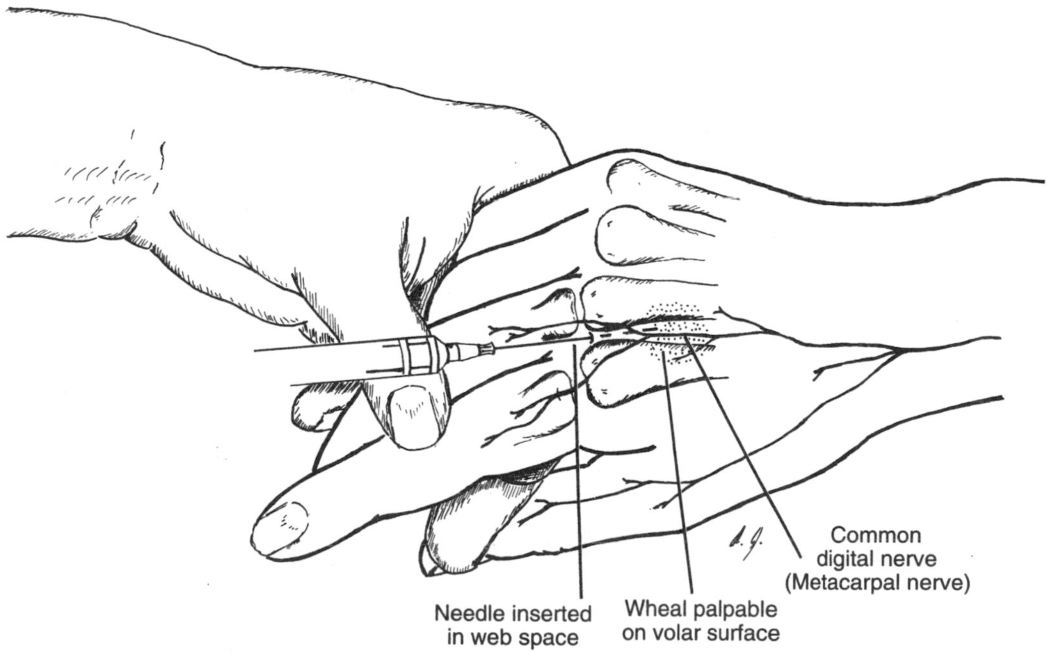

Figure 3.36. Block of the common digital nerve. See text for discussion.

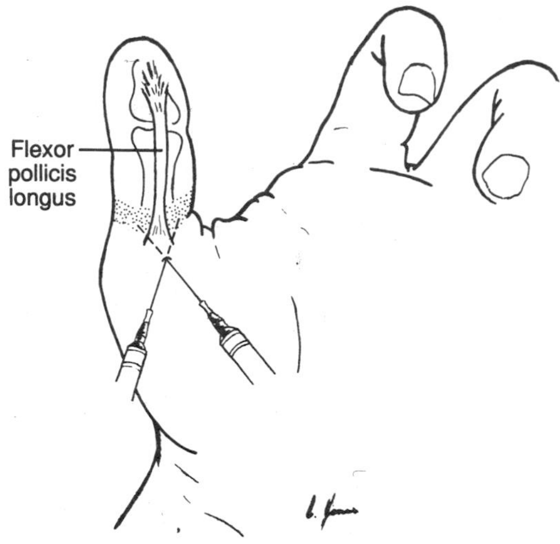

Figure 3.37. Nerve block of thumb.

lateral plantar branches, and these supply sensation to the sole of the foot.

TECHNIQUE (3, 6, 8, 23, 35)

Locate the base of the medial malleolus and the Achilles tendon, which serve as landmarks for the injection. Place the patient in a prone position when doing the procedure. Palpate the posterior tibial artery, and insert a 23-gauge, 2-inch needle perpendicular to the skin just medial to the Achilles tendon at the level of the upper border of the medial malleolus. Direct the needle immediately lateral to the artery, and advance it until it touches the tibia (Fig. 3.40*A*). Attempt to elicit paresthesias by moving the needle medially and laterally. When paresthesias are elicited in the sole, inject 5 mL of 1% lidocaine. If paresthesias are not elicited, inject 10 mL of solution along the posterior border of the tibia while the needle is slowly withdrawn. Anesthesia usually occurs in 5 to 10 minutes when paresthesia is elicited and in 20 to 30 minutes when paresthesia is not elicited. Almost the entire sole can be anesthetized with this block, with the exception of the proximal area, which is supplied by the sural nerve and the lateral portion.

SURAL AND SAPHENOUS NERVE BLOCKS

The sural and saphenous nerves supply sensation to the lateral and medial aspects of the foot, respectively. Figure 3.41 shows the level at which these two nerves are present. Notice that they are within the subcutaneous tissue on either side of the foot.

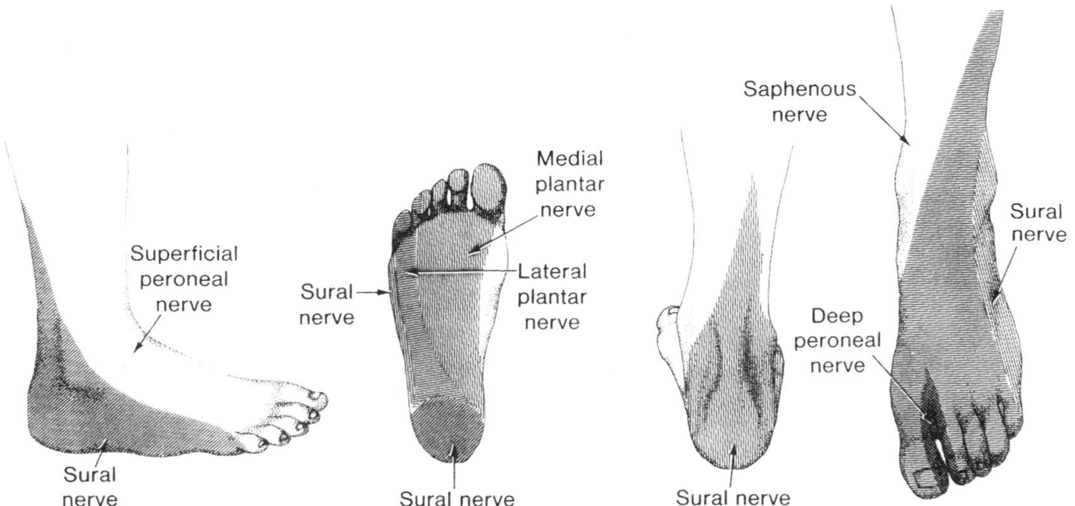

Figure 3.38. The sensory nerve supply to the foot.

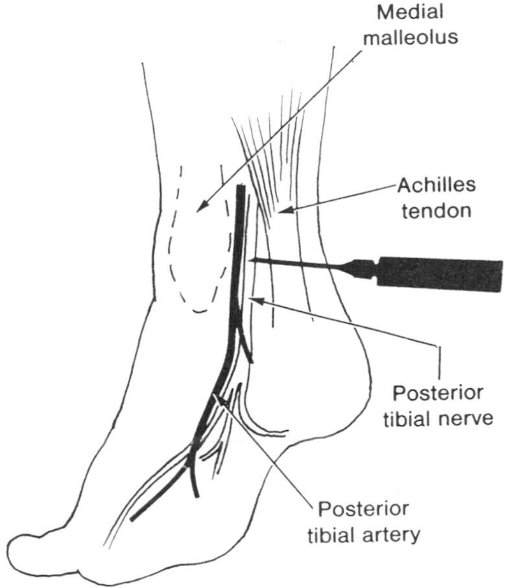

Figure 3.39. Posterior tibial nerve block. The nerve accompanies the posterior tibial artery and lies slightly deep and "lateral" to the artery.

The sural nerve can be blocked by inserting a needle adjacent and lateral to the Achilles tendon and depositing the anesthetic in the subcutaneous tissue, as shown (Fig. 3.42).

Sural Nerve Block

The sural nerve is a cutaneous nerve that becomes subcutaneous distal to the middle of the leg and courses along with the short saphenous vein behind the lateral malleolus to supply sensation to the posterior lateral aspect of the ankle and heel, and the lateral plantar aspect of the foot and fifth toe (Fig. 3.38). This nerve passes in the subcutaneous tissue just lateral to the Achilles tendon.

TECHNIQUE

This nerve is usually blocked along with blocking the posterior tibial nerve when complete anesthesia is desired for procedures performed at the heel of the foot. The landmarks for finding the sural nerve are the Achilles tendon and the outer border of the lateral malleolus. Place the patient in the prone position. Introduce a 23-gauge, 1.5-inch needle just lateral to the Achilles tendon, at a level of 1 cm above the lateral malleolus (Fig. 3.40*B*). Direct the needle toward a spot 1 cm superior to the malleolus of the fibula, and infiltrate 5 mL of 1% lidocaine as the needle is moved in a fanwise fashion within the subcutaneous tissue between the lateral malleolus and the Achilles tendon (Figs. 3.41 and 3.42).

Saphenous Nerve Block

The saphenous nerve runs parallel to the saphenous vein in the subcutaneous tissue on the anteromedial aspect of the ankle (35). It is one of the superficial nerves supplying the anterior aspect of the foot and is a sensory branch of the femoral nerve, becoming subcutaneous at the lateral side of the knee joint (Figs. 3.40*C*, 3.41, 3.42).

TECHNIQUE

Place the patient in the supine position, with a sandbag or pillow under the calf to relax the foot in a plantar-flexed posture (23). To block the nerve, infiltrate the anesthetic solution subcutaneously along a line extending from the medial malleolus to the tendon of the extensor hallucis longus (Fig. 3.43). Mark a line circumscribing the ankle, approximately 1 cm above the base of the medial malleolus. At a point on the line just medial to the extensor hallucis longus tendon, insert a 1.5-inch, 23-gauge needle perpendicular to the skin until it reaches the tibia, and then slightly withdraw the needle, and inject a small amount (2 mL) of anesthetic solution, followed by a subcutaneous injection toward the malleolus.

Superficial Peroneal Nerve Block

The superficial peroneal nerve runs subcutaneously along the dorsum of the foot, after piercing the fascia along the

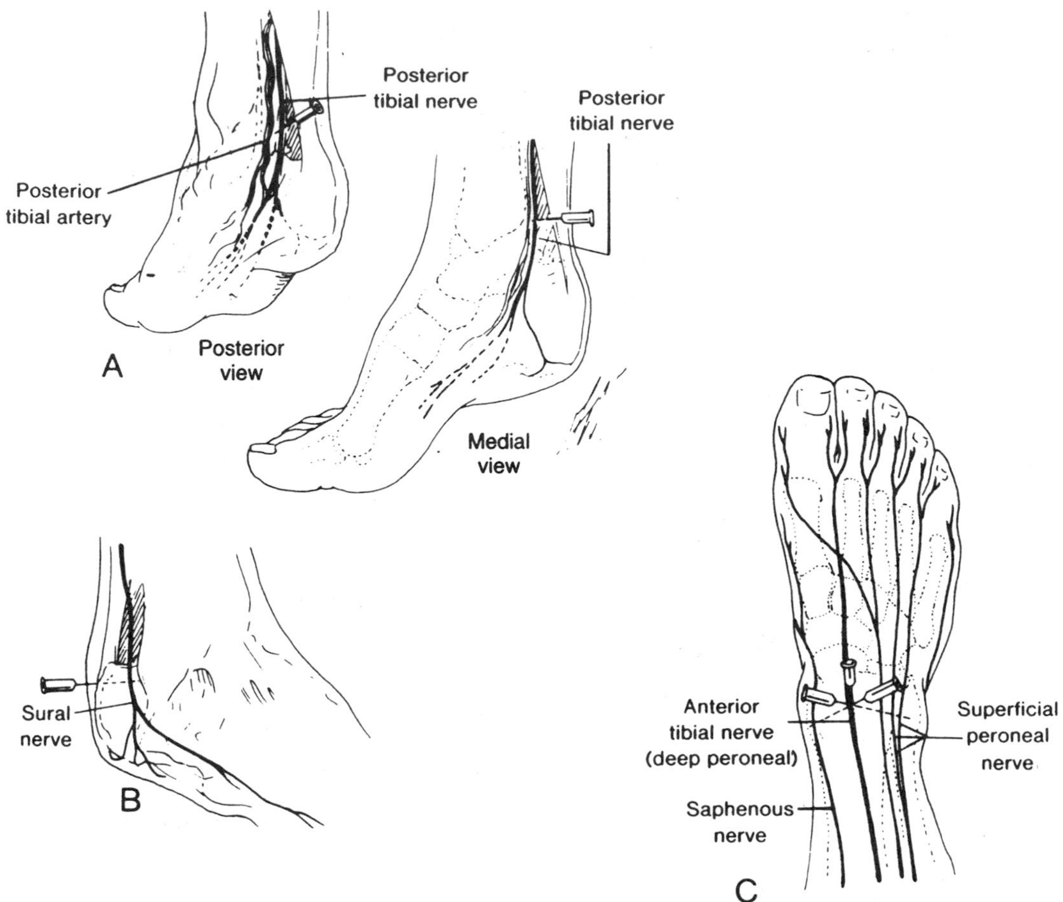

Figure 3.40. The technique of posterior tibial, sural, and anterior tibial nerve block. See text for details. (From Locke RK, Locke SE: Nerve blocks of the foot. JACEP 5:701, 1976, with permission.)

anterior aspect of the lower leg. It has a wide area of distribution, supplying the entire dorsum of the foot except for the small area between the first and second toe, which is innervated by the anterior tibial nerve (Figs. 3.38 and 3.40*C*).

TECHNIQUE

Block the superficial peroneal nerve by injecting 5 to 10 mL of 0.5% lidocaine subcutaneously in a line from the anterior border of the tibia to the lateral malleolus. This block and that of the saphenous nerve can often be performed from one injection site, as shown in Figs. 3.40 and 3.43 (23).

Anterior Tibial Nerve Block (Deep Peroneal Nerve Block)

The deep peroneal nerve is largely muscular in its innervation; however, it does supply sensation to the area between the first and second toes (Fig. 3.38). The origin of the nerve is the medial branch of the lateral popliteal nerve after it crosses the neck of the fibula. It passes deep to the flexor retinaculum at the ankle and emerges toward the base of the first and second toes, supplying a small area between these toes (8). The nerve is usually blocked when procedures are performed in the region of

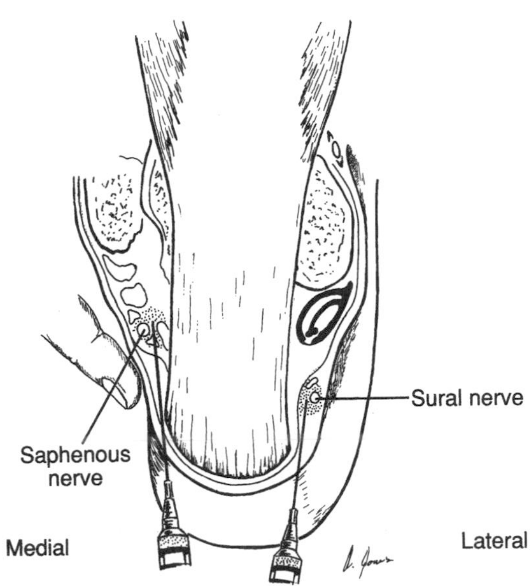

Figure 3.41. The depth of the sural and saphenous nerves. Note that the sural nerve is more posteriorly located. See text for discussion.

its sensation (3, 6). The deep peroneal nerve lies between the tendons of the tibialis anterior and the extensor hallucis longus.

TECHNIQUE

Insert a 2- to 3-cm needle dorsally on the foot, midway between the medial and lateral malleoli (Figs. 3.40*C* and 3.43). At less than 1 cm depth, the anterior aspect of the tibia is encountered, and at this point, deposit 3 to 4 mL of 0.5% lidocaine solution, which will spread between the flexor tendons and the bone (8). Paresthesias occasionally may be elicited. Alternatively, when the extensor hallucis longus muscle or the tibialis anterior can be identified, they serve as excellent landmarks for the point of injection. With the patient supine, insert the needle lateral to the tendon of the tibialis anterior until the tibia is encountered. Withdraw the needle approximately 3 mm, and inject 5 mL of 1% lidocaine into this area. Some authors have suggested that, in addition, the needle should be withdrawn and directed laterally between the extensor hallucis longus and extensor digitorum longus

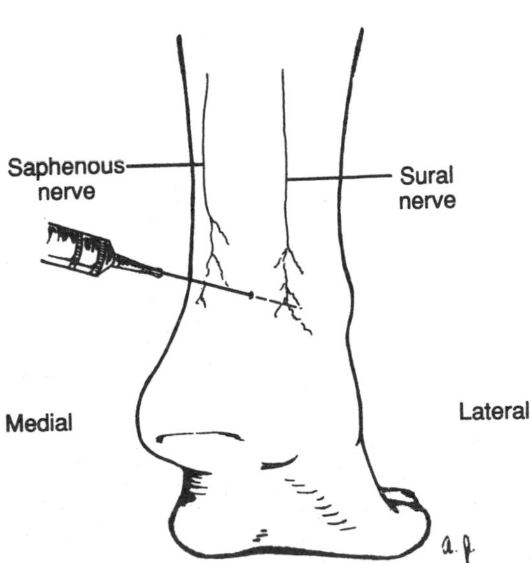

Figure 3.42. Infiltration of the branches of the sural and saphenous nerve with the posterior approach. See text for discussion.

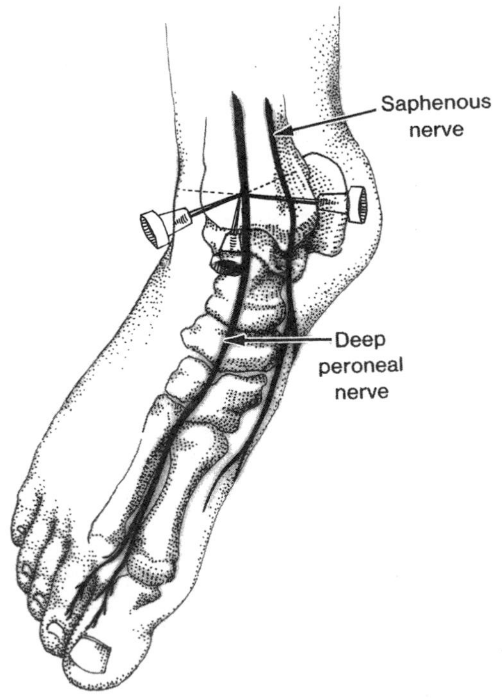

Figure 3.43. The saphenous and deep peroneal nerve blocks. See text for discussion.

tendons until the tibia is encountered, and additional anesthetic solution should be deposited here (3).

NOTE

A new approach to block the tibial nerve is described, based on applied anatomy of the osteofascial compartments of the leg and the constant position of the tibial nerve, located halfway between the medial border of the tibial and the fibula at the level of the tibial tubercle. The common peroneal nerve also may be blocked by a similar method. As the principal nerves of the leg are confined to the compartments, the duration of action of local anesthetic is prolonged, an advantage in postoperative pain relief. Continuous block is less traumatic than standard techniques because by aiming at a compartment, the nerve trunk is no longer in the target area for the needle point. Although much of the cutaneous innervation of the leg (supplied by the saphenous nerve and the sural nerve) is spared by compartmental block, these nerves can be dealt with simply by infiltration if necessary and have little significance in postoperative pain control for surgical procedures of the foot.

TECHNIQUE FOR COMPARTMENTAL BLOCK

Tibial Nerve (Posterior Compartment) Block

The tibial nerve lies under cover of the posterior intermuscular septum, forming part of a neurovascular bundle with the posterior tibial artery and veins, which run inferiorly in direct relation to the flexors of the toes. Introduce the needle approximately at a right angle to the medial surface of the tibia but aimed toward the fibula to a depth nearly equal to the width of the medial subcutaneous surface of the tibia or, alternatively, exactly equal to half the distance between the posterior border of the medial surface and the lateral surface of the fibula. At this depth, the tip of the needle lies very near to the tibial nerve in the deep subcompartment of the posterior compartment. A nerve stimulator always provokes a response at this position with an effective outcome for the operative field after injection of a local anesthetic.

Common Peroneal Nerve Block (Peroneal Compartment)

The common peroneal nerve may be blocked in the peroneal compartment before the nerve divides. With the leg to be anesthetized placed in a neutral position, palpate the head of the fibula with the insertion of the biceps femoris. After the usual preparation, introduce a nerve-block needle 2.5 cm below the head of the fibula in a horizontal direction, aiming at the lateral surface of the fibula and not at the nerve until contact is made with the bone. Then withdraw the needle 1 to 2 mm, and inject 5 to 7 mL of local anesthetic into the compartment. The block can be repeated at the bedside for postoperative pain relief (26).

NOTE

Slow injection of the local anesthetic is an important factor in reducing pain during penile block (38).

Sciatic Nerve Block

Most foot and ankle procedures can technically be performed in an outpatient setting. Postoperative pain usually limits what procedures can be done on an outpatient basis and is the most common reason for unanticipated hospital admissions. Therefore, pain management plays an important role in length of postoperative stay and the associated costs. Blocks of the lower extremity for surgery have become popular, and popliteal sciatic nerve blocks have been used for intraoperative anesthesia with generally good results. This also can be used in selected cases in emergency medicine.

TECHNIQUE

Place the patient in a prone position with the knee slightly flexed on a pillow. The landmarks of the popliteal fossa can then be identified. The horizontal skin crease divides the fossa into superior and inferior quadrants. The triangular superior quadrant is bordered medially by the semimembranosus and semitendinous muscles and laterally by the biceps femoris. Choose a point 7 to 8 cm (about four finger breadths) superior to the popliteal skin crease and 1 cm lateral to the midline. This location is just medial to the biceps femoris border, near the apex of the popliteal fossa. This is usually near the level where the common peroneal branch of the sciatic nerve leaves the tibial branch. Therefore blockade of both nerves is possible at this point. With this technique, a nerve stimulator is necessary (39). Thus because this is not readily available in the emergency department, this technique is less useful for the emergency physician.

Alternative Approach

The classic posterior approach to the sciatic nerve in the popliteal fossa requires placement of the patient in the prone position, which may be contraindicated in pregnant woman or impossible in selected trauma patients. Some clinicians prefer a lateral approach to the sciatic nerve in the popliteal fossa. With this approach, place the patient in a supine position, and palpate the upper edge of the patella and the groove between the lateral border of the vastus lateralis and the tendon of the biceps femoris, and draw them on the skin of the patient. To facilitate identification of the groove, ask the patient to flex the knee, and then straighten the leg again. Draw a line vertically from the upper border of the patella. The puncture site is located at the intersection of this line with the intermuscular groove. After standard skin preparation using a 22-gauge needle, insert the long 50-mm needle 20 to 30 degrees posterior to the horizontal plain with a slight caudal direction (43). Once again, this technique is not useful in the emergency setting but is described here for completeness.

Block of the Great Toe

To anesthetize the great toe, block the base of the toe circumferentially by depositing anesthetic solution subcutaneously. Insert a 1.5-inch, 25-gauge needle attached to a 10-mL syringe containing 1% lidocaine without epinephrine at the anterior lateral portion of the toe (point *A*, Fig. 3.44) and

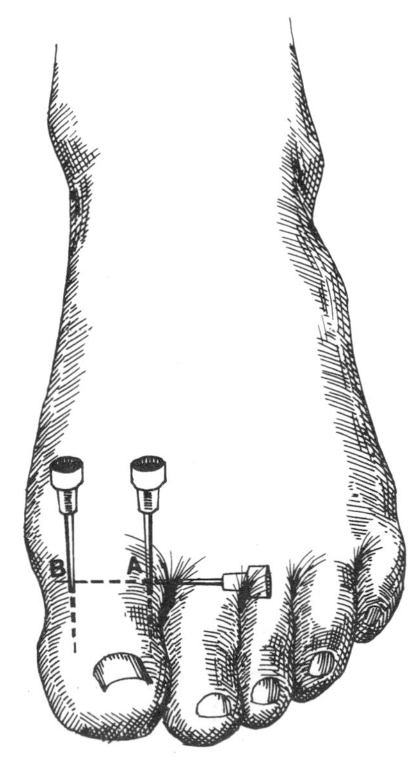

Figure 3.44. Block of the great toe. See text for discussion.

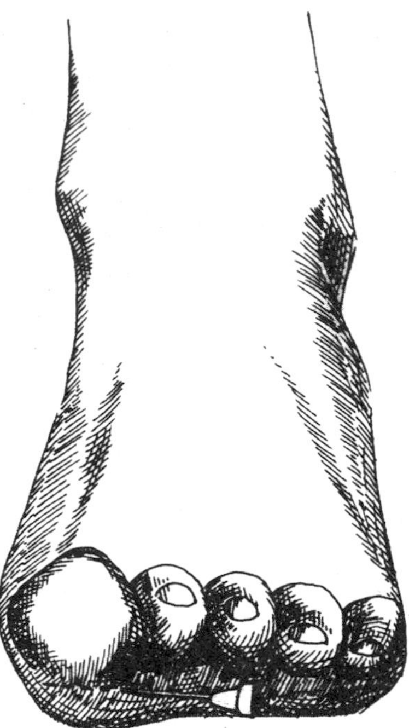

Figure 3.45. Block of the great toe. See text for discussion.

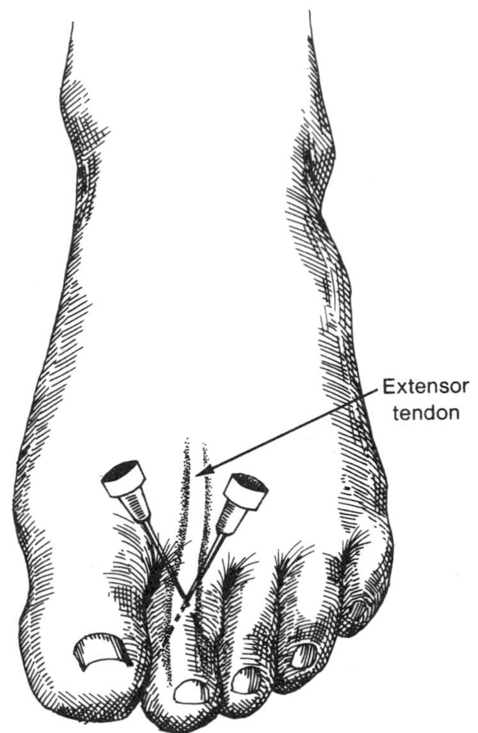

Figure 3.46. Block of the toes other than the great toe. The needle was inserted in the midline dorsally over the extensor tendon and directed to either side of the digit. See text for discussion.

direct it medially in the subcutaneous tissue. Deposit the anesthetic solution as the needle is advanced, and then redirect the needle posteriorly through the same puncture site, and deposit additional anesthetic solution in this area. Then introduce the needle at a second puncture site along the anterior medial portion of the great toe (point *B*, Fig. 3.44), and deposit the anesthetic solution posteriorly, as shown in Fig. 3.44. Finally, to complete the circumferential block, introduce the needle at the base of the toe over the volar aspect, as shown in Fig. 3.45, and direct it medially; anesthetic solution is deposited in this portion as well. The block usually takes 5 to 10 minutes to take effect.

Blocks of the Toes Other Than the Great Toe

To block the remainder of the toes of the foot, deposit anesthetic solution through one needle puncture at the dorsum of the toes in the midpoint, as shown in Fig. 3.46. Insert the needle at the midpoint of the dorsum of the foot, and direct it laterally and medially to the extensor tendon; deposit 2 mL of 1% lidocaine solution along each side of the toes. This technique provides good anesthesia for repairing lacerations of the toes, as well as for removing foreign bodies and dealing with nailbed injuries.

BLOCKS OF THE TORSO AND OTHER AREAS

Block of the Intercostal Nerves

The intercostal nerves course inferior to the ribs along with the intercostal artery and vein. The first six intercostal nerves carry sensation only to the chest, and the lower intercostals also carry sensation to the abdomen. The most common occasion necessitating intercostal nerve block in the emergency center is in the patient with rib fractures. This is particularly true in the elderly, in whom hypoventilation secondary to pain can result in serious complications, especially respiratory infections. Most of the patients with simple rib fractures who die do so of pneumonia, which has a fairly high incidence in the elderly (36). We advise that no attempt be made to immobilize the chest mechanically (strapping, taping, rib belts) in the elderly because of this complication. Rib blocks with long-acting anesthetics (bupivacaine; Marcaine) provide good anesthesia during the acute phase and permit good respiration and coughing, thus avoiding atelectasis and pneumonia (6, 36).

INDICATIONS

This is used in rib fractures for pain relief and to permit full inspiration without pain.

TECHNIQUE

The intercostal nerves can best be blocked in the area of the costal angles posteriorly, just lateral to the lateral border of the erector spinae muscles. This avoids the deep mass of paravertebral muscles in the middle of the back. In the average adult, this is about 3 inches from the midline. Place the patient in the sitting position, leaning forward over a pillow placed on the lap with the arms folded. This displaces the scapula laterally, permitting easier palpation of the rib borders. With the index finger of the left hand, palpate the rib or ribs to be injected, and pull the skin overlying the rib cephalad to tense it (Fig. 3.47). Insert at a right angle to the skin, a 23-gauge or smaller long needle attached to a 5-mL syringe filled with bupivacaine until it strikes the outer aspect of the rib (9). Cautiously walk the tip of the needle inferiorly until it slips off the edge of the rib, advance the needle 3 mm farther (half the thickness of the adult rib), and inject 5 mL of 1% lidocaine (Fig. 3.48) (35). Usually block the intercostal nerve above and below the affected rib to provide good anesthesia for rib pain.

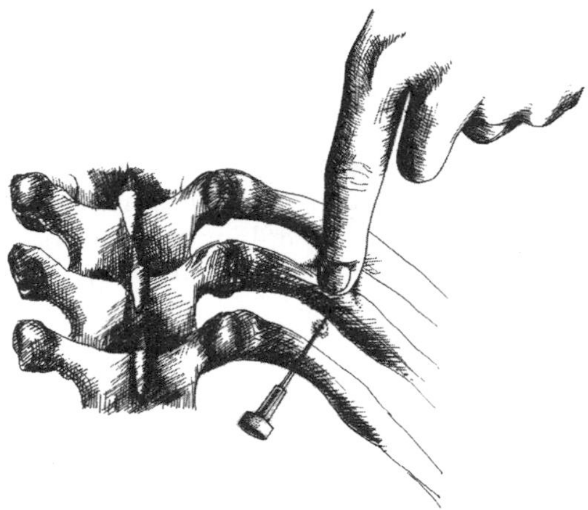

Figure 3.47. The intercostal nerve block. With the index finger of the left hand, palpate the rib to be injected and pull the skin overlying the rib cephalad. Insert the needle at a right angle to the skin and touch the rib.

COMPLICATIONS

1. **Pneumothorax.** Pneumothorax is the most frequent complication reported secondary to intercostal nerve block (9, 35, 36). The use of a small-gauge

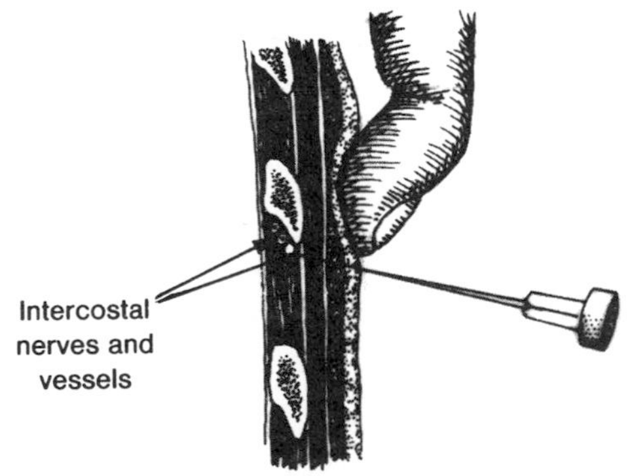

Figure 3.48. The intercostal nerves lie beneath the rib margin, accompanied by the intercostal arteries. "Walk" the needle cautiously down the rib until it passes just beneath the inferior margin. Deposit the anesthetic solution here. Exercise caution not to go too deeply when passing the needle beneath the rib margin.

needle and care in avoiding penetrating deeper than the distance indicated earlier should avoid this complication. If coughing is induced, discontinue the injection until the needle is properly placed, because coughing often indicates intrapleural penetration. All patients with an intercostal nerve block should have a chest radiograph performed after the procedure.

2. **Puncture of intercostal blood vessel** with a small hematoma. To avoid this complication, be certain to aspirate before injecting, as with all blocks.
3. **Cerebrospinal fluid aspiration.** This rare complication results from a severely misdirected needle (36). With proper care, this complication should not occur.

Transvaginal Pudendal Nerve Block

The pudendal nerve forms a single trunk 0.5 to 1 cm proximal to the ischial spine (21). It passes posterior to the spine, between the sacrospinous ligament anteriorly and the sacrotuberous ligament posteriorly to enter the lesser sciatic foramen (Fig. 3.49). The pudendal nerve arises from anterior divisions of S2, S3, and S4, and as the nerve crosses the spine of the ischium, it courses medial to the internal pudendal vessels to enter the pelvis. Two approaches for anesthetizing the pudendal nerve have been described in the literature: the transvaginal approach (Fig. 3.50) (5, 17, 22, 41) and the percutaneous extravaginal approach (Fig. 3.51) (21). The transvaginal approach is the procedure of choice because it is simpler to administer the anesthetic agent accurately to the region of the pudendal nerve and thereby reduce the trauma of injection. There are no complications such as infection or hemorrhage with this procedure, and there is no interference with uterine contractile ability (17). The incidence of postpartum hemorrhage is

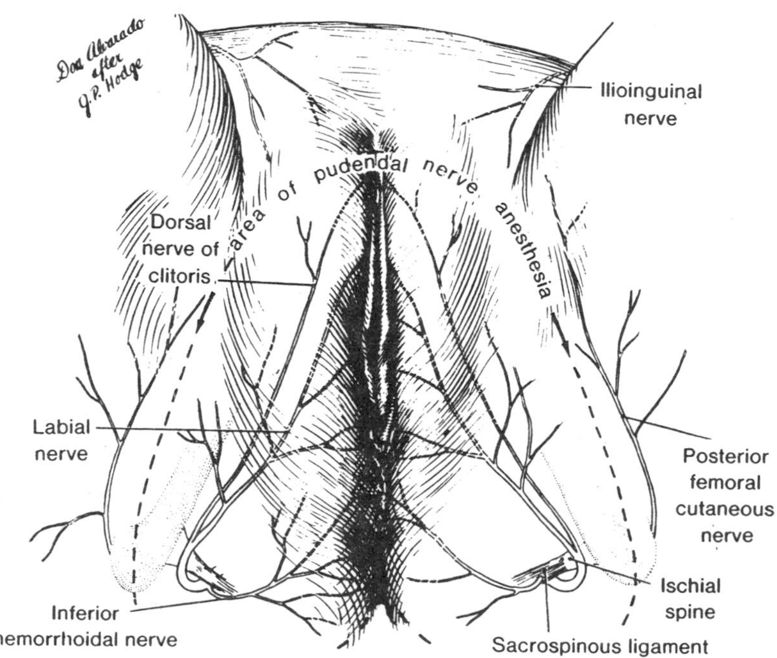

Figure 3.49. The pudendal nerve as it courses beneath the sacrospinous ligament. The inferior hemorrhoidal nerve and labial nerve are branches of the internal pudendal nerve, as shown. (From Wilds PL: Transvaginal pudendal nerve block. Obstet Gynecol 8:386, 1956, with permission.)

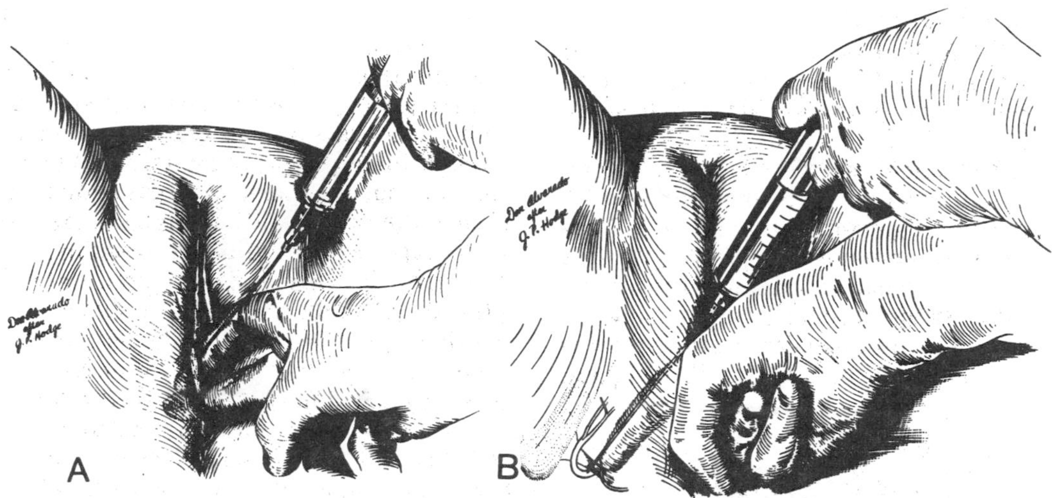

Figure 3.50. The transvaginal approach for internal pudendal nerve block. The technique of inserting the needle into the vagina *(A)*. The needle tip lies flat against the ball of the index finger during insertion. The sacrospinous ligament is pierced by the needle *(B)*. Deposit the anesthetic solution at this site. (From Wilds PL: Transvaginal pudendal nerve block. Obstet Gynecol 8:386, 1956, with permission.)

lessened, and there is no effect of the anesthetic on the fetus.

In the primiparous patient, the injection is withheld until the second stage of labor when there is complete cervical dilatation (5). In the multiparous patient, the injection is best withheld until 6 to 8 cm of cervical dilatation (22, 37).

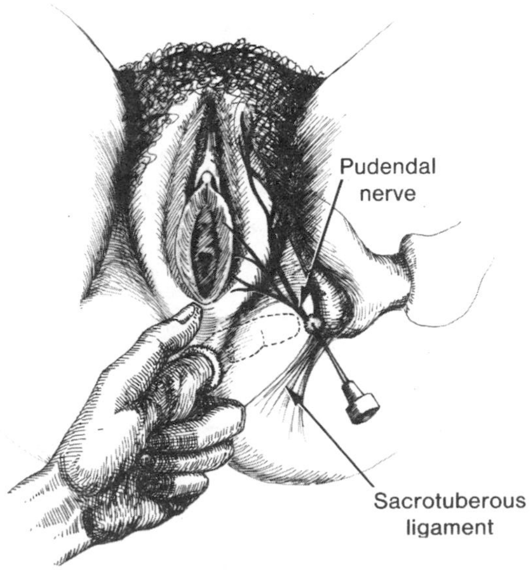

Figure 3.51. The percutaneous extravaginal approach. See text for discussion.

INDICATIONS

This procedure, when performed properly, provides good anesthesia for vaginal delivery, particularly in the multiparous patient. In the primiparous patient, more complete anesthesia may be necessary because of the greater pain experienced during delivery.

TECHNIQUE

A 6-inch, 20-gauge spinal needle with a 10-mL syringe is used for this procedure. Alternatively, a special needle is available with a needle guard that protects against advancing the needle too far. Prepare the patient for the delivery, but no vaginal preparation is necessary. Locate the ischial spines vaginally and hold the needle and attached syringe filled with 1% lidocaine with the tip of the needle pressed flatly against the ball of the index finger so that it is protected by and guided by the finger in its passage through the vagina (Fig. 3.50) (5, 37, 41). Alternatively, hold the needle between the index and middle fingers of the left hand (16). With the needle held parallel to the index finger and guided by the finger, carry it into the vagina to the tip of the ischial spine. Then pass the tip of the needle by lifting the finger and advancing it into the vaginal mucosa overlying the sacrospinous ligament, which is palpated just posterior and medial to the tip of the ischial spine.

NOTE

The most significant limiting factor in this technique is the occasional difficulty in identifying the sacrospinous ligament because it is so thin and relaxed in some multiparous patients at term. When this does occur, pass the needle just inferior and posterior to the ischial spine (22).

Infiltrate the ligament with 2 to 3 mL of 1% lidocaine; then the needle pierces the ligament and enters the loose tissue that contains the nerve. At this point, the resistance of the plunger decreases, and the fluid flows easily. Aspirate before injection to be certain the artery is not entered,

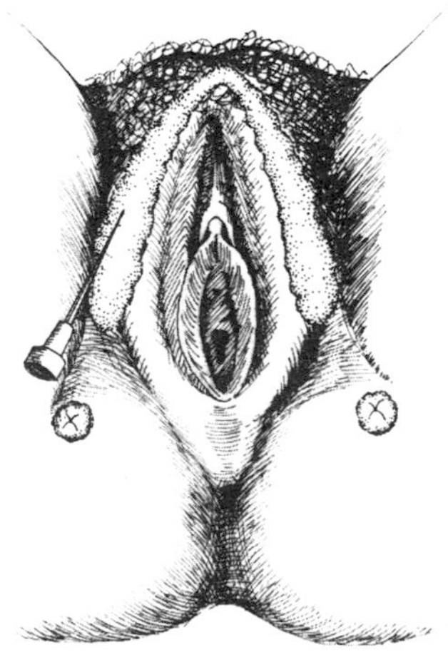

Figure 3.52. The points of insertion of the needle over the ischial tuberosities (*X*).

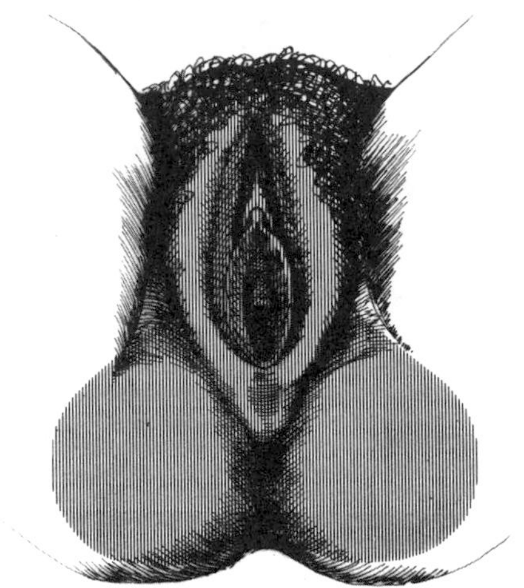

Figure 3.53. The area of anesthesia provided by a pudendal nerve block.

and deposit the fluid (5 mL) beneath the ligament. Repeat this same procedure on the opposite side.

With the extravaginal approach, the point of insertion of the needle is over the ischial tuberosities, as shown in Fig. 3.52. The procedure is similar to that of the intravaginal approach, with the exception that the physician places his index finger into the rectum, as shown in Fig. 3.51 and palpates the ischial spine, sacrospinous ligament, and sacrotuberous ligament per rectum. Then direct the needle toward the pudendal nerve, and infiltrate 5 to 10 mL of 1% lidocaine in this site. Repeat the procedure on the opposite side. The area of anesthesia provided by a bilateral pudendal nerve block is shown in Fig. 3.53.

Block of the Penis

Block of the penis can be easily performed. Inadequate anesthesia is usually secondary to poor infiltration of the anesthetic solution.

INDICATIONS

A block of the penis is used for repair of penile lacerations.

TECHNIQUE

With the patient supine, localize two points above the penis that are the sites of injection. Palpate the tubercles of the pubic bone, and locate the points 1/2-inch caudad and 1/2-inch medial to them. These points can be marked, because they are the two superior sites where the needle is to be inserted. The inferior site is on the median raphe of the scrotum at the base of the penis. Use a 25-gauge, 3-inch needle and 1% lidocaine with epinephrine for this block. Vigorous shaking of the penis will decrease the pain of injection. Carefully connect the two superior points with a linear infiltration of anesthetic deposited both intradermally and subcutaneously. Connect the site beneath the penis to the ends of the linear wheal just deposited superiorly, thereby forming a triangle (Fig. 3.54). Again, be careful to deposit the anesthetic both intradermally and subcutaneously. Finally, deposit a ring of anesthetic solution around the base of the penis, between the corpora cavernosa and the deep penile fascia (Fig. 3.55); otherwise, the small nerve filaments that innervate the posterolateral sides of the penis and the frenulum will not be anesthetized. Pass the needle through the "points of the triangle," and direct the solution as far as the corpus cavernosum each time, depositing a ring of anesthetic solution at the base of the penis in a fanlike fashion.

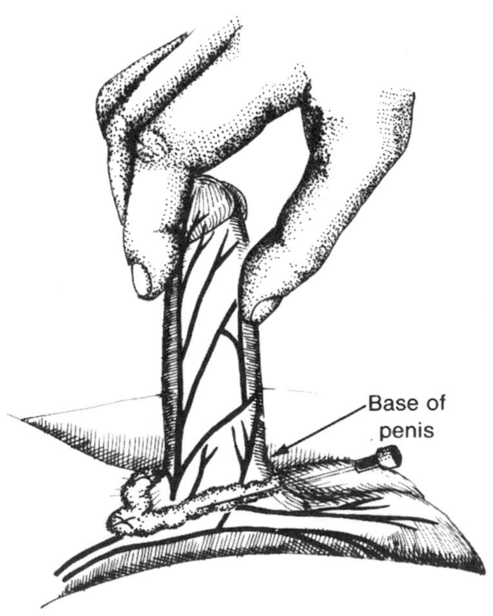

Figure 3.54. Deposit a subcutaneous wheal of anesthesia in a triangular fashion at the base of the penis.

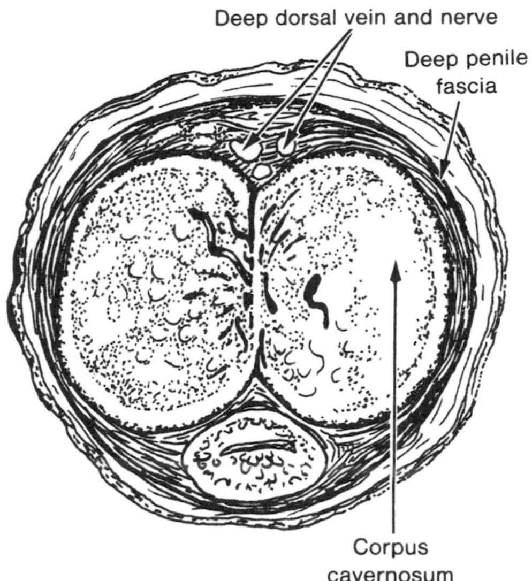

Figure 3.55. Deposit a ring of anesthetic around the base of the penis between the corpora cavernosa and the deep penile fascia to anesthetize the small nerve filaments.

NOTE

Slow injection of the local anesthetic is an important factor in reducing pain during penile block (38).

Urethral Anesthesia

Urethral anesthesia may be necessary for certain painful procedures involved with catheterization.

INDICATIONS

1. Catheterization.
2. Bougienage, if stricture is not too tight.

TECHNIQUE

Lidocaine gel is used in this procedure. Hold the penis firmly in the left hand, attach a plastic applicator to the tube of lidocaine gel, and insert it into the meatus. Express the gel gently from the tube into the urethra (9). Apply a penile clamp to prevent the gel from running out. Massage the gel backward into the posterior part of the urethra, and leave in place for 5 to 10 min for maximal effect.

Infiltration Anesthesia for Cesarean Section

The abdominal wall receives its sensory nerve supply from the lumbar nerves and the lower six intercostal nerves. These nerves give off cutaneous branches just lateral to the midline.

INDICATIONS

Emergency cesarean section.

TECHNIQUE

Infiltrate between the symphysis pubis and approximately 1 cm above the umbilicus to provide adequate anesthesia. The anesthetic solution should be 0.5% lidocaine with 1:200,000 epinephrine. Total dose should not exceed 100 mL. A 10-cm needle is used to infiltrate the abdominal wall. Hold the needle parallel to the surface of the skin. Inject the local agent during both insertion and withdrawal of the needle. This raises a wheal linearly parallel to and on both sides of the linea alba. This does not provide complete anesthesia for the patient and may have to be augmented. Nitrous oxide, when available, is a good agent to use.

Anesthesia of the Surface of the Cornea and Conjunctiva

Topical application of anesthetic solutions commercially available (Ophthaine) to the surface of the conjunctiva provides good surface anesthesia for some procedures (9). Deposit two drops in the conjunctival sac rather than directly on the cornea. This gives good analgesia for the cornea and conjunctiva but has no effect on any deeper structures (9).

The number of instillations is far more important than the amount administered at each instillation.

INDICATIONS

1. Tonometry. This procedure usually requires only one instillation of 2 to 3 drops of anesthetic solution.
2. Corneal foreign body removal. This generally requires repeated instillations, especially if the foreign body is situated in the area of the limbus where the blood vessels rapidly remove the anesthetic agent. Normally the first instillation causes a little pain and blepharospasm. When the discomfort has disappeared, usually within 30 seconds to 1 minute, a second instillation is made. If this should again cause pain, a third instillation may be necessary.
3. Conjunctival lacerations or foreign body. This requires more frequent instillations, repeated at short intervals. Conjunctival anesthesia is less effective than corneal anesthesia, especially when the conjunctiva is inflamed.

Hematoma Block for Reduction of a Fracture

Infiltration of a fracture hematoma is a useful block for reduction of some fractures, particularly in situations in which little manipulation is necessary. Palpate the site of the fracture, and puncture the fracture hematoma with a 21-gauge, 1.5-inch needle attached to a 10-mL syringe filled with 2% lidocaine without epinephrine. As the needle enters the hematoma around the fracture, aspirate blood into the syringe. At this point, inject the anesthetic solution slowly. Rapid injection may be quite painful. Wait approximately 10 to 15 minutes before proceeding with the reduction. Anesthesia obtained by this method is not comparable to that of nerve block or intravenous regional anesthesia; the latter are our preferred techniques for most fracture reductions. Hematoma block is not recommended for routine use and is indicated only in situations in which time does not permit performance of a regional block.

Intravenous Regional Analgesia (Bier Block)

The technique of intravenous regional anesthesia that involves the injection of a local anesthetic into a vein in an extremity after application of a tourniquet proximally was first described by Bier, but was largely reintroduced by Holmes (8). No knowledge of anatomy is required to perform this procedure. A suitable vein, preferably on the dorsum of the hand, is essential (8). Although this method of anesthesia can be used for both upper extremity and lower extremity procedures, intravenous regional anesthesia of the leg is not recommended by some authors (8) because the total amount of anesthetic needed for good analgesia is large, and the risk of cuff deflation is high. Cuff deflation would result in the release of a large volume of anesthesia into the circulation, producing toxicity. In addition, the anterior and posterior tibial vessels lie in the interosseous membrane, and a tourniquet applied beneath the knee would be ineffective in occluding these vessels and keeping the anesthetic from entering the circulation (8). This type of anesthesia is particularly useful for procedures involving the forearm and hand; however, it cannot be used for procedures involving the arm because the greater part of the cuff covers the arm. The primary indications in the emergency center for intravenous regional anesthesia are for soft tissue injuries and reduction of fractures involving the forearm and hand (8, 31).

TECHNIQUE

Preparatory Steps

1. Collect 40 mL of 0.5% lidocaine without epinephrine in a 50-mL syringe. Alternatively, a 20-mL bolus of 1% lidocaine, without epinephrine, can be injected.
2. Locate a suitable vein, preferably on the dorsum of the hand.
3. Begin a standard intravenous infusion in the contralateral arm for an intravenous route in case adverse reactions occur and the administration of emergency drugs becomes necessary (35).

Procedural Steps

1. With the patient in the supine position, place a sphygmomanometer cuff around the upper arm and inflate it to distend the vein distally. Insert a needle into the vein selected, and deflate the cuff (Fig. 3.56) (8).
2. Exsanguinate the arm with the application of an Esmarch bandage or, if this is impossible because of the nature of the lesion, elevate the arm for a few minutes to allow the blood to drain out of the vessels.
3. After the bandage has been applied, inflate the cuff to approximately 100 mm Hg above systolic pressure to prevent the arm from refilling with blood (8, 35). Lower the arm, and remove the bandage.
4. Inject 40 mL of 0.5% lidocaine without epinephrine into the vein. In procedures in the lower extremity, approximately 60 to 80 mL is required for the adult leg. Almost immediately there will be the onset of warmth, tingling, and numbness of the arm. Arm paralysis and analgesia is usually complete after 5 minutes. If analgesia is incomplete after 5 minutes, inject a further 5 to 10 mL of solution into the vein selected. As long as the tourniquet is in place, analgesia is maintained distal to it, and one can leave the tourniquet in place for 60 to 90

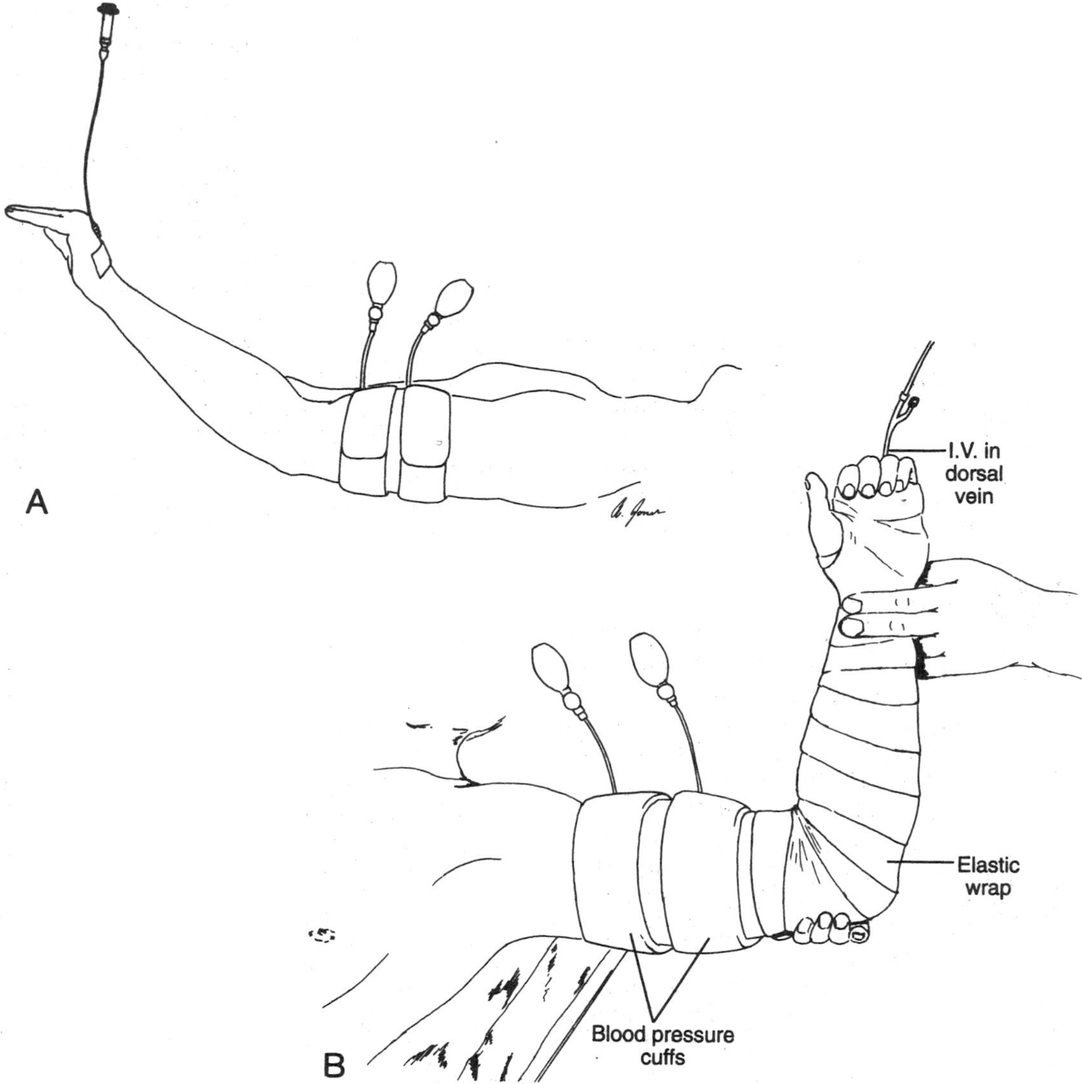

Figure 3.56. *A:* The Bier block. Insert a needle into a dorsal vein of the hand. *B:* Apply elastic wraps distally to proximally, to drain the blood from the superficial venous system in the hand and forearm, as follows. Attach two blood pressure cuffs along the arm as shown. Inflate the proximal cuff first. Then administer the anesthetic through the inserted needle into a dorsal vein of the hand. After anesthesia is obtained in the hand and forearm, inflate the more distal blood pressure cuff (as described in the text), and release the proximal one. This allows the blood pressure cuff to be inflated over anesthetized skin. See text for details.

minutes, permitting enough time to perform most necessary procedures.

CAUTION

The sphygmomanometer cuff used must be able to maintain pressure without leaking during the entire procedure. If the cuff is not capable of doing so, a large bolus of anesthetic will be released into the circulation and may cause a toxic reaction. A pneumatic tourniquet may be used instead of a sphygmomanometer and is applied to the limb proximal to the side of operation. Clamping the exit tubing with a hemostat may aid in preventing cuff leak.

---

5. The patient will experience ischemic pain under the tourniquet side in 15 to 20 minutes because this region is not anesthetized. A second tourniquet can be applied distal to the proximal tourniquet (provided that the proximal tourniquet is applied high on the arm) and inflated after adequate analgesia, and the proximal tourniquet can then be deflated, thus providing anesthesia at the tourniquet site. The same procedures can be performed in a lower extremity.
6. Deflate the cuff slowly. Repeated deflations and inflations of the cuff limit the amount of analgesic released into the general circulation and reduce the risk of complications. Do not deflate the cuff until 10 minutes after injection of a local anesthetic. Take care to avoid inadvertent deflations (8).

COMPLICATIONS

1. **Cardiac irregularities.** Because of the absorption of local analgesia after deflation of the cuff, cardiac irregularities, such as atrioventricular block, can occur (8).
2. **Transient loss of consciousness and seizures** have been reported (8).
3. Because of the rapid delivery of local anesthetic into the circulation after deflation of the cuff, **deafness or tinnitus** may occur (35).
4. **Thrombophlebitis** has been reported, and the procedure should not be used in patients with peripheral vascular disease.

TECHNIQUE FOR LUMBAR PUNCTURE ANESTHESIA

A field block has been described that produces anesthesia of the skin, interspinous ligaments, and muscles, as well as the periosteum, when performing lumbar punctures. This simple block makes this procedure virtually pain free.

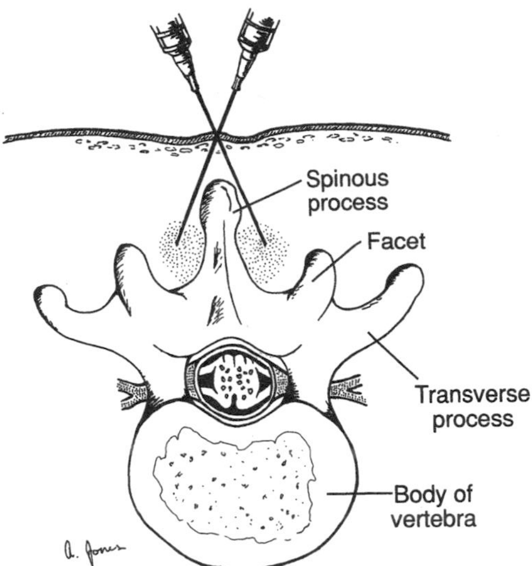

Figure 3.57. Anesthesia for lumbar spine puncture. See text for discussion.

The interspinous ligaments and the periosteum are supplied by the recurrent spinal nerves coming off the nerve roots exiting the spinal canal at the same level. In this procedure, lidocaine (1 mL of 1%) is deposited into the interspinous ligaments, between the tips of the spinous processes superior and inferior to the site of entrance of the spinal needle. In addition, lidocaine (2 mL of 1%) is deposited on either side of the interspinous space (Fig. 3.57).

REFERENCES

1. Accardo NJ, Adriani J: Brachial plexus block: a simplified technic using the axillary route. South Med J 42:920, 1949.
2. Adams RC: Regional anesthesia for operations about the neck and upper extremity. Anesthesiology 2:515, 1941.
3. Adriani J: Local and regional anesthesia for minor surgery. Surg Clin North Am 31:1507, 1951.
4. Adriani J: The clinical pharmacology of local anesthetics. Clin Pharmacol Ther 1:645, 1960.
5. Atkinson RS: Regional analgesia in obstetrics. Surg Gynecol Obstet 31:423, 1962.

6. Bone JR: Regional nerve block anesthesia. Anesthesiology 6:612, 1945.
7. Bonica JJ, Moore DC, Orlov M: Brachial plexus block anesthesia. Am J Surg 78:65, 1949.
8. Bryce-Smith R: Local analgesia of the limbs. In: Lee JA, Bryce-Smith R, eds. Practical Regional Anesthesia. Amsterdam: Excerpta medica; New York: American Elsevier Publishing Co., 1976.
9. Bryce-Smith R: Local analgesia of the trunk. In: Lee JA, Bryce-Smith R, eds. Practical Regional Anesthesia. Amsterdam: Excerpta Medica; New York: American Elsevier Publishing Co., 1976.
10. Bumsted RM, Ceilley RI: Surgical gems: Local anesthesia of the auricle. J Dermatol Surg Oncol 5:6, 1979.
11. Butterworth J, Ririe DG, et al: Differential onset of media nerve block: randomized, double blind comparison of mepivacaine and bupivacaine in healthy volunteers. Br J Anaesth 81:515–521, 1998.
12. Covino BG: Local anesthesia. N Engl J Med 286: 975, 1972.
13. Curatolo M, Perterson-Felix S, et al: Adding sodium bicarbonate to lidocaine enhances the depth of epidural blockade. Anesth Analg 86: 341–347, 1998.
14. Dagli G, Guzeldemir ME, Volkan Acar H: The effects and side effects of interscalene brachial plexus block by posterior approach. Reg Anesth Pain Med 23:87–91, 1998.
15. Dale HWL: Regional anesthesia for surgery of the nose and sinuses. Lancet 1:562, 1944.
16. DeJong RH: Axillary block of the brachial plexus. Anesthesiology 22:215, 1961.
17. Dugger JH, Kegel EE, Buckley JJ: Transvaginal pudendal nerve block: the safe anesthesia in obstetrics. Obstet Gynecol 8:393, 1956.
18. Hawkins JM, Isen D: Maxillary nerve block: The pterygopalatine canal approach. J Calif Dent Assoc 26:6, 58, 64, 1998.
19. Jones TM, Nandapalan V: Manipulation of the fractured nose: A comparison of local infiltration anaesthesia and topical local anaesthesia. Clin Otolaryngol 25:443–446, 1999.
20. Kasdan ML, Kleinert HE, Kasdan AP, et al. Axillary block anesthesia for surgery of the hand. Plast Reconstruct Surg 46:256, 1970.
21. Klink EW: Perineal nerve block: an anatomic and clinical study in the female. Obstet Gynecol 1: 137, 1953.
22. Kobak AJ, Sadove MS: Childbirth pain relieved by combined paracervical and pudendal nerve blocks. JAMA 183:931, 1963.
23. Locke RK, Locke SE: Nerve blocks of the foot. JACEP 5:698, 1976.
24. Macht SD, Thompson LW: Intraoral field block anesthesia for extraoral lesions. Surg Gynecol Obstet 146:87, 1978.
25. Mackay CA, Bowden DF: Axillary brachial plexus block: An underused technique in the accident and emergency department. J Accid Emerg Med 14:226–229, 1997.
26. Mansour NY: Compartment block for foot surgery: A new approach to tibial nerve and common peroneal nerve block. Reg Anesth 20: 95–99, 1995.
27. Moir DD: Axillary block of the brachial plexus. Anesthesia 17:274, 1962.
28. Molliex S, Navez M, et al: Regional anesthesia for outpatient nasal surgery. Br J Anaesth 76: 151–153, 1996.
29. Monsel LH: Regional anesthesia for operations about the head and neck. Anesthesiology 2:61, 1941.
30. Moore DC, Fridenbaugh LD, Bridenbaugh PO, et al: Bupivacaine: A review of 2,077 cases. JAMA 214:713, 1970.
31. Murphy MF: Local anesthetic agents. Emerg Med Clin North Am 6:769, 1988.
32. Murphy MF: Regional anesthesia in the emergency department. Emerg Med Clin North Am 6:783, 1988.
33. Nishiyama M, Nabanuma K, Amaki Y: A new approach for brachial plexus block under fluoroscopic guidance. Anesth Analg 88:91–97, 1999.
34. Olive-Perez A: Allergy during anesthetic procedures. Allergol Immunopathol (Madr) 25: 293–301, 1997.
35. Poulton TJ, Mims GR: Peripheral nerve blocks. Am Fam Physician 16:100, 1977.
36. Rovenstine EA, Byrd ML: The use of regional nerve block during treatment for fractured ribs. Am J Surg 46:303, 1939.
37. Sadove MS, Kobak AJ, Morch ET: Regional analgesia in obstetrics. Med Clin North Am 45:1743, 1961.
38. Serour F, Mandelpberg A, Mori J: Slow injection of local anaesthetic will decrease pain during dorsal penile nerve block. Acta Anaesthesiol Scand 42:926–928, 1998.
39. Sutherland ID: Continuous sciatic nerve infusion: Expanded case report describing a new approach. Reg Anesth Pain Med 23:496–501, 1998.
40. Sylaidis P, Logan A: Digital blocks with adrenaline: An old dogma refuted. J Hand Surg [Br] 23:17–19, 1998.
41. Wilds PL: Transvaginal pudendal nerve block. Obstet Gynecol 8:385, 1956.
42. Winne AO: Interscalene brachial plexus block. Anesth Analg 49:455, 1970.
43. Zetlaoui PJ, Bouaziz H: Lateral approach to the sciatic nerve in the popliteal fossa. Anesth Analg 87:79–82, 1998.

4

Cardiothoracic Procedures

PERICARDIOCENTESIS

Pericardiocentesis is a contraction of the phrase pericardial paracentesis and refers to the process of aspirating fluid from the pericardial space (39). Since the Viennese physician Franz Schuh first demonstrated it in 1840 (35), pericardiocentesis was performed blindly at the bedside until about the early 1970s. Use of more advanced technology has supplanted this approach and decreased the complication rate in the process. Its bedside emergency use and indications are controversial.

INDICATIONS

1. Diagnostic procedure during pulseless electrical activity (PEA) for a cardiac arrest.
2. Therapeutic procedure during PEA for a cardiac arrest.

In the emergency department setting, the sole indications for pericardiocentesis are first as a diagnostic and therapeutic procedure during PEA for a cardiac arrest patient, and second, as a temporizing measure for traumatic cardiac tamponade until a pericardial window can be performed. In these cases, bedside emergency pericardiocentesis could be life saving. All other patients, unless in severe hemodynamic extremis, would have the best results done under high-resolution fluoroscopy, such as in a cardiac catheterization laboratory and/or with echocardiographic guidance. Under echo, the ideal site for entry is the area of largest effusion that is closest to the transducer. In trauma, the patient with vital signs, but hemodynamically unstable, may represent a subset of patients that may benefit from pericardiocentesis as a temporizing measure before an emergency department or intraoperative thoracotomy. Removal of as little as 30 mL may be sufficient to relieve pericardial tamponade causing PEA.

Any patient who sustains injuries within the rectangle defined by the midclavicular line laterally, the clavicles superiorly, and the inferior margin of the rib cage must have pericardial penetration excluded (53). In trauma, the procedure has false-positive and false-negative results in approximately 50% of the cases (2, 34, 52). Attempted aspiration in the presence of clots in the pericardial space from acute bleeds may give a false-negative tap. Given its unacceptable false-negative and false-positive rate along with its potential for serious complications, it is *not* a very useful procedure in this setting. Thus a pericardial window is the procedure of choice, or if the patient is too unstable or in the presence of a loss of vital signs in the emergency department, a bedside thoracotomy is indicated.

DIAGNOSIS

Establishing the diagnosis in the emergency department can be difficult when relying only on clinical examination. Classically the findings of Beck's triad (distant heart sounds, neck vein distention, and hypotension) or pulsus paradoxus are absent more often than they are present. In a busy emergency department, muffled heart sounds are extremely difficult to hear, and decreased arterial pressures may be due to blood loss from other traumatic injuries. A study by Guberman et al. (26) found that the majority of patients with this condition had preserved blood pressure and heart sounds. Many of those with tamponade atypically manifest only fever, leukocytosis, or arrhythmias. Additionally, because of hypovolemia, the patient may not have distended neck veins. In addition, pulsus paradoxus does not readily develop among patients with aortic regurgitation, severe aortic stenosis, atrial septal defects, and severe left ventricular dysfunction (34). Other entities such as pulmonary emboli, right ventricular infarct, tense ascites, restrictive cardiomyopathy, chronic obstructive pulmonary disease (COPD), asthma, and shock can produce pulsus paradoxus (40). The electrocardiogram (ECG) and chest radiograph (CXR) also are rarely helpful; however, electrical alternans may be strongly suggestive of pericardial tamponade. The CXR is usually taken in a supine position in anteroposterior (AP) fashion, falsely enlarging the heart and mediastinum, simulating pericardial fluid.

Echocardiography remains the modality of choice for establishing the diagnosis. Swan–Ganz monitoring, if time permits, allows confirmation of the diagnosis as well as monitoring of treatment effectiveness (30).

RISKS AND COMPLICATIONS

In the hands of an experienced operator using fluoroscopy and echocardiography, the procedure has a complication rate of 5% (1, 11, 27, 33, 36, 43). However, blind, emergency pericardiocentesis has a very high complication rate. A rare complication of a successful pericardiocentesis can even be sudden ventricular dilatation and acute pulmonary edema (24, 40).

EQUIPMENT

Local anesthetic [lidocaine (Xylocaine) 1%, 10 mL]
10-mL syringe and 60-mL syringe with Luer lock
Three-way stopcock
9- to 15-cm 18-gauge spinal needle
Sterile double-ended alligator clip (sterile)
Iodinated prep solution
Sterile field with towels and clips
Sterile 4 × 4-inch sponges
1-inch adhesive tape
ECG machine (well grounded)
Defibrillator

THE BLIND AND ELECTROCARDIOGRAPHICALLY GUIDED PERCUTANEOUS PERICARDIOCENTESIS

In any procedure, preparation of equipment is essential. Simply needed are a 10-mL syringe, a three-way stopcock, a short-bevel 9- to 15-cm 18-gauge needle, a double-ended sterile alligator clip, and an ECG machine. The ECG should have equipotential grounding with no chance of a current wave that could induce ventricular fibrillation; if one is not available, do not use that ECG machine (32).

PREPARATORY STEPS

The patient also must be prepared. The patient is typically moribund and obtunded. Full cardiac monitoring, airway control, a resuscitation cart, and presence of a defibrillator are always needed. Other peripheral lines are needed for volume infusion. While the necessary equipment is being assembled, the patient should be hemodynamically supported to prevent collapse. Hemodynamic support should include volume expansion to delay the appearance of right ventricular diastolic collapse and hemodynamic deterioration (10). Use a balanced salt solution, plasma, or blood, in conjunction with norepinephrine and dobutamine, or combined with hydralazine or nitroprusside. Some have advocated isoproterenol as a single agent because of its β_1 and β_2 agonist effects (42). The goal is to increase cardiac output by either improving contractility or reducing elevated systemic resistance. β-Adrenergic blockade should be avoided, as should be positive pressure ventilation (3).

1. Prepare and drape in a sterile fashion.
2. When using the ECG machine, attach the limb leads before draping the patient.
3. Administer local anesthesia with lidocaine (Xylocaine) without epinephrine. However, the syringe is half filled with lidocaine to clear the needle as it passes through tissue. Spinal needles are often used; however, the long sharp bevel poses obvious additional hazards.

PROCEDURAL STEPS

1. Attach the syringe to the stopcock, and then connect this assembly to the needle. Attach the alligator clip to the base of the needle and the other end of the alligator clip to the V lead of the ECG machine. With the ECG running, the needle is inserted 1 cm inferior to the costal margin and left of the xiphoid at a 30-degree angle aiming toward the left or right shoulder (Figs. 4.1, 4.2, 4.3). Alternatively, the needle may be inserted in the fifth intercostal space on the left just above the sixth rib and within 1 cm of the sternal border (parasternal approach).
2. Advance the needle, with suction applied to the syringe, until aspiration of fluid is obtained or one sees sudden large ST-segment elevation indicative of epicardial injury. In addition, if a dysrhythmia ensues, slowly remove the needle, noting the depth, and aspirate on the way out. Remove the needle until the dysrhythmia ceases.

NOTE

The main issue confronting the operator is whether the needle is or was in the pericardial space, which is the reason it is called a blind procedure. When blood is suspected as the fluid in the pericardial sac, it is particularly difficult to ascertain one's position. On obtaining blood, the question arises as to whether the needle is in the pericardial space or in the right ventricle (or right atrium). One principle is to withdraw at least 30 mL regardless, and see if hemodynamics improve by monitoring the central venous pressure (CVP) waves, or blood pressure if an arterial line has been inserted. The aspirated blood's ability to clot may or may not be helpful in determining location. The often-used dictum "pericardial blood does not clot, whereas ventricular blood clots" does not frequently hold. Blood in the pericardium does frequently clot. Determination of pH, PCO_2, and PO_2 also can be used to distinguish pericardial fluid from central venous blood (PO_2 is lower and PCO_2 is higher in pericardial fluid) (48). This can be time consuming, and monitoring the hemodynamic response is the better immediate guide. If there is no improvement in the hemodynamic response, reposition the needle. Other possibilities are to inject fluorescein and look for a fluorescent "flush" under an ultraviolet light beneath the skin of the eyelid. If the needle is in the cardiac chamber, the test will be positive. Ventricular puncture is suggested by the hematocrit of the aspirated blood being the same as a peripheral hematocrit. In an alert patient, 3 mL of sodium dehydrocholate (Decholin) may be injected. The patient is then asked if he has a bitter taste, which indicates ventricular penetration of the needle.

Path of Pericardiocentesis Needle

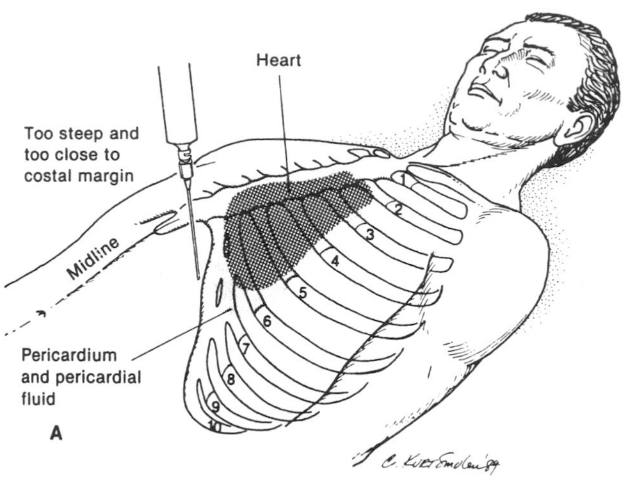

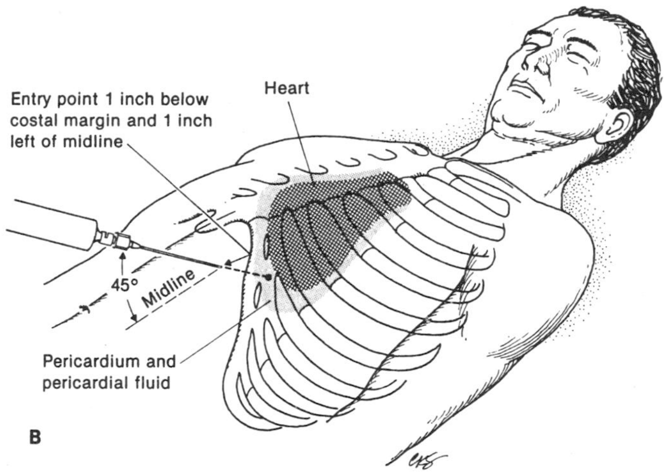

Figure 4.1. Path of pericardiocentesis needle. *A:* Sagittal view of the subcostal margin in the region of the pericardial needle entry point, indicating the difficulty that can transpire when the needle is introduced less than 1 inch below the left costal margin. *B:* Sagittal view of the subcostal margin in the region of the pericardial needle entry point, indicating that the introduction of the needle well below the left costal margin permits further insertion of the needle at the appropriate angle to the skin. (From Feliciano DV: Tube thoracostomy. In: Benumof JL, ed. Clinical Procedures in Anesthesia and Intensive Care. Philadelphia: Lippincott, 1992. Fig. 27-4, with permission.)

Relevant Pericardial Anatomy

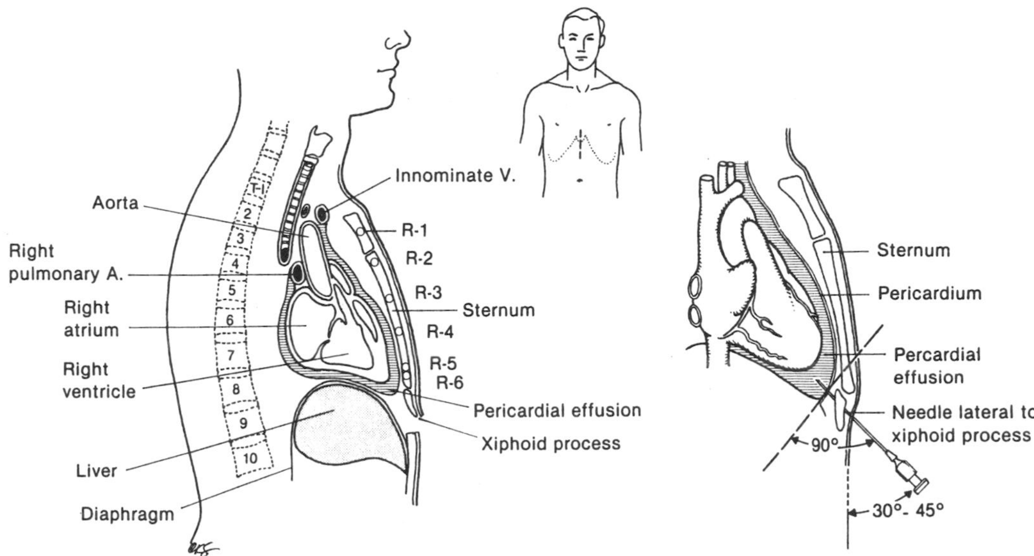

Figure 4.2. Sagittal view of the thorax indicating the orientation of the pericardial needle, introduced via the subxiphoid approach, relative to the surface of the pericardium. Note that the needle enters the skin to the left of the xiphoid (see Fig. 4.3), and that the needle enters the pericardial space at right angles to the pericardium when inserted with this approach. (From Feliciano DV: Tube Thoracostomy. In: Benumof JL, ed. Clinical Procedures in Anesthesia and Intensive Care. Philadelphia: Lippincott, 1992. Fig. 27-2, with permission.)

Optimal Entry Point for Pericardiocentesis Needle

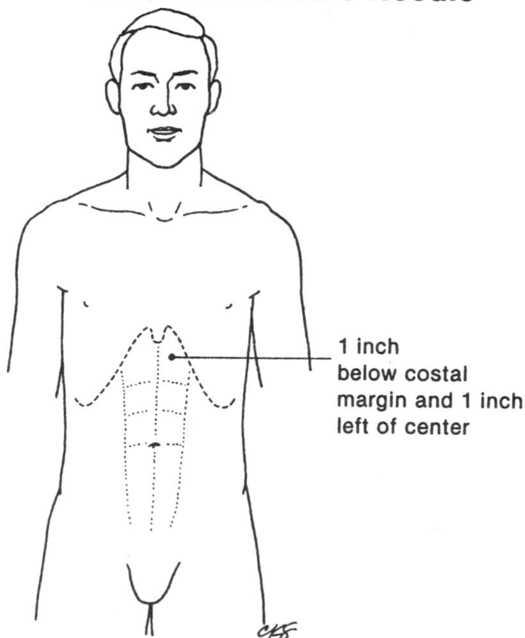

Figure 4.3. Anterior view of the xiphoid indicating the optimal entry point for the pericardiocentesis needle. Note that the optimal entry point is approximately 1 inch below the costal margin and 1 inch to the left of the midline. (From Feliciano DV: Tube thoracostomy. In: Benumof JL, ed. Clinical Procedures in Anesthesia and Intensive Care. Philadelphia: Lippincott, 1992. Fig. 27-3, with permission.)

CAUTION

On reaspiration in the new location, do not move the needle laterally. Respiration should be attempted with the same goals in mind.

3. The needle should not be used to drain the pericardial space completely. Use a guide wire–assisted catheter placement to drain the pericardial space to avoid injury to the heart. Then place the catheter under low continuous suction. However, never place a needle under continuous suction. Once hemodynamics have improved, take the patient immediately to the operating room for a definitive procedure to drain the pericardial space or repair the injury.

AFTERCARE

If the procedure is unsuccessful, withdraw the catheter and apply a sterile dressing and adhesive tape. Continue ECG monitoring of the patient. The patient, once stabilized, should have surgical consultation for pericardiotomy or pericardiectomy. Almost all patients will either go to the operating room or be admitted to an intensive care unit for further cardiac care management.

COMPLICATIONS

1. Laceration of the heart or of the coronary or internal mammary artery. The left anterior descending artery is especially vulnerable to injury from the advancing needle. The left parasternal approach is especially likely to injure this vessel. Aiming at the right shoulder after entering the left costosternal angle may avoid injury to this vessel. Always monitor the patient for any current injury during advance of the needle, and perform aspiration as the needle is advanced. Most patients with puncture of the myocardium secondary to a needle have no sequelae; the needle is simply withdrawn, and the patient is monitored and observed.
2. Pneumothorax, hemothorax, or hydrothorax. All patients with pericardiocentesis should have a follow-up CXR. When a pneumothorax is noted, depending on the size, a chest tube may be indicated.
3. Liver laceration.
4. Diaphragmatic tear.
5. Bowel puncture.
6. Hemopericardial tamponade.
7. Dysrhythmias. Asystole has been reported after this procedure. Ventricular fibrillation and vasovagal arrest also have been reported. If an arrhythmia occurs, withdraw the needle; if the arrhythmia persists, treat routinely (Table 4.1).

Table 4.1.
Complications of Pericardiocentesis

Complications of Pericardiocentesis
Perforation of the right ventricle
Laceration of the right coronary artery
Dysrhythmias
Pneumothorax
Pneumopericardium
Venous Embolism
Hemopericardium
Puncture/laceration of the liver and diaphragm
Ventricular dilatation with acute pulmonary edema

RESUSCITATIVE THORACOTOMY

There is little debate concerning the appropriateness of emergency department thoracotomy. Initially, all traumatic arrest patients were resuscitated with a thoracotomy procedure in the absence of massive head trauma. Much more selectivity has ensued after the review of the dismal results of this procedure on patients without vital signs at the scene. In a further refinement, patients with blunt trauma in arrest were found to have the worst outcomes, and in most places, no thoracotomy is performed unless vital signs are present in the emergency department for this subset of patients. Emergency department thoracotomy has the best results in patients with penetrating trauma as long as the patient has vital signs at least en route to the emergency department.

One issue concerns the training required to perform thoracotomy. Ideally, any physician should have done several thoracotomies in the operating room under controlled conditions and subsequently have accomplished some under supervision in the emergency department. This life-saving procedure can be initiated by emergency physicians or surgeons in the emergency department. The actual opening of the chest is just a small aspect of the resuscitative thoracotomy. Opening of the pericardium, repair of cardiac injuries, cross-clamping the aorta or pulmonary hilum, and controlling great vessel or lung hemorrhage are the major aspects of the procedure. Knowing the appropriate sequence to accomplish these tasks while in the chest also is vital. In addition, closure of the thorax requires a surgeon, and no resuscitative thoracotomies should be undertaken unless there is a trauma surgeon to complete this task. In this section, the decision tree is described. After this section is a more detailed description of each procedure.

INDICATIONS FOR RESUSCITATIVE THORACOTOMY

1. To control exsanguinating intrathoracic hemorrhage.
2. To manage a cardiac tamponade that cannot be decompressed via needle aspiration in a patient whose vital signs are rapidly deteriorating.
3. To cross-clamp the thoracic aorta to control intraabdominal exsanguination (1).
4. To perform internal cardiac massage.

There is some debate concerning the efficacy of emergency department thoracotomy for intraabdominal exsanguination. This probably is best reserved for patients about to undergo immediate celiotomy on the way to the operating room when proximal control is needed to support vital signs to ensure salvageable arrival to the operating room.

It is interesting to note that in the majority of cases, clotted blood was found within the pericardium in patients with cardiac wounds, thus dispelling the fallacy that a negative pericardiocentesis (i.e., clotted blood) is a reliable indicator of an uninjured heart. In 40% of patients with cardiac injuries, the blood within the pericardial sac was clotted; in 25% of cases, the pericardium contained both clotted and unclotted blood; and in only 20% was blood entirely unclotted within the pericardial sac (8).

OBJECTIVES

1. To stop lethal exsanguination by repair of injuries.
2. To relieve the pericardial tamponade with restoration of perfusion.
3. To cross-clamp the aorta for distal abdominal arterial vascular control.
4. To reestablish meaningful spontaneous cardiac contractions with signs of perfusion.

For the best outcome of the patient, it is imperative that these goals be kept firmly in mind, and that once accomplished, the patient be moved expeditiously to the operating room. The window of opportunity is slim and can be wasted by unnecessary time spent in the emergency department when the patient should be rapidly moved to a more controlled environment.

CONTRAINDICATIONS

1. Blunt trauma without vital signs at the scene or in transit to the emergency department.
2. Obvious massive intracranial trauma.

PREPARATION AND EQUIPMENT

The patient should have total airway control with either orotracheal intubation or intubation via cricothyrotomy, and a nasogastric tube should be placed. Short, large-bore catheter intravenous lines in the upper extremities or two Swan introducers placed in the subclavian or internal jugular veins are necessary to manage extreme hypovolemia adequately. A left anterolateral thoracotomy is the approach used, and several rolled sheets placed under the left scapula will give the best exposure, but they are not essential. No anesthesia or analgesia is necessary because these patients are moribund. Universal precautions must be used because there is no more invasive procedure than this in the emergency department, and staff can be readily exposed to blood.

All the following equipment ideally must be within arm's reach before beginning the procedure. Trying to perform the necessary repairs in a patient population with a 90% death rate with needless delays can only worsen the prognosis.

Povidone–iodine (Betadine)
Two Allis clamps
Tooth forceps
Sterile field
Scalpel with a no. 10 or 20 blade
Mayo scissors (curved), rib spreaders (Finochietto's chest retractor)
Lebsche's knife and hammer, hemostats
Satinsky's vascular clamps (two each large and small)
DeBakey tangential occlusion clamp (aortic clamp)
Tonsil clamps (four)
Needle holder (Hegar's) (two)
Various large silk sutures on large curved needles with Teflon pledgets (2-0, 0, 1, 2)
Adequate suction (two sources preferable)
Internal defibrillator paddles
Four towels
Thirty 4 × 4-inch sponges

TECHNIQUE AND SEQUENCE

1. With the patient intubated, apply povidone–iodine quickly over the anterolateral chest wall, and if time permits, the patient is draped.
2. A single large incision is made in the fourth or fifth intercostal space extending from the sternum (2-cm lateral to the sternum) to the posterior axillary line, preferably in one large stroke; the incision is extended below the nipple line in men and the inframammary line in women. The blade should incise through the skin, subcutaneous fat, and intercostal muscles.
3. To enter the chest cavity, use Mayo's, with care given to the underlying lung tissue. Use the Mayo's to separate the intercostals muscles not already severed with the scalpel while the second and third fingers separate the pleura of the lung from the chest wall.
4. Insert rib spreaders and crank them open for maximal exposure.
5. Move the lung manually out of the way; as mentioned earlier, evacuate clots for visual exposure (use an autotransfuser when removing blood from the thoracic cavity), and identify the pericardium. If blood is present, incise the pericardium.
   a. Using Allis clamps or hemostats (not forceps; they have a tendency to lose their "grip," thus wasting time), grasp the pericardium in a medial–lateral fashion and retract toward the operator.
   b. With the Metzenbaum scissors, incise the pericardium between the Allis clamps in a vertical fashion, with care given to not transect the left phrenic nerve. The phrenic nerve runs longitudinally along the pericardium; therefore the opening of the pericardium should be through a vertical incision but more anterior than the phrenic nerve. After the opening of the pericardium, the heart is easily exposed and brought out through the incised pericardium (Fig. 4.4). Then remove pericardial thrombi.

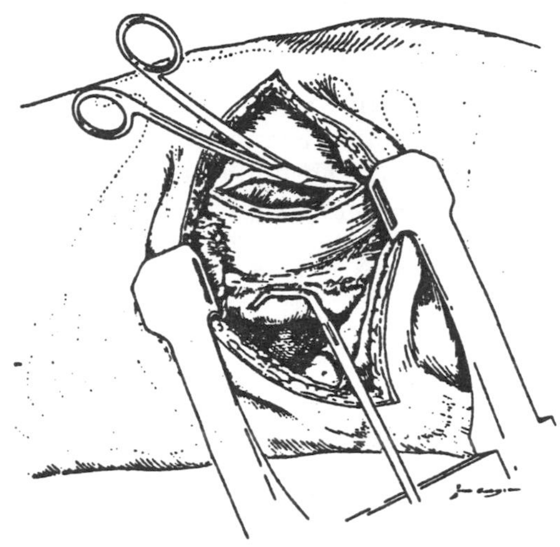

Figure 4.4. A vascular clamp is applied to the thoracic aorta inferior to the left pulmonary hilum. Pericardiotomy is done with scissors anterior to the phrenic nerve. (From Biffl WL, Moore EE, Harken AH: Emergency Department Thoracotomy. In: Mattox KL, Feliciano DV, Moore EE, eds. Trauma, 4th ed. New York: McGraw-Hill, 249, 2000. Fig. 13-2, with permission.)

CAUTION

An elevated hemidiaphragm is frequently mistaken for the pericardial sac. There have been cases in which the diaphragm was mistakenly incised instead of the pericardial sac. When identifying the pericardial sac and heart, sweep the hand inferiorly along the dome of the diaphragm and then come upward along the mediastinum medially.

---

c. Inspect the heart quickly for any injuries or wounds. Institute digital pressure and subsequent repair immediately if cardiac wounds are found. Numerous techniques have been described for repairing injuries including using digital pressure and suturing around the digitized wound, Foley insertion or balloon tamponade, or use of an occluding clamp, as is discussed later. Digital pressure is best when simultaneously performing open cardiac compressions to prevent blood from squirting out during manual systole.

d. If the wound location mandates better exposure for repair, continue the incision across the sternum, using the Lebsche knife, and continue in the right fourth or fifth intercostal space (clam-shell exposure). Reapply the rib spreaders at the sternum for maximal exposure.

1. If the pericardial sac is not showing evidence of tamponade (no blood in the pericardial sac), cross-clamp the aorta first. If so, then begin closed pericardial sac cardiac massage. Place the hand in the thoracotomy incision, and palpate the diaphragm posteriorly. As the fingers are brought to the midline, palpate the vertebral bodies, and the diaphragm will be below the hand. The first palpable structure alongside the vertebral bodies at this junction is the thoracic aorta. The thoracic aorta overlies the vertebral bodies and is separated from the esophagus. The esophagus courses anteriorly and medial to the aorta. The aorta is difficult to palpate in hypovolemic patients in whom the thoracic aorta may be collapsed. Furthermore with massive hemorrhage, it may be impossible to visualize the aorta. Thus this is most often a blind procedure, and the aorta is mobilized by freeing the pleura above and below, with care taken not to rupture the intercostal arteries. Identifying the esophagus (anterior to the aorta) by palpation of the nasogastric tube is helpful because of the poor visualization (which is usually the case, because this is mostly a blind procedure). Once the pleura are broached and the aorta is digitally freed, apply a DeBakey aortic occlusion clamp, but avoid the esophagus. Note verbally the time of cross clamp-

ing. A maximal time of cross clamping should be about 30 minutes to prevent sequelae, such as spinal cord, bowel, or renal ischemia.

2. Then open the pericardium, inspect the heart quickly for occult injuries, and continue cardiac massage. If ventricular fibrillation is present, apply 10 to 15 joules to convert the movements into more organized contractions. Volume resuscitation is essential if cardioversion is to have a better chance of success. Intracardiac epinephrine may be given to augment this and assist. Give no cardiac depressants. If there is asystole without evidence of spontaneous movement of heart muscle, then institute vigorous, but careful, cardiac massage along with restoration of intravascular red cell mass and intravascular volume. Again, use epinephrine in this setting to help establish return of spontaneous heartbeats or fibrillation, which can then be cardioverted. Once beating is resumed with signs of perfusion, and fair hemostasis achieved, take the patient expeditiously to the operating room for continued resuscitation and definitive repair.
3. In the course of performing the cardiac resuscitation, quickly inspect the lungs, hilum, aorta, and chest cavity for injuries. For control of bleeding, obtain proximal vascular occlusion for each injured organ. For the lung, this may mean cross-clamping the hilum. While performing this, recognize that hypoxia and pulmonary hypertension will ensue, with major stresses on an already ischemic heart.

Details of each procedure mentioned are given later. The important aspect is the decision sequence or tree. The critical moments are, first, when to perform and initiate a thoracotomy, and second, when to move the patient to the operating room.

CAUTION

Remember that when vital signs are restored suddenly after repair of the heart, anesthesia may abruptly be required because the patient may regain consciousness.

PERICARDIOTOMY

As mentioned earlier, the diaphragm can be mistaken for the pericardium, so care must be taken to identify the pericardium properly. This is made easy when spontaneous contractions are visible. If the heart is not beating, track the diaphragm medially to encounter the pericardial sac. Grasp the sac side by side with hemostats or Allis clamps, and retract away from the heart. Resist the attempt to use forceps for this procedure, because a good grip is often not maintained. Make a nick anterior to the left phrenic nerve with a scalpel or Metzenbaum scissors, and incise and open the pericardium in a parallel fashion to the phrenic nerve along the entire vertical axis of the pericardium. Bring the heart out through the incised pericardium and evaluate it. Note its fullness, color, presence or absence of spontaneous contractions (organized and unorganized), and any injuries. If no injuries are present and ineffectual contractions exist, initiate two-handed cardiac massage.

AORTIC OCCLUSION

The purpose of this procedure is to maximize blood flow preferentially to the heart and brain. Run a hand posteriorly along the diaphragm to the vertebral bodies; the aorta is the first structure encountered. While collapsed, the aorta may be difficult to identify readily. The nasogastric tube in the esophagus will aid in its location and differentiation. The pleura fold over the aorta and must be bluntly spread open and the aorta mobilized, but not retracted. Apply the occlusion clamp around this mobilized section of the aorta. Mark time verbally when this is accomplished. If difficulty is encountered with mobilizing the aorta, use 4 × 4-inch pad in the grasp of ring forceps to compress the aorta directly against the vertebral bodies (Rottman procedure, Fig. 4.5) (55). Release the compression every 10 minutes for 30 seconds to minimize the potential injuries from ischemia to the spine, liver, kidneys, and bowel. Minimize the time for occlusion of the aorta and keep it to a maximum of 30 minutes for reversible normothermic spinal ischemia. Cross-clamp times of up to 75 minutes with periodic releases have been described without spinal sequelae, but this should not be considered the norm (6). Blood flow to distal organs is reduced to 10% of normal with consequent anaerobic metabolism and secondary lactic acidemia development. This can contribute to the multiple organ failure seen in many of these patients (7). Release slowly to minimize any diminution of advances in hemodynamics achieved. Some practitioners have simply had an assistant apply manual posterior pressure over the vertebrae just superior to the diaphragm. This process saves time, avoids esophageal injury, and stops hemorrhage effectively. However, the value of this maneuver has not been evaluated and it does subject the assistant to increased risk of injury from sharp objects being used within the chest cavity.

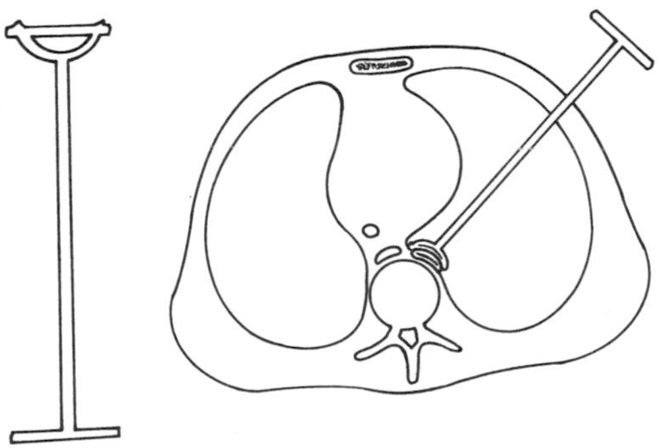

Figure 4.5. A solid metal aortic compression device can be made in any hospital maintenance shop. Rubber tubing placed across the base of the U-shaped device serves as an aortic compressor. This can be applied via a thoracotomy to compress the aorta, as shown in the diagram. (From Simon R, Brenner B. Emergency Procedures and Techniques. 3rd ed. Baltimore: Williams & Wilkins, 145, 1994. Fig. 4.24, with permission.)

OPEN CARDIAC MASSAGE

Cardiac massage can be performed in three different, but not equally efficacious, ways. The first and best is two-handed massage. This method causes the fewest injuries and greatest output (4, 18, 29). Hold the heart in the palms of the hands with the wrists at the apex and fingers at the base of the heart. Use a hinged clapping motion with ventricular compression proceeding from the apex to the base of the heart (5). Keep the fingers somewhat straight, never "digging" into the heart with the tips of the fingers. Open-chest massage approximately doubles cardiac output when compared with closed-chest massage, with values ranging from 35% to 55% of prearrest values in dogs. Coronary blood flow is 42% to 46% of the prearrest control flow and can increase to 55% with countermassage of the ascending aorta (28), with better survival from cardiac arrest noted in humans as well.

The second technique of internal cardiac massage is the one-handed technique using the sternum or the vertebral column. Compress the heart against the sternum (or vertebral column) from the apex to the base with one hand. Take care to be aware of sharp rib and sternal edges produced during the thoracotomy. This has the potential of injuring the heart during massage and compressions.

The third technique is the one-handed technique in which the thumb squeezes the heart against the fingers, with some palmar squeezing to help direct the flow to the base of the heart. This method has the potential for myocardial perforation with the thumb and has poorer cardiac output (5, 28). Use the other techniques instead of this one-handed technique.

Take care not to compress the coronary arteries while performing cardiac massage and allow time for filling of the ventricles.

CARDIAC REPAIR

Patients with penetrating cardiac injuries have a high mortality rate before reaching the hospital. From 60% to 80% die before reaching the emergency department of exsanguination or tamponade. DeGennaro (17) found cardiac injuries 62% of the time when wounds were found in the cardiac silhouette. In addition, Richardson et al. (47) found a 63% incidence of vital organ injury requiring thoracotomy in a series of transmediastinal gunshot wounds. Treat transmediastinal trajectories with the same outlook as those wounds within the cardiac silhouette.

There are some particulars concerning different anatomic structures of the heart.

VENTRICLES

The right ventricle (RV) is more often injured than the LV (35% to 24%) (50). There is greater survival when only the RV is injured. When the LV is involved alone or in conjunction with other chambers, the mortality is significantly greater. The incidence of chamber involvement is RV (42%), LV (33%), right atrium (RA) (15%), and LA (6%) with the great vessels constituting the remainder (Fig. 4.6) (46, 49, 52). Stab wounds with cardiac injuries often have cardiac tamponade (90%), but less so with gunshot wounds (20%). Those arriving alive are more likely to have tamponade than are those arriving dead to the emergency department (9, 19, 20).

Repair of the heart follows hemostatic control of the injuries. Most injuries can be repaired without bypass pumps (15, 54). For small lacerations, finger occlusion (finger is over, not into, the wound) is usually sufficient to achieve hemostasis with subsequent suture repair with Teflon-pledgeted 2-0 silk horizontal mattress sutures (Fig. 4.7). In the beating heart, it is often difficult to keep a finger on the wound because of the cardiac movement. Place an apical traction stitch, which is performed by placing a suture at the apex of the heart and holding the suture between the thumb and third finger of the left hand while the index finger is placed over the wound. The apex is selected because it is the region farthest from the major coronary arteries. The apical traction suture is commonly known as the *Beck's suture*. The suture placement should be at least 6 mm from the wound edge and not through the endocardium to avoid subsequent mural thrombi (55). Close the wound just tight enough to stop the bleeding without strangulating the myocardium.

Use of a Foley Catheter to Occlude the Rent in the Ventricle

A Foley catheter is inserted into the ventricular wound, inflate the balloon, and apply gentle traction to stop the bleeding (Fig. 4.8). Take care not to place too much traction so as to cause the wound to enlarge by inadvertent tear. This includes avoiding traction while placing knots during cardiac contraction. Again using Teflon–felt pledgeted 2-0 silk sutures, use a purse-string or multiple horizontal mattress suture to close the wound. When the suture ties are placed, deflate and remove the balloon of the Foley. Alternatively, Teflon–felt pledgeted sutures in a crossed suture technique may also allow control of wound bleeding (Fig. 4.9) (49). These involve horizontal mattress stitches on either side of the wound crossed to stop bleeding temporarily while a definitive repair is performed.

A secondary aspect of the use of the Foley is to infuse fluids and blood directly into the ventricular cavity. When repairing the ventricle, be aware of the potential for large air embolisms. Fill the Foley balloon with fluid and not air, to minimize

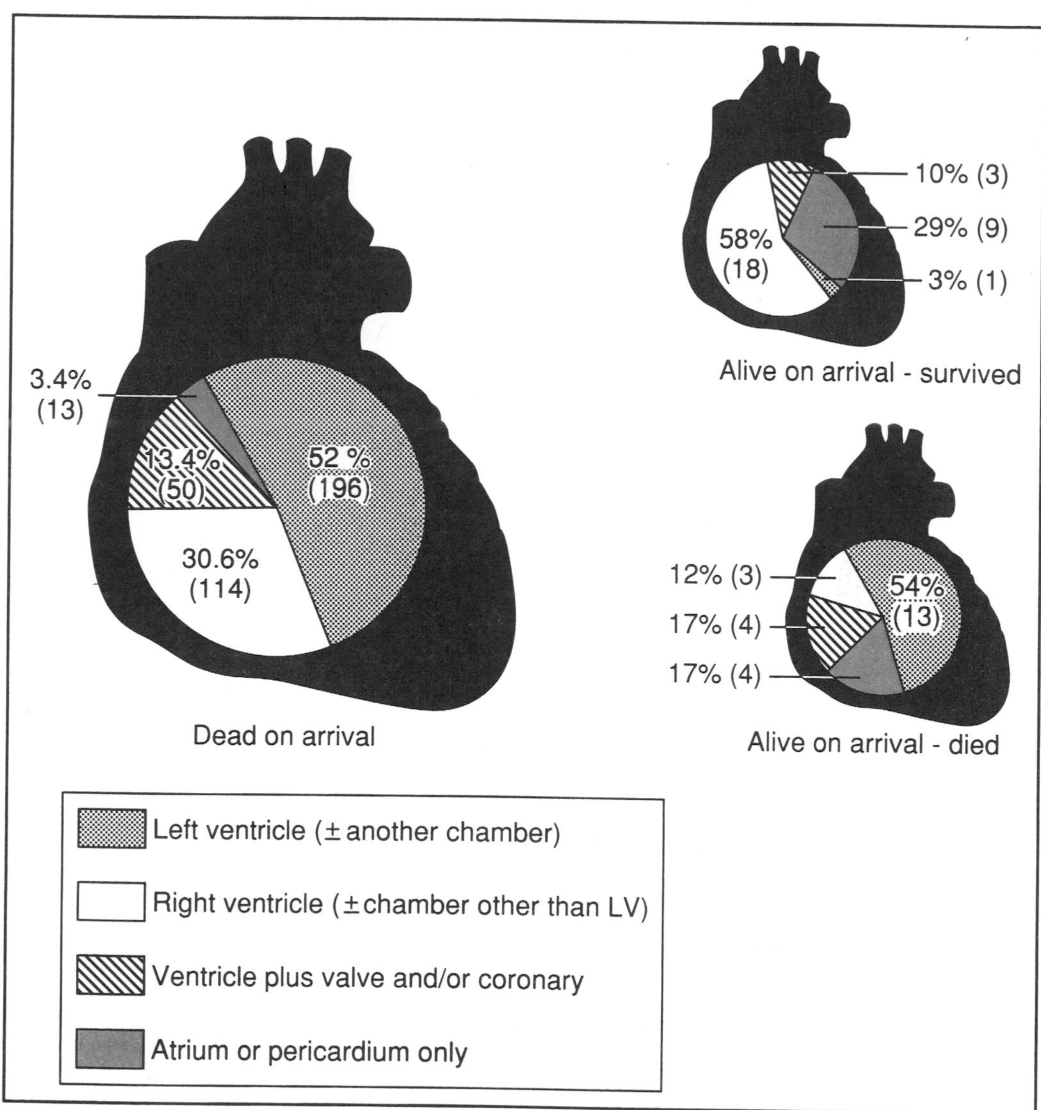

Figure 4.6. The overall distribution of cardiac wounds is shown for 459 patients with penetrating cardiac injuries. Comparisons are made for surviving and nonsurviving individuals, as well as for those with injured chambers. (From Sugg WL, Rea WJ, Ecker RR, et al: Penetrating wounds of the heart: An analysis of 459 cases. J Thorac Cardiovasc Surg 56:531–545, 1968; and Chitwood RW: Cardiac trauma: Penetrating and blunt. In: Moylan JA, ed. Principles of Trauma Surgery. New York: Gower Medical Publishing, Fig. 5.8, 1992, with permission.)

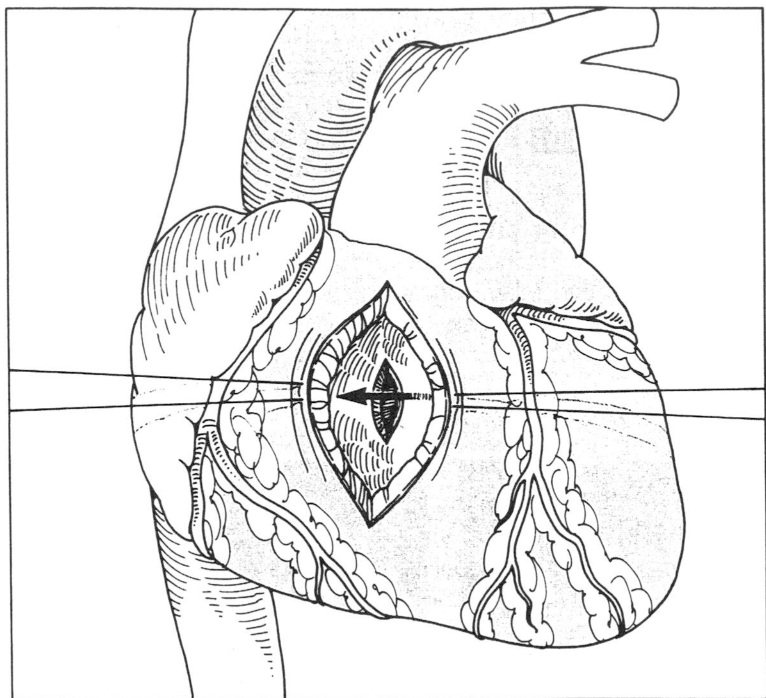

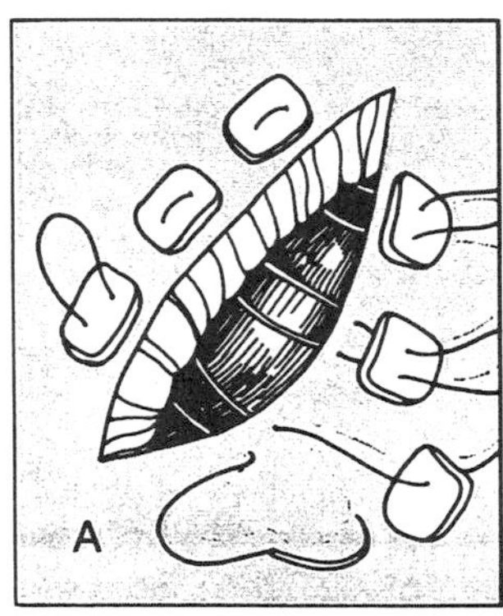

Figure 4.7. A ventricular septal defect resulting from a penetrating injury. Penetrating communications can often be closed by simple pledgeted mattress sutures. (Adapted from Whisennand HH, Van Pelt SA, Beall AC, et al: Surgical management of traumatic intracardiac injuries. Ann Thorac Surg 28:530–536, 1979; and Chitwood RW: Cardiac trauma: Penetrating and blunt. In: Moylan JA, ed. Principles of Trauma Surgery. New York: Gower Medical Publishing, 1992, Fig 5.29A, with permission.)

the risk of air embolism from an inadvertent puncture of the Foley balloon.

CORONARY ARTERIES

Coronary arteries are not usually involved with most wounds but may be in proximity to the wound, so take care not to catch the artery in the suture tie (Fig. 4.10) Direct the sutures beneath the arteries during approximation and closure of the wound. The incidence of injury to coronary arteries in penetrating cardiac trauma ranges from 4% to 12 % (21, 45, 46, 49). The most commonly injured is the left anterior descending (LAD; 62%) followed by the right coronary artery (RCA; 28%) and circumflex (10%). There is a 20% higher mortality when there is involvement of a coronary artery with penetrating cardiac trauma (45). If the two main arteries are transected, then bypass surgery is mandatory for survival. An attempt at repair of large arteries on a beating heart is nearly impossible, and thus bypass is required. Distal coronary arteries less than 1 mm can be safely ligated (45). A single coronary artery may be ligated and give a good chance at survival, but 90% of these patients have subsequent infarction

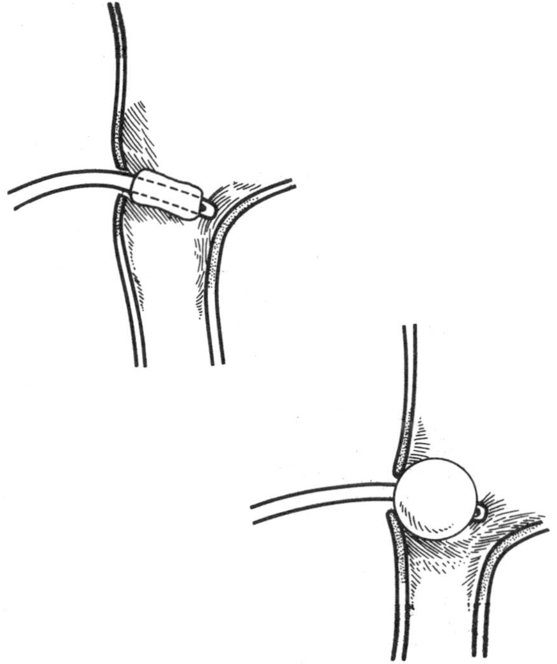

Figure 4.8. An atrial wound can be controlled by placing a Foley catheter into the perforation. Then inflate the Foley catheter with just enough saline to control bleeding from the site. Pull back the Foley catheter with enough pressure to control the bleeding. This will facilitate repair of the atrium when it is difficult to place a clamp around the site. (From Simon R, Brenner B. Emergency Procedures and Techniques, 3rd ed. Baltimore: Williams & Wilkins, 1994. Fig. 4.18, page 141, with permission.)

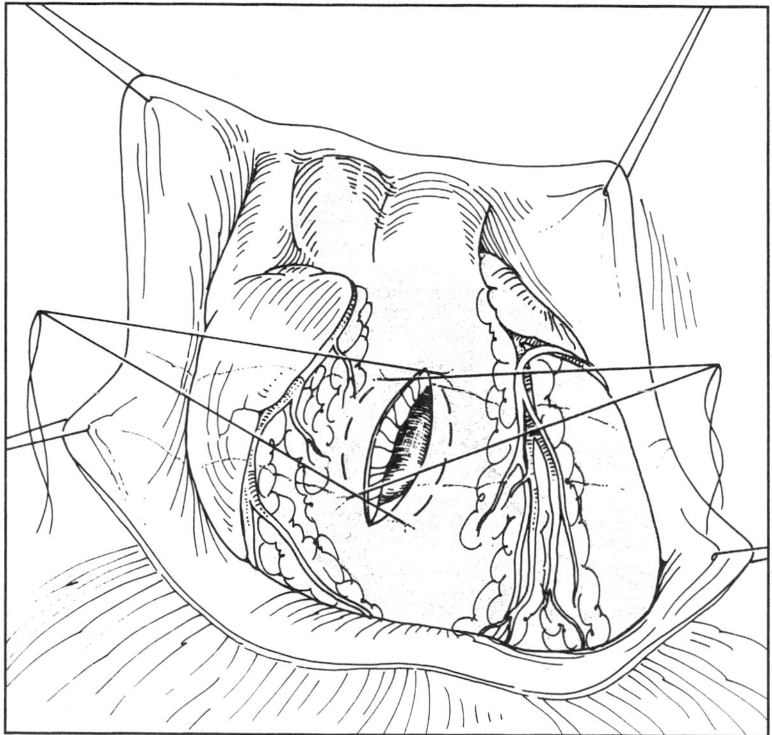

Figure 4.9. To relieve wall tension and control bleeding, apply the crossed-suture technique even for relatively large cardiac wounds. (Adapted from Symbas PN: Trauma to the heart and great vessels. In: Jamieson SW, ed. Rob & Smith's Operative Surgery. St. Louis: CV Mosby, 1986; and Chitwood RW: Cardiac Trauma: Penetrating and Blunt. In: Moylan JA, ed. Principles of Trauma Surgery. New York: Gower Medical Publishing, 1992, Fig 5.16, with permission.)

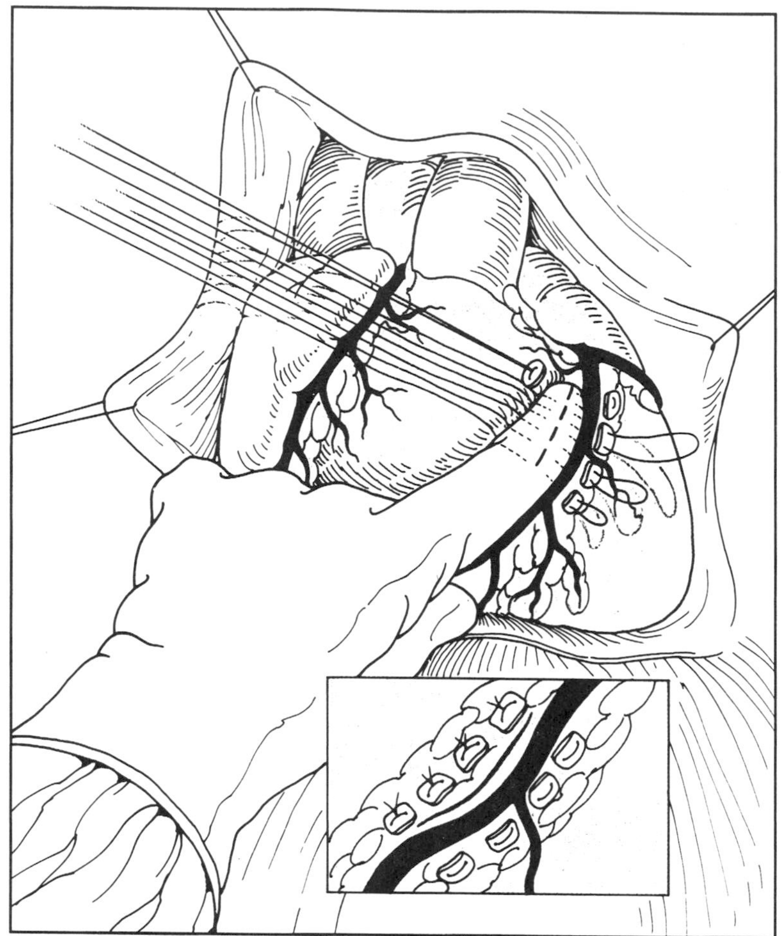

Figure 4.10. A ventricular laceration is present close to the left anterior descending coronary artery. Use pledgeted sutures to under-sew the coronary artery and close the laceration without creating myocardial ischemia. (Adapted from Symbas PN: Trauma to the heart and great vessels. In: Jamieson SW, ed. Rob & Smith's Operative Surgery. St. Louis: CV Mosby, 1986; and Chitwood RW: Cardiac Trauma: Penetrating and Blunt. In: Moylan JA, ed. Principles of Trauma Surgery. New York: Gower Medical Publishing, New York, 1992, Fig 5.19, page 5.15, with permission.)

secondary to the ligated artery (21, 45). If the patient is at a facility with bypass capability, do not use hemostats or other crushing instruments to achieve hemostasis. Sutures should be used to tamponade bleeding gently, even if this is difficult while the heart is beating. To assist in this process, use cold water placed on the myocardium, which can cause the local myocardium to fibrillate, creating a somewhat more quiescent field in which to accomplish the temporizing measure. Subsequently, DC countershock will restore the organized contractions (13).

ATRIAL REPAIR

The intraatrial pressures are much lower than those of the ventricles, and hence when wounded, the atria bleed much less vigorously. However, the wall of the atrium is thinner than that of the ventricles, and wounds of the atrium do not close spontaneously, as do those of the ventricles (13, 37). The bleeding is usually controllable with digital pressure if the wound is small and not located in the atrioventricular groove or coronary sinus. These latter wounds are treacherous to manage, often requiring cardiopulmonary bypass. Intraatrial stenting techniques have had success for these wounds when bypass was not available (14). For most atrial injuries, a noncrushing curved vascular clamp can occlude the tear, or use Allis clamps on either side of the wound and "tent them up" and criss-cross them, if needed, to stop the bleeding while repair is initiated. Smaller 3-0 or 4-0 silk suture is adequate for atrial repairs, but speed is of the essence, and larger suture is acceptable if immediately available. When dealing with a wound near the atriocaval junction, place a 12- to 14-French catheter into the laceration for temporary tamponade, and then repair as follows for atrial cannulation.

ATRIAL CANNULATION

When the cardiac chambers are "empty" and devoid of blood on opening the pericardium, an atrial line can be placed quickly to supply volume directly to the heart. In doing so, the intraatrial line should consist of either sterilized intravenous extension tubing with the tip cut off or, preferably, sterilized polyethylene tubing the size of intravenous tubing. This permits rapid volume replacement, which is desperately needed if the outcome is to be favorable. The right atrial appendage is the preferred site for an intraatrial line, because this area is usually accessible and thin walled and will permit blood to pass through the lungs for oxygenation before going into the central circulation, which does not occur with a left atrial line. In performing this procedure, use the following technique.

1. Place two small hemostats or Allis clamps with the tips opposing one another and securing the right atrial appendage. Lift the appendage and hold separated by these two hemostats by an assistant.
2. Place a small stab incision with a no. 11 blade between the opposing tips of the hemostats.
3. Pass the polyethylene tubing or intravenous tubing through the small opening, and apply a pursestring suture to secure the tubing. In this manner, volume infusion is initiated quickly while placing the pursestring suture and tying. Alternatively, apply a pursestring suture first in the atrial appendage and then make an incision within the center of the pursestring suture and, before tying, pass an atrial cannula. (The pursestring secured around the tubing avoids the bleeding that occurs during placement of a suture after the tubing has been passed). In either method, then take the ends of the suture, after tying the pursestring around the tubing, and make a second tie around the polyethylene tubing more proximally to secure its position.

The downside of this method is that it can be time consuming, interrupt cardiac massage, and can be associated with bleeding from the suture line in the pursestring.

INJURIES TO THE HILUM AND GREAT VESSELS

A major factor favoring survival after a major intrathoracic vascular injury is an intrapericardial location. It was not until 1958 that Perkins and Elchos (44, 56) were able to report the first successful repair of an acute penetrating wound of the aorta outside the pericardium. Stab wounds have a higher survival rate than do gunshot wounds.

VENA CAVAL INJURIES

Very few patients with superior vena cava injury live long enough to get treatment. Those that do survive long enough can have the caval injury repaired with a lateral venorrhaphy. Sudden clamping of either the superior or inferior vena cava can result in cardiac arrest because of the loss of venous return. Clamping of the descending aorta at the same time may help to maintain cardiac function. If cardiac arrest occurs, the opportunity to repair the vein quickly should be taken. Allowing the arrest to extend beyond 3 minutes is dangerous (56).

INNOMINATE OR SUBCLAVIAN VEINS

These two vessels may be ligated with impunity if unilateral (21). Ligation of both sides may produce a superior vena cava–like syndrome.

AZYGOUS AND HEMIAZYGOUS VEINS

These veins can be extremely difficult to control and not infrequently can cause exsanguination in spite of the best efforts to control them with multiple suture ligatures (21).

HILAR VESSELS

If the central lung vessels are injured, cross-clamp the hilum close to the pericardium (56). Clamp the corresponding pulmonary artery to prevent overload of the lung with blood and possible hypotension because blood is being sequestered in the clamped lung (Fig. 4.11). If a major pulmonary artery is clamped, clamp the corresponding bronchus because the involved lung would otherwise act as additional dead space (56).

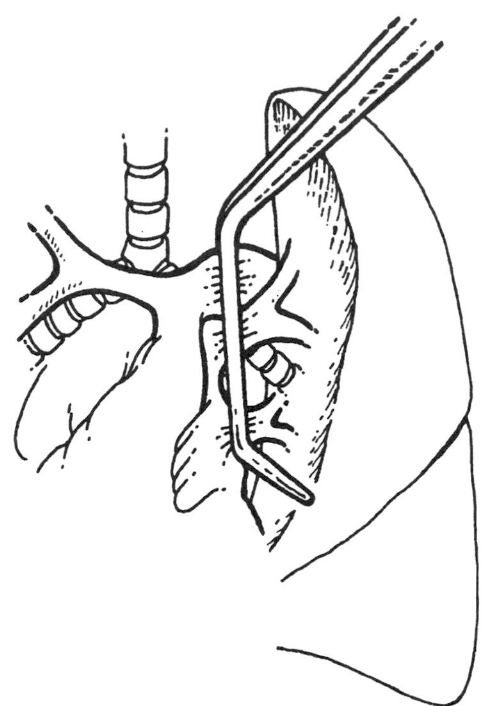

Figure 4.11. Occlusion of the pulmonary hilum with a Satin-sky clamp. (Reproduced from Rodriguez A, Thomas MD, Shillinglaw WRC: Lung and tracheobronchus. In: Ivatury RR, Catyen CG, eds. Textbook of Penetrating Trauma. Baltimore: Williams & Wilkins, 1996, 531–554; and Biffl WL, Moore EE, Harken AH: Emergency department thoracotomy. In: Mattox KL, Feliciano DV, Moore EE, eds. Trauma, 4th ed. New York: McGraw-Hill, 2000, Fig. 25.6, with permission.)

AORTA

In the ascending aorta or arch, lateral aortorrhaphy is usually easily accomplished. If this is not possible or practical, apply a side-clamp around the involved aorta. If this temporizes the exsanguination, then repair with cardiopulmonary bypass (56).

SUBCLAVIAN ARTERY

This is a very uncommon injury with difficult emergency department operative management. Frequently clamping the subclavian vessel or ligation is the best emergency department approach to this injury, until operative management in the operating room can be accomplished by using grafts (56). In the operating room, cardiopulmonary bypass with hypothermia may give the best approach to salvaging these patients.

CAROTID AND INNOMINATE ARTERY

The neurologic status of the patient and preservation of cerebral blood flow are imperative. The circle of Willis usually allows perfusion of the other side of the brain if the carotid is injured. Repair of these vessels in the emergency department is not feasible. Hemostasis and rapid transit to the operating room where cardiopulmonary bypass can assist the repair is the best choice. If there are already severe neurologic deficits, ligation in the emergency department can be a choice.

AIR EMBOLISM

Venous and systemic air embolisms result from penetrating wounds to the pulmonary vasculature. These can be life threatening both in a mechanical sense and by producing dysrhythmias. Serious morbidity from strokes and distal infarcts may occur. Venous emboli, if massive, may block the outflow tract of the RV causing shock and cardiac arrest. Manipulation of the patient's position to dislodge the air toward the apex and allow blood flow out of the RV is critical. Turning the patient on the left side and into the Trendelenburg position accomplishes this. Usually it is estimated that air entry of approximately 200 cc is needed to cause venous air embolism. Systemic or arterial air embolisms, if in the coronary arteries, may cause lethal dysrhythmias. Strokes also may ensue, and intubated patients with penetrating injuries to the chest and lungs are at risk. Usually the diagnosis is not thought of and is diagnosed at either surgery or autopsy. If, however, there is suspicion of systemic embolization, then place the patient immediately in Trendelenburg position (i.e., with the head down), and perform a resuscitative thoracotomy to seal off the injured vasculature proximal to the injured lung. Air in the LV and atrium can be released through aspiration. Bypass may be needed to manage coronary artery air embolisms (16, 25, 31, 51, 57; see Table 4.2).

Table 4.2.
Indications for Cardiopulmonary Bypass in Trauma

Penetrating
Major coronary artery injury
Valvular injury (aortic and mitral)
Foreign bodies in the left heart
Blunt
Chamber or septal rupture
Valvular injury (aortic and mitral)
Vascular trauma
Ascending aortic tear (acute or chronic)
Complex aortic arch, innominate or neck vessel injury
Descending thoracic aortic tears (usually left artrial-femoral bypass)
Miscellaneous
Severe hypothermia with hemodynamic instability
Inaccessible hepatic vein injury
Severe tracheobronchial injury with life-threatening hypoxia and hypercapnia
Hemodynamic collapse due to transient, reversible causes (contusion, drug toxicity, hyperkalemia, coronary air embolism) (12)

INTRACARDIAC INJECTION

This procedure is not commonly indicated in the emergency center because most medications can be given through a central venous line. However, when one is unable to give medications by the normal route, emergency drugs may have to be given through intracardiac injection.

TECHNIQUE

1. Prepare the chest wall with an iodinated preparation. The area of preparation should be in the precordial region around the fourth intercostal space and from the midclavicular line to the sternum and the xiphoid region.
2. With a long spinal needle, insert the needle in the left costosternal angle, aspirating while advancing the needle until the ventricular chamber is entered. Although the paraxiphoid approach is preferred, when entrance into the cardiac chamber is not possible by this method, place the needle through the anterior chest wall in the fourth intercostal space midway between the sternum and the midclavicular line.
3. Medications can be injected through the needle at this point.

COMPLICATIONS

1. Coronary artery injury. This is a less common problem with the paraxiphoid approach. With the anterior approach, the anterior descending coronary artery may be injured.
2. Pericardial hemorrhage and tamponade. This complication may be prevented by using a small-gauge spinal needle while performing the procedure and avoiding the anterior approach when possible.

NOTE

During internal massage, ECG monitoring is obscured; however, the heart can be observed and both atrial and ventricular action noted. The rates of the observed atrial and ventricular activity and their synchronization are as useful as the ECG. Treatment of dysrhythmias should follow standard Advanced Cardiac Life Support (ACLS) protocol. During internal massage, intracardiac injection may be performed with a 22-gauge needle inserted into the left ventricle or, preferably, the atrium. Care should be taken to avoid the coronary vessels. Intramyocardial injection of fluid can result in refractory ventricular fibrillation; therefore aspiration of blood should be performed before any injection into the heart.

NEEDLE DECOMPRESSION OF TENSION PNEUMOTHORAX

The use of needle decompression in the setting of tension pneumothorax can be life saving. It is simple, fast, and can be performed before the hospital, or by emergency or surgical department personnel.

The indication for needle decompression is evidence of a tension pneumothorax. The equipment needed is povidone–iodine solution, a 14-gauge needle, and anesthetic (1% lidocaine in a 5-mL syringe with a 25-gauge needle).

Prepare the second intercostal space in the midclavicular line on the affected side of the chest. Drapes are not necessary. Anesthetize the area in the middle of the intercostal space to avoid the intercostal arteries running above and below the interspace. Introduce the 14-gauge needle 90 degrees to the skin surface into the chest cavity. There will be a rush of air or fluid in the case of a tension hemopneumothorax. This will convert the tension pneumothorax into a simple pneumothorax and restore proper diastolic filling and improve cardiac output. Convert these into tube thoracostomy at the earliest opportunity. At this time the needle(s) are removed, but **not** before a functioning chest tube is in place.

TUBE THORACOSTOMY

Tube thoracostomy is one of the most common chest procedures performed in the emergency department. It is almost exclusively performed after spontaneous pneumothorax, trauma to the chest, or iatrogenic complications from invasive procedures. Some thought must go into whether to place a tube and the choice of the tube. This begins with the indications for placing a chest tube. The primary purpose of emergency tube placement is to restore the mechanical function of the lung and removal of air, blood, or pus that may currently or in the future restrict optimal pulmonary function.

There is no need to place a left chest tube if the patient requires an emergency thoracotomy. Adhesions of the lung to the chest wall also may preclude insertion of a chest tube at a particular site. Insertion of a chest tube at the site of a previous thoracostomy has some danger, that is, puncturing the lung with the chest tube during insertion. Other dangers include the issue of large blebs; these resemble pneumothoraces on CXR. Tube thoracostomy is not a treatment for large blebs. As with any invasive procedure, if time permits, correction of bleeding diatheses should precede the insertion of the tube. In addition, some simple and small nontraumatic pneumothoraces do not need a chest tube; they can be observed.

INDICATIONS

1. Tension pneumothorax. Perform needle aspiration of the pneumothorax first, because this could be life saving, followed by an anterior chest tube. In patients with asthma or COPD, the lung may be hyperinflated under pressure from auto-PEEP (positive end-expiratory pressure; see earlier under needle decompression of tension pneumothorax).
2. Hemothorax: posterolateral chest tube.
3. Hemopneumothorax: posterolateral chest tube and also may require an anterior chest tube for adequate drainage of a persistent pneumothorax.
4. Simple pneumothorax greater than 20%.
5. Chest trauma (penetrating) without evidence of a pneumothorax when the patient will be undergoing positive pressure ventilation.

Explain the procedure and its necessity if the patient is stable. Make sure the necessary equipment is present to have a smooth procedure.

EQUIPMENT

Antiseptic solution, drapes, and towel clips
1% lidocaine, 20 mL
25-gauge needle, 22-gauge needle, 10-mL syringe
No. 10 scalpel blade with handle, Kelly clamps (two), forceps
No. 36–40 French Argyle thoracostomy tube, 24–32 (nontraumatic pneumothorax), 20–24 (children), 18 thoracostomy tube in an infant
Pleurivac (collection bottle, underwater seal, suction control). Use only high-volume suction, such as wall suction, delivering at least 60 cm of water pressure with a flow of at least 15–20 L/min. Low-volume systems, such as Gomco, are not to be used.
Connecting tubing
Gauze pads, adhesive tape, 4 × 4-inch pads, Xeroform gauze dressing, antibacterial ointment
2, 1, or 0 suture (not 2-0 or 1-0), needle driver, and suture scissors

TECHNIQUE

Posterolateral Chest Tube: Preparatory steps

Five things help to ensure a smooth procedure:

1. The positioning of the patient. If the patient is in extremis with hypotension then perform the procedure with the patient supine. If the patient is more stable position the patient at least at a 30-degree angle, head up. In both instances with a posterolateral approach, the patient will have his upper extremity held above the head, allowing excellent exposure.
2. Adequate anesthesia. A patient writhing in pain will not well tolerate vocal assurances that "it is almost over." It is difficult to place a tube on a moving patient. Giving adequate anesthesia is the key to a successful and smooth placement.
3. Lay out all the instruments *in the sequence that each will be used.* Groping for instruments, suture materials, scalpels, and needles is time consuming, and with respect to infection control, can be dangerous. Have the needed items placed in sequence of use, and rid the area of the unnecessary clutter of rarely-to-be-used items.
4. Measure the chest tube against the chest wall. This is to determine how deep the chest tube will need to be inserted. Apply a Kelly to the tip to allow easy guidance and insertion into the chest.
5. Keep a backup chest tube ready in case of difficulty with the insertion of

the first tube, and this backup tube should usually be one size smaller.

In trauma in the adult, use a chest tube size 36 French or larger. In a spontaneous pneumothorax, use a smaller size (24 to 32 French) (22). The tube size chosen for children should be guided by the Broselow Tape for ease. Trocar-introduced chest tubes are no longer acceptable because of their excessive complication rates.

The patient should be at a 30-degree angle or higher (up to 90 degrees in stable patients) with the upper extremity placed above the head in as comfortable a position as possible. With hypotensive patients, the supine position is the only hemodynamically prudent position.

CAUTION

Beware when placing the chest tube, in that, with massive hemoperitoneum, the blood may push the diaphragm as high as the third intercostal space, and commonly into the fifth intercostal space (22). Insertion here may result in perforation of the liver or spleen. The patient should be receiving oxygen, as well as having a pulse oximeter and cardiac monitor. Resuscitation measures should also include, at a minimum, one large-bore, short intravenous line.

The choice of entry for the tube is the fourth or fifth intercostal space in the midaxillary line. Some prefer the posterior axillary line, but this may cause pain, as the patient lies against the tube and may even impair suction through kinking.

NOTE

Avoid old scars from a previous site or thoracotomy because underlying adhesions to the lung may have formed in proximity to these old scars.

This area should be devoid of pectoralis major muscle, thus making insertion of the chest tube easier. This is not the case when using the anterior approach (which we do not tend to use in the emergency department), where blunt dissection proceeds through the pectoralis major muscle. Short-fingered individuals may well have trouble exploring the insertion site because of the deeper layers of the chest wall.

Procedural Steps

1. Prepare and drape the area in a sterile fashion.
2. Anesthetize a 4-cm area on the skin along the axis one rib and interspace below your insertion point (sixth intercostal space or seventh rib) superficially with a wheal to be able to identify the incision point visually. (The idea is to have the tube tunnel underneath subcutaneous tissue for a short length before entering the chest cavity, so we start one space below). Next anesthetize the subcutaneous tissue along the tract from that incision point to the fifth or fourth intercostal space. Generously anesthetize the top of the fifth rib and intercostal muscles. Finally advance the needle to the pleura (anesthetizing generously) and the chest cavity. One may end up using the entire 20-mL in the process, but the patient will be infinitely more comfortable and cooperative. *No chest tube should be inserted without adequate local anesthesia if the patient is awake.* A simple skin wheal does not constitute adequate anesthesia nor does i.v. sedation with a narcotic. If time permits, give a small dose of a relatively hemodynamically neutral analgesic, such as fentanyl, *in addition to your local anesthesia.*
3. Incise along the rib axis through all skin layers and into the subcutaneous tissue. The length of the incision is dependent on the thickness of the chest wall. In very thin individuals, a 2-cm

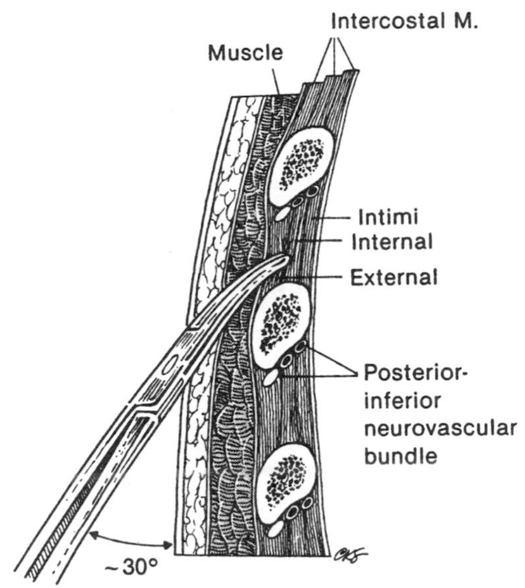

Figure 4.12. Perform blunt dissection through the subcutaneous tissues and intercostal muscles with a Kelly clamp. (From Feliciano DV: Tube thoracostomy. In: Benumof JL, ed. Clinical Procedures in Anesthesia and Intensive Care. Philadelphia: Lippincott, 1992, Fig. 15.2, with permission.)

incision is adequate, but in an obese patient, a larger incision must be made (4 to 5 cm). An inadequate incision will make placing the tube much more difficult. The working space in the chest wall cones down as one goes deeper and, if too small, can make the path too tight to advance the tube or even enter the chest cavity. So a good rule of thumb is to make the incision about 2 cm or slightly larger.

4. Dissect bluntly with the Kelly clamp the top of the rib at the chest tube insertion site (Fig. 4.12). Remain on the upper border of the rib in the interspace to avoid the neurovascular bundle that courses along the inferior rib margin. Then with one or two spreads of the intercostal muscles, close the Kelly, and use the tip to puncture the pleura in a controlled fashion (not plunging uncontrollably). With the tip of the Kelly near the pleural plane, open the Kelly and stretch the tissue to slightly larger than tube size.

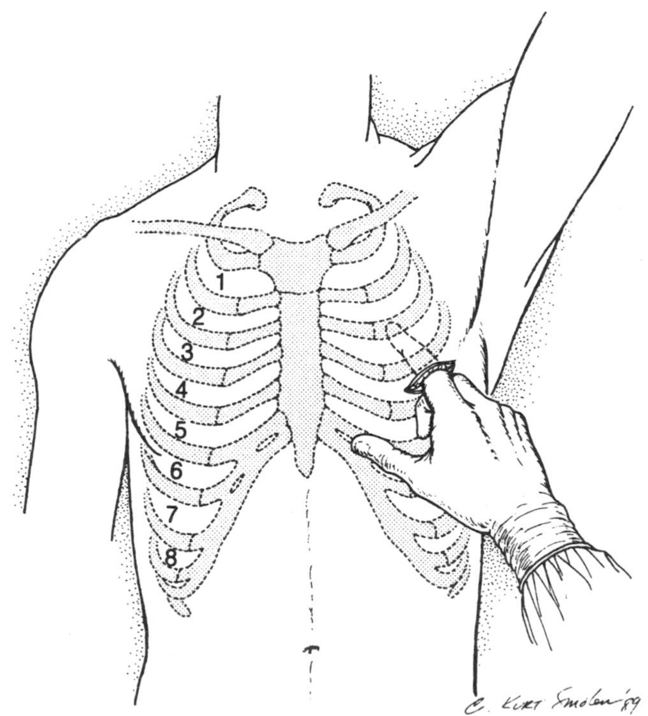

Figure 4.13. Perform finger thoracotomy before insertion of the thoracostomy tube. (From Feliciano DV: Tube thoracostomy. In: Benumof JL, ed. Clinical Procedures in Anesthesia and Intensive Care. Philadelphia, Lippincott, 1992, Fig. 15.3, with permission.)

5. Perform a "finger thoracostomy" (a sweep of the finger in the hole at the chest tube insertion site) with the objective to note any adhesions or diaphragm and to confirm the presence of the intrathoracic space (and not the intraperitoneal space noted by palpable liver or spleen) (Fig. 4.13). Pleural adhesions that cannot be easily separated by the finger should alert the operator that another site of insertion should be attempted. If a tear in the diaphragm is noted, then an operative repair is mandated.
6. Cover the pleural cutaneous opening with the hand before placing the tube into the pleural space.
7. Advance the chest tube with the Kelly clamped around the distal end into the chest wall tract and into the chest cavity. It is usually necessary to keep the puncture site open before advancing the tube. This can be done by inserting the Kelly clamp and spreading it apart. Direct it posteriorly and apically (Fig. 4.14). All the holes in the chest tube should be within the pleural space. Connect the tube immediately to the Pleurivac or suction apparatus under a water seal of negative 20 cm of H_2O to evacuate the pleural cavity and reexpand the lung.

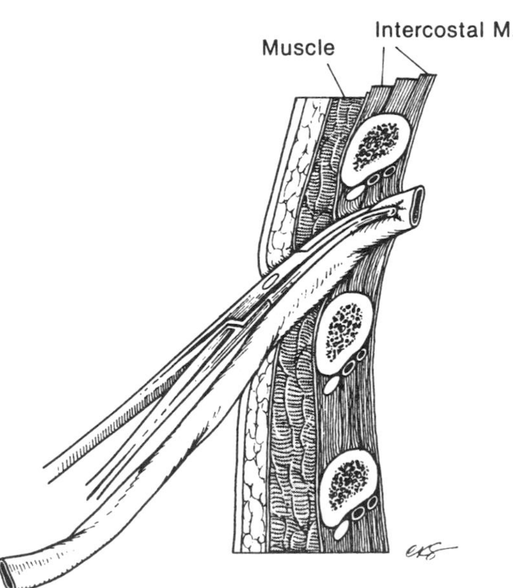

Figure 4.14. Direct the thoracostomy tube posteriorly and superiorly in patients with pleural effusions including hemothoraces. (From Feliciano DV: Tube thoracostomy. In: Benumof JL, ed. Clinical Procedures in Anesthesia and Intensive Care. Philadelphia, Lippincott, 1992, Fig. 15.4, with permission.)

NOTE

Once proper functioning of the tube setup is assessed, needles from any needle decompression of a tension pneumothorax should be removed to prevent laceration of the lung.

---

8. Secure the tube with sutures. Bring the sutures through both sides of the wound edge near the tube and tie. Wrap the two remaining ends multiple times around the tube, with each end wrapped in the opposite direction of the other. After multiple layers of the suture are wrapped, bunch them up at the entrance to the wound and tie tightly. Make a kink in the tube so that it wiil not slide in or out of the chest wall. Sutures superior and inferior to the tube along the wound will create a seal with the subcutaneous tissue.

CAUTION

Purse-string sutures may be used but may cause wound ischemia around the tube and possible necrosis at the entrance site.

---

9. Apply a sterile dressing with use of Xeroform *or* Vaseline-impregnated gauze placed around the wound covered by 4 × 4-inch gauze with Y incisions placed orthogonal to each other.

Tape the area with the tube enveloped in the tape for a few centimeters to prevent excessive movement at the skin/tube juncture, thus decreasing the pain experienced by the patient. The breath sounds of the patient should be heard well bilaterally; check the CXR immediately after for tube placement and evidence of reexpansion of the lung and evacuation of the fluid.

AFTERCARE

Check for leaks in the system. Reasons for failure to reexpand the lung are that there is a bronchial tear, a mucus plug in the chest tube, or the proximal hole is outside the chest cavity (22).

1. Leaks are indicated by persistent bubbling or failure to reexpand the lung. When a leak is found, this indicates one of the following causes.
   a. Leakage of air through a connection in the tubing. Check the connecting sites and make sure there is no leak. In addition, check for a hole in the tubing.
   b. One of the holes in the chest tube is not in the chest itself but in the subcutaneous tissue, and thus air is leaking out of the chest tube.
   c. Air is continuing to leak through a bronchiole with a bronchopleural fistula formed. If this continues, suspect a ruptured bronchus. When an air leak is massive and neither (a) nor (b) is the cause, then a rupture of the main stem bronchus or other larger bronchi should be suspected. Occasionally a small bronchopleural fistula may be "overpowered" and reduced by the insertion of two or three chest tubes.
   d. Rupture of the esophagus, although rare, is another possible cause of continuing air leak in the chest tube. With a ruptured esophagus, air dissects into the mediastinum and pleural spaces and is drained by the chest tube, causing a persistent air leak.
2. Close the remainder of the incision with simple interrupted vertical mattress sutures.
3. Apply antibacterial ointment to the incision site followed by a Xeroform dressing over the wound. After this, apply two sterile 4 × 4-inch dressings with a slit cut halfway across the center of the 4 × 4, and advance the pads around the chest tube via the slit so that two 4 × 4 dressings encircle the chest tube.
4. Secure the dressing in place with adhesive tape followed by an Elastoplast dressing. It is our preference to attach adhesive tape between the dressing and the chest tube, and spiral additional strips of 1-inch adhesive tape around the chest tube before application of the Elastoplast dressing to provide additional security against pulling the tube out.

Anterior Chest Tube

Only those differences between the insertion of the anterior and the posterolateral chest tube are discussed. An anterior chest tube is used only when dealing with a simple or tension pneumothorax in which there is no fluid to be drained. Remember, then, that when dealing with a tension pneumothorax, insert a needle before insertion of the anterior chest tube to relieve the tension pneumothorax.

1. The second and third intercostal space in the midclavicular line is the preferred site for placement of anterior chest tube.
2. In passing the tube, aim it anteriorly toward the apex of the lung. Locate the hole nearest to the proximal portion of the tube just behind the first rib, because this is where most air tends to accumulate in a pneumothorax.

COMPLICATIONS

1. Unilateral pulmonary edema. Unilateral pulmonary edema may occur from rapid expansion and excessive negative pressures. Rapid reexpansion causes a rapid increase in the pulmonary capillary pressure and blood flow, resulting in transudation of fluid across the capillary membrane, which in turn results in pulmonary edema. When dealing with a large hemothorax, interrupt drainage by clamping the tube after 200 to 300 mL has been evacuated, follow by intermittent release so that reexpansion can be in a staged, slow fashion. Anoxia may have also damaged these capillary membranes, facilitating the development of pulmonary edema. This phenomenon occurs 2 to 3 hours after thoracostomy (29, 31, 57).
2. Injury of the lung. The thoracostomy can be placed into the nonresilient lung fixed to the chest wall by pleural adhesions. This intrapulmonary insertion will cause a pneumothorax with persistent air leak and possibly hemoptysis (68). This complication is extremely common in neonates and has been reported in as many as 25% of cases of neonates with respiratory distress syndrome who require chest tubes (21). Laceration of the lung may also result from improper placement of the tube or the use of a trocar. This can be prevented by careful placement of the tube using the technique outlined in this section.
3. Bleeding from the chest wall. This complication may result from laceration of an intercostal artery in placing a posterolateral chest tube or laceration of an internal mammary vessel in placing an anterior chest tube. This complication may be prevented by inserting the chest tube along the superior edge of the rib below the interspace being entered to avoid the neurovascular bundle that courses under the ribs. With an anterior chest tube, do not place the tube any more medial than the midclavicular line to avoid the internal mammary vessels.
4. Continuing air leak. This was discussed earlier; check for holes in the tubing, loose connections, and chest tube holes being external to the pleural cavity. Prevent the problem of loose connections by taping the connection to the tubing.
5. Occlusion of the chest tube. Occlusion of the chest tube may occur from a large clot or kinking of the chest tube. Prevent this by inserting a sufficiently large chest tube when dealing with a hemothorax in the adult. Prevent kinking of the tube by inserting the chest tube at the midaxillary line rather than the posterior axillary line. In the latter position, the patient may kink the tube by lying on it.
6. Persistent pneumothorax. A persistent pneumothorax on repeated radiograph indicates that a large air leak is present, with failure of the lung to expand. The treatment of this is to increase suction; if this does not provide relief of the pneumothorax, then consider placing a second chest tube (anteriorly or laterally). In patients with a large air leak and a persistent pneumothorax, the defect usually involves a large bronchus, and surgical closure may be indicated.
7. Subcutaneous emphysema. This may result from continuing air leak into the subcutaneous space from a pneumothorax that is inadequately decompressed by the chest tube, resulting in leakage of air into the subcutaneous tissue. Another cause is that the skin may be too tightly sealed around the chest tube, resulting in air leakage into the subcutaneous tissue rather than through the skin incision. This is an unusual cause of this problem; however, when it occurs, it can be treated by removing the suture closest to the

chest tube at the incision site to permit venting of the subcutaneous tissue.

Other complications of this procedure include

1. Lung puncture with resultant hemothorax.
2. Diaphragmatic laceration with intraperitoneal placement.
3. Cardiac dysrhythmias from tube placement against the heart.
4. Extrapleural positioning of the tube.
5. Infection.
6. Erosion of the tip into extrapleural structures.
7. Tension pneumothorax after clamping the tube which should never be done; just leave it connected to the underwater seal.
8. Loss of tidal volume while on high suction due to a significant pulmonary air leak.

THORACENTESIS

Thoracentesis, or the placing of a needle in the pleural space, is performed in the emergency department for both diagnostic and therapeutic reasons. Patients entering with respiratory embarrassment will need removal of fluid from the pleural space to allow an increase in tidal volume. Fluid may accumulate from previous trauma, infections, metabolic processes (uremia, liver cirrhosis, or pancreatitis) and tumors. The tumors may be either primary (mesothelioma) or secondary (metastases from lung, breast, pancreas, or stomach) (23).

Typically the diagnosis is made by physical diagnosis and confirmed on plain CXR. To be evident on a chest film, the amount of fluid must usually be greater than 400 to 500 mL, depending on chest cavity size. Typically the fluid on the radiograph obscures the level of the diaphragm. The physical diagnosis clues include flatness to percussion and a change in lung sounds (Litten's sign: loss of resonance with respiration) (23).

EQUIPMENT

Many kits are available for thoracentesis. They have made the procedure effortless. In case there are no kits, the following can be assembled:

Povidone–iodine (Betadine) solution and drapes
1% lidocaine
25- and 22-gauge needles (one each), 10-mL syringe
50-mL syringe and three-way stopcock
Collection tubes or bags
16- or 18-gauge through-the-needle catheter or 18-gauge pigtail catheter with a guide wire
Vaseline gauze
Sterile connecting tubing (from stopcock to bag or bottle)

CONTRAINDICATIONS

1. Traumatic hemo- or pneumothorax. These need tube thoracostomy.
2. Coagulopathy
3. Tension pneumothorax

PROCEDURE

Position the patient. For fluid removal, use mainly the posterior approach, but if the fluid is anteriorly loculated, then of course use the anterior approach. Use plain films of the chest in upright and lateral decubitus positions to confirm the location of the fluid. The patient is sitting upright and leaning forward while resting the arms on an elevated bedside table for the posterior approach. The patient should be sitting upright on the stretcher for the anterior approach.

1. Determine the insertion site. For most purposes, use the seventh intercostal space in the midscapular line or at the angle of the rib, just lateral to the muscle mass of the erector spinae muscles. A frequently used safety rule for thoracentesis at any site is that a needle should never be inserted below the fifth rib in the midclavicular line, the

seventh rib in the midaxillary line, or the ninth rib in the scapular line (23). At each of these sites, the costophrenic angle lies three interspaces below, and damage to the diaphragm or intraabdominal structures is minimized. To aid in localizing the appropriate posterior interspace, it is helpful to remember that the inferior tip of the scapula overlies the seventh rib or interspace.
2. Prepare, drape in sterile fashion, and anesthetize. Make a wheal in the skin overlying the rib below the interspace to be used, by using the 25-gauge needle. With the 22-gauge longer needle, anesthetize and "walk" over the rib while continuing to infiltrate with lidocaine. Infiltrating as the needle is guided directly over the rib into the intercostal muscles, broach and infiltrate the intrapleural space. In the anterior approach, guide the needle through the mid second and third intercostal space, avoiding the vessels below and above the rib.
3. Aspirate to confirm the intrapleural space insertion, yielding the target fluid, if in the correct location. A hemostat may be placed on the needle to mark the depth of the 22-gauge needle. Remove the needle.
4. Advance through the established tract the 18-gauge through-the-needle catheter setup (attached to the 50-mL syringe and stopcock) with the depth marked by the hemostat (same depth marked by the hemostat used on the 22-gauge needle). Then advance this needle with negative suction. Once pleural fluid is noted, advance the catheter through the needle in a downward direction, and once good flow is established, withdraw the needle from the pleural cavity to avoid lung lacerations. Place the needle guard around the needle, and withdraw fluid until about 1,500 to 2,000 mL has been removed.
5. Monitor the patient's hemodynamic status while the fluid is removed. Respiratory embarrassment should improve as fluid is removed, as noted by the patient's decreased work of breathing and improved oxygen saturation.

NOTE

With a simple 2-inch Angiocath with an over-the-needle catheter, use the same setup. The only difference is that when the catheter is passed over the needle, the needle is again directed downward and the thumb or finger is used to occlude the port, thus avoiding a pneumothorax. Attach the 50-mL syringe with the stopcock to the hub of the catheter, and remove the fluid.

NOTE

If using the guide wire technique, advance the needle again into the pleural space where, pointing downward, a guide wire is advanced into the pleural cavity. Withdraw the needle, make a small skin incision, and advance the pigtail catheter over the guide wire. Occlude the catheter with the thumb until the stopcock is attached with the off position to the pleural cavity. Attach the 50-mL syringe, and aspirate fluid.

After the fluid has been removed, obtain a CXR to look for a pneumothorax, and send the fluid for diagnostic studies, if this is a diagnostic procedure.

COMPLICATIONS

1. Pneumothorax: persistent coughing by the patient can herald a newly created pneumothorax.
2. Lung laceration.
3. Hemopneumothorax.
4. Diaphragmatic tear.
5. Intraabdominal injuries from inadvertent needle puncture.
6. Infection.
7. Hypoxia and pulmonary edema. All

patients undergoing thoracentesis should have supplemental oxygen, as PO_2 may decrease by 10 to 16 mm Hg within 2 hours of the procedure because of an increase in ventilation/perfusion (V/Q) abnormalities.

8. Hypotension from removal of massive amounts of fluid.
9. Chest wall bleeding from lacerated intercostal artery.
10. Persistent localized anesthesia from injury to the intercostal nerve.
11. Loss of the guide wire into the pleural cavity.
12. Shearing off of the distal through-the-needle catheter into the pleural cavity.

The final step in a diagnostic thoracentesis is analyzing the fluid. The fluid is categorized into transudates and exudates. The exudate based on the biochemistry, and presence or absence of loculations is categorized as an empyema, a parapneumonic, or a nonparapneumonic effusion. The differences are listed later. If the effusion is a complicated parapneumonic effusion or empyema, a tube thoracostomy should be placed in addition to treatment with antibiotics. Thus the thoracentesis is followed by tube thoracostomy in several instances, depending on the results of the fluid analysis (38). The following represent fluid results that are best treated with both antibiotics and tube thoracostomy:

Simple complicated parapneumonic effusions (pH<7.00, glucose <40 mg/dL, or Gram stain positive or culture positive, but fluid, not frank pus or loculated).

Complex parapneumonic effusions (those previously mentioned plus loculations).

Simple empyema.

Complex empyema.

TRANSTHORACIC PACEMAKER INSERTION

This procedure has fallen out of favor and has been replaced with transcutaneous pacing and transvenous pacing. It was mainly used in the patient in cardiac arrest when there was failure of transvenous or transcutaneous pacing. When transcutaneous pacing is not producing results, a transvenous pacing wire is floated with a balloon. The problem is that in a cardiac arrest, there is no flow to direct the balloon. Without the aid of fluoroscopy, the wire position within the ventricle could not be assured or obtained quickly, as needed in a code. The advantage of transthoracic pacing is that it is quick, and the position is assured. No blood flow need be present to place a wire within the ventricle. Some of the reasons for falling out of favor include the potential complications, the most obvious of which is the creation of cardiac tamponade. In addition, it may injure the LAD coronary artery.

The indications are the same for transvenous pacing, with the exception that the patients must be unstable, moribund, or in cardiac arrest. Stable and awake patients should have transvenous pacing wires inserted.

EQUIPMENT

Elecath transthoracic pacemaker set (commercially available)

Povidone–iodine solution (Betadine)

ECG machine

1% lidocaine

10-mL syringe

25-gauge and 18-gauge needles

PROCEDURE

With the patient on the cardiac monitor defibrillator, prepare and drape the area of insertion in a sterile fashion. The areas of concern are the left fifth intercostal space and the xiphoid region. Either can be used as the approach. No anesthesia need be used in a patient who is obtunded, moribund, or in cardiac arrest. For the fifth intercostal space approach, direct the needle in the left parasternal fifth intercostal space, aiming slightly medially and cephalad. The needle should enter the intercostal space in the middle of interspace, not directly over or under the rib, to avoid intercostal arteries.

Once blood is aspirated, ventricular position is assumed; advance the wire through the needle's side port while the proximal leads are connected to the pacing box. When resistance is met or when capture is evident, advance the wire no farther. If no capture, bring out the entire needle and pacing wire as a unit to avoid shearing off the wire within the chest. Then repeat these steps.

Preparatory Steps

1. Prepare and drape the skin around the xiphoid process.
2. Keep the patient on an ECG monitor continuously throughout the procedure.
3. Infiltrate a local anesthetic to the left of the xiphoid process in the left costosternal angle.

Procedural Steps

1. Insert the 6-inch needle with the obturator in place in the left costosternal angle, as indicated in Fig. 4.15. After penetrating the skin, direct the needle toward the midclavicular line at an angle of 30 degrees to the skin. Alternately, aim the needle at either the right or the left shoulder.
2. Remove the obturator from the needle to ascertain entrance into the cardiac chamber (Fig. 4.16). A brisk flow of blood through the needle indicates that the ventricle has been entered. When ventricular pressures are too low to produce this rapid flow, attach a syringe to the needle and aspirate blood to ascertain entrance into the heart.
3. Pass a bipolar pacing stylet with a jacket around the J-shaped tip (to straighten the tip of the stylet to permit passage through the needle) (Fig. 4.17). Pass the stylet through the needle until well within the cardiac chamber.
4. Withdraw the needle over the stylet.
5. Pull the stylet back until its J-shaped tip enters the endocardial surface of the heart, at which point, resistance is met that prevents further withdrawal of the stylet (Fig. 4.18). The jacket

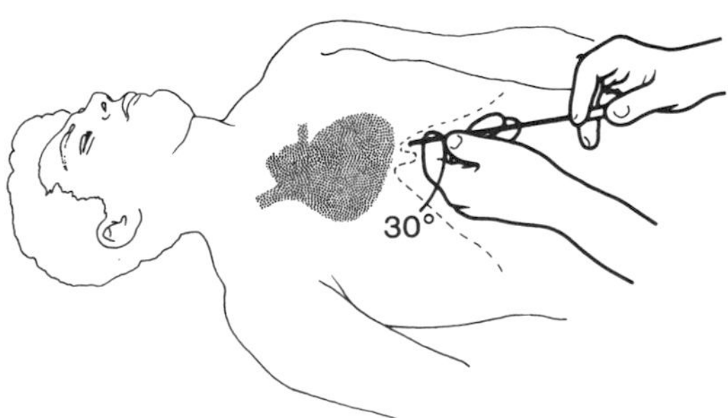

Figure 4.15. Passage of a transthoracic pacemaker. Insert the needle as shown above, directed toward the midclavicular line at an angle of 30 degrees to the skin. (From Simon R, Brenner B: Emergency Procedures and Techniques, 3rd ed. Baltimore: Williams & Wilkins, 1994. Fig. 4.34, page 157, with permission.)

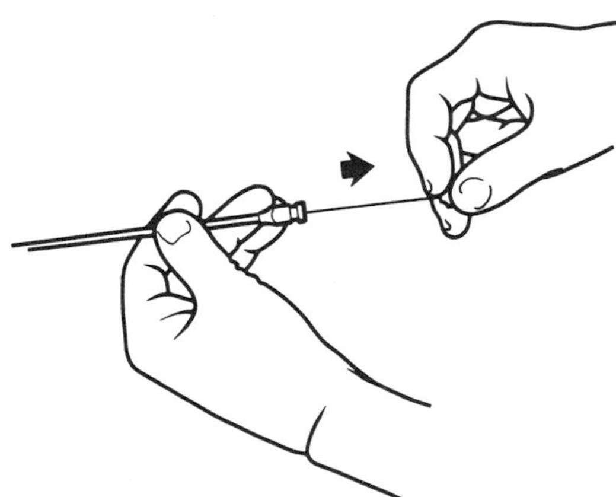

Figure 4.16. Remove the obturator from the needle to ascertain entrance into the cardiac chamber. A brisk flow of blood through the needle indicates the ventricle has been entered. When the procedure is being performed in a patient who has an asystole, aspiration intermittently performed during passage of the needle will indicate when the cardiac chamber has been entered. (From Simon R, Brenner B: Emergency Procedures and Techniques, 3rd ed. Baltimore: Williams & Wilkins, 1994. Fig. 4.35, page 157, with permission.)

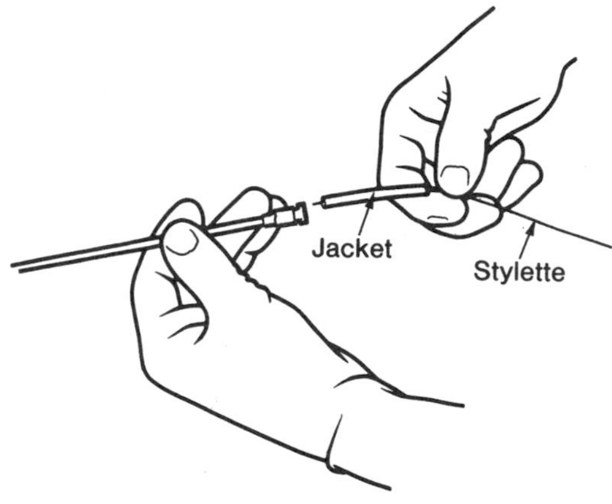

Figure 4.17. Pass a bipolar pacing stylet with a jacket around the J-shaped tip (to straighten the tip of the stylet to permit passage through the needle). The stylet should be passed through the needle until well within the cardiac chamber. (From Simon R, Brenner B: Emergency Procedures and Techniques, 3rd ed. Baltimore: Williams & Wilkins, 1994. Fig. 4.36, page 157, with permission.)

shown in Fig. 4.17 remains at the proximal end of the stylet and can be removed at this point.

6. Attach the stylet to the pacemaker unit via the connecting adaptor that is supplied in the set. The connecting adaptor has two leads extending from it, one marked distal, which is secured to the negative pole, and another marked proximal, which is attached to the positive pole of the pacemaker generator.
7. Set the pacemaker at 1.5 to 2 mA and at a rate of 70 beats/min and check for capture. The level of the current may have to be elevated over 2 mA for capture to occur.
8. Once capture occurs, suture the stylet to the chest wall, and apply a sterile dressing.

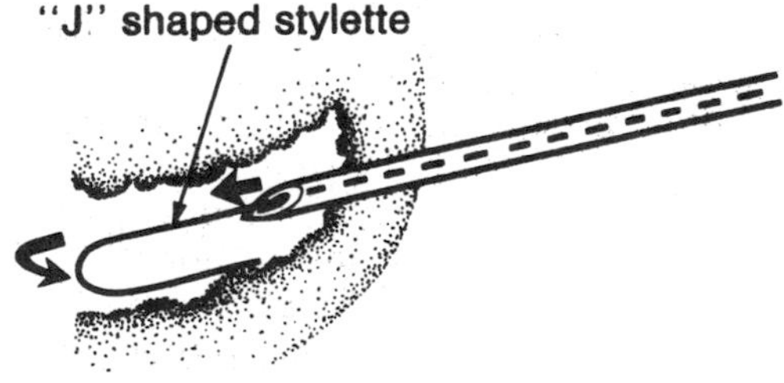

Figure 4.18. Pull the stylet back until its J-shaped tip enters the endocardial surface of the heart, at which point a resistance is met to withdrawal of the stylet. (From Simon R, Brenner B: Emergency Procedures and Techniques, 3rd ed. Baltimore: Williams & Wilkins, 1994. Fig. 4.37, page 157, with permission.)

Aftercare

Move the patient as little as possible to prevent inadvertent removal of the stylet or perforation of the heart.

COMPLICATIONS

1. Injury to the coronary arteries. This complication is extremely common and can be prevented by using the fourth intercostal space as recommended by some authors. By using the technique described and aiming the needle either at the midclavicular line or at the right shoulder, this problem generally can be avoided.
2. Pericardial hemorrhage and tamponade. This may result from puncture of a coronary vessel by the needle or from injury to the myocardium. There is very little, with the exception of exercising caution in performing the procedure, that one can do to prevent this complication.
3. Breakage of the stylet. This occurs from withdrawal of the stylet through the needle, which should never be done because it may shear when placing an Intracath. During cardiopulmonary resuscitation (CPR), external cardiac massage must be stopped, or the stylet may break. One author (B.B.) has seen such a case in which the stylet was retrievable only by open thoracotomy.
4. Failure to recognize underlying rhythm changes, such as ventricular fibrillation.

References

1. Armstrong NF, Feigenbaum H, Dillon JC: Acute right ventricular dilation and echocardiographic volume overload following pericardiocentesis for relief of cardiac tamponade. Am Heart J 107:1266, 1984.
2. Arom KV, Richardson J, Webb G, et al: Subxiphoid pericardial window in patients with suspected traumatic pericardial tamponade. Ann Thorac Surg 23:545–549, 1977.
3. Balakrishnan S, Hartman CW, Grinnan GL, et al: Pericardial fluid gas analysis in hemorrhagic pericardial tamponade. Ann Thorac Surg 27: 55–58, 1979.
4. Barnett WM: Comparison of open-chest cardiac massage techniques in dogs. Ann Emerg Med 15:408, 1986.
5. Biffl WL, Moore EE, Harken AH: Emergency department thoracotomy. In: Mattox KL, Feliciano DV, Moore EE, eds. Trauma, 4th ed. New York: McGraw-Hill, 250, 2000.
6. Biffl WL, Moore EE, Harken AH: Emergency department thoracotomy. In: Mattox KL, Feliciano DV, Moore EE, eds. Trauma, 4th ed. New York: McGraw-Hill, 248, 2000.
7. Biffl WL, Moore EE, Harken AH: Emergency department thoracotomy. In: Mattox KL, Feliciano DV, Moore EE, eds. Trauma, 4th ed. New York: McGraw-Hill, 247, 2000.
8. Borja AR, Lansing A, Randell H. Immediate operative treatment for stab wounds of the heart. J Thorac Cardiovasc Surg 59:662, 1970.
9. Breaux EP, Dupont JB, Albert HM, et al: cardiac tamponade following penetrating mediastinal injuries: improved survival with early pericardiocentesis. J Trauma 19:461–466, 1979.
10. Callaham M: Acute traumatic cardiac tamponade: diagnosis and treatment. JACEP 7:306, 1978.
11. Callahan JA, Seward JB, Nishimura RA, et al: Two-dimensional echocardiographically guided pericardiocentesis: Experience in 117 consecutive patients. Am J Cardiol 55:476, 1985.
12. Cameron DE, Shumway SJ, Borkon AM: Use of cardiopulmonary bypass in cardiovascular trauma. Trauma Q 4:44, 1988.
13. Casale AS, Borkon AM: Penetrating cardiac trauma. Trauma Q 4:39, 1988.
14. Chitwood RW: Cardiac trauma: Penetrating and blunt. In: Moylan JA, ed. Principles of Trauma Surgery. New York: Gower Medical Publishing, 5.16, 1992.
15. Chitwood RW: Cardiac trauma: Penetrating and blunt. In: Moylan JA, ed. Principles of Trauma Surgery. New York: Gower Medical Publishing, 5.13, 1992.
16. Cholankeril JV, Joshi RR, Cenizal JS, et al: Massive air embolism from the pulmonary artery. Radiology 142:33, 1982.
17. DeGennaro VA, Bonfils-Roberts EA, Ching N: Aggressive management of potential penetrating cardiac injuries. J Thorac Cardiovasc Surg 79:833–837, 1980.
18. Delguercio L, Feins N, Cohn J, et al: Comparison of blood flow during external and internal cardiac massage in man. Circulation 31(Suppl I): 171, 1965.
19. Demetriades D: Cardiac wounds: Experience with 70 patients. Ann Surg 203:315–317, 1986.
20. Demetriades D, Van Der Ven BW: Penetrating injuries of the heart: experience over two years in South Africa. J Trauma 23:1034–1041, 1983.
21. Espada R, Whisennand HH, Mattox KL, et al: Surgical management of penetrating injuries to the coronary arteries. Surgery 78:755–760, 1975.
22. Feliciano DV: Tube thoracostomy. In: Benumof JL, ed. Clinical Procedures in Anesthesia and Intensive Care. Philadelphia: Lippincott, 305–313, 1992.
23. Feliciano DV: Tube thoracentesis. In: Benumof JL, ed. Clinical Procedures in Anesthesia and Intensive Care. Philadelphia: Lippincott, 297–303, 1992.
24. Glasser F, Fein AM, Feinsilver SH, et al: Noncardiogenic pulmonary edema after pericardial drainage for cardiac tamponade. Chest 94:689, 1988.
25. Graham JM, Beall AC, Mattox KL, et al: Systemic air embolism following penetrating trauma to the lung. Chest 72:449, 1977.
26. Guberman BA, Fowler NO, Engel PJ, et al: Cardiac tamponade in medical patients. Circulation 64:633, 1981.
27. Heilerh B, Anderes U, Follath F: Diagnosis and therapy of cardiac tamponade: an analysis of 50 patients. Schweiz Med Wochenschr 111:735, 1981.
28. Jackson RE, Freeman SB: Hemodynamics of cardiac massage. Emerg Med Clin North Am 1: 501, 1983.
29. Johnson J, Kirby CK: An experimental study of cardiac massage. Surgery 26:472, 1949.
30. Kaiser E, Loewenneck H: Pericardial puncture: The most favorable anatomical approach. Munch Med Wochenschr 123:1697, 1981.
31. King MW, Aitchism JM, Nel JP: Fatal air embolism following penetrating lung trauma: An autopsy study. J Trauma 24:753, 1984.
32. Klopfenstein HS, Cogswell TL, Bernath GA, et al: Alternations in intravascular volume affect the relation between right ventricular diastolic collapse and the hemodynamic severity of cardiac tamponade. J Am Coll Cardiol 6:1057, 1985.
33. Krikorian JG, Hancock EW: Pericardiocentesis. Am J Med 65:808, 1978.
34. Leinbach RC, Goldstein J, Gold HK, et al: Percutaneous wire-guided balloon pumping. Am J Cardiol 49:1707, 1982.
35. Leonard DJ, Gens DR: Diagnosis of cardiac injury: Pericardiocentesis v diagnostic pericardial window. Trauma Q 4:29, 1988.
36. Levine MJ, Lorell BH, Diver DJ, et al: Implications of echocardiographically assisted diagnosis of pericardial tamponade in contemporary medical patients: Detection prior to hemodynamic embarrassment. Am J Coll Cardiol 17: 59, 1991.
37. Levitsky S: New insights in cardiac trauma. Surg Clin North Am 55:43–55, 1975.

38. Light RW: A new classification of parapneumonic effusions and empyema. Chest 108:299, 1995.
39. Lorell BH: Pericardial diseases. In: Braunwald E, ed. Heart Disease: A Textbook of Cardiovascular Medicine, 5th ed. Philadelphia: WB Saunders, 1493, 1997.
40. Lorell BH: Pericardial diseases. In: Braunwald E, ed. Heart Disease: A Textbook of Cardiovascular Medicine, 5th ed. Philadelphia: WB Saunders, 1494, 1997.
41. Lorell BH: Pericardial diseases. In: Braunwald E, ed. Heart Disease: A Textbook of Cardiovascular Medicine, 5th ed. Philadelphia: WB Saunders, 1492, 1997.
42. Moller CT, Schoonbee CG, Rosendorff C: Hemodynamics of cardiac tamponade during various modes of ventilation. Br J Anaesth 51:409, 1979.
43. Morgan CD, Marshall SA, Ross JR: Catheter drainage of the pericardium: Its safety and efficacy. Can J Surg 32:331, 1989.
44. Perkins R, Elchos T. Stab wound of the aortic arch. Ann Surg 147:83, 1958.
45. Rea WJ, Sugg WL, Wilson LC, et al: Coronary artery lacerations. Ann Thorac Surg 7:518–528, 1969.
46. Rich NM, Spencer FC: Wounds of the Heart in Vascular Trauma. Philadelphia: WB Saunders, 1978.
47. Richardson JD, Flint LM, Snow NJU, et al: Management of transmediastinal gunshot wounds. Surgery 90:671, 1981.
48. Scalea T, Sinert R, Duncan A, et al: Percutaneous central access for resuscitation in trauma. Acad Emer Med Nov-Dec: 6, 1994.
49. Symbas PN: Trauma to the heart and great vessels. New York: Grune & Stratton, 1978.
50. Symbas PN, Harlaftis N, Waldo WJ: Penetrating cardiac wounds: A comparison of different therapeutic methods. Ann Surg 183:377–381, 1976.
51. Thomas AN, Stephens BG: Air embolism: a cause of morbidity and death after penetrating chest trauma. J Trauma 14:633, 1974.
52. Trinkle JK, Franz J, Grover FL, et al: Affairs of the wounded heart: Penetrating cardiac wounds. J Trauma 19:467–472, 1979.
53. Trinkle JK, Marcos J, Grover FL, et al: Management of the wounded heart. Ann Thorac Surg 17:230–238, 1974.
54. Wall MJ, Mattox KL, Baldwin JC: Acute management of complex cardiac injuries. J Trauma 42:905, 1997.
55. Wasserberger J, Ordog GJ, Dang C: Emergency department thoracotomy. Emerg Med Clin North Am 7:107, 1989.
56. Wilson RF: Thoracic vascular trauma. In: Bongard FS, Wilson SE, Perry MO, eds. Vascular Injuries in Surgical Practice. Norwalk: Appleton & Lange, 107–116, 1991.
57. Yee ES, Verrier ED, Thomas AN: Management of air embolism in blunt and penetrating chest trauma. J Thorac Cardiovasc Surg 86:661, 1983.

5

Neurosurgical Procedures

BURR HOLES

Intracranial Hematomas in Severe Head Injury

More that 2 million patients are evaluated in the emergency department each year for acute head trauma (59, 61). Head injury is the leading cause of traumatic death in the under 25-years-old age group (52). The incidence of death from traumatic brain injury has a bimodal distribution and peaks again in the age group older than 65 years (52). Zimmerman et al. (63) noted that adults had a higher incidence of hemorrhagic contusions (33% vs. 16%) and subdural hematoma (20% vs. 5%) compared with children. In a study of 8,814 patients with head injuries of varying severity, subdural hematomas occurred in 6% of patients aged 0 to 4 years, in 3% of patients aged 5 to 14 years, and then steadily increased throughout adulthood to an incidence of approximately 30% in 70-year-old patients (35). In a study of 779 patients with severe head injury, Levin et al. (32) found a distribution of 20% subdural hematoma in patients aged 0 to 4 years, which decreased to 7% in patients aged 11 to 15 years, and increased to 25% in adults (32). Epidural hematomas occurred in 5% of all head injuries (35) and in 9% of severe head injuries in the 15- to 30-year-old group and then decreases with age (35).

Traumatic acute subdural hematoma is one of the most lethal forms of head injuries (62). Acute subdural hematoma may demonstrate abnormal neurologic signs. Although these signs are indicative of an organic lesion, they are frequently not of localizing value (15). In the series of 247 patients with subdural hematoma by Echlin et al. (15), 79 patients had localizing signs that correctly indicated the side of the hematoma; however, in 29 patients, the signs were the result of lesions on the side opposite that predicted. In 139 patients in this series, the neurologic findings were inconclusive in determining the side of the lesion. Unilateral motor weakness was present in a large number of patients. Inequality in the size of the pupils was noted in 115 of the patients with subdural hematoma before operative intervention. The large pupil was on the side of the hematoma in 74 of these patients and on the opposite side in 41. In 30 patients, there was a bilateral hematoma or a hematoma on one side and a laceration of the brain on the other side. Moreover, of 57 patients with a marked dilatation of one pupil, 36 demonstrated a hematoma on the same side, nine had a hematoma on the other side, and 12 had bilateral hematomas. These findings indicate that a fully dilated pupil is of some value in localization; however, a slight to moderate enlargement of one pupil is of no value.

An acute epidural hematoma is a true neurosurgical emergency. When a patient with the classic findings of an acute epidural hematoma is seen in the community hospital emergency center, death often ensues rapidly when there is no emergency decompression (8). If the patient is in a coma on presentation when the diagnosis is made, the mortality is approximately 20%. If the patient is not in a coma on diagnosis, the mortality is nearly zero (41). With rapid detection and evacuation, the prognosis is excellent (50).

Epidural hematomas are blood clots that form between the dura and the inner table of the skull. The source of the bleeding in 80% of cases is usually the middle meningeal artery or a dural sinus tear. After the artery courses through the foramen spinosum, it courses along the inner surface of the temporal bone. The main branch of this artery lies about one finger breadth anterior and superior to the external auditory meatus. This artery is usually torn by a linear fracture that passes through the temporal bone (Fig. 5.1). In many cases, the fracture may not be seen on routine radiographs of the skull (8). Temporal muscle edema overlying the fracture is an almost constant clinical finding with middle meningeal artery bleeding. Epidural hematomas are usually unilateral and develop rapidly when due to arterial bleeding and more slowly when due to injury of the dural sinus. About 30% of patients with epidural hematomas have a classic presentation of head trauma followed by a decreased level of consciousness, a "lucid interval," and a second episode of decreased consciousness. A lucid interval represents the period between recovery from concussion and lapse into coma as a result of increased intracranial pressure (ICP) secondary to the acute epidural hematoma. The lucid interval is not pathognomonic of an epidural hematoma and occurs with other expanding mass lesions (49). The duration of the lucid interval depends on the rate of recovery from initial concussion and the rapidity of development of cerebral compression from the accumulating hematoma. At this time, the patient may complain of severe headache on the side of the lesion. There also may be some nausea, vomiting, and lethargy. This is followed by a variable period after which is rapid development of unconsciousness, dilation of the ipsilateral pupil, and contralateral hemiplegia progressing to decerebrate rigidity (8). This development of unconsciousness is a terminal event, and unless immediate decompression is performed, changes in the brain will be irreversible, and death will ensue. Such a patient should never be transported from a community hospital to a distant neurosurgical facility without first decompressing the extradural space.

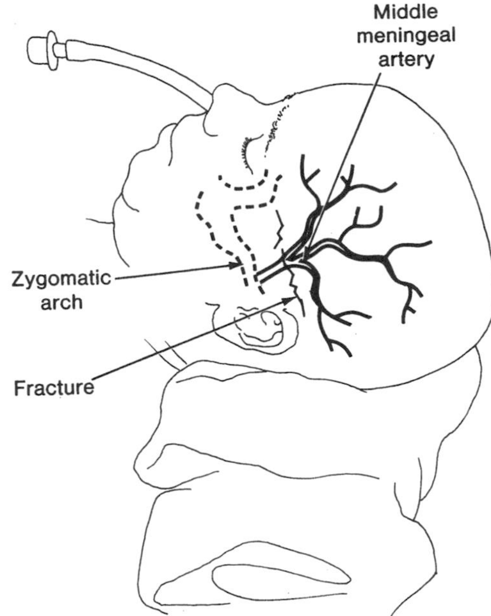

Figure 5.1. A fracture of the temporal bone and its relationship to the middle meningeal artery. A burr hole placed in the temporal area just superior to the zygomatic arch will relieve the pressure of a hematoma.

Treatment of the Patient Who Has Severe Head Injury

The overall mortality of severe head trauma is 40% (28). A number of measures must be taken in the patient with severe head injury to avoid death. The stuporous patient should be kept on his or her side to prevent airway obstruction by the tongue and aspiration of secretions. The airway must be protected, and oxygen should be administered. When necessary, endotracheal intubation should be performed (see Chapter 2 for indications) or even tracheostomy. Shock is almost never secondary to the head injury until the terminal stage and should be presumed to be due to injury elsewhere in the body. Shock must be corrected to treat the patient with severe head injury adequately. The most important adjuncts to the treatment of the patient with a severe head injury are the correction of hypovolemia, maintenance of the airway, and adequate oxygenation. Every unconscious patient also should be treated as if he or she had a fractured cervical spine until proven otherwise.

Patients who have sustained severe head injury and are suspected of having an intracranial hemorrhage may demonstrate signs of increased ICP. In addition to maintaining the airway and restricting fluids in these patients, a number of ancillary modalities that aid in decreasing ICP have been described.

Hyperventilation has an effect on reducing P_{CO_2}, which decreases cerebral blood flow markedly. A decrease in P_{CO_2} from 40 to 30 mm Hg decreases cerebral blood flow by one third. Hyperventilation has an onset of action almost immediately, making it the first choice in patients who are normotensive and who have increased ICP. A P_{CO_2} below 30 mm Hg may worsen the patient's condition by causing vasoconstriction and cerebral ischemia. Prophylactic hyperventilation is not recommended in patients unless there is evidence of increased ICP (38). The osmotic diuretic mannitol reduces cerebral edema and is an established treatment for intracranial hypertension (47). It has been used to decrease ICP preoperatively in many patients. In some cases, mannitol may increase bleeding by decreasing brain size and releasing the "tamponaded" cerebral vessels (53). The onset of action of mannitol is 20 to 30 minutes, and it reaches its peak effectiveness in 30 to 60 minutes.

The use of steroids in the treatment of severe brain injury has been controversial for many years; however, the most recent literature demonstrates that steroids do not reduce ICP secondary to cerebral edema in head trauma and may be harmful (increased risk of infection, altered fluid and glucose metabolism, adrenocortical suppression). Thus steroids are no longer recommended for improving outcome or reducing ICP in patients with severe traumatic brain injury (5, 12, 47).

Barbiturates have been shown to reduce intracranial hypertension refractory to less toxic therapeutic agents. They are ineffective as prophylactic agents against intracranial hypertension (47). The effects of barbiturates are delayed relative to other acute interventions for reducing ICP (50). Hypotension may be detrimental and offsets any beneficial effects of barbiturates (47). Barbiturates have no role during the early management of severe traumatic brain injury but may be used if other methods of reducing ICP are unsuccessful (50).

Cranial decompression in extreme circumstances may be life saving. Indications for surgical intervention in severe traumatic brain-injured patients include

Penetrating injury
Expanding mass
Epidural hematoma
Subdural hematoma
Focal contusions or intracranial hemorrhage
Compound depressed fractures

In general, emergency craniotomy is needed for two reasons: (a) to remove sources of mass effect or increasing ICP, and (b) to clear and debride contaminated open wounds in penetrating trauma (12).

INDICATIONS FOR BURR HOLES

Unilateral neurologic signs with deterioration despite usual therapy (hyperventilation, mannitol) and impending herniation with nonavailability of either a neurosurgeon or operating site are indications.

EQUIPMENT

Smedberg hand drill (Hudson hand drill or brace)
7/64-inch regular-angle carbon bit or a chisel-point bit
20-mL syringe
Anesthetic preparation (usually not necessary)
1% lidocaine (Xylocaine) with epinephrine, 1:100,000
10-mL syringe
25-gauge needle
18-gauge 1.5-inch needle
Prep solution
Medicine cups
Iodinated prep
4 × 4-inch gauze
Single-edge recessed-blade shaver
No. 11 Bard–Parker blade
No. 16 or 18 cone ventricular needle
Four curved hemostats
Drapes, mask, and gown
Frazier suction catheter
Self-retaining retractors

TECHNIQUE

Preparatory Steps

Several types of drills are available for performing trephination in the emergency center. A burr hole may be placed in the underlying skull by using either a standard drill or a drill bit with a chisel head (Fig. 5.2). A twist drill also is available for placing burr holes (Fig. 5.2)

Recently a new hollow screw drill has been introduced for placing burr holes with excellent results.

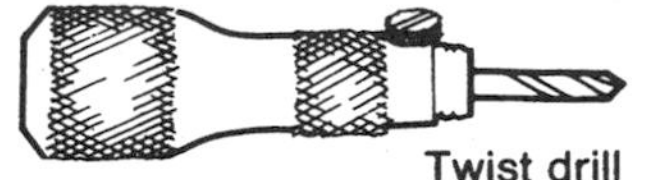

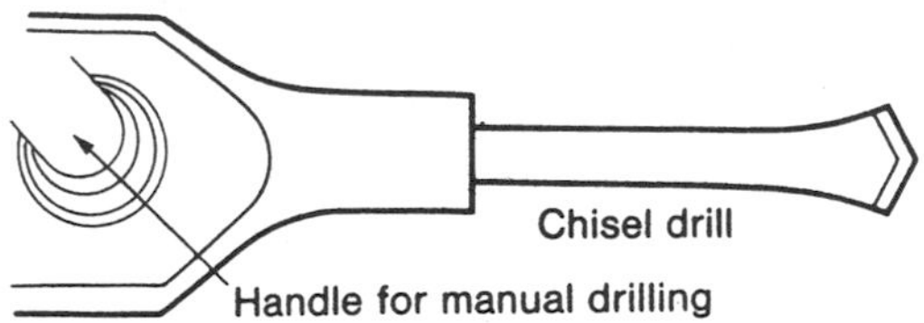

Figure 5.2. The twist drill and the chisel drill. See text for discussion.

NOTE

A twist drill is good for the evacuation of a chronic (i.e., watery) subdural hematoma; however, it may be useless for evacuation of solid or semisolid clotted blood. This is with either a subdural or an epidural hematoma. Such clots are too viscous for removal from such a small hole.

---

1. Place the patient in a supine position with the head of the bed elevated to 15 to 20 degrees.
2. Shave the scalp throughout, including the temporal areas.
3. Prepare the scalp with an iodinated solution.

NOTE

Endotracheally intubate the patient before the procedure is performed both to protect the airway should vomiting occur and for purposes of hyperventilating the patient. In addition, it is advisable that a nasogastric tube be inserted for decompression of the stomach and removal of gastric contents.

---

4. Drape the head of the patient with sterile towels, and wear a mask and gown when performing this procedure.

5. Locate the sites of trephination. In cases of trauma in which an epidural hematoma is highly suspected, place a temporal burr hole. If this is unsuccessful in localizing a hematoma, then place an anterior and a posterior burr hole on both sides of the midline, as shown in Fig. 5.3.

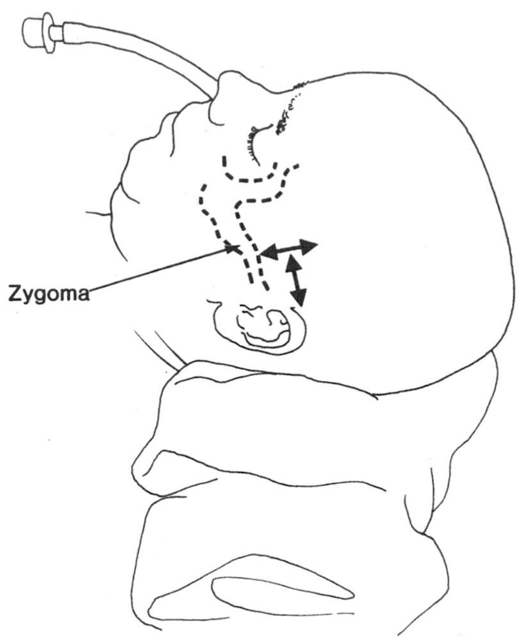

Figure 5.4. Place the temporal burr hole just above the midpoint of the zygomatic arch and one finger breadth anterior to the external auditory canal.

Temporal Burr Hole

Make a 3-cm vertical scalp incision and carry it through the temporalis muscle to the bone. The most common site for placing a burr hole to drain an epidural hematoma is just above the root of the zygoma and one finger breadth anterior to the external auditory canal (Fig. 5.4). When this successfully reduces ICP, the anterior and posterior holes are not necessary.

Anterior Burr Hole

Place the anterior burr hole just in front of the coronal suture and 4 to 5 cm lateral to the midline (Fig. 5.3).

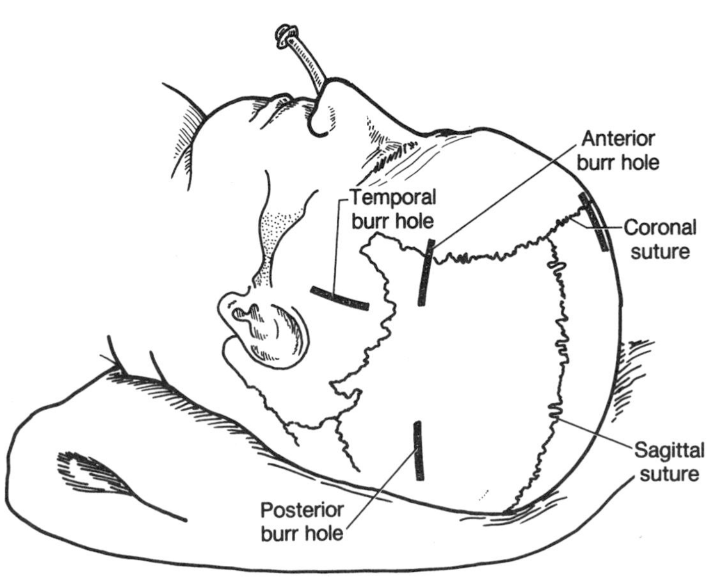

Figure 5.3. Place burr holes as shown above. The coronal suture and sagittal sutures aid in placing the burr holes. See text for discussion.

Posterior Burr Hole

Place the posterior or parietal burr hole over the parietal boss approximately 7 to 8 cm lateral to the midline (Fig. 5.3) (16, 32, 35, 62).

NOTE

The technique of manually measuring and calculating the burr hole site relative to the external occipital protuberance is prone to error. A new device is designed to improve this burr-hole selection process and to eliminate the need for hand measurements and subjective estimates of anatomic landmarks. A triangular frontal target-localizing device with bilateral supraorbital rim tabs is used to assist the surgeon in placing the midline scalp mark 2 cm above the line connecting the supraorbital rims (32). This procedure cannot be done in the emergency department and, thus, is given here only for those interested in learning more about the procedure.

Procedural Steps

1. When using the twist drill, make a small stab wound through the scalp and periosteum using a no. 11 Bard–Parker blade. When using the standard drill, make a linear incision as indicated in Fig. 5.3. When using the hollow screw drill, make a stab incision and percutaneous trephination. When a scalp bleeder is encountered, treat it by infiltrating anesthesia with epinephrine or by applying pressure. After the scalp incision has been made, place a self-retaining retractor in the wound.
2. *Twist drill:* Use a 7/64-inch regular-angle carbon bit driven by a Smedberg hand drill to perforate the skull. Insert it through the scalp incision perpendicular to the skull. When beginning the drill hole, be careful not to permit the drill point to "walk" by applying the drill firmly to the skull and drilling slowly. The dura is generally found to be tightly adherent to the inner table. The handle design of the twist drill provides for the maximal amount of control and force to be applied by alternately pronating and supinating the hand while the wrist is held in a neutral position. When the drill bit has penetrated the diploic space, turn the drill in a clockwise motion that will permit the bit to emerge through the inner table of the skull. The physician usually feels this as a definite end point.

   Standard hand-held drill: Introduce the drill bit perpendicular to the skull through the site of incision (Fig. 5.5). Penetrate the outer table; the drill often catches in the diploe between the inner and outer tables. Then penetrate the inner table.
3. Twist drill and standard drill: After carefully passing through the inner table, but no farther, remove the drill and irrigate the bone dust from the area. Palpate the dura then with a no. 16 or 18 cone ventricular needle. After placement of the burr hole, the physi-

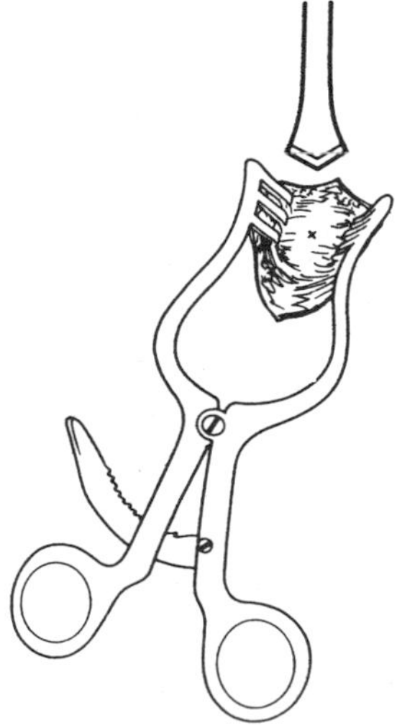

Figure 5.5. Introduce the standard hand-held drill through an incision. Center the drill along the periosteal surface of the outer table.

cian has access to the epidural and subdural spaces.

Hollow screw drill: After a stab incision and percutaneous trephination, place the screw in the bone, and remove the guide. After spontaneous drainage and irrigation, connect a closed drainage system with a collection bag with the screw (18).

Epidural hematoma: If a hematoma is obvious and the dura is not visible, and one is certain that perforation of the dura has not taken place, then one is generally dealing with an epidural hematoma. Aspiration can be attempted; however, the hematoma usually is clotted, making aspiration difficult. In such a case, enlarge the hole in the operating room with a rongeur to 4 cm and apply suction to remove the hematoma.

Subdural hematoma: When dealing with a subdural hematoma, one can see the blue dura bulging through the burr hole. Ballot the hematoma with the cone needle, and, if fluctuant, incise the dura with a scalpel (no. 11 blade). Aspirate the hematoma with a suction catheter (Fig. 5.6). When the pressure is relieved, the convolutions of the underlying brain may be visualized (Fig. 5.7). Aspiration of a chronic subdural hematoma seen acutely to the emergency center is performed easily through a simple burr hole, and the hematoma can be removed by needle aspiration through either a twist drill hole, a standard drill burr hole, or a hollow screw drill. However, when an acute or subacute subdural hematoma is encountered, further surgical intervention may be warranted. In a study that evaluated hemodynamic changes of the middle cerebral artery and their clinical significance before and after surgical aspiration in patients with chronic subdural hematomas, 19 patients with this condition who received transcranial Doppler sonography examination demonstrated the lesions within 5 days after the neurosurgical treatment (30, 39).

4. Standard hand-held drill: Once the epidural space is entered, a hematoma may be noted and suctioned (Fig. 5.6). After the clot is evacuated, search for a bleeding point and, if found, ligate or coagulate it. When this is not possible, loosely pack the epidural space, permitting some bleeding to the outside to continue decompression. In

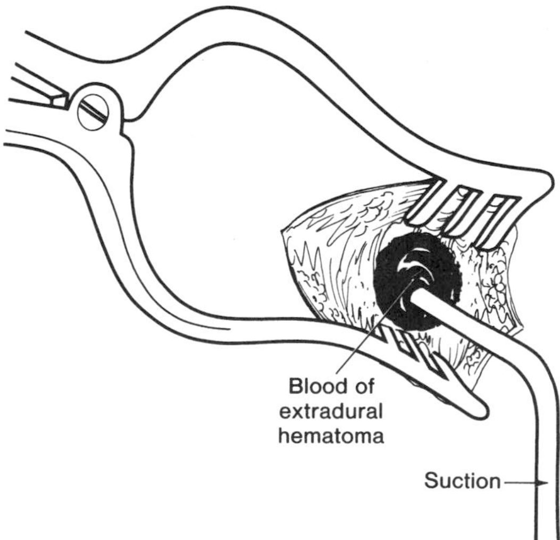

Figure 5.6. Once the extradural space is entered, a hematoma may be noted. Suction the partially clotted or gelled or liquid hematoma.

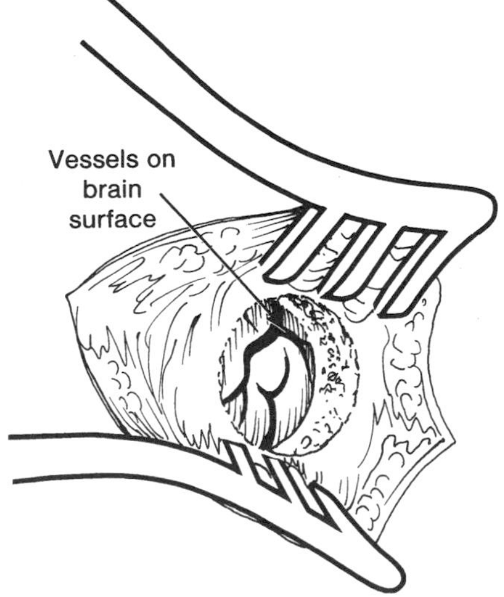

Figure 5.7. Once the pressure is relieved, swelling of the brain will cause the convolutions of the underlying cortex as well as overlying vessels to be visualized.

some cases in which the hematoma cannot be evacuated by this procedure, enlarge the hole with a rongeur in the operating room in a radial fashion to a diameter of approximately 4 cm, thus permitting evacuation.
5. Apply a loose dressing over the area, and transport the patient then to a neurosurgical center.

NOTE

Brain decompression, although ideally performed in the operating room by a neurosurgeon, may have to be performed in the emergency department in a rapidly deteriorating patient. Where time is of the essence, burr or twist drill holes offer access to the intracranial cavity and permit decompression by the removal of fluid contents as a prelude to formal surgery. Immediate decompression in these situations may prevent further irreversible neurologic deterioration and may be life saving (6).

COMPLICATIONS

1. Penetration of the sagittal sinus. This complication has been reported to occur in use of the twist drill (46). One must be certain to stay several centimeters from the midline, as indicated earlier.
2. Broken twist drill point in the skull. Keeping the drill perpendicular to the skull and avoiding angulating the drill, which may cause breaking of the bit, can avoid this complication.
3. Subdural empyema. Avoid this complication by maintaining sterile conditions. The physician should wear a mask and gown as with any major surgical procedure.
4. Superficial intracerebral hematoma mistaken for a subdural hematoma. This complication was reported as occurring in three cases in a large series (46).
5. False-positive or false-negative taps. A false-positive or false-negative tap has been reported to occur with use of the twist drill (6, 46). When one considers the total number of complications with use of this instrument, false negatives account for one third of all the complications seen in the series by Rand et al. (46).
6. Laceration of an afferent middle meningeal artery.

CAUTION

Be very careful to avoid penetration beyond the inner table. We recommend looking at the lateral radiograph of the skull and determining the location of the meningeal vessel by looking for the grooves in the skull radiograph. Note the position of these grooves in relation to the external auditory meatus and avoid them in performing the temporal burr-hole procedure.

---

7. Local skin infection after implantation of the hollow screw.

LUMBAR PUNCTURE

Infections of the nervous system are a continuing diagnostic and therapeutic challenge. Successful treatment of diseases depends on rapid and accurate diagnosis. Lumbar puncture (LP; cerebrospinal fluid; CSF) evaluation provides specific identification of infectious agents, and microbiologic testing now offers multiple techniques ranging from culture to identification of nucleic acid or protein components of pathologic organisms (42). The usual information obtained from examination of the spinal fluid is opening pressure, glucose level, protein level, cell count and differential, Gram stain, smear for acid-fast organisms, India ink, culture, and cytologic testing for malignancies. This information is important in establishing a diagnosis of meningitis and other inflammatory conditions affecting the brain and spinal canal. In addition to routine studies, specific diagnostic tests are indicated by clinical impression, such as cultures for bacteria, fungi, viruses, and *Mycobacterium tuberculosis.* Microbial assays for cryptococcus, coccidioidomycoses, pneumococcus, haemophilus, meningococcus, and group B streptococcal antigens are available. CSF VDRL test for neurosyphilis and CSF Lyme index for neuroboreliosis can be done. Polymerase chain reaction (PCR) testing *for Borrelia burgdorferi, M. tuberculosis,* herpes simplex virus (HSV), and varicella zoster virus (VZV) (45) are available. In addition, when performing a microscopic examination on the fluid, one must not only determine the number of lymphocytes, polymorphonuclear cells, and red blood cells, but also search for abnormal cells such as fat-laden histiocytes, indicative of acute brain damage, tumor cells, or lupus. Immunofluorescent techniques aid in the identification of cells coated by antigen in herpes simplex encephalitis and in *Haemophilus influenzae* meningoencephalitis. Antigens to bacteria in CSF can be demonstrated rapidly by counterimmunoelectrophoresis (CIE), diagnosing partially treated bacterial meningitis.

When a spontaneous subarachnoid hemorrhage is suspected, an LP may be performed to confirm the diagnosis. In this situation, an experienced physician should do the LP. A number of situations have occurred in which many questions could have been avoided, if it were not for a traumatic LP.

INDICATIONS

1. Diagnosis of suspected meningitis or encephalitis in patients with headache, fever, nuchal rigidity, and acutely altered mental status.
2. Diagnosis of acute or chronic inflammatory demyelinating polyradiculoneuropathy (IDP; i.e., Guillain–Barré syndrome) and CNS demyelinating diseases (e.g., multiple sclerosis).
3. Diagnosis of carcinomatous meningitis, lymphomatous meningitis, and central nervous system (CNS) leukemia.
4. Diagnosis of subarachnoid hemorrhage.
5. Diagnosis and relief of intracranial hypertension (e.g., pseudotumor cerebri).

CONTRAINDICATIONS

1. Signs of increased ICP. With the advent of computerized axial tomography (CT), the indications for LP in patients with suspected intracranial mass lesions have decreased markedly. When the suspicion is high, a CT scan should be obtained before performing LP. With intracranial mass lesions, it is rare that an LP will give enough information to justify the risk (19).

There is a significant amount of controversy surrounding the issue of LP in patients with intracranial mass lesions. In one series, reported by Lubic and Marotta (34), of 401 patients with histologically verified brain tumors in whom LP was performed, it was found that only one patient showed evidence indicating an untoward effect of the LP. Papilledema and increased CSF pressure were present in 32% of the patients. Mass lesions were located in the temporal lobe in 14% of the patients and in the posterior fossa in 18.5%. Even with this extraordinarily low complication rate, Lubic and Marotta (34) emphasized that the procedure should not be performed routinely on such patients. In a study involving 30 patients with increased ICP, Duffy (14) showed that their condition worsened after LP was performed. In half the cases, deterioration occurred immediately and was dramatic; in the other half, it occurred within 12 hours after LP. The overall mortality rate in Duffy's series was 40%.

A history of progressively increasing headache associated with mental status changes and the development of localizing neurologic signs is highly suggestive of increased ICP due to a mass lesion (14).

In a study by Korein et al. (26) involving 129 patients with increased CSF pressure in which 70 of the patients had papilledema and 59 did not, it was found that the incidence of complications after LP was significantly higher in the group without papilledema. From their extensive review of the literature, Korein et al. stated that the actual complication rate of LP in the presence of papilledema is less than 1.2%. They further stated that careful LP in the diagnosis and management of patients with papilledema is of definite value and may prevent unnecessary surgical intervention. This is no longer relevant in the days of CT scanning. In a study regarding cranial CT before LP, investigators found that the most common radiographic finding was a normal or unchanged CT scan in 84% of patients (24). The frequency of new radiographically documented lesions was 15.3% with a mass in eight, hemorrhage in three, and stroke in two patients. The data identified three statistically significant predictors of new intracranial lesions: (a) the specific findings of papilledema, focal neurologic examination, and altered mental status; (b) the physician's overall impression was the strongest positive predictor of CT-identified lesions contraindicating LP; and (c) the presence of one or more positive responses on a screening questionnaire (24).

We believe that when the following features are present, an LP should not be performed before obtaining neuroimaging of the head:

a. History of progressively increasing headache.
b. Presence of localizing neurologic signs or symptoms.
c. History of progressive deterioration in mental status.
d. Presence of papilledema.

2. Presence of severe bleeding diathesis is a relative contraindication to LP and an increased risk of spinal epidural hematoma has been demonstrated. However, with adequate factor replacement an LP can be done safely in patients with hemophilia (54).

In patients with coagulation defects or with anticoagulant therapy, LP is a relative contraindication (increased risk of spinal subdural hematoma). Although careful LP seldom induces complications in these patients, Edelson et al. (16) described eight patients with thrombocytopenia in whom a lumbar subdural hematoma developed after LP. When LP is indicated in such patients, an experienced physician must do it with extreme care and with a small-gauge needle. All reported patients with spinal epidural hematomas (a rare complication of LP) were receiving anticoagulant therapy before performance of the procedure (29). Thus patients with thrombocytopenia, leukemia, hemophilia, or advanced liver disease and those receiving anticoagulant therapy pose a significant danger with regard to intraspinal bleeding after this procedure (36).

3. Local infection at the proposed site of needle entry due to risk of infectious seeding of meninges.

EQUIPMENT

Standard LP kits are available for performing LP in both children and adults. These kits contain all of the materials needed.

Local anesthetic (i.e., 10 mL 1% lidocaine)
25-gauge 5/8-inch and 22-gauge 1.5-inch needles
3-mL syringe
Skin prep
Iodinated solution
4 × 4-inch sponges
Sterile towels and barrier
Spinal needles with stylet

NOTE

Although a number of authors have used 18- and 20-gauge spinal needles in performing this procedure, we advocate the use of the smallest needle possible. In the adult, the commonly used needle is a 20- or 22-gauge 3-inch spinal needle with a stylet. We advocate the use of a 25-gauge 2.5-inch needle for performing this procedure. This needle has been found to reduce greatly the incidence of headache after LP (31, 37, 60). A common fallacy is that a 25-gauge needle is more prone to breakage than is a 20- or 22-gauge needle. In a study by Dessloch (13), it was found that the breakage rate of a 20- or 22-gauge needle was higher than that of a 24- or 25-gauge needle. The advantages of a 25-gauge needle are as follows (60):

1. Loss of spinal fluid is negligible.
2. There is a small puncture hole in the dura and skin, providing for a smaller portal of entry.
3. Headache after LP is decreased markedly.
4. Needle breakage is less than that with a larger size needle.
5. Needle insertion is both rapid and relatively painless to the patient. In the child, a 25-gauge needle also is used.

Three-way stopcock
Manometer
Four specimen-collection tubes
Band-Aid
Sterile sponges

TECHNIQUE

Preparatory Steps

1. Position the patient in a lateral decubitus position with the back flexed maximally. Unless the lumbar spinous processes are "separated" by a spinal flexion and the patient's back is positioned perpendicular to the examining table, the chances are increased of painfully snagging the periosteum or a nerve root as well as an unsuccessful attempt (19). The following position should be used (Fig. 5.8).
   a. The back should be at the edge of the table with the knees and hips flexed maximally.
   b. Place a small pillow under the head of the patient.
   c. Check the shoulders and the pelvis to be certain they are perpendicular to the examining table.

   Alternate position: In patients who have scoliosis or ankylosing spondylitis or those who are very obese, the midline may be difficult to localize in the position indicated. In these patients, the midline is more accurately found by placing the patient in the sitting position at the edge of a table with his head and arms leaning over a pillow on a bedside stand. Once the midline of the spinal column is localized, change the patient to the position indicated.

2. Localize the site for needle insertion. The site for needle puncture is in the L4–L5 or L5–S1 interspace. Palpate the posterior aspect of the iliac crest

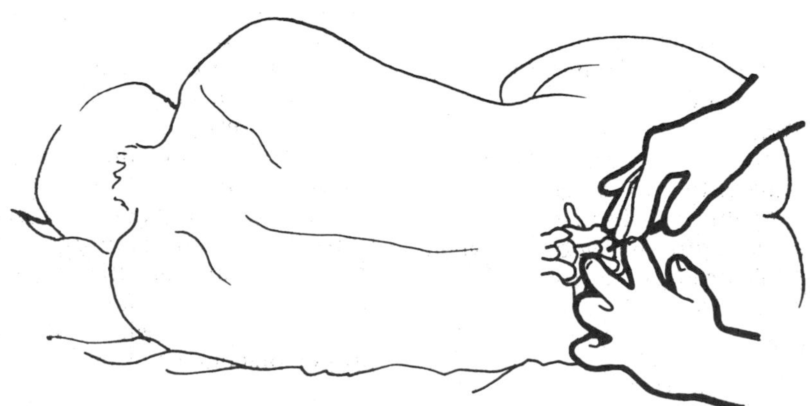

Figure 5.8. The position for a patient for a lumbar puncture. The back should be at the edge of the table with the knees, hips, and neck flexed maximally. Place a small pillow under the head of the patient. The shoulders and the pelvis should be perpendicular to the examining table. Then introduce the needle in the midline with the bevel directed in the horizontal plane.

bilaterally, and draw an imaginary line connecting the two. The spinous process of L4 is at the level of the iliac crest, and such a line traverses this point. The optimal site of needle puncture is in the midline in the L4–L5 interspace. Alternatively, use the L5–S1 or the L3–L4 interspace.

3. Prepare the patient's back with iodinated solution, beginning at the site of needle puncture and working outward in the routine fashion, and drape the area at the puncture site.
4. Locally infiltrate 1% lidocaine into the skin and subcutaneous tissue with a 25-gauge needle. A 22-gauge needle can be used to infiltrate the interspinous region between the spinous process of the areas selected.

Procedural Steps

1. Insert the needle in the midline with the bevel directed in the horizontal plane parallel to the axis of the spine (this allows the needle to split rather than cut the ligamentous fibers), which is likely to reduce the incidence of post-LP headaches (31, 37). Accurate puncture requires keeping the needlepoint in the midline during advancement. Patients often can aid in this procedure by reporting whether the needle is going to the left or to the right, because this can be felt by the patient (19). Hold the needle as shown in Fig. 5.8, and advance it through the interspinous ligament, directing it at an angle of approximately 10 degrees cephalad and toward the umbilicus. A "pop" may be noted as the needle passes through the ligamentum flavum.

Once the subarachnoid space is approached, there is a real danger that one will advance the needle too far rather than not far enough. The sharp needles contained in disposable LP sets reduce the dural "pop" markedly. Thus, as the physician advances the needle beyond this point, the stylet must be removed after every 1- to 2-mm advance of the needle to avoid going through the subarachnoid space and penetrating the ventral epidural space, which is richly endowed with a venous plexus and is responsible for most traumatic LPs (19). A second "pop" may be felt as the needle advances through the dura mater and into the subarachnoid space. If this second "pop" is felt, remove the stylet and check for CSF immediately because one is almost certain to be in the subarachnoid space at this point.

NOTE

Once the spinal needle is engaged in the interspinous ligament, a technique described by Livingston (33) aids in determining when the subarachnoid space has been entered. Remove the stylet, and place a drop of sterile saline in the adaptor of the needle once the needle is in the interspinous ligament. As the tip of the needle is advanced, it displaces the dura, thus creating a negative pressure in the extradural space that "sucks" the drop inward. Advancing the needle only slightly at this point is likely to penetrate the subarachnoid space, which contains the CSF. This maneuver is often used by anesthesiologists in guiding proper placement of epidural anesthesia. Because overpenetration can be a significant problem in LPs and has a risk of nerve root impingement, pain, and inducing a traumatic tap, this procedure is indicated whenever one is involved with a case that may be difficult.

Traumatic tap versus intracranial bleed: It may be difficult to interpret the meaning of a bloody tap in some patients. One must distinguish between intrinsic bleeding and that caused by trauma of the LP. If bloody fluid is obtained, note closely if it clears as more fluid is withdrawn. In addition, obtain cell counts in the first and the last tubes of fluid to aid in determining and quantifying this value. Examine the supernatant of the centrifuged sample of fluid.

The supernatant should be crystal clear when red cells are present for less than 2 hours, and the red cell count should be decreased from the first to the last tube if the LP is traumatic. Remember when looking at the supernatant that nonhemorrhagic fluid can be mildly to moderately xanthochromic when the patient is deeply jaundiced or if the CSF protein is greater than 150 mg/dL (58). Tourtellotte et al. (56) observed that if a traumatic tap contains more than 12,000 red cells/mL, the oxyhemoglobin would stain the fluid within half an hour after puncture. In most patients, the absence of xanthochromia and a declining cell count are the two most reliable criteria for determining if a LP is traumatic. In general, for every 700 RBCs found in the CSF, 1 WBC is also expected, and the ratio of these cells in the peripheral blood can be used to calculate the expected WBCs in the CSF for a given number of RBCs.

When bone is encountered during advancement of the needle, withdraw the needle to the subcutaneous tissue, and change the angle. Puncturing bone is usually caused by directing the needle away from the midline during advancement.

2. Attach the manometer and three-way stopcock to the needle after CSF is noted at the hub (Fig. 5.9). The zero point in measuring the CSF pressure is the needle itself. The normal range of CSF pressure is 70 to 180 mm of water.

NOTE

Forced deep breathing is contraindicated because this results in hypocapnia and induces a false low CSF pressure reading as a result of cerebral vasoconstriction. Dessloch (13) found that increased cerebral intraventricular pressure may decrease to normal within 1 minute after introduction of a spinal needle before withdrawal of fluid. Thus one should not wait more than a minute before checking the pressure of the fluid in the canal.

---

3. Once the subarachnoid sac is punctured, a manometer is applied to the needle after the stylet is removed. At this time, ask the patient to at least relax his legs and neck to decrease intraabdominal pressure (19, 33).
4. Collect four samples of CSF (Fig. 5.10). In the first tube, collect 1 to 2 mL of fluid for Gram stain, culture, and sensitivity. In the second tube, collect 1 mL of fluid for glucose and protein determination. In a third tube, collect 2 mL of CSF to send to the laboratory for antibodies and antigens, if

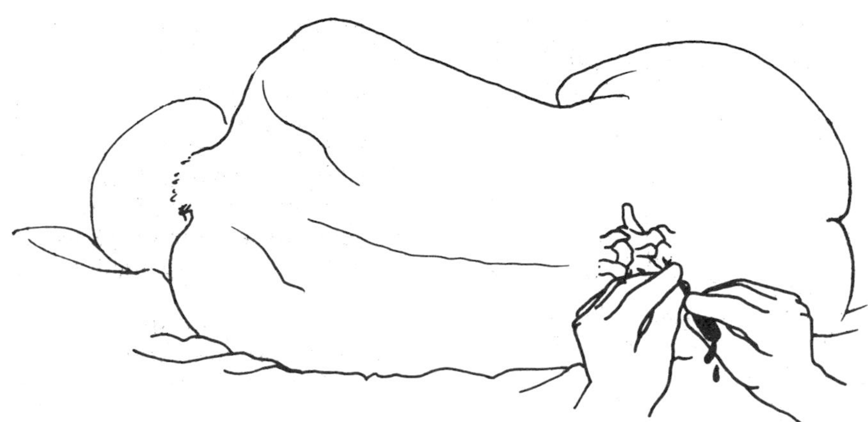

Figure 5.9. Once cerebrospinal fluid is noted at the hub of the needle, attach a manometer and three-way stopcock.

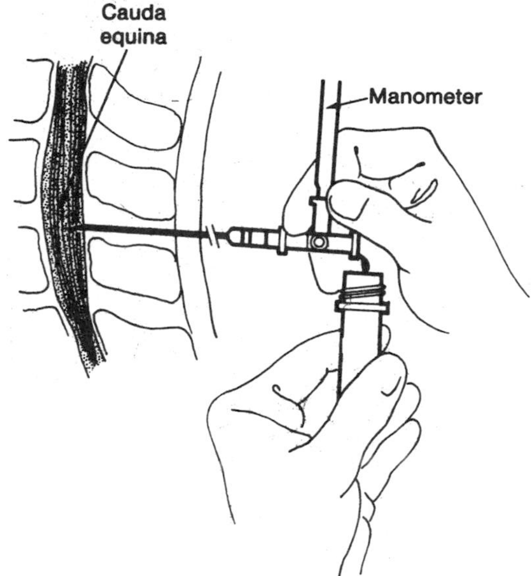

Figure 5.10. Collect four samples of cerebrospinal fluid.

indicated. In the fourth tube, collect 1 mL of fluid cell count. If needed, collect a sample for cytology in a fifth tube; approximately 10 mL should be collected if possible. Yield is proportionate to the amount of CSF collected and availability of a cytospin.

NOTE

If the flow rate decreases while collecting samples, rotate the needle 180 degrees, or slightly withdraw the needle. This decrease may be due to a nerve root that is impinging on the orifice of the needle.

Remove the needle after reinserting the stylet. The stylet should be reinserted before withdrawal of the needle because this will protect the patient from nerve root herniation (13, 33). Rapid withdrawal of a spinal needle may initiate enough suction to herniate a spinal nerve root and adjacent arachnoid and fix them into the epidural space (57).

AFTERCARE

1. Apply a Band-Aid over the puncture site.
2. Instruct the patient to lie in the prone position for several hours. In a large study by Brocker (58), 894 patients were placed on their abdomens for 3 hours before ambulation after LP was performed in the routine position. Only four patients developed post-LP headache (an incidence of less than 0.5%). In a control group of 200 patients in whom LP was performed with the same size needle in the decubitus position, but who were placed in the supine position for a period of 3 hours, the incidence of post-LP headache was 36.5%. It is believed that the dural, arachnoid, and ligamentum flavum holes are "staggered" during extension of the spine in the prone position, thereby decreasing CSF leak and decreasing post-LP headache (2).

COMPLICATIONS

1. Post-LP headache. Spinal headaches caused significant discomfort to the patient. The incidence of LP headaches in the literature is approximately 41% (2, 20). The headache is worse in the erect position and diminishes or disappears completely in the supine position. Post–dural puncture headaches are directly correlated with the patient's age. Reports are much higher in adults younger than 50 years than in the elderly. In addition, these headaches are seldom reported in children younger than 10 years (22). The headache may also decrease after applying epigastric pressure to compress the inferior vena cava while the patient is sitting. To do this, push the right fist beneath the right costal margin and place the left hand on the patient's back for 1 minute (21). The success rate for using epidural blood patch is about 85% after one injection

and near 98% after a second. The patch is performed by slowly injecting 10 to 20 mL of the patient's blood into the lumbar epidural space at the same interspace or the interspace below the prior puncture. After the procedure, the patient should stay in the decubitus position for at least 1 hour and preferably for 2 hours to obtain maximal benefits (21). The pain is attributed to intracranial hypotension. The possible cause of the headache may be traction on pain-sensitive structures such as sensory cranial nerves (V, VIII, and X) and the upper cervical nerves related to downward displacement of the brain. Another explanation of post-LP headaches is venous engorgement in the meninges as a consequence of reduced CSF volume. Magnetic resonance imaging (MRI) findings reported in patients with intracranial hypotension show downward displacement of the cerebellar tonsils and the optic chiasma with anterior displacement of the pons (27). The size of the tear left in the dura is the most important factor in the production of these headaches; be careful to produce only one hole and to use the smallest possible needle (2, 19, 60). Postspinodural arachnoid rents can occasionally persist for months, with accompanying leakage of CSF and persisting headaches (56). Four key points with regard to preventing LP headaches deserve emphasis here.

   a. Use a small (25-gauge) nontraumatic needle (2, 19, 31, 37, 60).
   b. Place the patient in the prone position for a period of 3 hours after the procedure.
   c. Place the bevel of the needle parallel to the long axis of the spine (31, 37).
   d. Reinsert the stylet before removing the needle (55).

2. Intraspinal epidermoid tumors (1). Intraspinal epidermoid tumors may be induced by LPs performed with needles without a stylet or with an ill-fitting stylet. This results from the implantation of epidermal fragments into the spinal canal. The most common symptoms are pain in the back or lower extremities, which may appear months later in these patients. MRI should be considered in every patient who has pain in the lower extremities or back and who has had a previous LP (1, 20).
3. Spinal subdural hematoma (11, 17). This complication has been reported in patients with thrombocytopenia in whom LP was performed. The symptoms of a spinal subdural hematoma in some patients are weakness and sensory loss in the lower extremities. Some patients may have bladder dysfunction. Removal of large volumes of CSF in an elderly patient also may cause a subdural hematoma, as a result of low CSF pressure, resulting in traction on the meninges and tearing of dural vessels. Prevent this problem by correcting coagulopathies before the procedure is performed (54). When performing the procedure in the elderly, remove the fluid slowly and in small volumes.
4. Spinal epidural hematoma. This is a rare complication of LP (20, 44, 51). All reported patients were receiving anticoagulant therapy or had severe hepatic dysfunction. The complication is usually due to laceration of the ventral epidural venous plexus. Such bleeding may result in paraplegia (36). Needle aspiration of the clot or laminectomy may or may not be beneficial in these patients. Avoid this complication by avoiding deep penetration of the needle during LP, and maintain the needle in the midline during advancement, because lateral displacement also will cause injury to the venous plexus anteriorly. When performing LP on a patient who has a blood dyscrasia or who is taking anti-

coagulants, place a drop of sterile saline at the hub of the needle after penetrating the interspinous ligament to aid in determining when the extradural space is penetrated (as indicated earlier in the section on technique). This procedure will aid in avoiding deep penetration in such patients.

5. Herniation of the spinal cord. This complication results from the removal of CSF from below the foramen magnum in patients in whom there is a site of neural impaction and increased CSF pressure proximally, resulting in a pressure gradient and herniation. LP distal to an intraspinal mass should not be performed.
6. Exacerbation of peripheral neurologic symptoms secondary to an intraspinal tumor. After the removal of CSF distal to a complete intraspinal block (usually due to a tumor), the patient may experience exacerbation of symptoms, secondary to a tumor or to herniation of the spinal cord. Remove small volumes of CSF slowly.
7. Dry tap. This is most commonly due to lateral displacement of the tip of the needle. Keep the needle in the midline during advancement, as indicated earlier, to avoid this problem.
8. Cranial neuropathies are due to removal of large volumes of CSF, resulting typically in traction of the cranial nerves IV or VI and less likely of other cranial nerves. The symptoms are usually transient. CSF should be removed slowly and in only those quantities that are needed.
9. Injury to the annulus fibrosus or rupture of the nucleus pulposus is due to excessively deep penetration of the spinal needle, resulting in injury to the intervertebral disc. Avoid further advancement of the needle when it is obvious that it has gone beyond the subarachnoid space.
10. Infection. Epidural or subdural empyema has occurred after LP. Meningitis also has been reported. Introduction of organisms into the epidural, subdural, or subarachnoid space from a contaminated needle is the cause. This may be due to inadequate skin preparation or to puncture placed in the presence of focal skin infection. Avoid puncturing skin that is infected, macerated, or involved in any skin disease. In addition, follow strict aseptic technique.
11. Subarachnoid hematoma. Hematomas can occur in the epidural, subdural, or subarachnoid spaces, or within the spinal cord after LP. Bleeding within the spinal subarachnoid space usually produces a clinical syndrome characterized by the sudden onset of intense back pain followed by neck stiffness and headache (20, 44). A subarachnoid hematoma after an LP can cause compression of the cauda equina, resulting in neurologic deficits to the legs, urinary bladder, and anus. When such a deficit is encountered, particularly in a patient who was previously taking anticoagulants, suspect this rare complication (4).
12. Stylet injury syndrome. Insert a stylet before withdrawing a spinal puncture needle to avoid aspiration of the lumbar nerve root and adjacent arachnoid tissue, thus fixing the nerve in the epidural space. This syndrome is characterized by pain that requires laminectomy and replacement of the nerve root within the subarachnoid space (20, 57).
13. Herniation as a result of LP; an infrequent but potentially lethal complication. Korien et al. (26) reported a 1.2% complication rate in a series of patients with papilledema and increased ICP from a variety of causes.
14. Intracranial bleeding is a rare complication of LP that can occur in healthy patients without bleeding disorders. A typical post-LP headache is present initially. The age of reported patients ranges from 22 to 79 years. The sub-

dural hematoma, which can be unilateral or bilateral, may be diagnosed after an interval from 3 days to several months. The mechanism of this may be low CSF pressure, resulting in traction of the meninges and tearing of the dural vessels. Similarly, traction of the vessels can result in a tear of a saccular aneurysm. Thus if the patient reports a headache that is persistent for 1 week after the tap or resolves and then recurs, be suspicious.

15. Nerve root irritation and low back pain. During LP, contact with the sensory roots causing transient electric shocks or dysesthesias is commonly reported in approximately 13% of patients. Permanent sensory and motor loss can rarely occur.

Lumbar Puncture in the Neonate

The performance of an LP in the young infant and neonate is often difficult. Greensher and Mofensen (25) introduced a simplified technique for performing LPs in the neonate. Perform the puncture by using a butterfly needle (21 gauge) produced by Abbott Laboratories. This needle has a 20-gauge bore, is thin walled, and has a plastic tubing approximately 30 cm long attached to its end. The dead-space volume of the tubing is 0.25 mL. One of the problems routinely encountered in performing punctures on neonates is that fluid is lost, and the pressure is difficult to obtain because the infant is squirming and difficult to handle. Insert the needle in the third, fourth, or fifth lumbar interspace and advance it into the spinal canal in the routine manner. When spinal fluid flows into the plastic tubing, elevate the tube and take a pressure measurement, as shown in Fig. 5.11. After this, lower the plastic tubing, and collect samples in collecting tubs. The advantages of this technique are that it is simple, and the spinal fluid is easily visualized through the tube. If the tap becomes traumatic, then remove the needle before contamination of previously collected specimens.

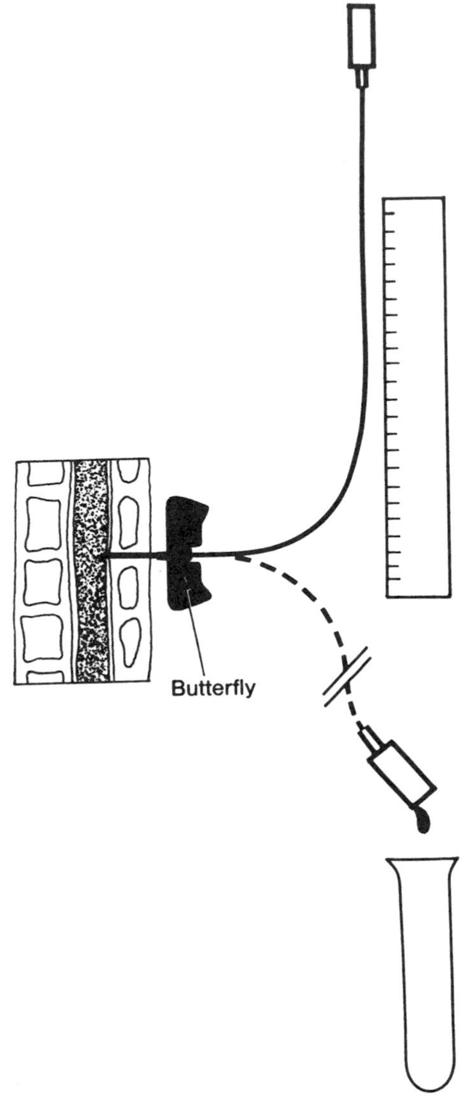

Figure 5.11. Lumbar puncture in the neonate. Insert the needle in the third, fourth, or fifth lumbar interspace. A 21-gauge butterfly is excellent for performing this procedure in the neonate. Introduce the butterfly into the spinal canal and once fluid is noted to be advancing into the catheter tubing of the butterfly, lift the catheter vertically and measure the pressure with a standard centimeter ruler. After the pressure is measured, take the samples.

In a study by Naidoo (40) involving 136 newborn infants, no complications were found with this type of needle without a stylet. The discomfort of LP should not be minimized, because the stimulation may cause tonic seizures in the asphyxiated newborn or even vagal cardiac arrest in children with cardiopulmonary disease (4). Hold the child firmly but not tightly flexed, because this can embarrass respiration and cause restriction in venous return from the head. Local anesthesia or conscious sedation may be a great assistance in decreasing the degree of struggling and is a help to the child and physician rather than a hindrance (7, 43).

In a study aimed at providing a practical guide that would help eliminate correct depth of insertion using a child's age, height, and weight, the results showed that the depth of the LP needle insertion to obtain uncontaminated CSF correlates best with the child's height. Calculate the main depth of insertion by using the graph: mean depth equals 0.03 cm × height in centimeters (8).

SKELETAL TRACTION FOR CERVICAL SPINE DISLOCATIONS AND FRACTURES

Immediate treatment in the emergency department may be indicated for patients with severe dislocations of the cervical spine without evidence of spinal cord compression. The need for treatment depends largely on the degree of displacement. Fractures and dislocations of the cervical spine requiring tongs within the emergency department are those that are accompanied by neurologic compromise on initial evaluation or those in which minimal motion of the cervical spine produces paresthesias. Those fractures and dislocations that are so unstable as to make movement of the patient dangerous also should be placed in tongs before moving the patient. Collars and braces are often of no value in treating these patients because immobilization of the cervical spine is not achieved (10). Crutchfield (10) first introduced the Crutchfield tong, which was inserted into the calvarium and provided traction for patients with cervical spine fractures and dislocations. Since then, a number of devices have been introduced on the market, including the Gardner tong, Heifetz tong, Vinke tong, and Blackburn tong. Two of these devices are described here. Both devices can be applied in the emergency department with very little difficulty.

Gardner–Wells Tong (63)

This tong consists of a rigid member that follows the coronal contour of the calvarium. A threaded hole that accommodates a screw for the advancement of the cone-shaped points is retractable by an enclosed spring that is calibrated to indicate when a squeeze pressure of 30 pounds is reached. The instrument is designed for emergency bedside application under antiseptic rather than aseptic conditions. This makes its utility in the emergency department excellent.

TECHNIQUE OF APPLICATION

Shave the hair around the site where the tong is to be applied. This will decrease the chance of osteomyelitis of the skull. Prepare the scalp then with an antiseptic solution. Inject 1% lidocaine at the sites where the points of the tong will be applied. Insert the points of the tong above the ears and below the "equator" (Fig. 5.12). Obtain flexion and extension of the

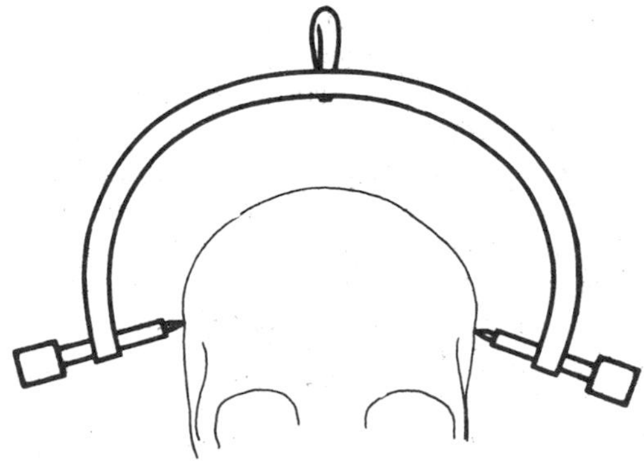

Figure 5.12. The Gardner tong. This tong consists of a rigid member and two cone-shaped points. See text for discussion.

head by adjusting the height of the pulley. Advance the tapered points into the skin. Because the points are directed upward, as they advance, the skin is stretched increasingly snugly about them. This seals the point of entry and prevents bleeding. When bone is encountered, the stiff spring yields until the posterior end of the spring-loaded point just protrudes out of the casing. This indicates that the spring is fully compressed and is exerting 30 pounds of squeeze between the points. Then tilt the tong back and forth to ensure proper seating, after which, retighten it if the posterior end of the spring-loaded point has recessed. The total excursion of the spring is approximately 5 mm, thus avoiding the possibility of penetrating too deeply and causing pressure atrophy. The points of the tong, when applied properly, rarely pull out because of their angle. The points should be just below the temporal ridges. The tong will tolerate easily traction of 65 pounds, if necessary. In the first 24 hours, tighten the points. With the patient supine, placing a sandbag under such projecting end of the points prevents rotation of the head. This is especially important when dealing with fractures of the odontoid.

Heifetz Tong

The Heifetz tong has the advantage of being able to maintain constant position of the patient's head and neck in flexion or extension when dealing with fractures or dislocations of the cervical spine. The Gardner tong and other tongs available will permit flexion, extension, or "swivel" of the skull within the tong. The Heifetz tong can be applied without the use of drills or incisions. The device consists of a rigid stainless steel arc with three self-drilling bolt drills providing for skull fixation (Fig. 5.13). The three-pronged principle avoids the tendency to swivel that occurs in other tongs. The traction device literally becomes an integral part of the patient's head. The physician is able to drill into the skull with simple hand rotation of the bolt drill, similar to the technique used with the Gardner tong. The depth of penetration of the bolt is easily determined because there are 2-mm increment markings on the side of the bolt drill.

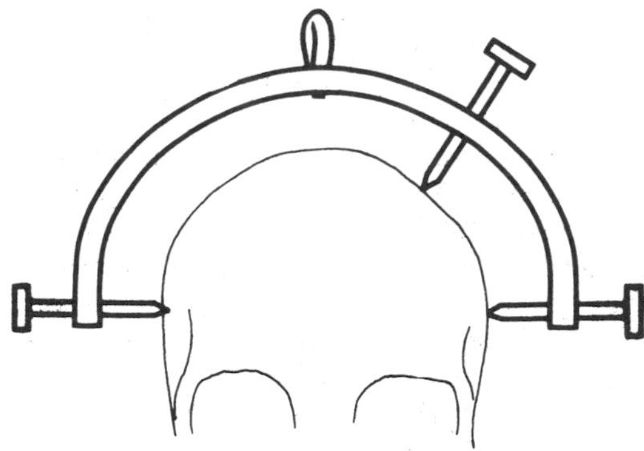

Figure 5.13. The Heifetz tong. This tong consists of a rigid stainless steel arc with three self-drilling bolt drills, providing firm fixation of the skull. See text for discussion.

TECHNIQUE OF APPLICATION

The site of penetration is along the lateral aspect of the calvarium. The optimal angle of insertion is perpendicular to the plane of traction desired. Cleanse and prepare the area of insertion along the scalp, and inject a local anesthetic. Place the arc containing the three bolt drills in position along the parietal fossa. Advance the bitemporal bolt drills into the scalp until they firmly impinge on the skull. At this point, note the millimeter markings on the bolts. Advance the temporal bolt drills into the skull alternately, by using the following technique: turning it clockwise three complete revolutions advances one bolt drill. Then retract the bolt drill by unscrewing it two complete revolutions. Then advance the opposite bolt drill three turns and retract it two turns. With this maneuver of alternately advancing and then retracting the temporal bolt drills, continue until each drill has penetrated the outer table by 2 to 3 mm, as determined by notches on the drill. When insertion is complete, rotate the bolt so that the flat edge of the bolt is facing the patient's feet. Then tighten the locked bolt at the end of the arc (Fig. 5.13) to maintain the temporal bolts in their position. Then tighten the parietal bolt and apply traction.

Subdural Aspiration

Subdural aspiration may be necessary in the infant for diagnostic purposes. The procedure is indicated when a subdural hematoma is suspected in an infant. The procedure is safe as long as the physician remains away from the midline, thus avoiding the sagittal sinus. The procedure should be performed bilaterally even when one side is positive, because a bilateral subdural hematoma is often present in these patients. Remember that a negative subdural tap does not rule out the presence of a subdural hematoma.

TECHNIQUE (FIG. 5.14)

1. Restrain the child, and have an assistant immobilize the head. Place the child's head at the edge of the examining table.
2. Shave the top of the scalp over the region of the fontanelle.
3. Prepare the scalp with an iodinated solution, and drape the area of the fontanelle.
4. Locate the point of puncture. The point of puncture is in the anterior fontanelle at the junction of the coronal suture with the fontanelle. This point must be 3 cm lateral to the midline to avoid the sagittal sinus.
5. Anesthetize the area of puncture with a 25-gauge needle and 1% lidocaine with epinephrine.
6. Insert a 20-gauge needle at the point selected. Direct the needle laterally after it has penetrated the skin. A "pop" will be felt as the subdural space is entered. In addition, there is a decrease in resistance to advancement of the needle when the space is entered.
7. Then remove the stylet from the spinal needle and permit the fluid to drip from the needle spontaneously. Never use a syringe to aspirate. This may injure pial vessels. If a subdural hematoma is present, the fluid will appear usually as a brown or pale yellow color.
8. Remove the needle, and apply pressure at the puncture site. Apply a sterile dressing to the scalp.

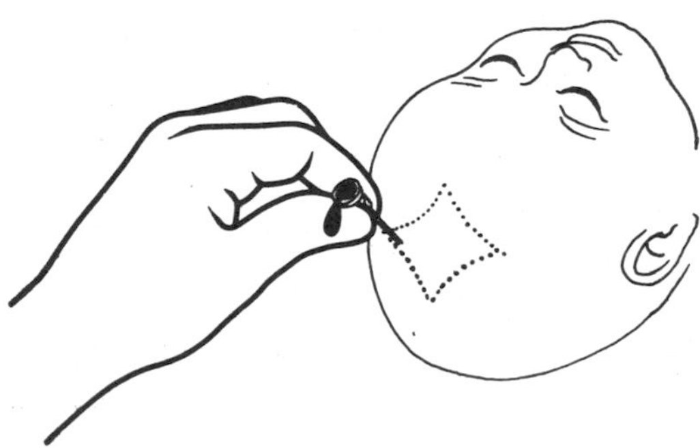

Figure 5.14. Subdural aspiration in the infant. See text for discussion.

REFERENCES

1. Batnitzky S, Keucher TR, Mealey J, et al: Iatrogenic intraspinal epidermoid tumors. JAMA 237:148, 1977.
2. Brocker RJ: Technique to avoid spinal tap headache. JAMA 168:261, 1958.
3. Brown BA, Jones OW Jr: Prolonged headache following spinal puncture: Response to surgical treatment. J Neurosurg 19:349, 1962.
4. Brown JK: Lumbar puncture and its hazards. Dev Med Child Neurol 18:803, 1976.
5. Bullock R, et al: Joint Section on Neurotrauma on Critical Care Guidelines for the Management of Severe Head Injury. Washington: The Brain Trauma Foundation, 30:18, 1995.
6. Burton C, Blacker HM: A compact hand drill for emergency brain decompression. J Trauma 5: 643, 1965.
7. Carroccio C. Lidocaine for lumbar puncture. Arch Pediatr Adolesc Med 150:1044, 1996.
8. Craig F, Stroobant J, Winrow A, Davies H: Depth of insertion of a lumbar puncture needle. Arch Dis Child 77:450, 1997.
9. Craig TV, Hunt WE: Emergency care of extradural hematoma. JAMA 171:405, 1959.
10. Crutchfield WG: Skeletal traction for dislocation of the cervical spine. South Surg 2:156, 1933.
11. DeAngelis J: Hazards of subdural and epidural anesthesia during anticoagulant therapy: A case report and review. Anesth Analg 51:676, 1972.

12. Dearden NM, Gibson JS, McDowall DG, et al: Effects of high-dose dexamethasone on outcome from severe head injury. J Neurosurg 64:81, 1986.
13. Dessloch JC: Problem of broken needles in spinal anesthesia: A survey. Anesth Analg 18: 353, 1939.
14. Duffy GP: Lumbar puncture in the presence of a raised intracranial pressure. Br Med J 1:407, 1969.
15. Echlin FA, Sordillo SVR, Garvey TQ Jr: Acute, subacute and chronic subdural hematoma. JAMA 161:1345, 1956.
16. Edelson RN, Chernik NL, Posner JB: Spinal subdural hematoma complicating lumbar puncture. Arch Neurol 31:134, 1974.
17. Egede LE, Moses H, Wans H: Spinal subdural hematoma: A rare complication of lumbar puncture. Md Med J 48:15, 1999.
18. Emonds N, Hassler WE: New device to treat chronic subdural hematoma hollow screw. Neurol Res 21:77, 1999.
19. Petito F, Plum F: The lumbar puncture [Letter]. N Engl J Med 290:225, 1974.
20. Evans RW: Complications of lumbar puncture. Neurol Clin 16:30, 1998.
21. Evans RW: Complications of lumbar puncture. Neurol Clin 16:83, 1998.
22. Flaatten H, Krakenes J, Vedeler C: Post-dural puncture related complications after diagnostic lumbar puncture, myelography and spinal anaesthesia. Acta Neurol Scand 98:445, 1998.
23. Garell PC, Mirsky R, Noh MD, et al.: Posterior ventricular catheter burr-hole localizer: Technical note. J Neurosurg 89:157, 1998.
24. Gopal AK, Whitehouse JD, Simel DL, et al.: Cranial computed tomography before lumbar puncture: A prospective clinical evaluation. Arch Intern Med 159:2681, 1999.
25. Greensher J, Mofensen HC: Lumbar puncture in neonate: A simplified technique. J Pediatr 78: 1034, 1971.
26. Korein J, Cravioto H, Leicach M: Reevaluation of lumbar puncture: A study of 129 patients with papilledema or intracranial hypertension. Neurology 9:290, 1959.
27. Krause I, Kornreich L, Waldman D, et al.: MRI meningeal enhancement with intracranial hypotension caused by lumbar puncture. Pediatr Neurol 16:163, 1997
28. Krause RJ: Epidemiology of head injury. In: Cooper PR, ed. Head Injury, 3rd ed. Baltimore: Williams & Wilkins, 1993.
29. Laglia AG, Eisenberg RL, Weinstein PR, et al: Spinal epidural hematoma after lumbar puncture in liver disease. Ann Intern Med 86:515, 1978.
30. Lee EJ, Lee MY, Hung YC: The application of transcranial Doppler sonography in patients with chronic subdural haematoma. Acta Neurochir (Wein) 141:835, 1999.
31. Leibold RA, Yealy DM, Coppolam Cantees RK: Post dural puncture headache: Characteristics, management, and prevention. Ann Emerg Med. 22:1863, 1993.
32. Levin HS, Aldrich EF, Saydjar C, et al: Severe head injury in children: Experience of traumatic coma data bank. Neurosurgery 31: 435, 1992.
33. Livingstone KE: Technique of lumbar puncture [Letter]. N Engl J Med 287:724, 1974.
34. Lubic LG, Marotta JT: Brain tumor and lumbar puncture. Arch Neurol Psychiatry 72:568, 1954.
35. Luersenn T, Klauber M, Marshal L: Outcome from head injury related to patient's age. J Neurosurg 68: 409, 1988.
36. Messer HD, Forshan VR, Brust JCM, et al: Transient paraplegia from hematoma after lumbar puncture: A consequence of anticoagulant therapy. JAMA 235:529, 1976.
37. Morewood GH: A rational approach to the cause, prevention and treatment of postdural puncture headaches. Can Med Assoc J 149: 1087, 1993.
38. Muizelaar JP, Marmarou A, Ward JD, et al: Adverse effects of prolonged hyperventilation: A randomized clinical trial. J Neurosurg 75:731, 1999.
39. Muller M, Merkelbach S, Hermes M, et al: Transcranial Doppler sonography at the early stage of acute nervous system infections in adults. Ultrasound Med Biol 22:173, 1996.
40. Naidoo BT: The cerebrospinal fluid in the healthy newborn infant. South Afr Med J 42: 933, 1968.
41. Narayan RK: Closed head injury. In: Rengachary SS, Wilkens RH, eds. Principles of Neurosurgery, London: Wolfe Publishing, 1994.
42. Narinder KM, Stratton CW: Laboratory tests in critical care. Crit Care Clin 14:1, 1998.
43. Pinheiro JM, Furdon S, Ochoa LF. Role of local anesthesia during lumbar puncture in neonates. Pediatrics 91:379, 1993.
44. Prieto A Jr, Cantu RC: Spinal subarachnoid hemorrhage and associated neurofibroma of the cauda equina. J Neurosurg 27:63, 1968.
45. Pruitt AA: Infections of the nervous system. Neurol Clin 16:2, 1998.
46. Rand BO, Ward AA, White LE Jr. The use of the twist drill to evaluate head trauma. J Neurosurg 25:410, 1966.
47. Randal M, Chestnut MD: The management of severe traumatic brain injury. Emerg Med Clin North Am 15:30, 1997.
48. Rengachary SS, Murphy D: Subarachnoid hematoma following lumbar puncture causing compression of the cauda equina: Case report. J Neurosurg 41:252, 1974.
49. Rockswold GL, Leonard PR, Nagib MG: Analysis of 33 closed head trauma patients who talked and deteriorated. Neurosurgery 21:51, 1987.
50. Rosen P, Barkin R. Emergency Medicine: Concepts and Clinical Practice, 4th ed. St. Louis: Mosby, 30, 1998.
51. Senelick RC, Norwood CW, Cohen GH: "Painless" spinal epidural hematoma during anticoagulant therapy. Neurology 26:213, 1976.
52. Shack Ford SR, MacKenrsie RC, Holbrook TL, et al: The epidemiology of traumatic death: A population based analysis. Arch Surg 128:571, 1993.

53. Shenkin HA, Bouzarth WF: Clinical methods of reducing intracranial pressure: Role of the cerebral circulation. N Engl J Med 282:1465, 1970.
54. Silverman R, Kwatkowski T, Bernstein S, et al: Safety of lumbar puncture in patients with hemophilia. Ann Emerg Med 22:1739, 1993.
55. Stupp M, Brandt T, Muller A: The incidence of post lumbar puncture syndrome reduced by reinserting the stylet: A randomized prospective study of 600 patients. J Neurol 245:589, 1998.
56. Tourtellotte WW, Somers JF, Parker JA, et al: A study on traumatic lumbar punctures. Neurology 8:129, 1958.
57. Trupp M: Stylet injury syndrome. JAMA 237: 2424, 1977.
58. Vastola EF: Non-hemorrhagic xanthochromia of cerebrospinal fluid. J Neuropathol Exp Neurol 19:292, 1960.
59. Waxweiler RJ, Thurman D, Sniezek J, et al: Monitoring the impact of traumatic brain injury: A review and update. J Neurotrauma 12: 509, 1995.
60. Wetchler BV, Brace DE: A technique to minimize the occurrence of headache after lumbar puncture by use of small bore spinal needles. Anesthesiology 16:270, 1955.
61. White RJ, Likavec MJ: The diagnosis and initial management of head injury. N Engl J Med 327: 1507, 1992.
62. Wilberger JE Jr, Harris M, Diamond DL: Acute subdural hematoma: morbidity, mortality, and operative timing. J Neurosurg 74:212, 1991
63. Zimmerman R, Bilaniuk L: Computed tomography in pediatric head trauma. J Neuroradiol 8: 257, 1981.

6

Obstetric and Gynecologic Procedures

NORMAL DELIVERY OF THE INFANT

Infrequently the emergency physician is called on to deliver an infant when the obstetrician is not available or when the mother is brought in with the cervix completely dilated and the delivery imminent. He or she must be capable of performing a normal delivery and a breech extraction. The occiput or vertex presentation occurs in approximately 95% of all labors. The fetus may enter the pelvis in either an occiput anterior position or an occiput posterior position, the former being by far the most common. A detailed discussion of the various steps and stages of labor is beyond the scope of this chapter. The reader is referred to any one of a number of excellent obstetric texts available (24).

History

It is important for the physician to obtain certain information rapidly when a woman arrives in the emergency department in active labor and delivery is imminent. One needs to know the patient's gravidity, parity, number of weeks of gestation, whether the pregnancy is a singleton or multiple, any complications during the pregnancy, and previous pregnancies, delivery history, and prenatal care status. This information can help predict the final outcome and prepare the physician and staff for possible complications. Inquiry also must be made as to the frequency and intensity of the uterine contractions. Finally, the patient must be asked if rupture of the membranes with leakage of fluid vaginally has occurred and whether there has been any significant vaginal bleeding in excess of a bloody show.

PREMATURE RUPTURE OF MEMBRANES

If the patient has given a history of premature rupture of membranes (PROM), which is defined as ruptured membranes occurring more than 12 hours before the onset of uterine contractions, then appropriate intravenous antibiotics (ampicillin or erythromycin) should be given prophylactically on maternal presentation to the emergency department. The dosage of ampicillin is a 2-g bolus and then 1 g every 4 hours. For the penicillin-allergic patient, the dose of erythromycin is 500 mg every 4 hours.

Examination

Evaluate the heart rate, presentation, and size of the fetus abdominally. Check the fetal heart rate at the end of a contraction and immediately thereafter to identify any pathologic bradycardia that may foretell danger to the fetus.

RUPTURE OF MEMBRANES

A diagnosis of ruptured membrane is not always easy to make unless amniotic fluid is seen escaping from the cervical os by the examiner. Three tests are commonly used to document rupture of membranes. Although a phenaphthazine (Nitrazine) test is commonly performed to ascertain rupture of membranes, it is not completely reliable. The basis of the test is that normally the pH of the vagina ranges from 4.5 to 5.5, and if amniotic fluid has leaked into the vagina, the pH of the amniotic fluid is usually 7.0 to 7.5.

Insert phenaphthazine-impregnated paper into the vagina, and interpret the color of the reaction by comparison with a standard color chart. Intact membranes generally result in a color ranging from yellow to olive green. When ruptured membranes have occurred, the color of the paper changes from blue–green to deep blue, depending on the pH.

In a second test, place fluid on a microscope slide and permit it to dry. If the fluid crystallizes as it dries, this is a positive "ferning" test.

Finally, the accumulation of fluid in the posterior vagina is known as pooling, and this also is indicative of rupture of the membranes. To minimize bacterial contamination if there is a question of rupture of the membranes, carefully insert a sterile speculum, and look for fluid in the posterior vaginal fornix. Observe the fluid for vernix, meconium, and frank blood. No speculum examination is done if the patient is bleeding more than a bloody show.

EFFACEMENT AND DILATATION

Palpate the cervix for softness and effacement as well as for dilatation. The degree of effacement of the cervix is expressed in terms of the length of the cervical canal compared with that of an uneffaced cervix (Fig. 6.1*A*). When its length is only 1 cm, the cervix is usually said to be 50% effaced, because the normal uneffaced cervix averages approximately 2 cm in length. At the point when the cervix becomes essentially a thin ring of tissue flush to the vaginal fornix, it is termed "completely effaced" or 100% effaced (Fig. 6.1*C*). Ascertain the amount of dilatation of the cervix by estimating the average diameter of the cervical opening. Place a finger within the margins of the cervix, and express the diameter traversed in centimeters. When the diameter of the

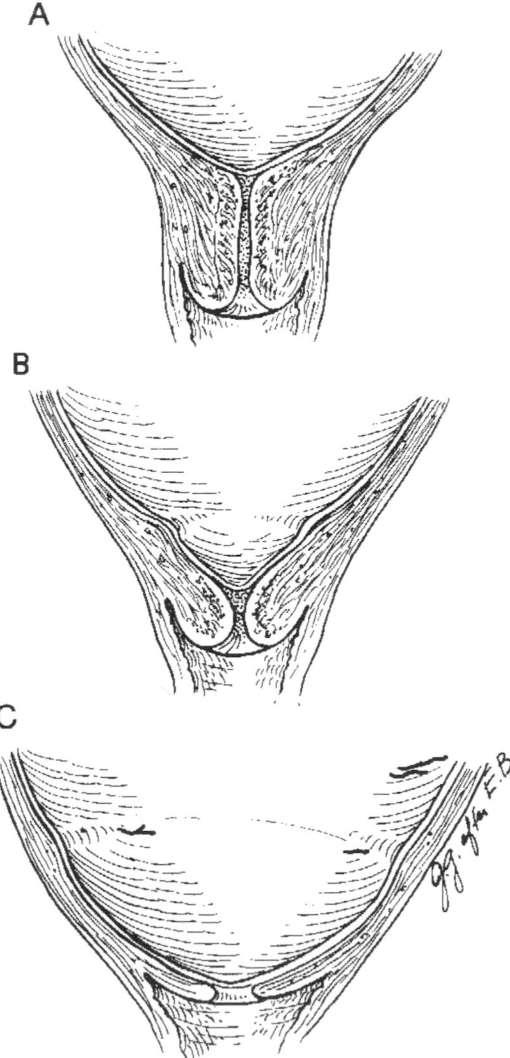

Figure 6.1. Cervical effacement.

opening measures 10 cm, the presenting part can usually pass through the cervix without difficulty, and this is termed "fully dilated."

It is important to note that the emergency physician should not perform digital or speculum examinations in patients with frank vaginal bleeding in their third trimester until placenta previa has been ruled out and obstetrical backup is available.

The onset of the second stage of labor is indicated by full dilatation of the cervix. The duration of the second stage of labor from complete dilatation of the cervix to delivery of the fetus is highly variable between patients; however, on the average, in the nulliparous woman, it is 50 minutes, and in the multiparous woman, it is approximately 20 minutes. It is imperative that the status of the fetus be monitored closely during this critical period, because the force of contraction during labor may significantly reduce the placental blood flow. Determine the presenting part positively, and identify its position.

STATION

It is important to identify the level of the presenting part within the birth canal. The ischial spines are approximately halfway between the pelvic inlet and the pelvic outlet. When the lowermost portion of the presenting part is at the level of the ischial spines, it is designated as being at zero station. The birth canal above the ischial spines is arbitrarily divided into thirds. If the presenting part is at the level of the pelvic inlet, it is at −3 station. If it has descended one third of the distance from the pelvic inlet to the ischial spines, it is termed a −2 station. Finally, two thirds of the distance from the inlet to the spines is termed a −1 station. Similarly, the birth canal is divided into thirds below the ischial spines. When the presenting part is one third of the distance between the ischial spines and the pelvic outlet, this is termed a +1 station; two thirds of the distance is termed a +2 station. When the presenting part reaches the perineum, delivery may be imminent, and the station is termed +3. A few of the preparatory steps taken in normal delivery are bypassed in the emergency center when delivery is imminent; this is the only time that the emergency physician performs delivery in the emergency center.

FETAL DISTRESS

It is important to ascertain the fetal heart rate with either a DeLee/Hillis fetoscope or a Doppler ultrasonic device. Fetal distress is suggested if the fetal heart rate immediately after a contraction decreases below 120 beats/min or increases above 160 beats/min. The diagnosis is definite if fetal distress is anticipated; the fetus is at high risk, and the obstetrician should be contacted immediately. Simultaneous notification of a pediatrician and/or a neonatologist for care of the neonate is necessary.

ULTRASOUND EVALUATION

With the availability of ultrasound devices in most emergency departments today, it is important to mention a timely manner in which to evaluate the infant before delivery. Identify the presenting part by using the abdominal probe placed on the patient's gravid abdomen with proper conducting medium. Is the infant cephalic or breech? If the infant is cephalic, then normal spontaneous delivery will be imminent in 95% of obstetrical cases. If the infant is breech, then determine if it is feet first (footling breech) or true breech (complete or frank). If the fetus is footling breech, routine vaginal delivery is contraindicated, and immediate obstetrical backup should be arranged for an eventual cesarean section. If an obstetrical service is not available, then use the method of breech extraction discussed further in this chapter.

Once the presentation has been determined, use the abdominal ultrasound probe to locate the four-chambered heart of the fetus, and measure the fetal heart rate during and after contractions. This method allows the emergency physician to establish the presence or absence of fetal distress and to summon immediate obstetrical and neonatology backup when indicated.

Ultrasound evaluation also can aid in making the diagnosis of placenta previa, characterized by the presence of placenta in front of the fetal presenting part, partially or completely covering the cervical os. This diagnosis also requires immediate obstetrical consultation because of the potential for severe hemorrhage.

Preparation for Delivery in the Emergency Department (3)

Check the mother's temperature initially and blood pressure periodically. Place an 18- to 19-gauge intravenous line, and draw blood hemoglobin, hematocrit, and typing. If the patient is high risk, include a blood sample for cross-matching. If the membranes have been ruptured previously, many hours before arrival at the emergency center, the pregnancy is considered high risk. All oral intake should be withheld during labor and delivery because gastric emptying time is prolonged once labor is established. Empty the bladder either spontaneously with the mother voiding in a bedpan or, if this is not possible, by catheterization of the bladder. Test the urine for the presence of protein, and if it is present and the patient has increased blood pressure, preeclampsia should be assumed and treated appropriately with magnesium sulfate. The dose is a 4-g bolus intravenously and then 2 g per hour until delivery of the infant and the blood pressure and proteinuria have resolved. This patient also requires an obstetrical consult as soon as possible. The emergency physician may also desire to have intravenous calcium gluconate at the bedside during magnesium sulfate infusion to reverse the rare but potentially fatal magnesium toxicity.

Scrub the vulva, perineum, and adjacent areas with povidone–iodine (Betadine) or soap, and apply sterile drapes in preparation for delivery. An obstetric kit containing the necessary items for delivery is then opened. The physician should scrub his or her hands and wear sterile rubber gloves.

Use a transvaginal pudendal nerve block in the emergency center as discussed in Chapter 3: Anesthesia and Regional Blocks. As the head descends through the vaginal canal, the perineum begins to bulge. The scalp of the fetus may be seen through a slit-like vulvar opening at this time.

Spontaneous Cephalic Delivery

As the head descends with each contraction, the perineum bulges, and the vulvar opening becomes more and more dilated. Its shape changes from an oval to an almost circular opening. With the cessation of each contraction, the head recedes, and the opening becomes smaller. As labor progresses, the vulva is stretched farther and ultimately encircles the baby's head, a condition known as "crowning."

An *episiotomy* can be performed at, but not before, crowning. Although a medial lateral episiotomy has been described, the midline episiotomy is more commonly used. The more common practice is to begin the episiotomy in the midline and to direct it downward toward the rectum. Be careful not to incise the fibers of the external sphincter or ani muscle. To avoid this, remain in the subcutaneous tissue, and avoid anal musculature. This episiotomy is the simplest to make and easiest to repair. It also heals with the least discomfort (28). The key point is to avoid extension into the rectum, which can lead to rectovaginal fistula (28). Episiotomies are performed to prevent irregular or jagged tears of the perineum that may extend into the rectum. In addition, episiotomies serve to prevent excessive stretch of the pelvic diaphragm, to protect the fetal head, and to shorten the second stage of labor (19).

When an episiotomy is performed too early, bleeding from the wound may be significant. It is common practice to perform an episiotomy when the head of the fetus is visible for a diameter of 3 to 4 cm with a contraction. The episiotomy is generally not repaired until after the placenta has been delivered.

The perineum now may be extremely thin and in danger of rupture with subsequent contractions. In multiparous women, an episiotomy may not be necessary. The anus becomes greatly stretched and protuberant, and, if an episiotomy is not performed, perineal and rectal lacerations may occur during passage of the head. This may lead to permanent relaxation of the pelvic floor and the possibility of cystocele and uterine prolapse. Perform an episiotomy by making a midline incision with a sharp scissors to relax the tense perineum, as shown in Fig. 6.2*A*.

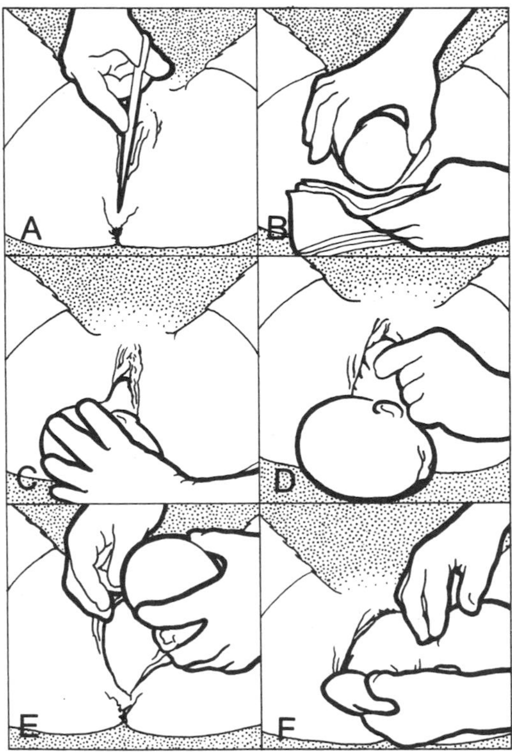

Figure 6.2. The normal vaginal delivery of an infant. See text for discussion.

When making the incision, protect the fetal presenting part from accidental injury by placing two fingers (index and middle finger) inside the vaginal introitus, between the presenting part and the scissors. As the vertex of the head appears, or hair is seen on the perineum in the absence of a uterine contraction through the perineum, drape a towel over the physician's hand to protect the fetus from the anus and fecal excretions and to exert forward pressure against the forehead of the fetus (Fig. 6.2*B*). This procedure is called a modified Ritgen maneuver and permits the physician to control the delivery of the head. Use the physician's other hand, draped with a sterile towel, to provide counterpressure and support to the perineum to prevent or minimize perineal damage or lacerations. This known as "hands-on care." Deliver the head slowly by using continuous downward pressure on the fetal head until the anterior shoulder appears at the introitus and with the base of the occiput rotating around the lower margin of the symphysis pubis. On delivery of the head, pass the physician's finger along the neck of the fetus to ascertain if there are any encircling coils of umbilical cord. Although these commonly are noted and usually cause no harm, they may occasionally be so tight as to constrict the cord vessels and result in hypoxia. If the coil is loose, slip it over the infant's head; however, if it is too tightly applied to the neck, and the probability of constriction is present, clamp the cord and cut between the two clamps, and then deliver the infant immediately.

After the head is delivered, it generally rotates laterally to the right occipitoanterior or left occipitotransverse (Fig. 6.2*C*). Usually the shoulders appear in the vulva in anteroposterior position. Grasp the sides of the head with both hands, and apply gentle downward traction until the anterior shoulder is delivered under the pubic symphysis. Completion of delivery of the anterior shoulder can be performed before delivery of the posterior shoulder (Fig. 6.2*D*). After this, apply an upward movement to deliver the posterior shoulder (Fig. 6.2*E* and *F*). The remainder of the body almost always follows the delivery of the shoulders without difficulty.

SHOULDER DYSTOCIA

A child presenting with shoulder dystocia cannot be predicted by examination or careful history. Shoulder dystocia occurs in 2.23% to 2.09% of all vaginal deliveries and is a true obstetrical emergency. Thus the emergency physician confronted with this problem must be prepared for the appropriate intervention. Woods (27) reported that, by progressively rotating the posterior shoulder 180 degrees in a corkscrew fashion, the impacted anterior shoulder could be released. This frequently is referred to as the "Woods corkscrew maneuver" (Fig. 6.3).

Deliver the posterior shoulder by carefully sweeping the posterior arm across the chest of the fetus, followed by delivery of the arm (Fig. 6.4). Then rotate the shoulder girdle into the oblique diameter of the pelvis with subsequent delivery of the anterior shoulder.

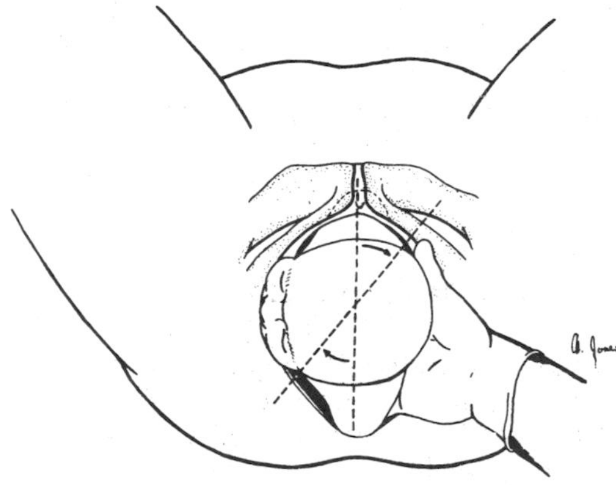

Figure 6.3. In the Woods' Maneuver, place the hand behind the posterior shoulder of the fetus. Then progressively rotate the posterior approximately 180 degrees clockwise in a corkscrew manner so that the impacted anterior shoulder is released.

Another method used to deliver an infant with a shoulder dystocia involves bending the patient's legs and displacing them cephalad (exaggerated hyperflexion), spreading them maximally apart to open the pelvis, straighten the maternal sacrum and rotate the pubis symphysis in the cephalad direction. This is known as the McRobert's maneuver. At this time, apply pressure to the uterine fundus during contractions to dislodge the infant's shoulder. Both of these maneuvers assume that the physician has at least two assistants at the time of delivery.

The Zavanelli maneuver involves manually replacing the head of the fetus back into the uterus during a period of relaxation or absence of contractions, then followed by an emergency cesarean section. At some point, the uterine relaxation must be provided, and inhaled amyl nitrate is preferable to intravenous nitroglycerine.

DELIVERY OF THE PLACENTA

Two clamps are applied to the cord, and the cord is cut between the clamps. The cord should be cut approximately 2 cm from the abdomen of the fetus. A sample of cord blood from the placenta should be taken for VDRL and Coombs test. After delivery of the infant, ascertain the consistency and height of the uterus. As long as there is minimal bleeding, never pull the placenta manually to accomplish delivery; rather, patient waiting is advised. When the placenta is to be delivered, the uterus becomes globular and firm. This is the earliest sign of placental delivery. The umbilical cord protrudes farther out of the vagina, indicating that the placenta has descended; this is often preceded by a sudden gush of blood. These signs generally appear within 5 to 15 minutes after delivery of the infant (maximally 30 minutes unless bleeding is profuse).

After delivery of the placenta, one enters a critical period with regard to postpartum hemorrhage. Postpartum hemorrhage due to uterine atony is most likely to

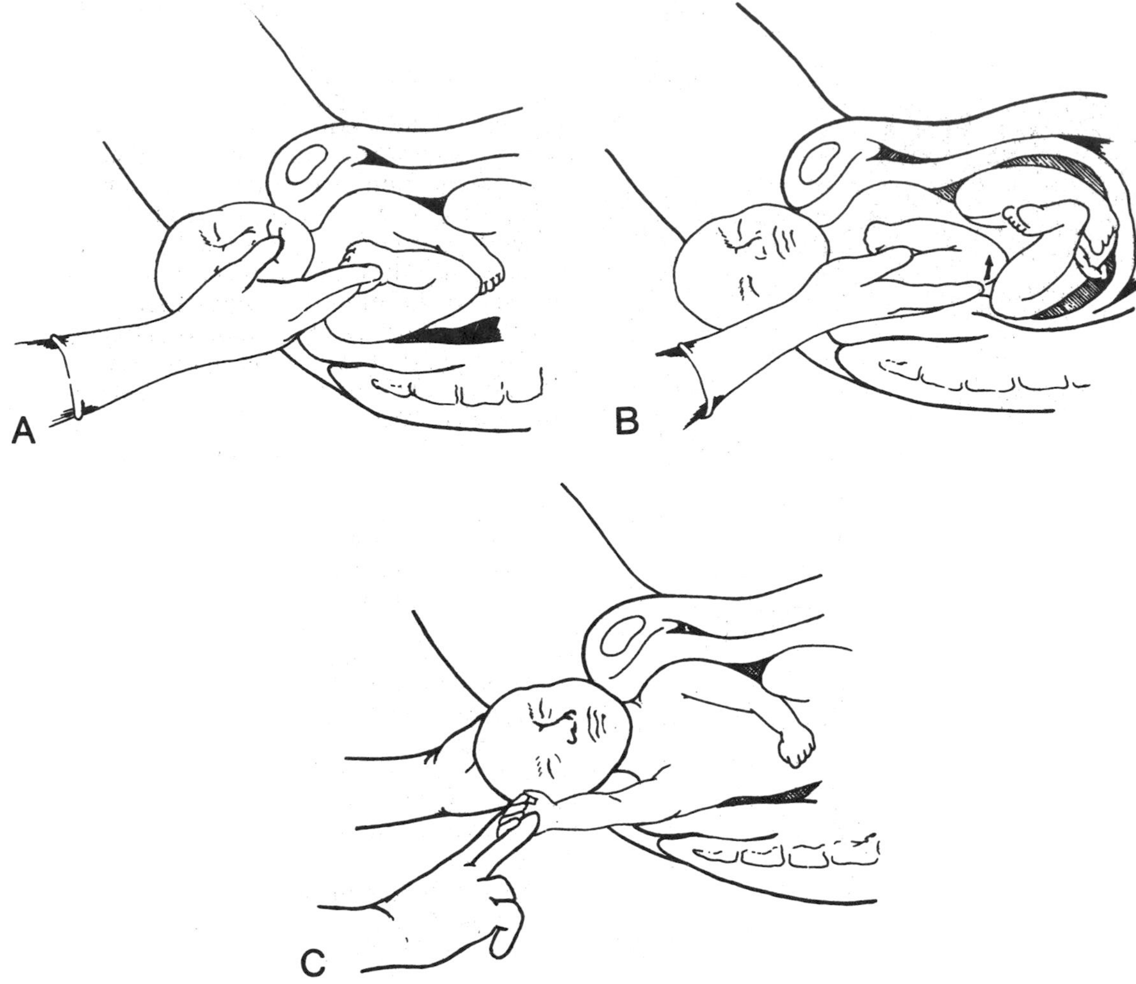

Figure 6.4. Shoulder dystocia with an impacted anterior shoulder of the fetus *(A)*. The posterior humerus is "splinted" by the physician's hand as the posterior arm is swept across the chest, while keeping the arm flexed at the elbow *(B)*. Grasp the hand of the fetus just under the pubic symphysis, with the arm extended along the side of the fetus's face (as shown above, *C*). Then deliver the posterior arm from the vagina (as shown above), which then allows delivery of the anterior shoulder.

occur at this time. It is mandatory that the patient be observed constantly throughout this period. Oxytocin is often placed in the intravenous solution and infused at this point; place 20 units of oxytocin in 1 L of intravenous fluid and administer at a rate of 10 mL/min over a few minutes until the uterus remains firmly contracted and the bleeding is controlled. After this, reduce the infusion rate to 60 to 120 mL/h. Bimanual uterine massage also may decrease bleeding resulting from postpartum uterine atony. If the oxytocin infusion and bimanual uterine massage do not stop the bleeding, then give 0.2 mg of methylergonovine (Methergine) intramuscularly, provided that the patient is not hypertensive. If the patient is hypertensive or the methylergonovine has failed to stop the hemorrhage, then use intramuscular carboprost (Hemabate). In the event that this does not stop the bleeding, then obtain an immediate obstetrical consult, and transfer the patient to the operating room for

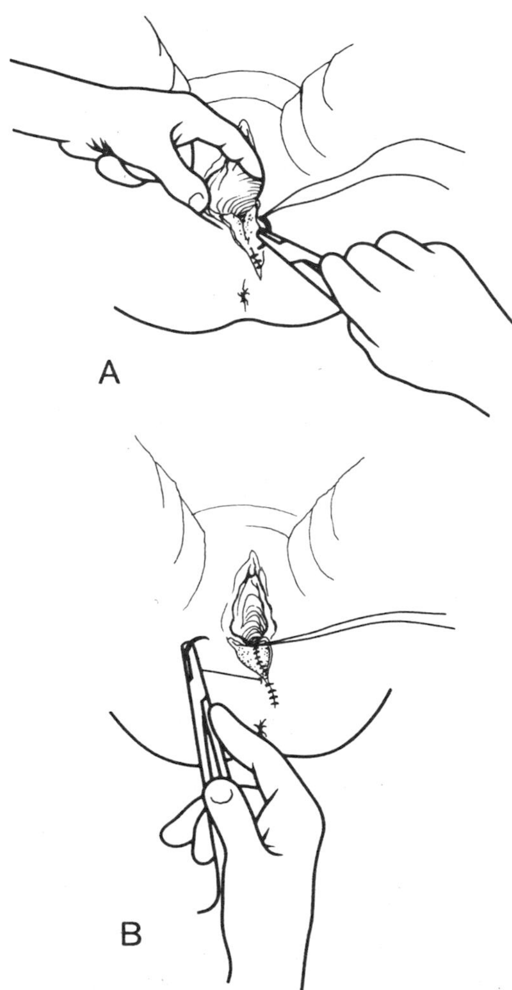

Figure 6.5. Repair of an episiotomy incision. First close the vaginal mucosa with a continuous suture. After this, place three or four interrupted sutures of 2-0 catgut in the fascia and muscle layers of the perineum *(A)*. Repair the episiotomy from posterior to anterior. Use a continuous suture to repair the skin and subcutaneous fascia *(B)*.

immediate suction curettage or uterine artery ligation. Examine for cervical and vaginal wall lacerations at this point, and be sure that all sponges that have been used are removed.

Retained placenta is defined as a placenta that has not separated within 30 minutes after delivery of the infant. This condition necessitates an obstetrical consult for manual extraction or surgical extraction in the operating room.

REPAIR OF EPISIOTOMY INCISION

Repair of the episiotomy should be performed with 2-0 absorbable suture material [i.e., catgut, chromic, or polyglactin (Vicryl)]. First close the vaginal epithelium with a continuous interlocking suture. After this, place three or four interrupted sutures in the fascia and muscle layer of the perineum with care to avoid the underlying rectum (Fig. 6.5*A*). Then use a continuous suture to close the subcutaneous tissue. Use a subcuticular stitch to close the skin, or place several interrupted sutures through the skin to close the skin and subcutaneous tissue loosely (Fig. 6.5*B*) (4, 5, 8, 21).

BREECH EXTRACTION

Three types of breech deliveries are possible: a **spontaneous breech delivery,** in which the entire infant is expelled without manipulation; **partial breech extraction,** in which the infant is delivered spontaneously as far as the umbilicus and the remainder of the body must be extracted manually; and **total breech extraction,** in which the entire body of the infant is extracted by the physician. Fortunately, breech extraction is an uncommon procedure for the emergency physician to perform. It should be performed only in the instance of a complete or frank breech presentation (fetal buttocks are the presenting part). Strongly consider cesarean section for a footling breech presentation because of the risk of an entrapped aftercoming head. In the case of twin gestation and twin A is breech and twin B is cephalic, emergency cesarean section is indicated. Do not attempt vaginal delivery in this case unless obstetrical services are not available. If the twins present in any other way, vaginal delivery can be attempted. It is best to allow a breech fetus to deliver spontaneously to the umbilicus and then to extract it. However, if fetal distress develops, a decision must be made as to whether to perform a total breech extraction or a cesarean section. For breech extraction to be performed vaginally, the birth canal must be sufficiently large to permit passage of the fetus without trauma, and the cervix must be effaced and fully dilated. If these conditions are not present, cesarean section is often necessary (1).

A breech delivery should be done by the emergency physician when vaginal delivery is likely before the obstetrician arrives and when acute fetal distress occurs and breech extraction is possible and cesarean section is impossible (because of prolapsed cord, etc.). The ideal anesthesia for breech extraction is epidural spinal anesthesia, with the ability to use general anesthesia with halothane after delivery to the umbilicus. This is usually not available to the emergency physician.

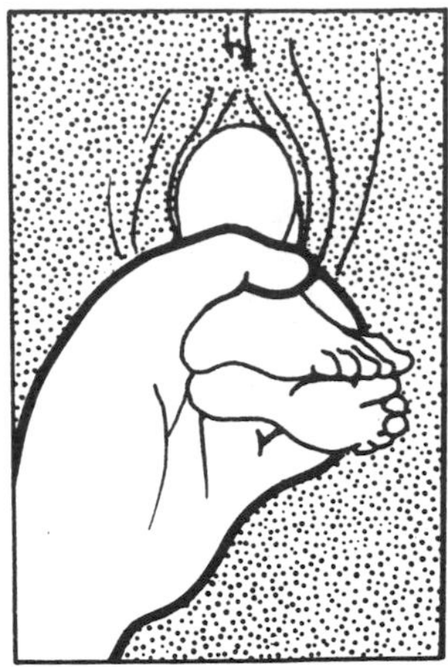

Figure 6.6. Breech extraction. Bring down the feet by gentle traction until they appear at the vulva.

TECHNIQUE

Prepare for extraction when the buttocks or the feet of the fetus appear at the vulva. Introduce the physician's hand into the vagina, and grasp both feet of the fetus. Hold the ankles of the fetus, with the second finger of the physician lying between them. Then bring down the feet by gentle traction until they appear at the vulva (Fig. 6.6) (5) Perform a midline episiotomy at this time, before delivery of any larger parts. Once the feet are drawn through the vulva, wrap them in a sterile towel to obtain a firmer grasp, because vernix caseosa makes them slippery and difficult to hold. Apply continuous downward traction, and grasp the legs and then the thighs. When the buttocks appear at the vulva, apply gentle traction until the hips are delivered. Place the physician's thumbs over the posterior iliac spines and sacroiliac area, as shown in Fig. 6.7. With the fingers

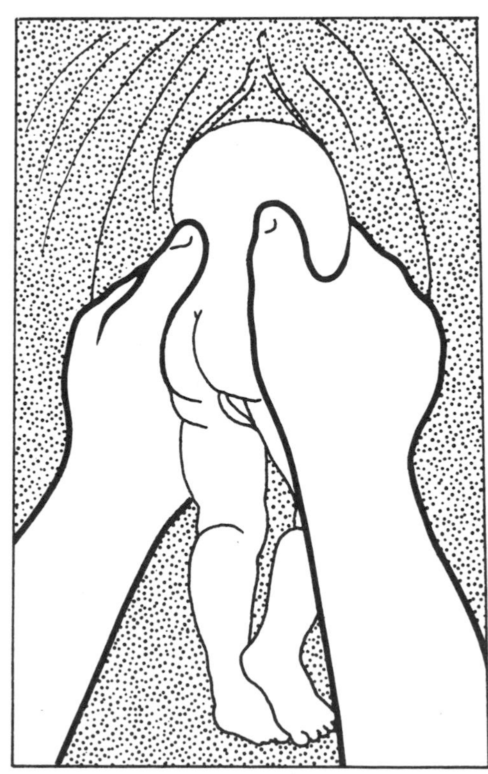

Figure 6.7. Place the physician's thumbs over the posterior iliac spines and sacroiliac area, with the hands around the infant's pelvis anteriorly. Apply downward traction until the rib cage is visualized.

Cox WL: The technique of breech delivery. J Obstet Gynaecol 62: 395–403, 1955; and Crichton D, Seedat ED, et al: The technique of symphysiotomy. South Afr Med J 37: 227–234, 1963.

of the physician encircling the hips, continue downward traction until the rib cage is visible. Further downward traction produces the scapulas. Once the buttocks are delivered, the back of the child generally faces upward; however, as further traction is exerted, the child tends to rotate spontaneously. If rotation does not occur during traction, add slight rotation while traction is maintained to bring the bisacromial diameter of the child into an anteroposterior position with the outlet and the back of the fetus facing laterally. Do not attempt to deliver the shoulders and arms until one axilla becomes visible during downward traction. Once one of the axillae appears through the vulva, deliver the shoulder. There are two methods of delivering the shoulders:

1. Rotate the infant's trunk in such a way that the anterior shoulder and arm appear at the vulva and can easily be released and delivered first. This can be accomplished by rotating the trunk of the infant in a clockwise direction to deliver the anterior shoulder and arm. Then rotate the body of the infant in the reverse direction to deliver the other shoulder. Generally extract the arm by sweeping it across the chest.
2. If this method of trunk rotation is not successful, deliver the posterior shoulder first because the posterior and lateral portions of the normal pelvis are wider. Grasp the feet in one hand, and draw them upward (Fig. 6.8). In this way, exert leverage on the posterior shoulder, which slips out over the perineal margin and is followed by the arm and hand (Fig. 6.9). After this, depress the body of the infant, and delivered the anterior shoulder beneath the pubic arch, followed by the arm (Fig. 6.10). After this, the back generally rotates spontaneously and faces the pubic symphysis of the mother. If rotation does not occur, effect it by manual rotation of the body.

Once the shoulders are delivered, the head rotates in the pelvis so that the chin is directed posteriorly, and extract the head by the Mauriceau maneuver.

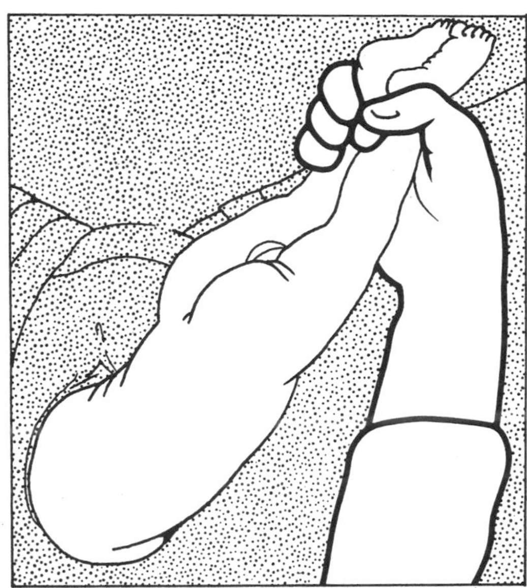

Figure 6.8. Deliver the posterior shoulder first. Exert leverage superiorly so that the shoulder slips out over the perineal margin, followed by the arm and the hand.

Mauriceau Maneuver (1)

Introduce the index finger of one hand into the mouth of the child while the body rests on the palm and forearm of the hand,

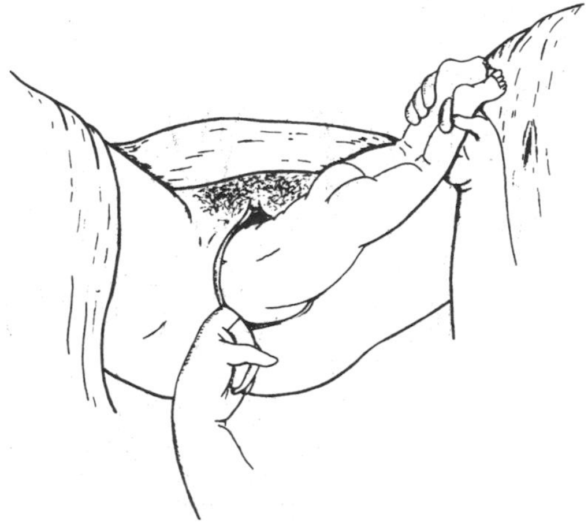

Figure 6.9. Insert the finger to aid in the passage of the posterior shoulder.

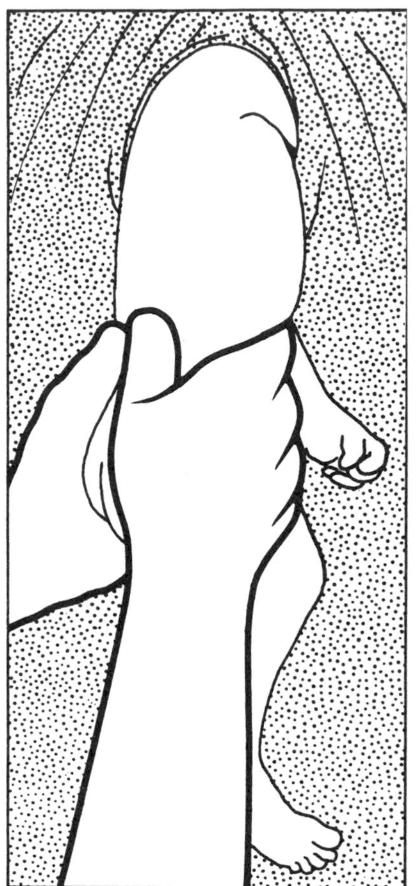

Figure 6.10. Depress the body of the infant as shown, and deliver the anterior shoulder beneath the pubic arch.

as shown in Fig. 6.11. Then place the index and long fingers of the other hand around the neck posteriorly, grasping the shoulders, and apply downward traction until the suboccipital region appears under the symphysis. An assistant applies downward suprapubic pressure at this point. The body of the infant is now elevated toward the mother's abdomen, and the mouth, nose, brow, and occiput emerge successively over the perineum. Exert downward traction during this procedure only by the fingers over the shoulders and not by the fingers placed in the infant's mouth.

Use total breech extraction or cesarean section to deal with a prolapsed cord. When the head is not deliverable by routine methods, use suprapubic pressure as well as a Piper forceps, as shown in Fig. 6.11*B* (4, 5, 8, 21).

SYMPHYSIOTOMY AND ITS USE FOR THE TRAPPED FETUS IN A BREECH DELIVERY AND SEVERE SHOULDER DYSTOCIA

Symphysiotomy has very few indications. However, when needed, it can save the life of a fetus and possibly that of the mother and is an alternative to cesarean section or traumatic vaginal delivery, and should be understood by all emergency physicians (7, 10, 14, 15).

Use this procedure in patients with trapped after-coming parts of a breech delivery or a presentation of shoulder dystocia refractory to the other mentioned methods and fetal distress. The most dreaded complication of a vaginal breech delivery is entrapment of the after-coming head of the fetus. This problem is due to pelvic–fetal disproportion. In this situation, persistent attempts at vaginal extraction are likely to result in a dead or damaged baby, still without extracting the fetus.

A largely unknown but superb solution to this desperate predicament is to enlarge the pelvis surgically by means of a symphysiotomy. A review of the literature shows that this procedure to free the entrapped after-coming head typically re-

Figure 6.11. Mauriceau maneuver. *A:* Introduce the index finger of the left hand into the mouth of the child to open the mouth. The remainder of the infant's body rests on the palm and forearm of the left hand as shown. Then place the index and long fingers of the right hand around the neck posteriorly, grasping the shoulders, and apply downward traction until the suboccipital region appears under the symphysis. *B:* Use the Piper forceps for extracting a breech pregnancy. Inserting the forceps gently, placing the forceps as shown above. Gentle traction permits the head to be more easily extracted.

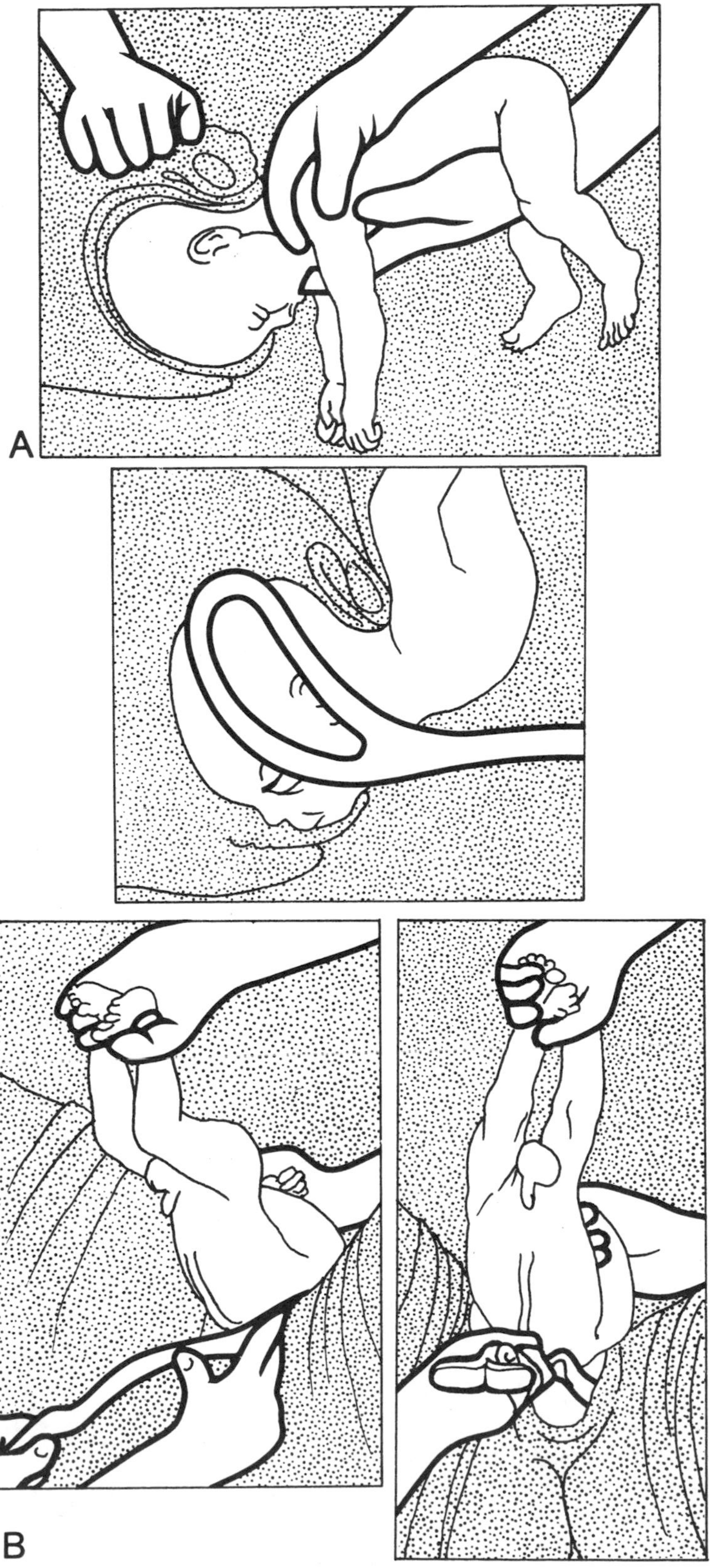
A
B

sults in an 80% survival rate of the babies (10, 23). Most symphysiotomies are undertaken for cephalopelvic disproportion with the vertex presenting and a live fetus. Thus it is an alternative to cesarean section or traumatic vaginal delivery. When improperly done, the trauma inflicted with this procedure may cause severe soft tissue problems for the mother.

Do not undertake symphysiotomy unless the fetal head has entered the pelvic brim. If the fetal head has reached the maximal distance that the head can pass, either labor has not progressed far enough, or there is severe cephalopelvic disproportion (16).

Equipment

No. 10 scalpel
Finger guard
Drapes
Urethral catheter set
Local anesthesia setup
Hemostats (2)
Mayo scissors

Technique

When assistants are available, hold the patient's thighs at an angle of no greater than 90 degrees to each other or 45 degrees to the bed. With no assistants, maintain this lithotomy position with bandages tied between the knees to prevent overabduction, which is a major problem after separation of the pubic symphysis.

Catheterize the urethra using an indwelling Foley catheter.

Identify the symphysis pubis, which in labor is a softer fibrocartilaginous structure and is wider than that in the normal situation (Fig. 6.12).

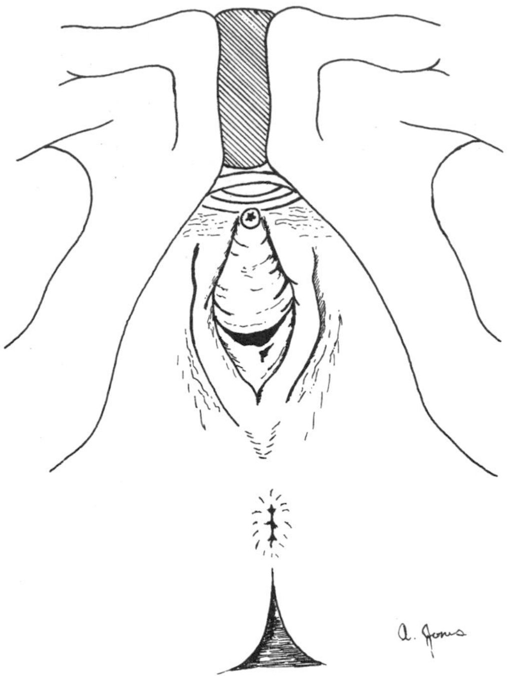

Figure 6.12. The symphysis pubis.

Deposit local anesthesia over the skin and tissues in front of, above, and below the pubic symphysis (Fig. 6.13). Introduce the index finger of the left hand, palm surface up, into the vagina between the fetal upper back and the posterior aspect of the symphysis. Use the index finger to push the Foley catheter and urethra to the side (Fig. 6.14). Next, insert the middle finger on the posterior aspect of the pubic joint to monitor the action of the scalpel (Fig. 6.15). Note that a finger guard is placed over the index finger, which is directly under the symphysis pubis, to protect the physician's finger from injury by the

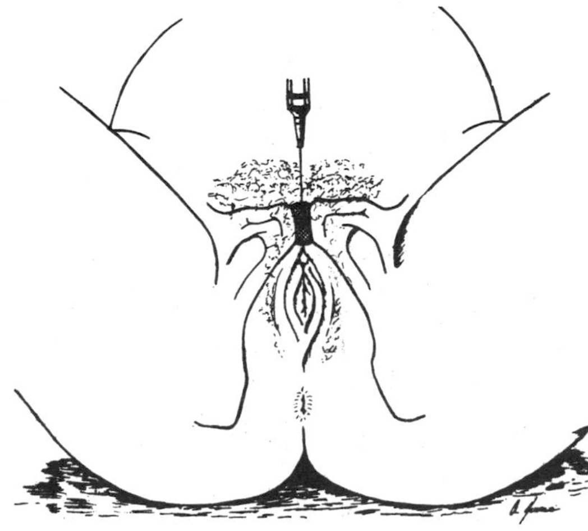

Figure 6.13. Infiltration of anesthetic solution over the symphysis pubis. See text for discussion.

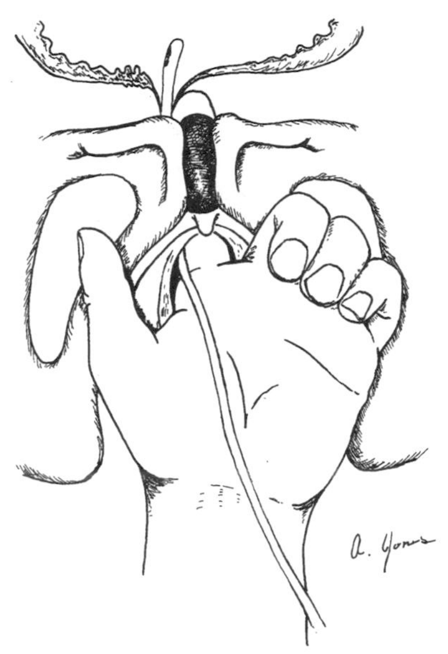

Figure 6.14. Insert a Foley catheter into the urethra. The index finger then displaces the Foley catheter and the urethra laterally away from the symphysis pubis.

scalpel. Stand between the patient's legs. Grasp the scalpel, with a no. 10 blade, like a pencil, and keep it in strict sagittal plane. Incise the symphysis then by a stab incision into the center of the joint, with the blade pointing downward (Fig. 6.15). There should be little resistance. If there is resistance while inserting the blade, then it has deviated laterally and should be reinserted. When the tip of the scalpel is felt through the posterior vaginal wall, which must not be pierced, lower the knife handle toward the maternal abdomen by using the upper part of the pubic symphysis as a fulcrum. Then remove the scalpel, turn it 180 degrees, and reinsert it so that the cutting edge faces away from the operator, and then incise the upper part of the pubic symphysis.

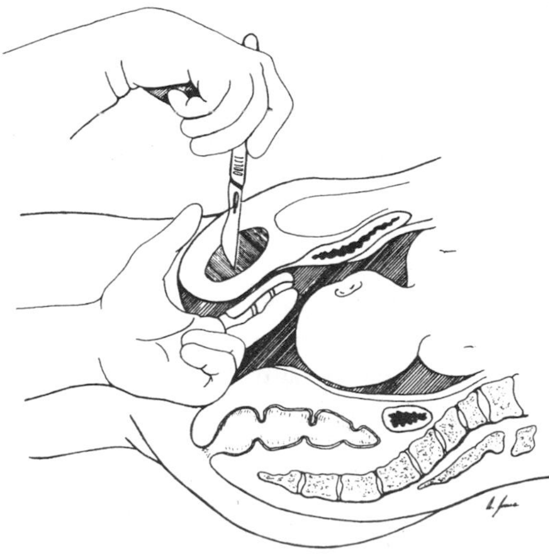

Figure 6.15. Make an incision into the symphysis pubis with a no. 10 blade. See text for discussion.

The joint will then begin to separate and allow delivery of the entrapped fetal head. After delivery and administration of any urgent treatment required by the infant, repair this skin incision. One suture is usually sufficient. Insert the suture fairly deeply because the edges of the skin incision usually bleed freely. Repair the episiotomy at this time.

Ambulation can occur within 8 hours after the procedure is done. Immediate complications of this procedure are uncommon. Hemorrhage from the vascular area over the pubic symphysis is sometimes substantial. However, this almost always stops as soon as the baby is born. If the bleeding continues, control it initially with direct pressure by an assistant and later suture it.

Cesarean section remains the best treatment for breech extraction. However, if one encounters a vaginal delivery in which the infant's head is not able to pass and one cannot perform cesarean section in that setting, use this procedure. Systemic analgesia such as fentanyl should be considered to augment local anesthesia. In this dangerous situation, a speedy symphysiotomy, undertaken for the delivery of the aftercoming head, may eliminate difficulty and save the lives of the mother and child.

CESAREAN SECTION

The emergency physician is rarely called on to perform a cesarean section in the emergency center. Most obstetricians would feel that this should be done for maternal indications only. The risk of saving the fetus may impose incredible maternal risk. Four indications for performing a cesarean section in the emergency center are

1. A postmortem (maternal) cesarean section (for example, if a mother has been involved in automobile accident and is severely injured, with impending death).
2. Severe traumatic abruptio placentae or bleeding from placenta previa, when blood loss is greater than the ability to transfuse the patient.
3. Suspected uterine rupture.
4. Questionable fetal indications such as continuous bradycardia and acute cord prolapse.

Perform an emergency cesarean section in the operating room by the obstetrician or general surgeon whenever possible; however, in the situations indicated earlier, it may become necessary for the emergency physician to perform this procedure. Although there is continuing controversy over this issue, we believe that the procedure should at least be known to the emergency physician should a case arise in which the mother's life is in jeopardy, and the fetus is viable.

EQUIPMENT

12 Kelly clamps
20 hemostats
ring forceps
Eight towel clips
Six Allis forceps
Four Babcock forceps
12 Pennington forceps
Six straight Kocher clamps
One bandage scissors
1 Metzenbaum scissors forceps
Two suture scissors
One curved Mayo scissors
Three needle holders, 8 inch
One needle holder, 6 inch
Two knife holders
Two Adson forceps
One dressing forceps, 10 inch
One dressing forceps, 5.5 inch
Two Russian forceps, 5.5 inch
One DeBakey forceps, 8 inch
One bladder retractor
Two Goulet retractors
One Richardson retractor, large
One Richardson retractor, medium
Two tonsil suction tips
Two clip applicators
Two sets skin clips
Two cord clamps
Two red-top tubes
One Steri-Strip
One no. 10 scalpel and blade
Drapes
Gloves
1% lidocaine anesthesia with epinephrine
One baby de Lee forceps
One Bovie tip
One Bovie cord
One bulb syringe
Three suction tubing sets

TECHNIQUE

In performing an emergency cesarean section in the emergency center, one may have to eliminate a number of the steps detailed later. We believe that to perform a procedure such as this as an emergency, one must be aware of the steps to follow in performing the procedure somewhat more electively. It then becomes obvious which steps can be excluded. In performing the emergency cesarean section, those steps that are preceded by an asterisk are regarded as the essential steps in performing the procedure in the emergency center (18).

Preparatory Steps

1. Provide anesthesia for this procedure by epidural or spinal anesthesia. If this is not possible, local infiltration will suffice.

2. Shave the hair from the abdominal wall, from the mons pubis to above the umbilicus in the midline and laterally to the length of the abdomen.
3. Prepare the area with iodinated solution.
4. Empty the bladder through an indwelling catheter, which should remain in place during the entire procedure.
5. Apply sterile drapes to the area bounded by the mons pubis below and 4 to 6 cm above the umbilicus and 2 to 3 cm to each side of the midline. Use a mask and gown, as for any major operative procedure.

Procedural Steps

*1. Make an infraumbilical vertical incision, because this is the quickest technique for entering the abdomen. Extend the incision from just above the upper margin of the pubic symphysis to just below the umbilicus.
2. Dissect the subcutaneous fat away from the anterior rectus sheath to expose a strip of fascia in the midline approximately 2 cm wide.
*3. Make a small opening in the rectus sheath with a no. 11 scalpel and then insert a scissors and incise the fascia in the midline vertically to expose the uterus. Do not incise the rectus sheath with a scalpel or without being able to visualize it adequately; to do so risks inadvertently entering the bowel, which might be lying beneath the peritoneum. Separate the rectus muscles in the midline and expose the underlying transversalis fascia and the peritoneum.
4. Treat any bleeding encountered along the abdominal incision by clamping with hemostats rather than by ligation. Ligation usually is performed later, unless the hemostat is in the way.
5. Carefully dissect the transversalis fascia and the properitoneal fat to reach the underlying peritoneum.
*6. At the upper end of the incision, pick up the peritoneum with two hemostats placed approximately 2 cm apart in the midline. Palpate the fold of peritoneum between the clamps to rule out inclusion of bowel, bladder, or mesentery. Make an incision between the hemostats, and carry it superiorly to the upper pole of the abdominal incision and inferiorly to just above the peritoneal reflection over the bladder.
*7. Place a retractor firmly against the pubic symphysis.
*8. Identify the bladder, and grasp the serosa overlying the upper margin of it and extending along the anterior aspect of the lower uterine segment in the midline with forceps, as shown in Fig. 6.16. Insert scissors between the edge of the serosa of the bladder and the myometrium over the lower uterine segment, and separate a 2-cm wide strip of serosa from the uterus by blunt dissection with the scissors. Extend the dissection laterally along both sides of the bladder–uterus inter-

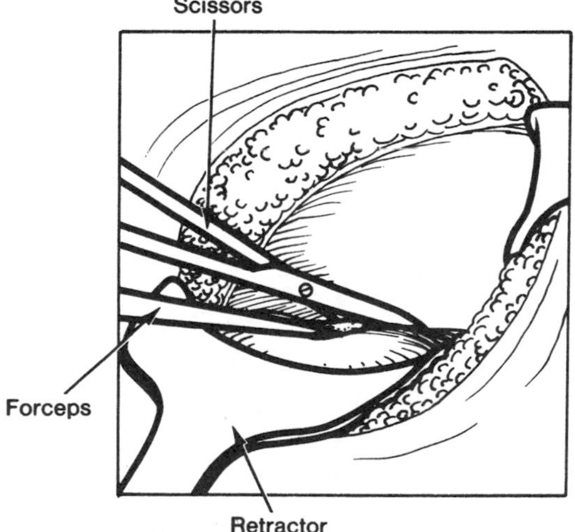

Figure 6.16. Cesarean section. Identify the bladder, separate it from the lower uterine segment, and retract inferiorly. See text for discussion.

face. Then incise the area dissected with the scissors, and separate the bladder gently by blunt dissection from the underlying uterus. Do not separate the bladder more than 5 cm from the uterus.

*9. Then retract the bladder inferiorly beneath the pubic symphysis with a bladder retractor.

10. Palpate the uterus quickly to identify the size of the presenting part of the fetus.

NOTE

The uterus is usually rotated to the right so that the left round ligament is more anterior and closer to the midline than is the right.

---

*11. Then make a transverse uterine incision with the no. 10 scalpel into the exposed lower uterine segment midway between the lateral margins of the uterus (Fig. 6.17). As the initial incision is made into the uterus, note a spurt of amniotic fluid as the uterine cavity is entered. This aids in determining the depth of the incision. The incision should be approximately 2 cm long. Perform the transverse incision carefully so as not to cut completely through the uterine wall and injure the underlying fetus. Suction is very important during this procedure and should be carried out by an assistant. Once the uterus is opened, extend the incision by either placing the index fingers into the wound and applying lateral pressure as shown in Fig. 6.18 or, preferably, by using either a bandage or blunt-pointed scissors to extend the incision laterally. Make the uterine incision large enough to allow delivery of the head and trunk of the fetus without tearing the uterus and cutting the uterine arteries, which course along the lateral margins of the uterus. When this is a possibility, curve the uterine incision upward bilaterally, rather than extending it farther laterally.

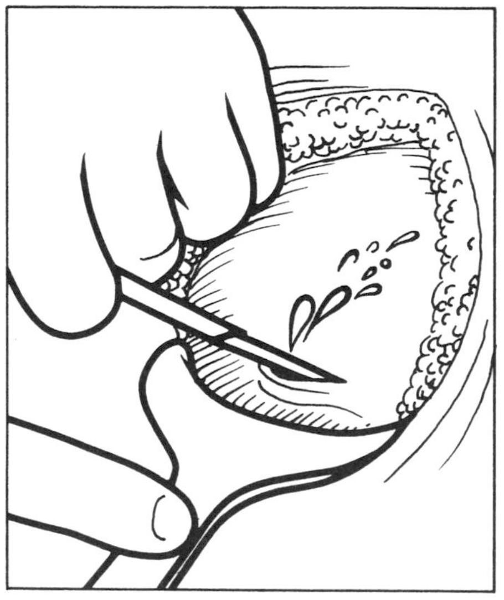

Figure 6.17. Make a small, 2-cm transverse incision over the exposed lower uterine segment. Amniotic fluid will spurt out of the wound, once the uterine cavity is entered. This guides the physician as to the depth of the incision to avoid injury to the fetus.

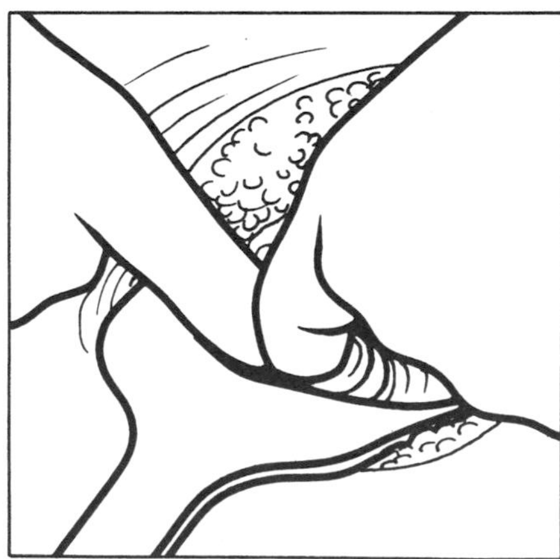

Figure 6.18. Once the uterus is opened, extend the incision by placing the index fingers into the wound and applying lateral pressure. Use a bandage or blunt-pointed scissors alternately to extend the incision laterally.

CAUTION

Uterine arteries and veins, both of which are quite large, course along the lateral margins of the uterus. When extending the transverse uterine incision, take care to avoid these veins and arteries.

NOTE

The uterus can be opened by either a vertical or a transverse incision; however, the vertical incision that extends into the uterine fundus is not very commonly used in cesarean sections. The transverse incision over the lower uterine segment has the advantage of requiring very little dissection of the bladder as compared with the vertical incision. The vertical incision has the advantage that it avoids the laterally placed uterine vessels. Another disadvantage of the vertical incision is that if it extends too far inferiorly, it may tear through the cervix and vagina.

NOTE

Place a Richardson retractor into the wound to retract the abdominal wall laterally when performing the uterine incision.

*12. Incise the membranes at this time, and if the placenta is encountered during the incision, detach it. If the placenta is incised, fetal hemorrhage may be severe. In this situation, clamp the umbilical cord as soon as possible.

*13. Then place the hand into the uterus between the symphysis pubis and the head of the fetus. Gently elevate the fetal head, and lift it out of the uterus (Fig. 6.19). Aspirate the nares and mouth with a bulb syringe to minimize aspiration of amniotic fluid before delivery of the thorax of the infant. Then deliver the shoulders by using gentle traction along with fundal pressure (Fig. 6.20). Once the shoulders are delivered, the remainder of the body follows without any problem.

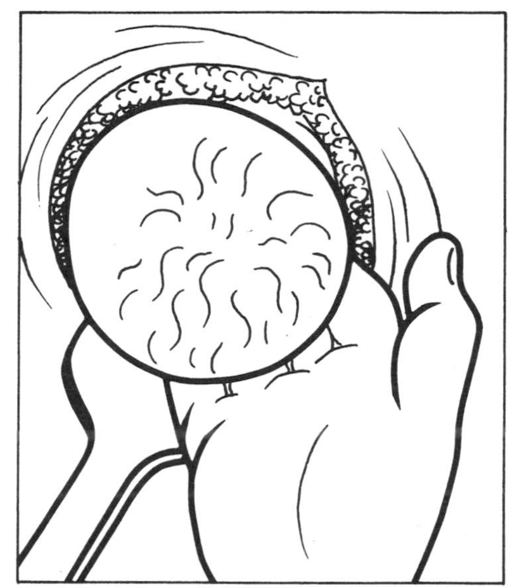

Figure 6.19. Place the hand into the uterus after the membranes have been incised, and withdraw the head of the fetus.

14. Begin an intravenous infusion containing approximately 20 units of oxytocin per liter at the rate of approximately 10 mL/min until the uterus contracts satisfactorily, at which time the rate can be reduced to 2 to 4 mL/min. Begin this infusion after the shoulders are delivered.
15. Then clamp the cord, and place the infant in an incubator; an attendant continues suctioning and any necessary resuscitative maneuvers. Obtain a sample of cord blood at this time.
16. As the uterus contracts, the placenta will bulge through the uterine incision and will be delivered.

Repair of the Uterus

1. Search the uterine incision at this time for any major bleeding points, and clamp and ligate them. Examine the placenta to be certain that there

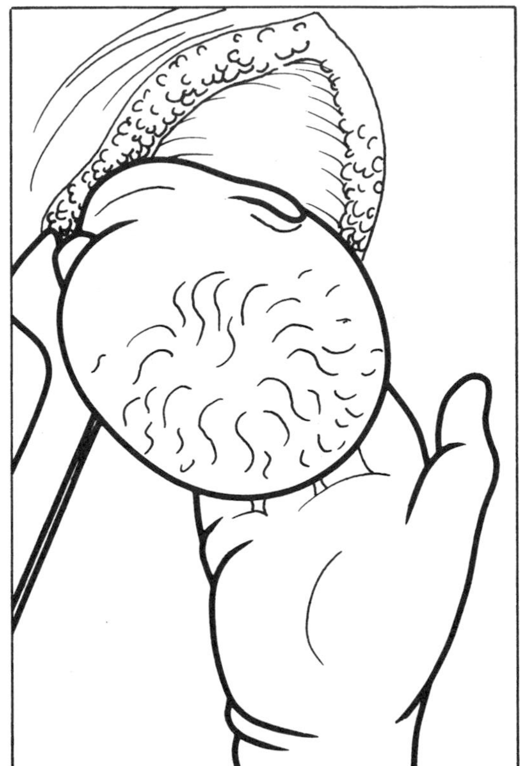

Figure 6.20. Deliver the shoulders by using gentle traction along with fundal pressure.

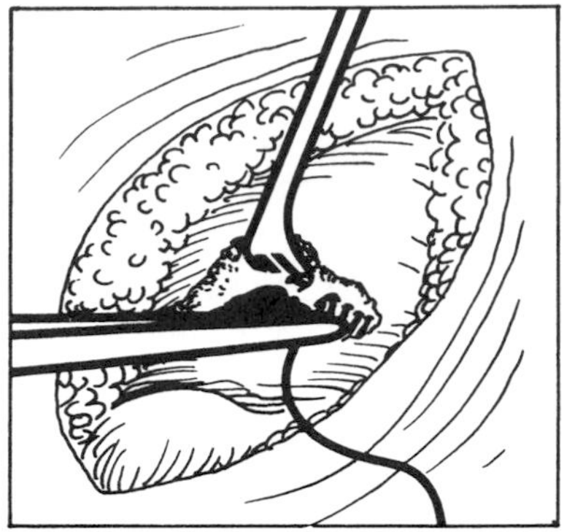

Figure 6.21. A two-layer closure of the uterus. A one-layer closure will suffice in which a continuous running locked suture is used.

are no retained fragments within the uterus. If this is suspected, use a gauze pack to wipe out the uterine cavity.

2. Then close the uterine incision with a continuous chromic suture. Use a running lock suture begun just beyond the end of the uterine incision. Place each stitch in the full thickness of the myometrium. Pass the sutures through the myometrium carefully, and continue the running lock suture just beyond the opposite angle of the incision. Use either a one- or a two-layer closure (Fig. 6.21). The one-layer closure generally is preferred when dealing with the very thin-walled lower uterine segment. Search for bleeding sites before closing the abdominal wall; when encountered, ligate them.
3. Then approximate the serosa overlying the bladder to its original location with 2-0 chromic catgut suture. Close the abdominal wound in a layer-by-layer fashion.

SUCTION CURETTAGE

Women with incomplete and inevitable spontaneous abortions can receive definitive treatment in the emergency department. The treatment of choice is suction curettage to evacuate the remaining products of conception from the uterine cavity. This outpatient treatment in the emergency department was first introduced in the 1970s, and subsequent studies in 1982 proved it to be a successful and safe procedure for emergency physicians (2, 12, 13, 20). This procedure is completed in about 10 to 20 minutes and should be followed by a 2- to 3-hour observation period with intravenous infusion of oxytocin (Pitocin).

The rationale for suction curettage to be an emergency department procedure is to control the hemodynamics of the patient and to give relief for the associated discomfort of spontaneous abortion. Immediate treatment also will assist in the prevention of subsequent endometritis and expedite the patient's movement to the most comfortable and supportive surroundings, which in most instances is the home. This procedure done in the emergency department also represents a significant cost-savings to the patient by eliminating the expense of an operating room and anesthesiologist.

INDICATIONS

It is indicated for all first trimester inevitable or incomplete spontaneous abortions. These are diagnosed on the basis of physical findings and a positive pregnancy test.

CONTRAINDICATIONS

1. A history of coagulopathy or the clinical suspicion of such should be correlated with appropriate laboratory studies.
2. Evidence of endometrial infection and or sepsis. In such cases, treat the patient with appropriate intravenous antibiotics (either with 2 g of ceftriaxone or 3 g of piperacillin and tazobactam (Unasyn); if the patient is allergic, use both 2 mg/kg of gentamicin and 600 mg of clindamycin). The patient also should receive a gynecologic consultation. An infected uterus can easily be perforated and should be evacuated by an experienced operator or gynecologist.
3. A closed cervical os also is a contraindication because it indicates a complete, missed, or threatened abortion, or a possible ectopic pregnancy. These patients should receive ultrasonic evaluation, and if products of conception are present in the absence of cardiac activity or ectopic pregnancy, the patient should receive a dilatation and curettage in the operating room by a consulting gynecologist. Never force a suction curette through a closed cervical os.
4. Any peritoneal signs or evidence of ectopic pregnancy also are contraindications and indicate immediate consultation with a gynecologist.

EQUIPMENT

The equipment used is simple and inexpensive and should include (Figs. 6.22, 6.23) an instrument tray containing:

Gauze sponges
Vaginal speculum
Ring forceps
Single-tooth tenaculum
Sharp uterine curette
Plastic suction curettes (8 to 11 mm)
Vacuum curette pump
Collecting container

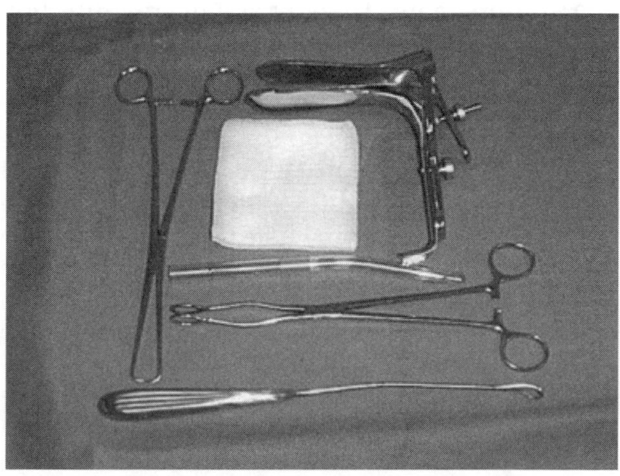

Figure 6.22. Suction curettage equipment.

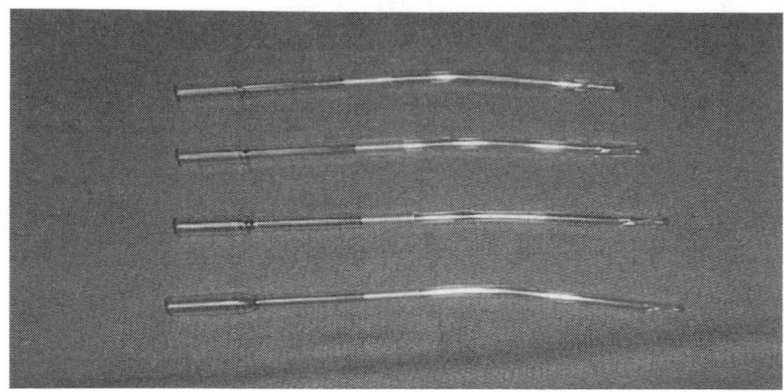

Figure 6.23. Plastic suction curettes, 8 to 11 mm.

TECHNIQUE

Preparatory Steps

Give an explanation of the procedure to the patient and obtain informed consent. Maintain intravenous access with lactated Ringer's or normal saline running at maintenance levels during the procedure and then with 20 units of oxytocin to be infused over a 2- to 3-hour period after the procedure is completed. Provide intravenous antibiotics as previously discussed to prevent subsequent endometritis or bacteremia. Give the patient supplemental oxygen to keep oxygen saturation above 95% during the procedure, and use cardiac, blood pressure, and oxygen saturation monitors.

Anesthesia and Analgesia

Both can be obtained quite easily with the administration of 5 to 10 mg of diazepam by mouth approximately 20 to 30 minutes before the procedure and then a short-acting narcotic such as fentanyl (100 to 200 μg) intravenously. Fentanyl is relatively safe, rapidly metabolized, and will be effectively eliminated in 45 minutes to 1 hour. It also can be easily reversed with naloxone as needed. After sedation and analgesia, obtain local anesthesia by using a paracervical block in the following manner. First insert a vaginal speculum and locate the cervix, and then grasp the inferior aspect of the cervix with the single-tooth tenaculum and lift superiorly. With a 19-gauge needle, inject 20 mL of 1% lidocaine in a 20-mL syringe into the cervix in the 3-, 5-, 7-, and 9-o'clock positions in the area where the vaginal mucosa reflects into the cervical mucosa, with 4 to 5 mL of lidocaine in each position. Remove the tenaculum and allow 5 to 10 minutes for anesthesia to occur before proceeding.

Procedural Steps

After adequate sedation and anesthesia is achieved, reinsert the vaginal speculum and once again locate the cervix. Attach the tenaculum to the superior aspect of the cervix, and pass the largest suction cannula through the os. The tenaculum also provides countertraction during the procedure. The curve of the cannula should follow the flexion of the uterine canal in either the anteflexed or retroflexed position. There should be no active suctioning while inserting or removing the cannula through the endocervix. Use suction only while inside the uterine cavity. With a gentle rotating motion and slowly moving curette in a superior and inferior direction 180 degrees clockwise and counterclockwise, administer proper suctioning. Remember never to push the cannula or curette through a resistance, because uterine perforations can occur easily. Sound the uterine fundus with the suction curette and vacuum line attached. Then turn the suction pump to 50 to 75 mm Hg. Release the suction by a slip ring on the vacuum line on insertion of the curette through the endocervical withdrawal canal. This procedure is repeated 2 to 3 times until no tissue can be retrieved; do not apply suction to the endocervical canal.

Next insert a sharp uterine curette and feel for remaining tissue inside the uterine cavity. The curette glides smoothly over retained products of conception and scrapes over normal endometrial tissue. Reinsert the suction cannula and use the same method as described previously. Avoid vigorous scraping, and remember to never push through resistance to avoid uterine perforation. After completion of curettage, remove all instruments from the vaginal vault and use a bimanual uterine massage to stimulate contractions and begin the previously mentioned oxytocin infusion. Send all specimens to the pathology laboratory in 10% formalin. Continue to observe the patient for 2 to 3 hours during infusion, and discharge home if there is no significant cramping, pain, vaginal bleeding, or fever, and the patient is hemodynamically stable.

Provide for appropriate gynecologic follow-up, and instruct the patient to observe strict bed and pelvic rest until proper follow-up with a gynecologist.

Rh Sensitization

Protect the patient from Rh sensitization. If the patient does not know her Rh type, and it cannot be obtained from the medical records, or if it is known to be negative, then an Rh antibody titer must be sent to the laboratory. If a negative result is confirmed, and no antibodies are present, then the patient must be given Rh immune globulin within 72 hours of the miscarriage and must be provided with appropriate gynecologic follow-up.

Also, provide the patient with appropriate and sometimes much needed emotional support either from social services, religious representatives, or psychiatric services available at the facility.

Discharge Medications

Discharge the patient to her home with methylergonovine, 0.2 mg by mouth, 4 times per day for 2 days, appropriate analgesia, ferrous sulfate ($FeSO_4$), 325 mg by mouth, twice per day for 1 month. Discuss complications such as retained products of conception, endometritis, bleeding, pain, and fever with the patient, and give proper instructions.

CULDOCENTESIS

Culdocentesis is used to identify blood or pus within the peritoneal cavity (5, 17, 22, 26). Its most common application is in the diagnosis of a ruptured ectopic pregnancy or ruptured ovarian cyst. Some authors stated that culdocentesis is more reliable in the adult female than is peritoneal lavage in determining if there is intraabdominal bleeding after blunt abdominal trauma (25). Gravity places small amounts of intraabdominal fluid or blood within the pouch of Douglas, where it can be aspirated with a single needle puncture. In addition, the pouch of Douglas normally contains a small amount of clear peritoneal fluid that, on aspiration, is very valuable in ascertaining a negative lavage.

INDICATIONS

Perform culdocentesis to identify the presence of peritoneal fluid, blood, or pus within the peritoneal cavity. This is most useful in the diagnosis of ectopic pregnancy, although diagnostically this test has been replaced by transvaginal ultrasound.

CONTRAINDICATIONS

1. Mass in the cul-de-sac (especially if there is a possibility of a tuboovarian abscess or ovarian neoplasm).
2. Cases in which the introduction of intraperitoneal air may confuse the radiologic diagnosis.

EQUIPMENT

Graves' bivalve vaginal speculum
Tenaculum
18-gauge spinal needle

10-mL glass syringe
Iodinated prep: 5-mL syringe, 1% lidocaine with epinephrine
25-gauge spinal needle

TECHNIQUE

Preparatory Steps

Place the patient in the lithotomy position.

Procedural Steps (Fig. 6.24)

1. Insert Graves' bivalve vaginal speculum, and identify the cervix.
2. Grasp the posterior lip of the cervix with the tenaculum.
3. Cleanse the posterior vaginal fornix with an antiseptic solution.
4. Deposit anesthetic solution at the point of puncture, although this is usually unnecessary.
5. Puncture the cul-de-sac with an 18-gauge spinal needle attached to a 10-mL syringe. Make this puncture in the midline of the posterior fornix, 1 to 1.5 cm posterior to the cervix. Insert the needle, but not more than 2 cm, while gentle suction is applied. Have an assistant seat the patient slightly upright at this point to permit the pooling of blood in the cul-de-sac. The aspiration of unclotted blood indicates a positive tap. If no aspiration of blood is noted, then there is no diagnostic value to the procedure. When a serosanguinous aspirate is obtained, the rupture of an ovarian cyst should be considered. If purulent material is obtained, this often indicates a ruptured tuboovarian abscess or ruptured appendix. Thus a *positive* tap is indicated when nonclotting blood is obtained. This indicates either a ruptured ectopic pregnancy, a ruptured ovarian cyst, or a ruptured spleen. A *negative* tap is indicated when pus is withdrawn into the syringe or a clear straw-colored peritoneal or cystic fluid is withdrawn. A *nondiagnostic* tap is indicated when there is no return of blood or when clotting blood is obtained. If the clotting blood is less than 1 to 2 mL, this usually comes from the vaginal epithelium or small vessels. More than 2 mL indicates the possibility of an intraperitoneal bleed.

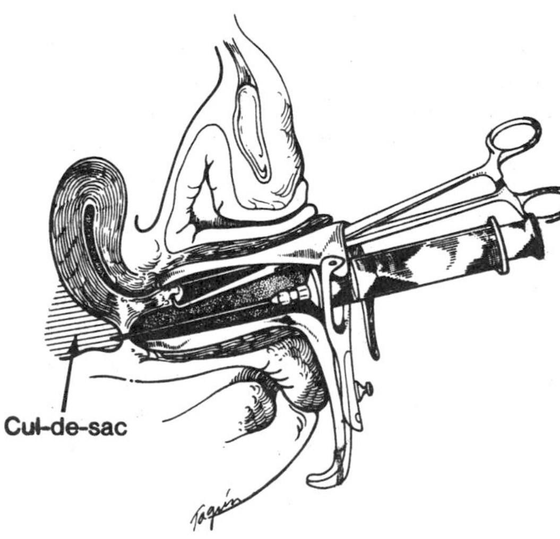

Figure 6.24. Culdocentesis. See text for discussion.

Bartholin's Abscess

Bartholin's gland and duct may become obstructed, resulting in a Bartholin's cyst or abscess. This obstruction may be secondary to infections, and abscess formation may occur primarily with the cyst.

TECHNIQUE OF DRAINAGE AND MARSUPIALIZATION

Incision and drainage of a Bartholin's abscess, while providing immediate relief of symptoms, is occasionally followed by a recurrence of a cyst or abscess. When an abscess occurs, it is best drained after local anesthesia by vertical incision of the mucocutaneous junction of the labia minora, followed by culture, lysis of loculations, and then packing or insertion of a wound catheter (Fig. 6.25). Definitive treatment then can be delayed, and the patient referred for follow-up. When a painless Bartholin's cyst is the presenting com-

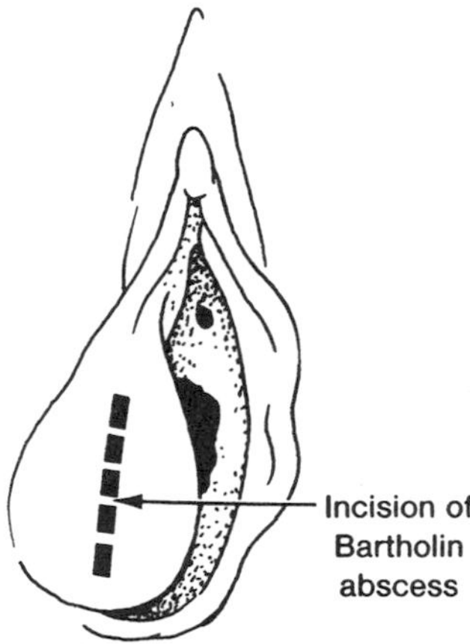

Figure 6.25. Incision and drainage of a Bartholin's cyst or abscess. Marsupialization of the gland involves suturing the inner layer of the cyst to the outside to keep the cavity open, promoting granulation and healing from within outward.

plaint, refer the patient. Marsupialization involves opening the Bartholin's abscess and emptying its contents; then the edges of the abscess are stitched to the edges of the external incision. This keeps the cavity open while the interior of the cyst suppurates and closes by granulation.

For treatment of a Bartholin's abscess, infiltrate a small amount of 1% lidocaine vertically along the mucocutaneous junction at the incision site. Make an incision, and extend it vertically, as shown in Fig. 6.25. Drain the contents of the cyst, and irrigate the cavity with saline. After irrigation, place a Ward catheter, which has a balloon tip, in the cavity to allow drainage of the abscess. If this catheter is not readily available, pack the cavity with iodoform gauze. Encourage sitz baths, twice daily, after the first day. Remove the Ward catheter or gauze packing within 48 to 72 hours.

REMOVAL OF AN INTRAUTERINE DEVICE (IUD)

Intrauterine devices are a common method of contraception in the United States, and it may become incumbent on an emergency physician to remove such a device. The use of these devices can increase the incidence of infection and inflammation in certain populations of women. These are usually young sexually active women with multiple partners. On removal of these devices, the inflammatory process quickly resolves or improves, and the patient generally becomes fertile again. A 2% pregnancy rate is associated with the use of an IUD, and therefore, rule out pregnancy before removal of the device.

If the patient is indeed pregnant, arrange for a gynecologic consultation.

INDICATIONS FOR REMOVAL

The most common reasons for removal of an IUD are pain and bleeding, and it is usually requested in the first 6 months after insertion. The patient also may have an acute pelvic, uterine, or vaginal infection and need to be treated with appropriate antibiotics and IUD removal.

EQUIPMENT

The equipment is relatively simple to use and inexpensive. Stock an equipment tray with a vaginal speculum, a uterine sound, a single-tooth tenaculum, Bozeman's forceps, sponge (ring) forceps, and if available, an IUD extraction device (Fig 6.26).

TECHNIQUE

Explain the procedure to the patient, discuss complications, and obtain informed consent before beginning the procedure. This procedure is generally easier, quicker, and safer when done in the emergency department by emergency physicians.

Procedural Steps

First insert the vaginal speculum and locate the cervix. The IUD string should be readily visible and easily grasped with the Bozeman's forceps. A slow traction or pull

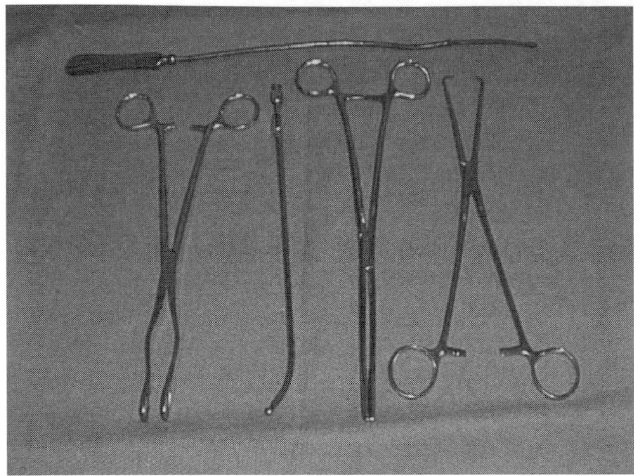

Figure 6.26. Intrauterine device removal set.

on the string with the forceps is usually successful in removing the device. Do not suddenly jerk on the string, because it may break and render the procedure more complicated. If easy dislodging of the intrauterine device is not achieved with this method, then use the uterine sound to probe gently for the IUD, but do not push against resistance to avoid uterine perforation. If this is unsuccessful, then progressively dilate the cervix (by a gynecologist secondary to the time constraints on the emergency physician and the possible complications involved).

If the string is not visible at the os, then pregnancy must be excluded and the IUD can be located by radiographs or more easily by ultrasound. Again, consult a gynecologist at this time. If the patient is pregnant, then she should be referred for routine but timely consultation with a gynecologist.

COMPLICATIONS

Commonly pain, cramping, and bleeding can follow an IUD extraction and, if severe, may indicate rare but possible uterine perforation. If the patient shows signs of peritonitis or sepsis, then one should consider perforation; in either case, consult a gynecologist. If perforation indeed has occurred, then infuse the patient with broad-spectrum antibiotics, and send a type and screen to the laboratory. Immediate gynecologic consultation is mandatory at this time.

In the event of IUD removal secondary to pelvic inflammatory disease, give the patient antibiotics by mouth for 2 weeks; she may need intravenous antibiotics in the emergency department to prevent bacteremia or sepsis. Some physicians recommend routine antibiotic therapy before IUD removal, and it should always be done in women with valvular heart disease. It should be mentioned that endometritis is difficult to exclude in these patients, and borderline cases should be treated prophylactically with broad-spectrum antibiotics. Usually, only mild analgesia is indicated and should be provided; provide an alternative means of pregnancy prevention.

REFERENCES

1. Baskett TF: Essential Management of Obstetric Emergencies. Chichester: John Wiley and Sons, 109–117, 1985.
2. Brennan DB, Caldwell M: Dilatation and evacuation performed in the emergency department for miscarriage. J Emerg Nursing 13:144, 1987.
3. Brunette DD, Sterner SP: Prehospital and emergency department delivery: A review of eight years' experience. Ann Emerg Med 18:149–151, 1989.
4. Burns JW: Breech: A method of dealing with the aftercoming head. J Obstet Gynaecol 41:923–929, 1934.
5. Clarke JM: Culdocentesis in the evaluation of

blunt abdominal trauma. Surg Gynecol Obstet 129:809, 1969.
6. Cox WL: The technique of breech. J Obstet Gynecol 62:395–403, 1955.
7. Crichton D, Seedat ED: The technique of symphysiotomy. S Afr Med J 37:227–234, 1963.
8. Cunningham FG, MacDonald PC, Gant NF: Dystocia due to abnormalities in presentation, position, or development of the fetus: Abnormalities of labor and delivery. In: Pritchard J, MacDonald PC, eds. Williams' Obstetrics, 18th ed. Norwalk, CT: Appleton & Lange, 349–382, 1989.
9. Cunningham FG, MacDonald PC, Gant NF: Techniques for breech delivery: Abnormalities of labor and delivery. In: Pritchard J, MacDonald PC, eds. Williams' Obstetrics, 18th ed. Norwalk, CT: Appleton & Lange, 393–403, 1989.
10. Cunningham GF, MacDonald PC, Gant NF, et al: Conduct of normal labor and delivery. In: Pritchard J, MacDonald PC, eds. Williams' Obstetrics, 18th ed. Norwalk, CT: Appleton & Lange, 322–335, 1989.
11. Dudley H, Carter DC, Russell RCG, et al: Operative surgery. Gynaecol Obstet 256–273, 1987.
12. Farrel RG, Stonington DT, Ridgeway RA: Incomplete and inevitable abortion: Treatment by suction curettage in the emergency department. Ann Emerg Med 11:652, 1982.
13. Filshie GM, Sanders RR, O'Brien PM, et al: Evacuation of retained products of conception in a treatment room with and without general anesthesia. Br J Obstet Gynecol 84:514, 1977.
14. Gebbie DAM: Symphysiotomy. Clin Obstet Gynaecol 9:663–683, 1982.
15. Gebbie DAM: Symphysiotomy. Obstet Care 2: 69–75, 1974.
16. Gebbie DAM: Symphysiotomy. Trop Doct 4: 69–75, 1974.
17. Generelly P, Moore TA III, LeMay JT: Delayed splenic rupture. JACEP 6:369, 1977.
18. Goodlin RC: An incision technique for emergency cesarean section. Surg Gynecol Obstet 165:544–546, 1987.
19. Harris RE: An evaluation of the median episiotomy. Am J Obstet Gynecol 106:660, 1970.
20. Hill DL: Management of incomplete abortion with suction curettage. Minn Med 54:225, 1971.
21. Jotkowitz MW, Picton FCR: An appraisal of an anatomically and physiologically correct method of breech delivery: The Bracht manoeuvre. J Obstet Gynaecol 10:151–159, 1970.
22. Lucas C, Hassim AM: Place of culdocentesis in the diagnosis of ectopic pregnancy. Br Med J 1: 200, 1970.
23. Menicoglou SM: Symphysiotomy for the trapped aftercoming parts of the breech: A review of the literature and a plea for its use. Obstet Gynaecol 30:1–19, 1990.
24. Pritchard J, MacDonald PC, eds.: Williams' Obstetrics. New York: Appleton-Century-Crofts, 1976.
25. Rothenberg D, Quattlebaum FW: Blunt maternal trauma: a review of 103 cases. J Trauma 18: 173, 1978.
26. Webb MJ: Culdocentesis. JACEP 7:451, 1978.
27. Woods CE: A principle of physics as applicable to shoulder delivery. Am J Obstet Gynecol 45:776, 1959.
28. Zuspan FP, Quilligan EJ: Management of delivery trauma. Operative Obstetrics. Norwalk, CT: Appleton & Lange, 527–566, 1988.
29. Zuspan FP, Quilligan EJ, et al: The technique of symphysiotomy. South Afr Med J 15:455–472, 1988.

7

Orthopedic Procedures

This chapter on orthopedic procedures for the emergency physician is divided into five sections:

Arthrocentesis
Fracture Principles, Casting Techniques, and Common Splints
Reduction of Selected Common Fractures
Reduction of Selected Common Dislocations
Injection and Aspiration of Selected Soft Tissue Disorders

A detailed presentation of each of the disorders discussed is beyond the scope of this text. A number of excellent orthopedic texts give a detailed discussion of the mechanism of injury, clinical findings, and complications of each of the disorders (50). Some of the key features that are pertinent to the procedure being discussed are, however, presented briefly. In the sections on reductions of selected fractures and dislocations, only those procedures that should be performed by the emergency physician are discussed. Some of the procedures that are discussed are not routinely performed by the emergency physician; nevertheless, the emergency physician must be familiar with the procedure if an urgent indication for the procedure arises.

ARTHROCENTESIS (14, 17)

The optimal site for arthrocentesis is usually over the extensor surface of the joint, where the synovial pouch is close to the skin and is as removed as possible from major nerves, arteries, and veins (22, 38, 39, 58). The flexor surfaces of the joints generally have a high concentration of periarticular nerves, vascular structures, and tendons, making aspiration of the flexor side more difficult (38, 58).

Techniques of aspiration based on absolute measurements are unreliable because there is a striking variation between individuals and races (38). In this section, few measurements are offered; instead, the size and the position of each anatomic structure are used to aid in the localization of the injection site. Bony prominences are more readily palpable, constant, and closely related to each articulation. Palpable bony landmarks are usually available in the immediate vicinity of the injection site (38, 39). If the landmarks are not easily palpable when the joint is placed in the best position for aspiration, these landmarks may become more readily palpable by changing the position of the joint and subsequently moving it to a more optimal position for aspiration (39).

Two points are critical in performing arthrocentesis in any joint: *positioning* and *traction on the joint.* Proper positioning enlarges the target area of a joint that is to be aspirated. This almost always involves placing the joint in 20 to 30 degrees of flexion. Because arthrocentesis is usually performed on the *extensor surface* of the joint, flexion enlarges the joint space. The application of traction along the long axis of the bone distal to the joint opens the joint space and is especially important in small joints. Traction of the metacarpophalangeal joint is applied by pulling on the digit, which opens the metacarpophalangeal joint space. These techniques stretch the capsule and any supporting ligaments that might be penetrated by the needle (39). To enlarge the target area, the technique of traction can be used most effectively in the wrist and metacarpophalangeal and interphalangeal articulations, where the joint capsules are sufficiently loose to permit this technique (38, 39). The technique of positioning also may be used to enlarge the target area and is especially helpful in aspirations of the knee, because of the shape of the femoral condyles in which the vertical extent of the joint cavity is largest when the knee is flexed. Proper positioning, as is discussed, also aids in enlarging the target area for aspiration of the first carpometacarpal articulation. Medial rotation of the thigh facilitates palpation of the greater trochanter of the femur by moving it out from under the gluteus maximus, thus aiding in hip arthrocentesis. When a joint is aspirated, the direction at which the needle enters should be such as to minimize the damage to the articular cartilage from scoring with the needle tip, because hyaline cartilage regenerates poorly (38, 39). In the discussion that follows, the angle at which to pass the needle is not discussed because it varies and is easily forgotten. By knowing the space to enter and the osseous anatomy, the angle at which to pass the needle is obvious.

If the site of aspiration is properly prepared, the incidence of infection is reduced to 1:15,000 (62). After preparation, in some patients with a markedly distended joint capsule, there is no need to raise a wheal with lidocaine (Xylocaine), and only a brief spray with ethyl chloride solution gives sufficient anesthesia to perform the procedure (22). When the synovial lining is entered, the folds of synovium or cellular debris may act as a flap valve on the end of the needle, preventing easy withdrawal of fluid (22). When this is suspected, move the needle about gently and reinject a little fluid already withdrawn to push the tissue or clot away from the tip of the needle. When aspiration must be performed in joints with little fluid (e.g., for the detection of septic arthritis), aspiration may be facilitated by wrapping the joint, except for the site of aspiration, with an elastic bandage to compress the free fluid into that portion of the sac being punctured (22). In general, always aspirate all readily accessible fluid at the time of aspiration.

In summary, three points should be stressed:

1. Arthrocentesis is usually performed on the extensor surface of a joint.
2. The joint usually is placed in 20 to 30 degrees of flexion.
3. Traction is important to open the joint space, especially in smaller joints.

Synovial Analysis

Synovial fluid is an ultradialysate of plasma. Joints may be swollen in disorders such as protein-losing syndrome, nephrotic syndrome, and congestive heart failure, but these are usually not very painful or inflamed and pose little problem in differentiation.

One of the major concerns relating to an unnecessary arthrocentesis is the introduction of infection. In properly prepared patients, the incidence of infection is extremely low and occurs in fewer than 1 in 15,000 procedures (62).

Joint fluid varies in composition, depending on the cellular responses, which can be classified into three groups: minimal inflammatory reactions as can occur in mild trauma; mild inflammatory reactions as can occur in rheumatic fever, systemic lupus erythematosus, and viral arthritides; and severe inflammatory reactions as can occur in septic arthritis, acute gout, and acute rheumatoid arthritis. Normally joint fluid is straw colored; as an inflammatory reaction occurs, it changes to a lemon yellow or a greenish hue. In some conditions, such as osteoarthritis and osteochondritis dissecans with a joint effusion, the color remains normal. Hemorrhagic fluid suggests trauma to the joint; however, one must remember that there are four causes of a hemorrhagic effusion: trauma, coagulation defects, hemangiomas of the synovium, and villonodular synovitis. In the normal knee, the most common site for a joint effusion, there is 0.5 to 2 mL of fluid (63). The total protein is 1.8 g/dL, and glucose is normally 10 mg/dL less than it is in the serum. A very low joint-fluid glucose suggests septic arthritis. Noninflammatory arthritides usually have less than 2.5 g/dL protein, whereas inflammatory fluids show a protein concentration of 6 to 8 mg/dL.

Viscosity is a function of the concentration and quality of hyaluronic acid in the fluid. The **mucin clot test** can be performed on all joint aspirates by adding glacial acetic acid, drop by drop, to a small amount of joint fluid in a test tube. In the normal synovial aspirate, the fluid will form a white clot. A clot that breaks up easily on agitation is indicative of an inflammatory or an infected fluid. Mucin clots of noninflammatory fluids do not break when agitated. An alternative method of checking for viscosity is placing a drop of joint fluid between the thumb and index finger and separating the fingers. In normally viscous fluid, "stringing" of the fluid between the fingers reflects a noninflammatory condition. In inflammatory conditions, the synovial fluid will not "stretch" between the fingers.

The turbidity of the fluid is proportional to the number of cells present and is influenced by the presence of crystals and cartilage debris in the effusion (58). Normally the synovial fluid contains 10 to 200 cells/mL. A high white cell count can occur with acute gout, in which case, uric acid crystals can be seen under a polarizing light within the white cells or even free in the synovial fluid. Infectious arthritis usually contains leukocyte counts in excess of 50,000 cells/mL, accompanied by a variable blood sugar that is less than half the serum sugar and a high protein count. Other forms of arthritis that are accompanied by high cell count include acute pseudogout, acute gout, and rheumatic fever. In patients with rheumatoid arthritis, mononuclear cells predominate in the first 6 weeks. Later, with acute exacerbations, the fluid may contain 65% to 85% neutrophils, many of which appear degenerated.

Joint aspiration is done either for therapy of an acutely swollen joint or for diagnostic purposes within the emergency center. Relief of joint pain is achieved rapidly, whether the joint aspirate is due to a traumatic, gouty, infectious, or rheumatoid arthritis. The only time one should attempt to aspirate a joint that does not contain an effusion is when there is a suspicion of septic arthritis (54). This relief varies directly with the rapidity with which the fluid has accumulated. Table 7.1 indicates the findings in different joint effusions. The tests that should be performed on aspirated joint fluid include a leukocyte count with differential, a search under polarizing light for crystals, a mucin clot test or "string test," a Gram stain in patients suspected of having septic arthritis, and a synovial fluid glucose and protein test.

EQUIPMENT

Prep solution povidone–iodine (Betadine)
Anesthetic prep
18-gauge, 1.5-inch needle
23-gauge, 3/8-inch needle
3-mL syringe
1% lidocaine with epinephrine
Assortment of 1.5-inch needles: 18, 22, and 23 gauge (specific needle sizes and lengths are indicated in the description

Table 7.1.
Characteristics of Synovial Fluid Effusions

	Color	Clarity	Viscosity	Leukocytes/mL	Protein
Normal	Clear	Transparent	High	200	3.5
Noninflammatory	Yellow	Transparent	High	200–2,000	3.5
Degenerative joint disease, osteochondritis dessicans					
Inflammatory	Yellow–green	Opaque	Low	2,000–50,000	3.5
Acute gout, pseudogout, rheumatic fever, rheumatoid arthritis, Reiter's syndrome[a]					
Septic					
Bacterial infections	Yellow–green	Opaque	Low	50,000–200,000	3.5

[a]Synovial fluid complement is high in Reiter's syndrome but is low in other acute inflammatory arthritides.

of the specific procedure, especially when longer needles are required)
10-mL syringe
20-mL syringe
Sterile gloves and towels
4 × 4-inch gauze
Sample tubes for specimens

SURGICAL PREPARATION OF A JOINT SURFACE

Perform arthrocentesis under sterile conditions. When a joint surface is prepared properly, the incidence of infection is extremely low. Scrub the site of aspiration with povidone–iodine for a 5-minute preparation. Drape the area with sterile towels, and perform the procedure under sterile conditions. When performing arthrocentesis over the sites indicated for the various joints, avoid vessels and nerves.

Metacarpophalangeal And Interphalangeal Joint Aspiration

The metacarpophalangeal and interphalangeal joints of the hand have a wide range of motion that makes traction an effective means of increasing the target area, especially when aspirating the joints of the thumb and little finger. This technique is least effective in cases involving the third and fourth fingers. The volar surface of the joint contains the volar plate, nerves, and vessels, all of which contraindicate aspiration on the volar surface. Therefore, the optimal site for aspiration is over the dorsal surface on either side of the extensor tendons (38). The best landmark of aspiration of the metacarpophalangeal joints is at the head of the metacarpal with the fingers flexed. If the first metacarpophalangeal joint is passively flexed and traction is applied, there is a separation noted between the metacarpal and the proximal phalanx that is accentuated by this technique, making penetration easier. The interphalangeal joints are best aspirated by distracting the joint as shown in Figs. 7.1 and 7.2. Insert the needle tip in the dorsal crease line at the joint as shown in Fig. 7.1. Note that the dorsal crease line is an imaginary line connecting the dorsal points of the proximal and distal interphalangeal skin creases. "Lift up" the extensor tendon, trying to insert the needle tip under the tendon (Fig. 7.2). The undersurface of the tendon is attached to the dorsal surface of the joint capsule in both interphalangeal joints, and being just under the tendon with the

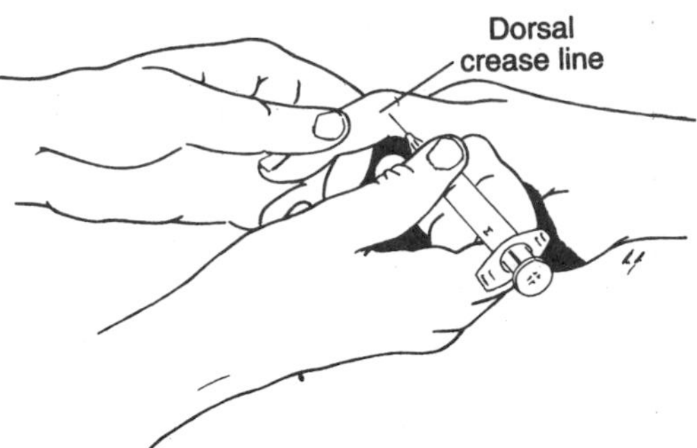

Figure 7.1. To perform arthrocentesis of the interphalangeal joints, place the needle in the dorsal crease line produced by the joint as shown. Attempt to lift up the tendon, inserting the needle underneath it.

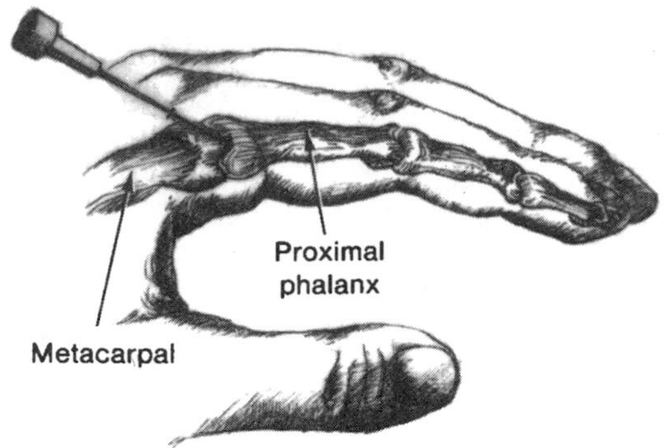

Figure 7.3. Metacarpophalangeal joint aspiration. Enter the joint immediately medial or lateral to the extensor tendon, where a small depression or "pit" often is seen when traction is applied. Traction is critical in aspiration of this joint. Flex the joint in the position shown and open by traction performed by an assistant.

needle means that the needle must be in the joint space.

To aspirate the metacarpophalangeal joints, locate the head of the metacarpal and place the needle adjacent to the extensor tendon either laterally or medially in the fossa created by distraction of this joint (Fig. 7.3) (22, 37).

To perform arthrocentesis of the thumb metacarpophalangeal joint, place the needle on the radial side of the joint as shown in Fig. 7.4. Insert the needle just radial to the extensor pollicis longus tendon as shown in Fig. 7.4.

Carpometacarpal Aspiration of the Thumb

This small joint is a common site of arthritides that may require aspiration for diagnostic purposes. The best site from which to enter this point is the dorsal aspect over the radial side of the hand (Fig. 7.5) (22). Traction of the thumb and flexion of the wrist and thumb with the hand held in slight ulnar deviation will aid in increasing the target area.

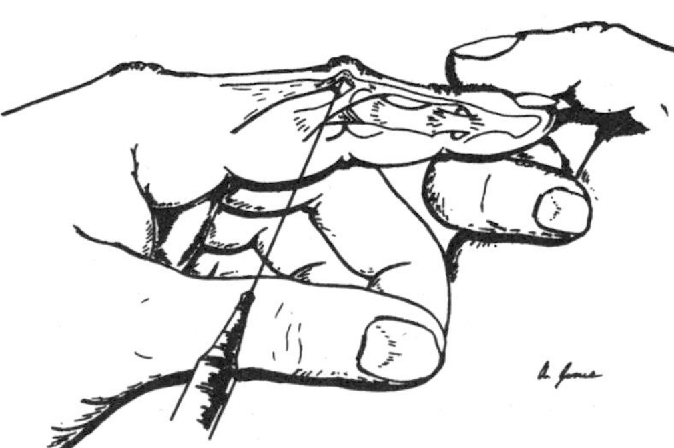

Figure 7.2. To perform arthrocentesis of this joint, be sure to distract the joint and "lift up" the extensor tendon with the needle tip. The undersurface of the extensor tendon is attached to the dorsal surface of the joint capsule.

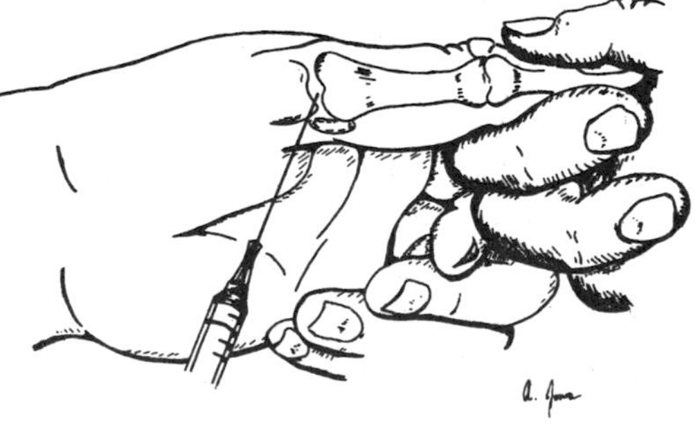

Figure 7.4. Arthrocentesis of the metacarpophalangeal joint of the thumb. To perform this arthrocentesis, be sure to distract the thumb as shown and insert the needle laterally along the radial border of the joint, once again attempting to lift the extensor pollicis.

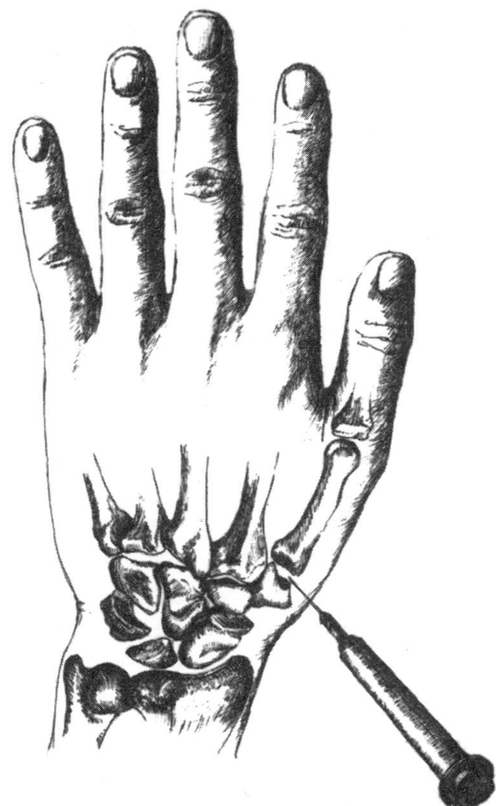

Figure 7.5. Carpometacarpal aspiration of the thumb. See text for details.

Radiocarpal Arthrocentesis (Wrist Arthrocentesis)

The joint line of the radiocarpal joint runs between the radial and ulnar styloid processes. The best site for aspirating the radiocarpal joint is dorsally, because the volar aspect contains numerous tendons, vessels, and nerves. Although it might appear at first glance that the radial side of the dorsum of the wrist would be the optimal site for aspiration, this area should be avoided. From lateral to medial, the following structures criss-cross that region: the abductor pollicis longus tendon; the extensor pollicis brevis tendon (which forms the radial side of the anatomic snuffbox); the radial artery, which in the snuffbox branches into a dorsocarpal branch and a first dorsometacarpal branch; the extensor pollicis longus tendon, forming the ulnar border of the snuffbox; and the extensor carpi radialis brevis tendon (Fig. 7.6). Thus although one can enter the joint through the anatomic snuffbox, better sites can be selected. Between the ulnar border of the anatomic snuffbox and the common extensor tendons is a space containing no large vessels, nerves,

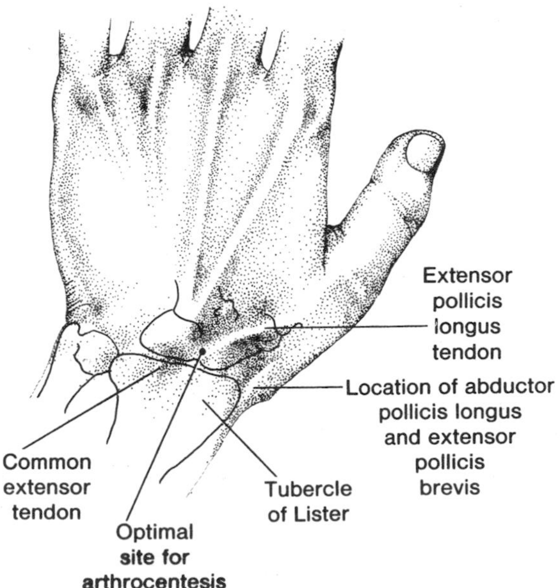

Figure 7.6. Radiocarpal arthrocentesis. The optimal site for arthrocentesis is shown and is discussed in the text. A depression can be palpated just ulnar to the course of the extensor pollicis longus tendon distal and ulnar to Lister's tubercle. This is the site of aspiration.

or tendons. This space is just ulnar and distal to a bony landmark on the dorsal aspect of the radius called the tubercle of Lister (Fig. 7.6). Extending the thumb makes the extensor pollicis longus tendon stand out and defines the ulnar border of the anatomic snuffbox. It will be noted that the extensor pollicis longus tendon courses around Lister's tubercle. *Relax* the wrist in a flexed position and palpate Lister's tubercle with the index finger. With the wrist extended slightly, one can feel the extensor carpi radialis brevis tendon stand out as it courses just distal to the tubercle and almost obliterating it as the wrist is extended. With the wrist relaxed, a slight depression will be noted just ulnar to the extensor carpi radialis brevis tendon at a point just distal to the dorsal rim of the radius. This depression marks the site of choice for arthrocentesis of the radiocarpal joint. It should be noted that this depression lies between the extensor carpi radialis tendon and the common extensor tendon. An index finger placed in the depression will always point directly at the head of the third metacarpal. This depression can be easily palpated in most patients; insert the needle at that site (Fig. 7.7). Flexion and ulnar deviation open the joint cavity dorsally and stretch the capsule and the extensor retinaculum. Traction on the hand may further increase the radiocarpal joint space (22, 38, 58). Insert a needle just distal to the rim of the radius in the depression. Direct the needle between the radius and the lunate (the bone that lies at the floor of the depression).

A technique has been described for arthrocentesis of the wrist (ulnocarpal) joint, when there is marked bulging noted over the ulnar surface of that joint. Enter the ulnar surface of this joint by insertion of the needle just distal to the ulnar styloid process and dorsal to the pisiform bone (Fig. 7.8) (22). This is not the optimal site for routine aspiration of this joint because tendons course through this area through which the needle must pass. We prefer the radiocarpal approach.

Because the joint cavities of the *intercarpal* joints usually communicate freely through a common synovial space, a single site for either aspiration or injection is usually adequate (37). In performing intercarpal arthrocentesis, palpate Lister's tubercle with the patient clenching the fist. Place the examining finger just distal and ulnar to the tubercle between the tendons of the extensor carpi radialis brevis and the extensor digitorum communis. As the patient flexes the wrist, the dorsum of the lunate bone becomes palpable, and just distal to it is a depression between the lunate and the capitate. This is the optimal site for intercarpal aspiration (37). Thus radiocarpal arthrocentesis is performed in the depression proximal to the lunate (be-

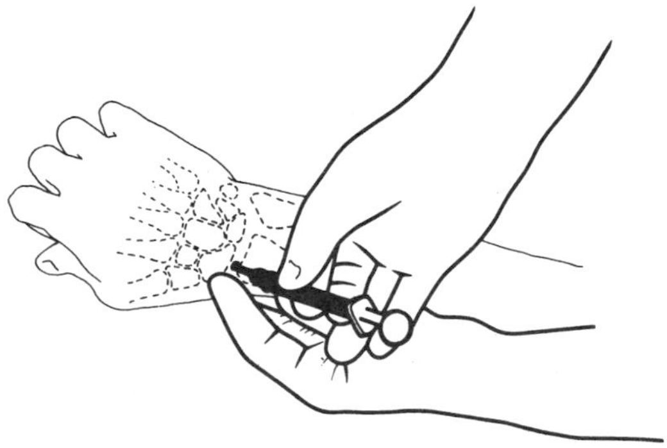

Figure 7.7. Radiocarpal arthrocentesis. Palpate Lister's tubercle and enter the joint with the wrist in 15 to 20 degrees of flexion over the fossa shown in Figure 7.6.

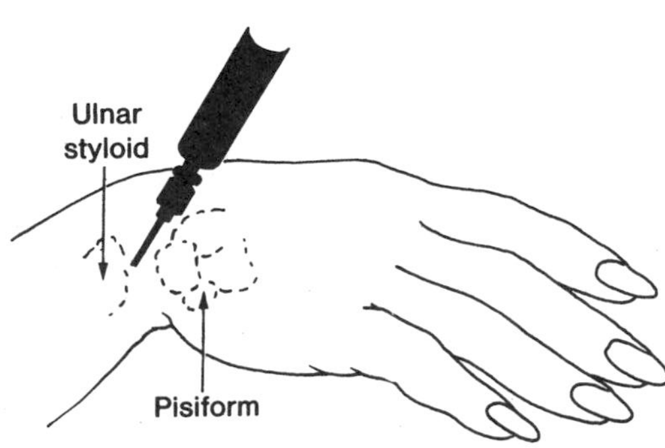

Figure 7.8. Ulnocarpal joint arthrocentesis. See text for discussion.

tween it and the distal radius), and intercarpal arthrocentesis is performed distal to the lunate with the wrist more acutely flexed.

Elbow Arthrocentesis

Aspiration of the elbow joint is one of the easiest procedures to perform in the emergency center. Arthrocentesis of the elbow joint medial to the olecranon is not recommended (22, 38, 58). Although a number of techniques have been described (22, 38, 58) for arthrocentesis over the lateral aspect of this joint, the optimal site is through the anconeus muscle. With the elbow extended, three bony landmarks are readily palpable on the lateral side of this joint: the lateral epicondyle, the head of the radius, and the tip of the olecranon process. Identify the radial head by supinating and pronating the forearm. Extend the elbow to approximately 135 degrees with the forearm held midway between pronation and supination after identifying the three bony landmarks (58). Then insert the needle in the middle of a triangle formed by connecting these three points (Fig. 7.9), with the needle entering the joint posteriorly at a 90-degree angle to the humerus, traversing the skin and anconeus muscle to enter the joint space between the olecranon and lateral epicondyle (38). No major nerves or vessels traverse this area of the joint.

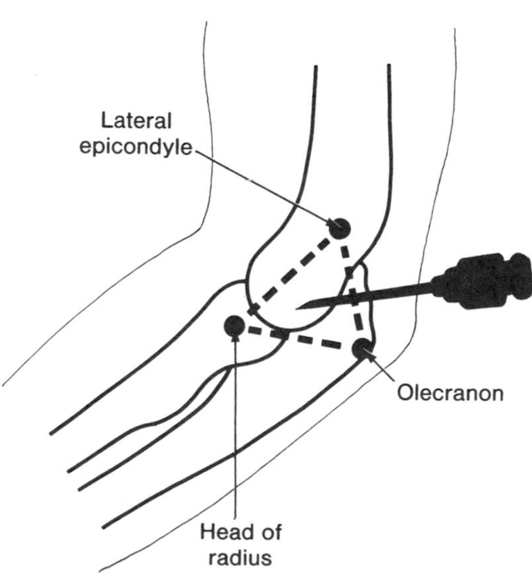

Figure 7.9. Elbow joint arthrocentesis. See text for discussion.

Shoulder Aspiration

ANTERIOR APPROACH

Aspiration of the shoulder (glenohumeral) joint through the anterior approach is the most common method. The bony landmarks are readily palpable and include the coracoid process and the head of the humerus, which is palpable just medial to the lesser tuberosity. Abduct the arm 15 to 20 degrees, and relax the capsule (58). Obtain further opening of the joint space by an assistant applying gentle downward traction on the arm. The patient may be either sitting or supine; however, the procedure is more easily performed with the patient in the sitting position. Then insert the needle just medial to the head of the humerus between it and the tip of the coracoid process (Fig. 7.10) (22).

POSTERIOR APPROACH

We prefer the posterior approach. One advantage of the posterior approach over the anterior approach is that, to reach the synovial cavity by the anterior approach, the needle must pass through the tendons of the coracobrachialis and the subscapularis, whereas with the posterior approach, the needle passes through the posterior fibers of the deltoid only. In addition, the anterior portion of the capsule is strengthened by the glenohumeral ligaments, which must be pierced by the needle in the anterior approach to enter the joint cavity. In addition, the patient sees the needle with the anterior approach. We prefer the posterior approach to shoulder arthrocentesis. Figure 7.11 shows the position of the arm in abduction with the examiner's hand held behind the arm and the patient

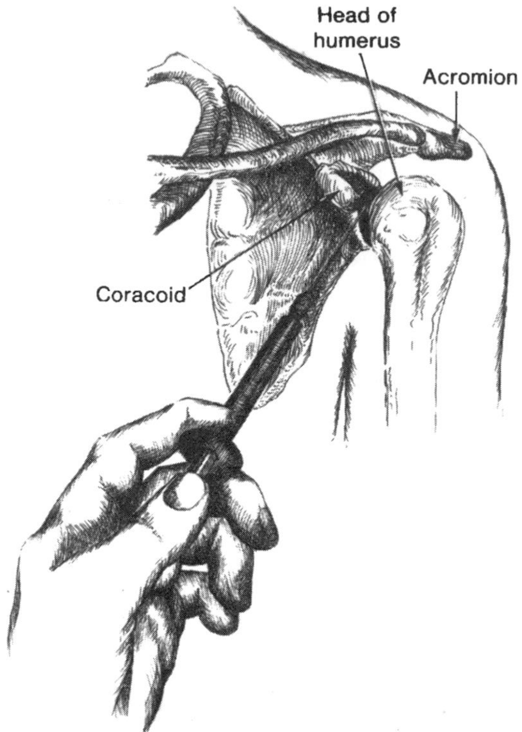

Figure 7.10. The anterior approach for shoulder arthrocentesis. See text for discussion.

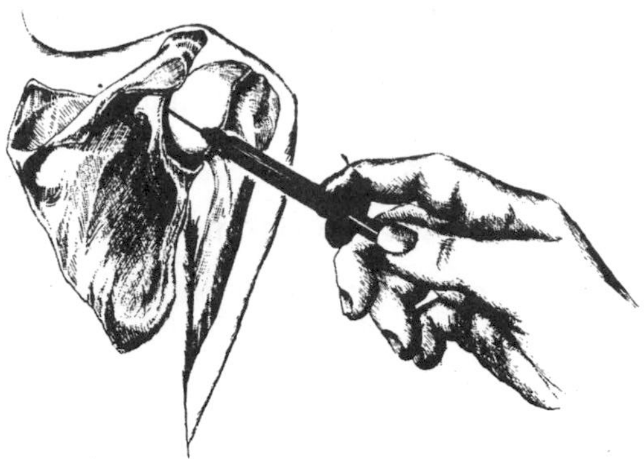

Figure 7.12. The posterior approach for shoulder arthrocentesis. Insert the needle one finger breadth below the angle of the acromion, which is easily palpable posteriorly at the junction of the spine of the scapula and acromial process. Position the patient so that the humerus is internally rotated to tighten the posterior capsule.

pushing against the examiner's hand. This brings out a "fossa or indentation" produced by the deltoid and infraspinatus. Insert the needle in this fossa while the shoulder is internally rotated to separate the humeral head from the glenoid fossa, as shown in Fig. 7.12 (38).

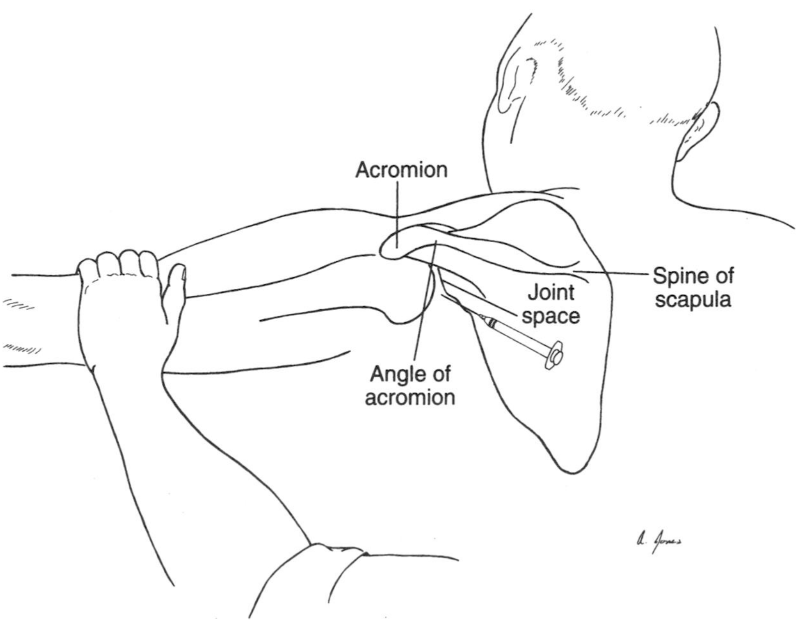

Figure 7.11. Posterior approach to shoulder arthrocentesis. The needle is placed in the "fossa" or indentation between the inferior border of the infraspinatus and deltoid (see Figure 7.12).

Aspiration of the Sternoclavicular Joint

This joint is the most common site for septic arthritis and osteoarthritis in patients who abuse intravenous drugs (24, 46). The sternoclavicular joint is difficult to enter from directly anterior because of the fibrocartilaginous articular disc that lies within the joint (22). It is a rather difficult joint to aspirate or inject unless it is distended. For this procedure, place the patient in a supine position with the arm on the side to be aspirated abducted to 90 degrees and dropped backward over the edge of the table. This brings the clavicle forward and permits insertion of the needle from a medial position (adjacent to the suprasternal notch) and avoids the articular disc. Insert the needle into the joint just adjacent to the suprasternal notch, aiming the needle posteriorly. Enter the joint after a few millimeters (Fig. 7.13).

Hip Arthrocentesis

The hip joint is the most difficult to aspirate or inject because of the large amount of soft tissue around this joint (22). In patients with osteoarthritis, it may be impossible to enter the joint space with certainty even with fluoroscopic guidance. In the best of hands, a more than 50% failure rate is reported with hip arthrocentesis (20, 21, 23, 39). The anterior approach is the most frequently used for performing this procedure (43, 52), although some authors prefer to use the lateral approach (33, 34, 57). We prefer the anterior approach, and primarily discuss it here.

ANTERIOR APPROACH

The head of the femur lies halfway between the anterior superior iliac spine and the lateral tubercle of the pubis and approximately 1 to 1.5 inches distal to the inguinal ligament (Fig. 7.14). Use a 19- or 20-gauge needle that is approximately 2.5 to 4 inches long, depending on the size of the individual patient (22, 58). Enter the joint at approximately 2 to 3 cm below the anterior superior iliac spine and 2 to 3 cm lateral to the femoral pulse, depending on the size of the patient (Fig. 7.14). Locate this point by palpating the femoral pulse and going approximately 2 cm lateral to it, entering the skin 1 to 1.5 inches distal to the inguinal ligament or measuring out the distances as indicated earlier. Insert the needle at a 60-degree angle with the skin,

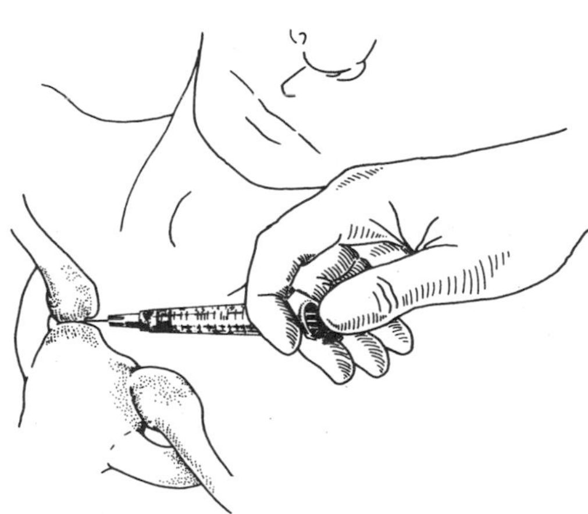

Figure 7.13. Sternoclavicular joint arthrocentesis. Insert the needle adjacent to the suprasternal notch, and aim it posteriorly.

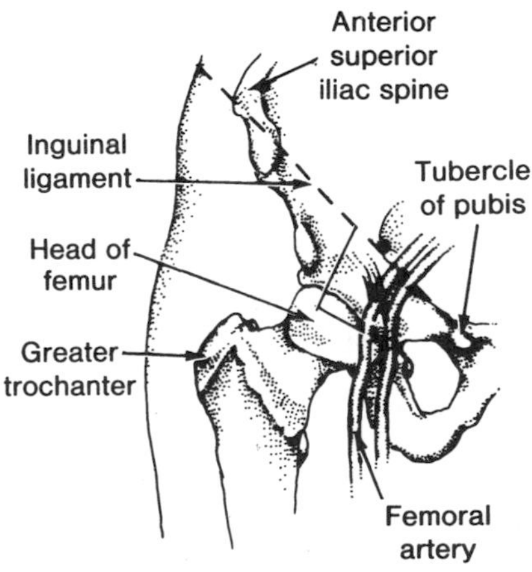

Figure 7.14. Hip arthrocentesis anterior approach. The point of entrance is approximately 2 to 3 cm below the anterior superior iliac spine and 2 to 3 cm lateral to the femoral pulse, depending on the size of the patient.

aiming it posteromedially through the capsular ligaments until the bone is reached (22). Then withdraw the tip slightly, and aspirate to check the position and be certain the needle is not in a vein or artery. Nothing may be aspirated even though the joint has been entered, so use fluoroscopic guidance to ascertain entrance into the joint. In this procedure, it is easiest to enter the joint with the hip in maximal extension and internally rotated, which brings the greater trochanter out from under the gluteus maximus and brings the neck of the femur in a plane parallel to the table (39).

LATERAL APPROACH

The landmark to localize in using this approach is the greater trochanter. Place the patient in the supine position, and rotate the thigh medially (internally) to bring the greater trochanter out from under the gluteus maximus muscle and to bring the neck of the femur into a plane parallel to the table. Place the thumb and index finger on the greater trochanter, and insert a 4-inch, 20-gauge needle superior to the middle of the upper margin of the trochanter, parallel to the table, and at right angles to the femur (39). The needle will pass through the gluteus medius and will contact bone at a nonarticular surface. Injections here will be intrasynovial, because the capsule extends laterally if the needle is passed slightly superiorly over the head of the femur. Perform this procedure under fluoroscopic control; it has the advantage that there are no large vessels or nerves in the vicinity. The largest vessels in the area are the inferior branches of the superior gluteal artery and vein.

Knee Aspiration

The knee contains the largest synovial cavity in the body and is the largest weight-bearing structure. It is also one of the most common sites of synovial inflammation and the most commonly aspirated joint in the emergency center for various pathologic processes. Because of the size of this joint and its relatively superficial nature, it is the easiest joint to aspirate, particularly when it is tightly distended with an effusion (22). Suprapatellar, infrapatellar, and parapatellar approaches have been advocated by various authors (20–22, 39, 57, 58). The suprapatellar approach is a good method if large volumes of fluid are present in the suprapatellar bursa; however, this approach has the disadvantage that the suprapatellar bursa is not always continuous with the joint cavity. This problem is especially likely in patients with multilocular joint effusions, such as patients with chronic arthritis. If a small effusion or no effusion is present, the bursa may be little more than a potential space and is an irregular structure in patients with arthritis (39). The two approaches advocated here are the medial parapatellar approach by Hollander (22) and the infrapatellar approach (39). A tightly distended knee can be aspirated from almost any angle without difficulty; however, the techniques described later will allow ready entrance into the joint even if little fluid is present.

PARAPATELLAR APPROACH (MEDIAL OR LATERAL APPROACH)

Place the patient in a supine position on the examining table with the knee fully extended. Prepare the medial surface of the knee adequately with an iodinated solution. The site of puncture is on the medial border of the patella 1 to 2 cm proximal to the inferior pole. Insert the needle between the inferior surface of the patella and the patellar groove of the femur (22, 58). Place the knee in 20 degrees of flexion to relax the quadriceps muscle completely for the needle to advance readily and without difficulty (Fig. 7.15) (58). The needle tip may produce crepitance on the undersurface of the patella, demonstrating entrance into the joint space even with very little fluid (22). The

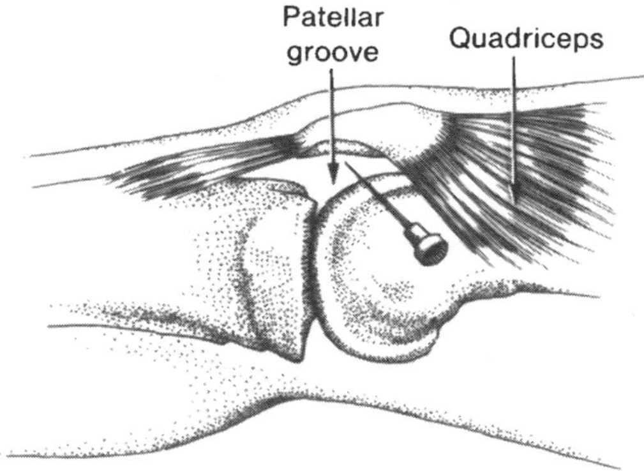

Figure 7.15. Medial view of the knee showing the parapatellar approach to knee arthrocentesis.

advantages of this approach are that synovial membrane folds are seldom encountered. This is the preferred approach with a distended knee.

INFRAPATELLAR APPROACH

The medial parapatellar approach advocated earlier has the disadvantage that the needle tip can easily contact the cartilaginous surface, which some authors believe is a major disadvantage because contacting the cartilage may result in damage (39). If the patella is ankylosed, the optimal site for aspiration is in the infrapatellar region, coursing through the fat pad into the knee joint space between the condyles of the femur (22). In performing the aspiration, use an 18- or 20-gauge needle on a 10-mL syringe, except when performing the procedure for purposes of aspirating a hemarthrosis, in which case, use a 16- to 18-gauge needle on a 20-mL syringe. In addition, if the knee has a flexion deformity limiting extension or has a small effusion, the medial approach may not be optimal. The infrapatellar approach has the advantage of a good landmark, the patellar tendon. In addition, no major vessels or nerves course through the area through which the needle may penetrate. Because of the shape of the femoral condyles, flexion in the infrapatellar approach greatly enlarges the vertical dimensions of the joint and stretches the patellar ligament, permitting easy entrance into the joint space without scoring the articular surface. In addition, there are very few pain fibers in the patellar ligament, making the procedure relatively painless; some authors regard it as the best approach of all (39).

To perform knee aspiration by the infrapatellar approach, insert the needle immediately below the apex of the inferior pole of the patella, through the middle of the patellar ligament, and pass through the fat pad and into the intercondylar fossa. Hold the knee at 90 degrees of flexion (the patient can be sitting with the legs hanging over the edge of the table), and direct the needle perpendicular to the patellar tendon as shown in Fig. 7.16 (39). Access to the joint can be readily demonstrated by aspiration.

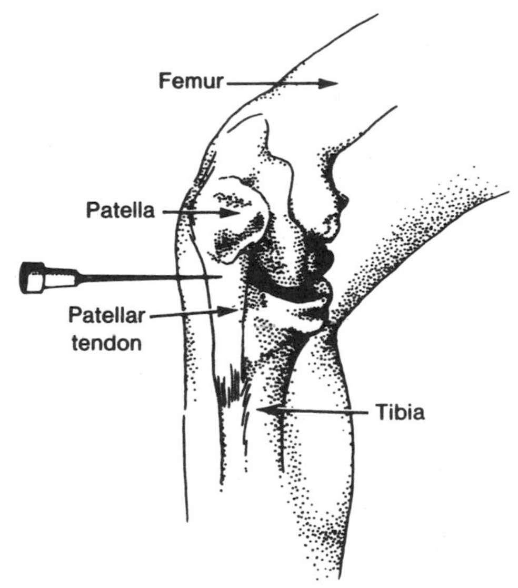

Figure 7.16. The infrapatellar approach for knee arthrocentesis. The anterior oblique view of the knee is shown with the needle inserted just inferior to the inferior pole of the patella, through the patellar tendon, and into the joint space after traversing the fat pad behind the patellar tendon. Flex the knee to 90 degrees with this approach, to avoid striking the articular surface.

Ankle Aspiration (Tibiotalar Joint Aspiration)

Enter the ankle joint from either an anteromedial or an anterolateral approach. Most authors prefer the anteromedial approach (22, 39, 58) because there is slightly more space for insertion of the needle between the joint surfaces with this approach.

ANTEROMEDIAL APPROACH

As indicated earlier, this is the procedure of choice for ankle aspiration. Locate the medial malleolus and palpate the sulcus between the medial malleolus and the most distal articular surface of the tibia. With the foot plantar flexed, palpate this sulcus medial to the tendon of the tibialis anterior. Inversion of the foot aids in tensing the tibialis anterior and helps in locating the point of entrance (39). A more easily noted landmark for performing the procedure is the extensor hallucis longus tendon, which can be palpated and visualized by asking the patient alternately to flex and extend the great toe (22, 39, 59). This tendon is more laterally placed than is the tibialis anterior tendon; however, the extensor hallucis longus tendon is a more readily visible structure and allows easy entrance into the joint space (Fig. 7.17). Place the patient in a supine position with the ankle plantar flexed to permit a wider area for entrance into the joint. Insert the needle just medial to the extensor hallucis longus tendon, directing it perpendicular to the floor (in the supine patient) and in line with the medial malleolus. The point of insertion should be just distal to the edge of the tibia. The tibialis anterior tendon is easily palpable and can be used as a reference point and landmark for insertion of the needle in the same fashion as the extensor hallucis longus tendon. Using the anterior approach, insert the needle just lateral to the extensor hallucis tendon under the inferior edge of the tibia with the foot in plantar flexion as shown in Fig. 7.18. The medial approach allows insertion of the needle just medial to the extensor hallucis longus tendon, again under the inferior border of the tibia. If the patient inverts the foot against resistance, a "fossa" will be seen, which is the site of insertion of the needle (39).

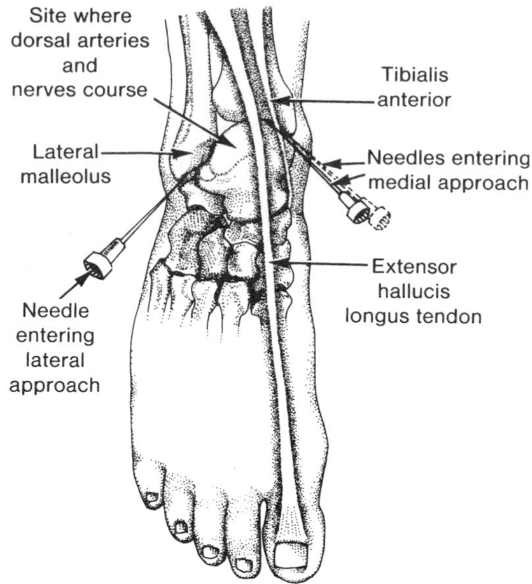

Figure 7.17. Arthrocentesis of the ankle. See text for discussion.

ANTEROLATERAL APPROACH

To perform ankle arthrocentesis with the anterolateral approach, palpate the medial margin of the lateral malleolus (Fig. 7.17). After asking the patient to extend the toes, palpate the extensor digitorum communis tendons. The point of entry is between the lateral margin of the extensor digitorum communis tendon and the medial margin of the fibular malleolus (Fig. 7.17) (58). The patient should be supine when this procedure is performed. Identify the point of entrance, and then plantar flex the ankle. A depression can be palpated at the site of entrance, adjacent to the medial margin of the fibular malleolus. This is not our preferred approach; however, in cases in which the medial approach is not feasible (cellulitis, rupture of the deltoid ligament), it may have to be used.

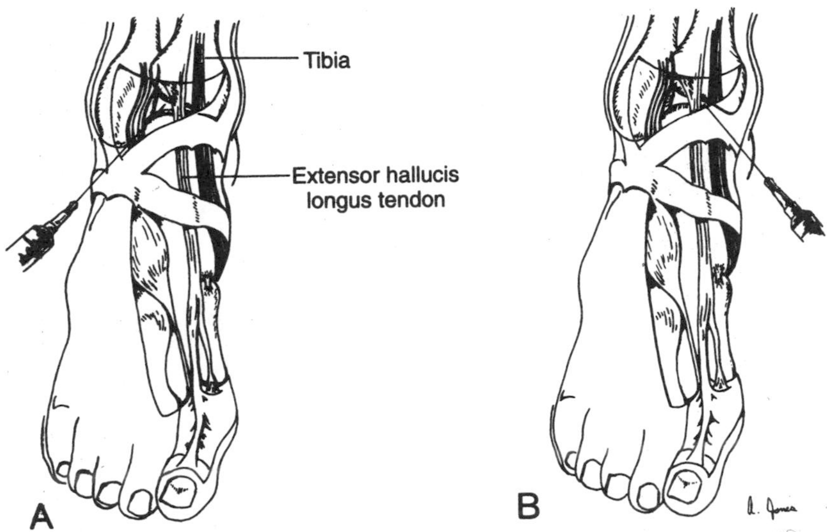

Figure 7.18. Arthrocentesis of the ankle. To perform the arthrocentesis of the ankle, two approaches are shown. In the first, the anterior approach is shown with the extensor hallucis identified. Insert the needle underneath the inferior border of the tibia with the foot in plantar flexion just lateral to the extensor hallucis tendon (*A*). In the second approach (*B*), insert the needle medial to the extensor hallucis tendon, between that tendon and the end of the tibia. One usually finds that, by inverting the foot against resistance, the tibialis anterior tendon will stand out, revealing a "fossa" inferior to this tendon at the distal end of the medial malleolus. This "fossa" is the site for insertion of the needle.

Subtalar Arthrocentesis

The subtalar joint is very difficult to enter, and arthrocentesis of this joint is not commonly performed in the emergency center. When an effusion is present within the subtalar joint, swelling will be noted below the lateral malleolus. This joint space, which lies between the talus and the calcaneus, may be widened as a result of an effusion. When an effusion is present and one needs to aspirate it for diagnostic purposes, perform the procedure while the patient is supine with the foot held perpendicular to the leg. Enter the joint by inserting a needle just below the lateral malleolus, perpendicular to the skin (58). The site of injection should be just proximal to the sinus tarsi (Fig. 7.19) (58). The major indications for performing this procedure in the emergency center are suspected septic arthritis in this joint or suspected crystalline arthritides involving the joint.

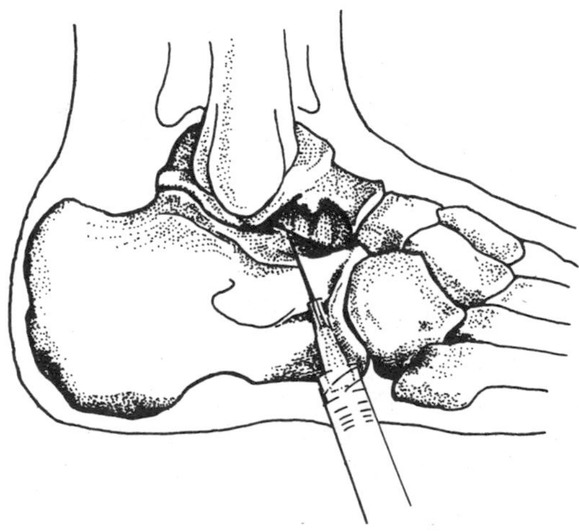

Figure 7.19. Subtalar arthrocentesis. The site of injection should be just proximal to the sinus tarsi.

Metatarsophalangeal Joint Aspiration

The first metatarsophalangeal joint is a frequent site of involvement in gouty arthritis. Aspiration is easily performed in the patient with a joint distended by an effusion. After linear traction is applied, insert the needle between the metatarsal head and the base of the first phalanx, perpendicular to the toe from the dorsal surface of the foot (Fig. 7.20). Linear traction on the toe opens the space and facilitates entry into the joint (58). The point of entry into the dorsal surface should be just medial to the extensor hallucis longus tendon, as shown in Fig. 7.21. Enter the remainder of the metatarsophalangeal joints in a similar manner. Use a 22-gauge needle attached to a 5-mL syringe in performing this procedure.

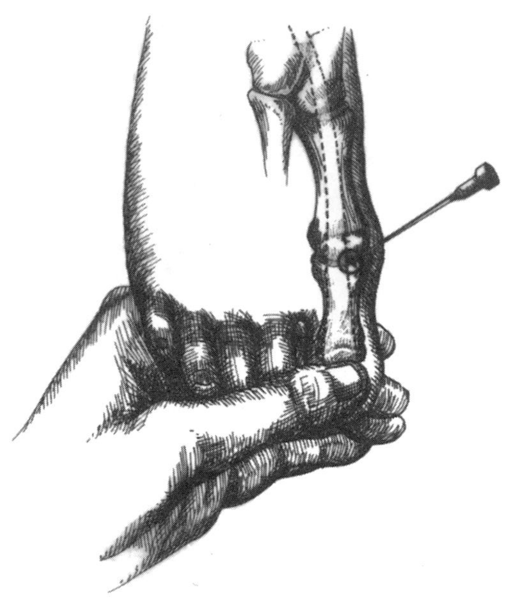

Figure 7.21. To enter the metatarsophalangeal joint, insert the needle just medial to the extensor hallucis longus tendon over the point marked *X*.

Interphalangeal Joint Aspiration

Use a 22-gauge needle in performing interphalangeal joint aspiration of the toes (22). Insert the needle over the dorsal surface from either a medial or a lateral direction, slipping the needle beneath the extensor tendon between the cartilaginous surfaces forming the joint (22, 58). Traction of the toe may facilitate entry into the joint.

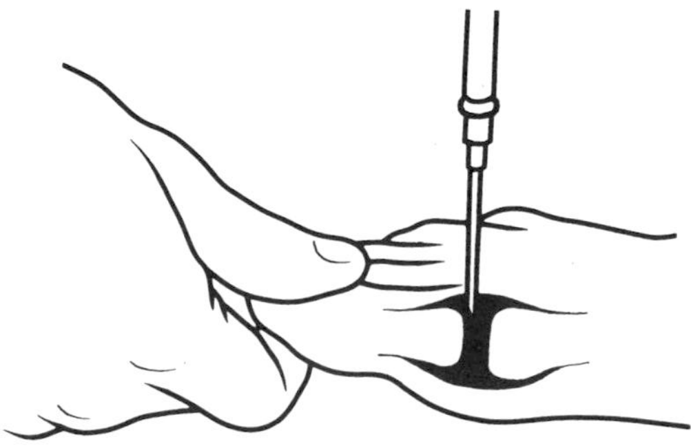

Figure 7.20. Metatarsophalangeal joint aspiration. Enter the joint from the dorsal surface, just medial or lateral to the extensor hallucis longus tendon. Distraction is crucial in entering this joint.

Temporomandibular Joint Aspiration (19)

Temporomandibular joint (TMJ) injections may be indicated in the emergency center in patients with rheumatoid arthritis involving this joint or in patients with TMJ syndrome, in which case, injections of anesthetic and a steroid are both diagnostic and therapeutic in selected cases (22). Anesthetic deposited in this joint is useful in reduction of TMJ dislocations. A fibrocartilaginous disc in the joint space makes it difficult to be certain that the needle is properly placed within the joint in some cases. Use a small needle, preferably a 23 or 24 gauge. The point of insertion should be well anterior to the tragus of the ear to avoid damage to the facial nerve and the superficial temporal artery (Fig. 7.22). Insert the needle at a point just below the zygomatic arch, approximately 1.3 cm anterior to the tragus of the ear (22). Direct the needle slightly posteriorly and superiorly until it has penetrated to a depth of approximately 1.5 cm and one

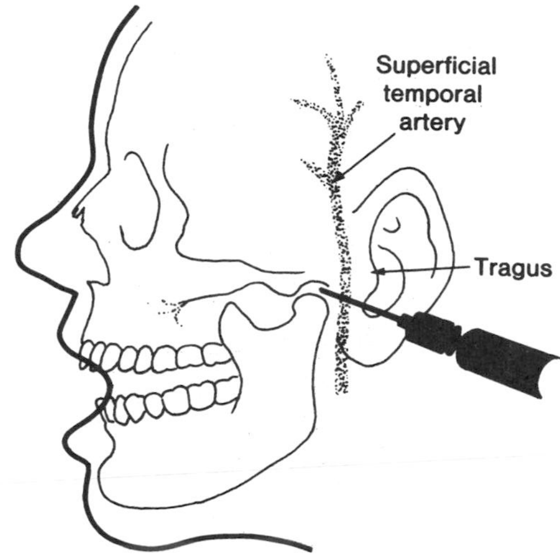

Figure 7.22. Temporomandibular joint aspiration. Enter the joint just anterior to the tragus of the ear and anterior to the superficial temporal artery. The patient's mouth should be slightly open when this procedure is performed, to make entrance into the joint easier.

feels the needle freely in the joint space. Locate the joint by placing the finger over the site of insertion before performance of the procedure and asking the patient to open and close the mouth.

FRACTURE PRINCIPLES, CASTING TECHNIQUES, AND COMMON SPLINTS

Initial Management

In the initial assessment of a fracture, a number of important questions must be answered. Is the fracture stable or unstable? If it is unstable, it must be stabilized by some form of external splinting or traction before any movement or transportation of the patient. There must be an assessment as to whether there is any associated injury involving the surrounding vessels, viscera, skin, or nerves. A well-documented neurovascular examination must be performed before any assessment is made of the patient with suspected or clinically obvious fracture. As a general rule, elevation is crucial when dealing with extremity injuries to promote adequate drainage and to permit healing without swelling. In the noncompliant patient, particularly in children, apply a much larger dressing than is necessary so that the involved extremity will be adequately immobilized. The adult patient will be reluctant to remove and redress a large complicated dressing, and the pediatric patient will forget about the existence of the injured part under a bulky dressing; both patient types will be less likely to unravel the dressing and move the injured extremity. Table 7.2 indicates the commonly used splints and casts that are described in detail in this section.

EMERGENCY SPLINTING

The purposes of emergency splinting are threefold: to prevent further soft tissue injury by the fracture fragments, to provide pain relief, and to decrease the incidence of clinical fat embolism. Perhaps the most commonly known splint is the Thomas splint, which is a half-ring splint used for femoral fractures. A modification of this splint is the Hare traction splint, based on the same principle of applying continuous traction to the fracture to stabilize it and to prevent further soft tissue injury (Fig. 7.23). These splints are practical and safe to use and provide good support for the patient in transport. Once a splint is applied, it should not be removed before radiographic evaluation. A new splint that is becoming popular is the Sager traction splint. This splint has many advantages over the Thomas splint, Hare traction splint, and other half-ring splints, including its relative ease of application and ability to provide stability of the femoral fracture without angulating the proximal femoral fractured segment, as occurs with use of the Thomas splint. The Sager traction splint (Fig. 7.24) is our preference in emergency stabilization of all proximal femoral and shaft fractures of the femur in both children and adults. The splint can be applied to the outer side or inner side of

Table 7.2.
Commonly Used Splints

Splints	Indications	Comments
Dorsal distal phalanx splint	Avulsion fracture involving the extensor tendon of the distal phalanx	This must be maintained in position for 6 weeks. Splint must not interfere with motion at the PIP joint
Hairpin splint	Comminuted fracture of the distal phalanx of a finger	This should remain in place until pain and swelling subside
Volar and dorsal finger splints	Collateral ligament injuries of the PIP, DIP, or MP joint[a]	Place the MP joint in 50 to 90 degrees of flexion and the IP joint at 15 to 20 degrees of flexion
Long-arm posterior splint	Stable fractures of the forearm, fractures of the elbow, sprains and dislocations of the elbow	Apply a posterior slab with the elbow at 90 degrees and wrist in neutral position (unless contraindicated due to vascular compromise). Use sling after splint is applied
Anterior–posterior splint of the forearm or arm	Fractures of the wrist and distal forearm in which more immobilization is necessary because of instability	With unstable fractures of the forearm, splints should extend above the elbow and thus be an anterior–posterior splint, immobilizing both the wrist and the elbow joint
Sugar-tong splint of the forearm	Fractures of the distal radius, wrist, and forearm	This splint permits immobilization in supination or pronation
Sugar-tong splint of the arm	Fractures of the humeral shaft	For stable fractures with no displacement, this splint along with a collar and cuff is all that is necessary. For unstable fractures, immobilize the fracture with this splint and refer the patient for definitive care
Common sling	Used in numerous situations in which one desires immobilization of the upper extremity	
Collar and cuff	With a sugar-tong splint of the arm for stable humeral fractures	
Stockinette valpeau	For immobilization of unstable fractures of the proximal humerus, which have a tendency to displace because of the pull of the pectoralis major	This splint relaxes the pectoralis major, which has a tendency to displace fractures of the proximal humerus
Posterior splint of the ankle	Complex ankle sprains, initial treatment for immobilization of fractures of the ankles, initial management of foot fractures and distal tibial fractures	
Gutter splint	Stable phalangeal and metacarpal fractures	Splints should be applied so that the MP joint is at 50 to 90 degrees, depending on pain, and the IP joints are at 15 to 20 degrees
Thumb spica	Scaphoid fractures	
Short-arm cast	Simple fractures of the forearm, particularly incomplete fractures in children, stable distal forearm and metacarpal fractures	
Dynamic finger splint	Sprain of IP or MP joints of fingers or toes	

[a]PIP, proximal interphalangeal; DIP, distal interphalangeal; MP, metacarpophalangeal; IP, interphalangeal.

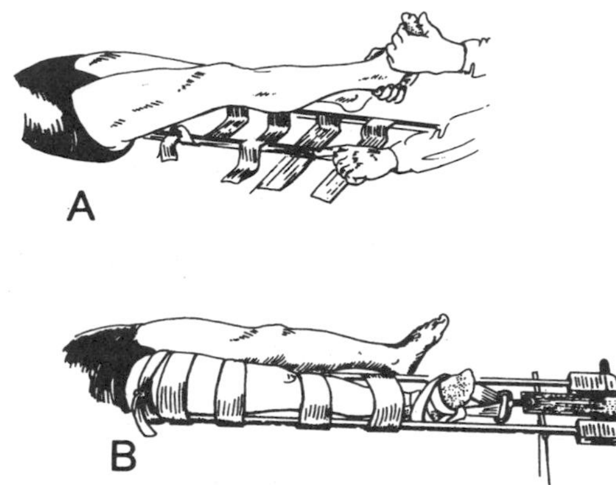

Figure 7.23. A half-ring fracture splint. The two most commonly used are the Hare and the Thomas splints. *A*: Apply traction to the patient's extremity in which there is a fractured femur, and lift the leg while an assistant places the half-ring splint beneath the involved leg as shown. *B*: With the splint in position, apply the ankle straps as well as straps along the thigh and leg, and apply traction through the ankle straps.

the leg, as shown and described in Figs. 7.25 through 7.27. The splint does not have a half-ring posteriorly, which eliminates any pressure on the sciatic nerve and, most important, eliminates the angulation of the fracture site that occurs with half-ring splints. The advantages of this splint are listed in Table 7.3.

Inflatable splints, made of a double-walled polyvinyl jacket with a zipper fastener, placed around the injured limb, are quite popular. Although they afford the advantages of easy application and control of swelling, disadvantages to using them must be recognized. They are useful only for fractures of the forearm, wrist, and ankle. All too often one sees patients with fractures in sites other than those indicated who have been given an inflatable splint before they reach the hospital. This splint provides little or no support. When inflated at two pressures of 40 mm Hg, they markedly reduce the blood flow to

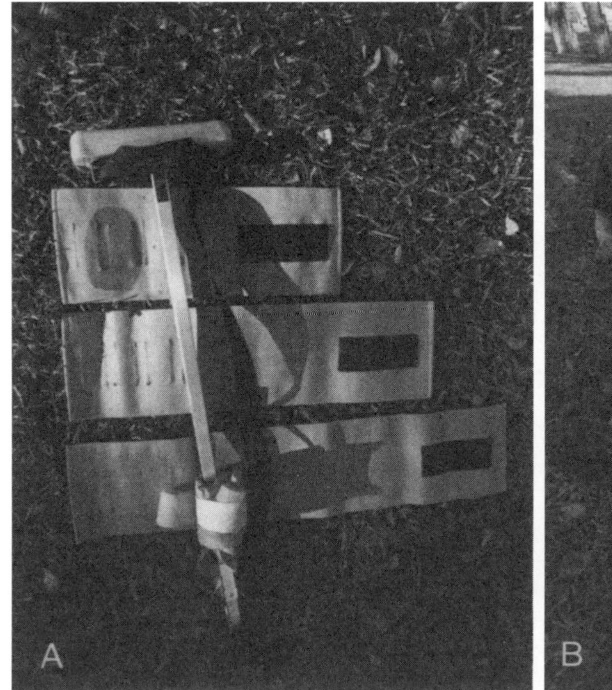

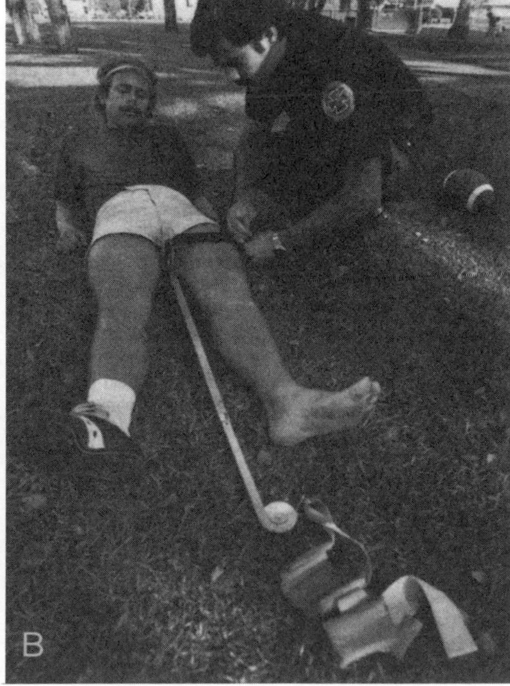

Figure 7.24. *A*: The various parts of the Sager traction splint. *B*: Application of the Sager splint.

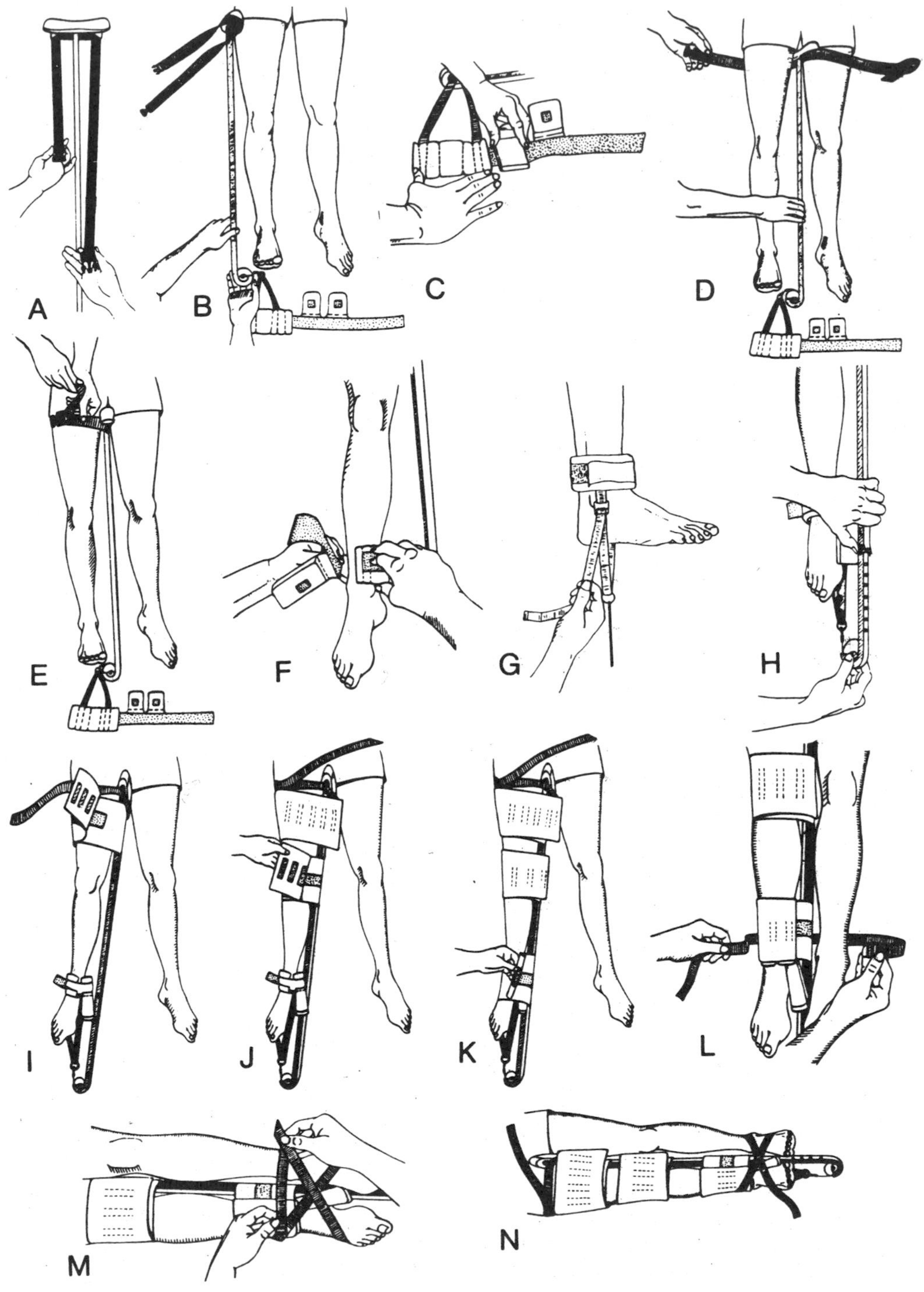
A
B
C
D
E
F
G
H
I
J
K
L
M
N

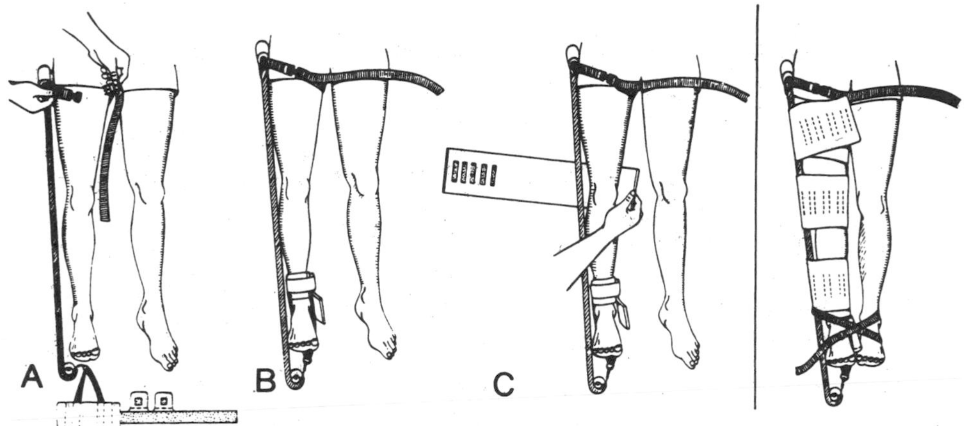

Figure 7.26. Application of Sager splint on the outside of the leg. *A*: Application of Sager splint on the outside of thigh is appropriate if perineal injuries or pelvic fractures are encountered. Carry out steps *A* through *C* shown in Figure 7.25, and then apply the splint on the outside of the leg. *B*: Leave the Kydex buckle thigh strap loose so that it makes a sling around the upper thigh and forms an angle of about 55 degrees with the shaft of the splint. Pad the strap as needed. *C*: Apply the thigh straps in sequence. *D*: Add figure-of-eight strap as last step before securing the patient on the spine board.

the limb and may even cause complete cessation of blood flow in some patients. Thus circulatory embarrassment may occur at high pressures, and at lower pressures, they may be ineffective in providing support. These splints should not be applied over clothing, because they may cause skin blisters. The application of these splints is shown in Fig. 7.28. The pillow splint is an alternative type of splint that can be used before reaching the hospital and can be fashioned by wrapping an ordinary pillow tightly around a lower extremity fracture and securing it

Figure 7.25. Standard application of the Sager emergency traction splint. *A*: Before applying the splint to the leg, slide the Kydex plastic buckle so that, when it is closed, it will be located on the anterior (top) surface of the thigh. *B*: Before application of the splint, obtain a rough measure of the length of splint needed. Extend the splint so that the wheel is at the heel. NOTE: Patients wearing tight jeans or tight underclothing, especially males, will find the splint uncomfortable to wear unless clothing is removed or cut open, which, of course, should be done as part of the secondary evaluation before application of the splint. *C*: Roughly estimate the size of the ankle, and fold a number of gauze pads as needed to provide padding all around the leg. *D*: Grasp the Kydex buckle, and slide the thigh strap up under the leg so that the perineal cushion is snug against the perineum and ischial tuberosity. *E*: Tighten the Kydex buckle thigh strap, drawing the perineal–ischial pad to the lateral portion of the crotch. *F*: Apply the ankle harness tightly around the ankle, above the medial and lateral malleoli of the ankle. Check posterior tibial and dorsalis pedis pulses before hitch application and after traction is established. *G*: Shorten the loop of the harness connected to the cable ring by pulling on the strap threaded through the square "D" buckle. *H*: Extend the inner shaft of the splint by opening the shaft lock and pulling the inner shaft out until the desired amount of traction is noted on the calibrated wheel. As a rough guide to determine amount of traction needed, apply traction equal to 10% of body weight to a maximum of 22 to 25 pounds (10 to 12 kg) of traction. *I*: Apply the longest 6-inch-wide thigh strap as high up the thigh as possible. *J*: Apply the second longest thigh strap around the knee. Use padding if needed. *K*: Apply the shortest 6-inch-wide strap over the ankle harness and lower leg. *L*: Apply figure-of-eight strap around both ankles by slipping the strap under the ankles. *M*: Cross strap over the feet as noted. Secure buckle snugly. *N*: Patient's leg is now secured, traction is controlled, and medial and lateral shift of distal fragment and internal and external rotation are prevented. Patient is ready for strapping to spine board for transport.

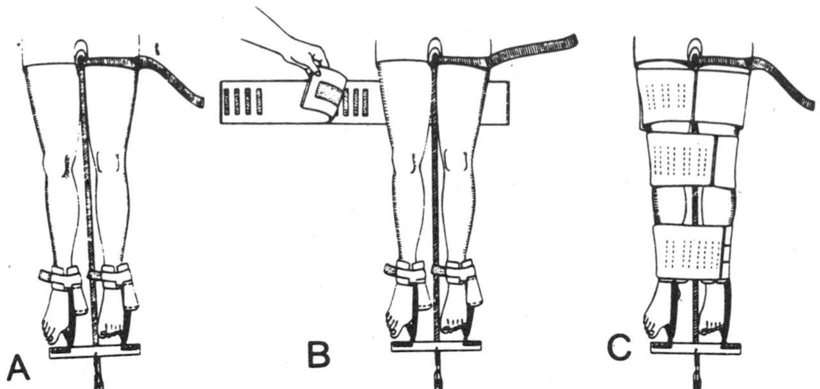

Figure 7.27. Application of the bilateral Sager splint. *A*: Application of double splint is accomplished in the same manner as with the single splint. Modify step *B* of Figure 7.25 by lengthening splint so that the harness bar is adjacent to the patient's heels. *B*: Apply the 6-inch-wide thigh straps, hooking together more than one thigh strap to give a proper length for wrapping strap around both thighs. *C*: Apply all three sections of leg strapping to secure the legs together. A figure-of-eight strap may be used around both ankles and feet, if needed.

Table 7.3.
Advantages of the Sager Traction Splint

1. No sciatic nerve compression as may occur with half-ring splint devices
2. Flexion of the proximal femoral segment (as occurs with half-ring splint devices with midshaft and especially proximal one third femoral fractures) is eliminated. This results in a more perfect bony alignment
3. Overtraction, common with half-ring devices, resulting in knee edema and injury to epiphyseal growth centers in children, is eliminated. The precise weight of traction, based on 10% of body weight of the patient and not to exceed 22 pounds, can be applied. The amount of traction applied is shown on the circular metered wheel
4. The same splint can be used for pediatric and for adult patients
5. This splint can be used with most trousers in place
6. The splint can be used in patients with groin injuries by strapping it to the outer side of the leg
7. The splint can be used in patients with severe pelvic fractures
8. The ankle straps are so placed that one can monitor dorsalis pedis pulse with the splint in place
9. The splint comes with a cross bar that permits splinting of bilateral femoral fractures with one splint between the legs
10. Splints of the fracture are in a more anatomic position, so there is no rotation of the proximal fragment outward

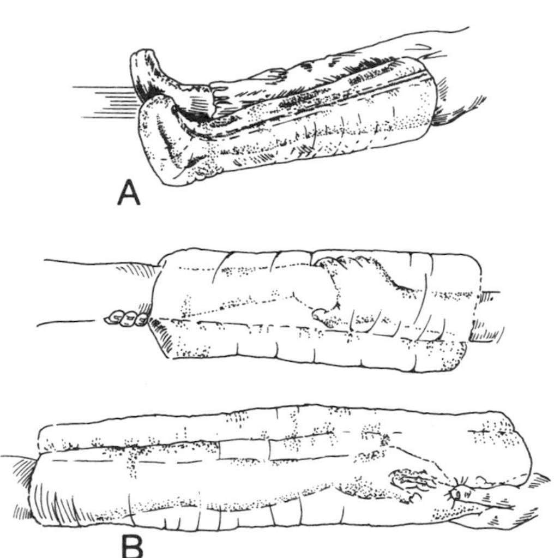

Figure 7.28. Inflatable splints are commonly used in field emergency care. *A*: An inflatable splint is shown applied over the leg and thigh in a patient with a fractured ankle. *B*: Apply the deflated splint by applying traction to the injured extremity and then feeding the splint from over the physician's forearm and hand onto the injured extremity. While traction is maintained, inflate the splint.

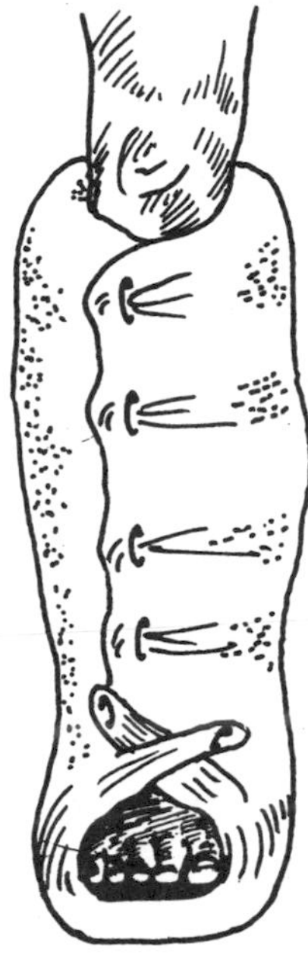

Figure 7.29. A pillow splint.

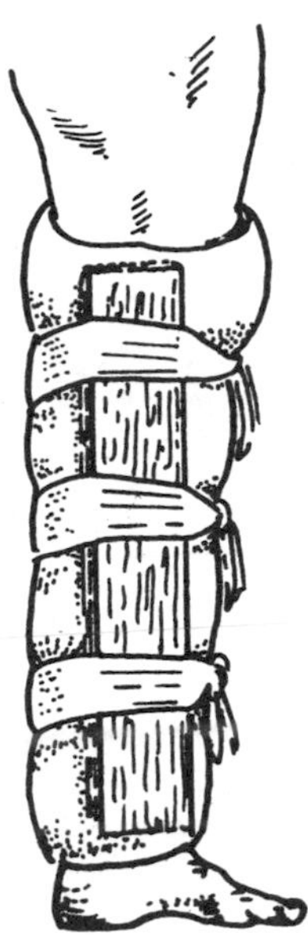

Figure 7.30. A splint fashioned from towels and wooden splints. Wrap towels to protect the involved extremity, and apply wooden slabs to both sides of the extremity; secure the entire device with rags or pieces of towel as noted.

with safety pins, as shown in Fig. 7.29. A splint can be made from towels wrapped around a limb and supported on either side by wooden splints, as demonstrated in Fig. 7.30. This type of splint can be used for fractures of the forearm, as well as those of the lower extremity. The only additional support necessary when applying such a splint to the upper extremity is a sling. Patients who are seen before arriving at the hospital with an open fracture can be splinted in a manner similar to these. However, cover the site of skin puncture with a sterile dressing, and be careful not to reposition any exposed bony fragments through the skin back into the wound, because this will cause further contamination.

SELECTION OF DEFINITIVE TREATMENT

The selection of the definitive treatment of a fracture is a joint effort between the emergency physician and the referring doctor. Table 7.4 shows some of the common fractures, dislocations, and sprains and gives general guidelines as to the initial splint or sling to use. Some fractures can be treated safely and followed up by the emergency physician, whereas others need urgent consultation for operative intervention. These are discussed in the individual sections of the text. Closed treatment of fractures may include some form of manipulative reduction, which should be performed in the first 6 to 12 hours, because swelling rapidly ensues and makes reduction more difficult. A displaced fracture usually leaves the periosteum intact on one side. Without this intact periosteal bridge, reduction would be difficult to maintain (Fig. 7.31). To reduce a fracture, apply traction in the long axis of the bone and reverse the mechanism that produced the fracture (Fig. 7.31*B* and *C*). Align the fragment that can be manually maneuvered with the one that cannot. An intact periosteal bridge may help align the traction for reduction; however, soft tissue in-

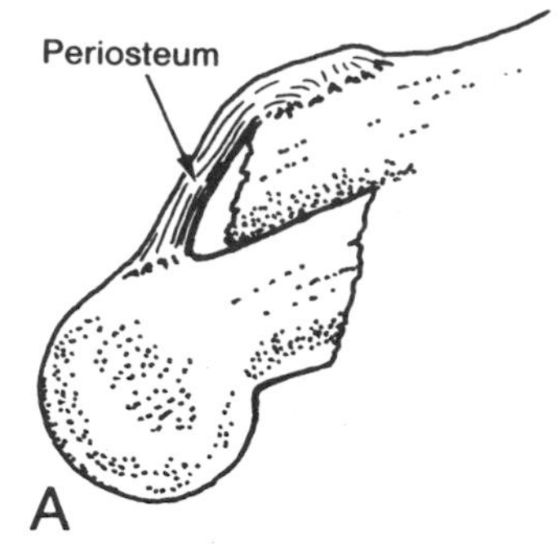

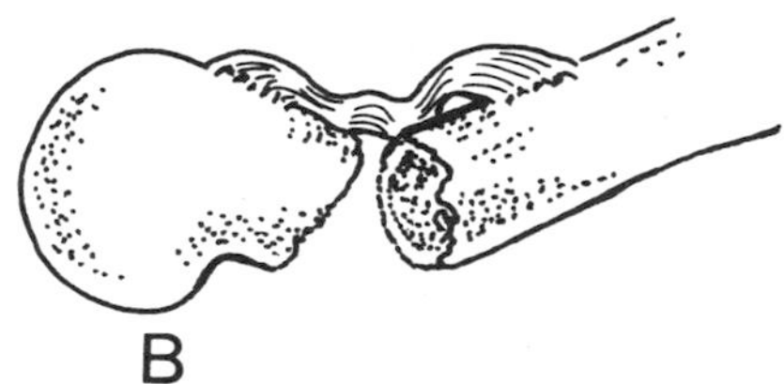

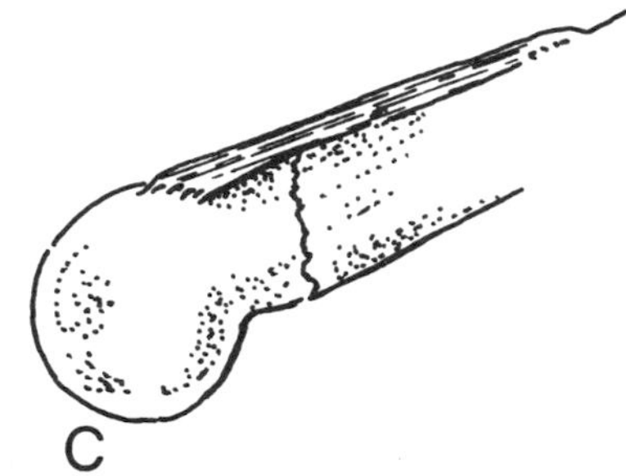

Figure 7.31. *A*: The intact periosteal bridge aids in reducing a displaced fracture. *B*: To reduce a fracture, apply traction in the long axis of the bone, and reduce the fracture by reversing the mechanism that produced it. *C*: Maintain the reduction by the intact periosteal sleeve as shown.

terposition or a large hematoma may make reduction by closed means impossible. Once reduction is accomplished, immobilization with plaster, continuous traction, or some form of splint is required to hold the position.

Traction is a good means for immobilization of some fractures. Use skin traction primarily, and usually temporarily, in children. When skin traction is used in adults, it should always be temporary and should never be applied with adhesive tape to the skin but rather with moleskin tape (Fig. 7.32). Tape the limb and apply traction to the tape via a block of wood suspended from the end of the tape. Be careful to protect all bony prominence with cotton wads. Skeletal traction applied through a pin placed through a bony prominence distal to the fracture site is a good form of immobilization, especially in comminuted fractures that cannot be held by plaster fixation. Skeletal traction is used most frequently in fractures of the femur and is also used in some humeral fractures.

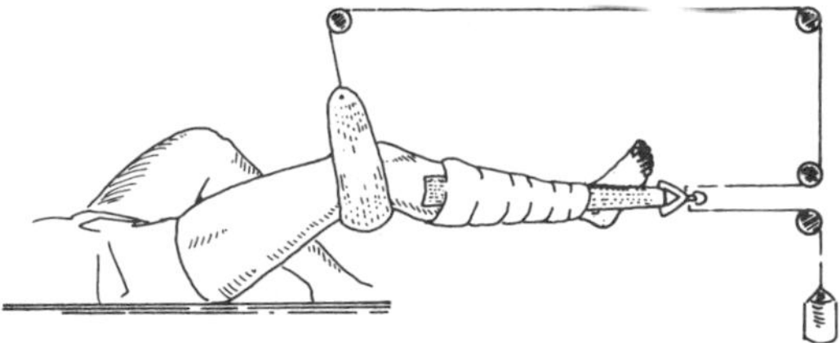

Figure 7.32. Apply skin traction to the leg. This type of traction is often provided in dealing with fractures of the distal femur and some distal humeral fractures.

Fractures through the metaphysis of a long bone have a good blood supply and heal well, as a general rule, whereas diaphyseal fractures heal more slowly and need more attention because of the poor blood supply at this portion of the bone.

INDICATIONS FOR OPERATIVE TREATMENT OF FRACTURES

Be aware of the indications for operative intervention in fractures; these are discussed in the individual sections, but some general guidelines can be stated here. Operative intervention is indicated in the following circumstances:

1. In displaced intraarticular fractures.
2. When arterial injury is associated with the fracture.
3. When experience shows that open treatment yields better results.

Table 7.4.
Common Fractures, Dislocations, and Sprains and Their Treatment

Fracture, dislocation, or sprain[a]	Treatment	Page
Comminuted fracture of distal phalanx, hand	Hairpin splint	265
Mallet fracture of distal phalanx, hand	Dorsal distal phalanx splint	265
Fracture of middle or proximal phalanx	Ulnar or radial gutter splint	262
Fracture of metacarpals	Ulnar or radial gutter splint	262
Suspected fracture of scaphoid	Sugar-tong splint of forearm	269
Suspected fracture of dorsal chip of carpal	Thumb spica cast, volar splint	264
Stable fracture of distal radius	Sugar-tong splint of forearm	269
Unstable distal radius fracture	Anterior–posterior splint (short arm) or long arm	268
Fracture of radius and ulna	Long-arm anterior and posterior splint	268
Fracture of distal humerus	Long-arm anterior and posterior splint	268
Fracture of humerus shaft	U-shaped coaptation splint of arm	269
Fracture of proximal humerus	Sugar-tong splint of arm, sling and swathe, sling and valpeau	270
Fracture of femur	Sager traction splint	253–255
Fracture of ankle	Posterior splint, ankle	270
Fracture of phalanges, foot	Dynamic "toe" splint	229
Collateral ligament sprain of IP or MP joints		
1° or mild 2°	Dynamic finger splint	266
Severe 2°	Dorsal or volar finger splint	265
Complete rupture 3°	Gutter splint	262
Elbow sprain	Posterior splint, elbow	268
Elbow dislocation	Posterior splint, elbow	268
Shoulder dislocation	Sling and swathe	233
Collateral ligament sprain, knee		
Mild or swelling	Jones compression dressing	271
Moderate or severe	Posterior splint, knee	
Patella dislocation	Posterior splint, knee	
Knee dislocation	Posterior splint, knee	
Ankle sprain	Posterior splint, ankle	270
Tibiotalar dislocation	Posterior splint, ankle	270
Sprain of IP joints of foot	Dynamic "toe" splint	229

[a]IP, interphalangeal; MP, metacarpophalangeal.

4. When closed methods fail to heal.
5. When the fracture is through a metastatic lesion (open treatment is usually indicated).
6. In patients in whom continued confinement in bed would be undesirable (open reduction and internal fixation may be indicated).

Casting

Do not equate the presence of a fracture with the need for casting. Casts are used for three reasons: to immobilize a fracture to permit healing, to relieve pain by rest, and to stabilize an unstable fracture.

The plaster rolls or slabs used in casting are rolls of muslin stiffened by dextrose or starch and impregnated with a hemihydrate of calcium sulfate. When water is added, the calcium sulfate takes up the water, and a reaction occurs that liberates heat; this heat is noted by both the patient and the physician applying the cast. Accelerator substances are added to the bandages to allow them to set at differing rates. Common table salt can be used to retard the setting of the plaster, if this is desired, simply by adding the salt to the water. Acceleration of the setting occurs by increasing the temperature of the water or by adding alum to the water. The colder the water temperature, the longer the plaster takes to set. There are several methods of applying plaster.

Skin-tight casts applied directly over the skin, although advocated by some in the past, are no longer used because of the complications of pressure sores and the circulatory embarrassment that may ensue. Most commonly used today is a stockinette applied at the locations of the ends of the cast (Fig. 7.33*A*), followed by a sheet of cotton padding (Webril); apply the padding from the distal to the proximal end of the limb (Fig. 7.33*B*). Too much padding reduces the efficacy of the cast and permits excessive motion. Generally the more padding used, the more plaster is needed. The cotton padding interposed between the skin and the plaster provides elastic pressure and enhances the fixation of the limb by compensating for slight shrinkage in the tissues after the application of the cast. Next apply the plaster. Roll the plaster bandage in the same direction as the padding so that each turn overlaps the preceding layer of plaster by half the width. Always lay the plaster on the limb transversely, keeping the roll of plaster in contact with the surface of the limb almost continuously. Instead of being lightly guided around the limb, shape and smooth the roll with pressure applied by the thenar eminence. Apply this thenar pressure to the middle of the plaster roll, which permits no excessive pressure to fall on either edge of the bandage so that no sharp ridges occur. Smooth each turn with the thenar eminence of the left hand as the right hand guides the roll around the limb. As the limb tapers, make the bandage lie evenly by small tucks made with the index finger and thumb of the left hand before smoothing each turn into position (Fig. 7.33*C*). As the cast is applied, smooth it with the palms and the thenar eminences of both hands (Fig. 7.33*D*). Remember that the durability and strength of the cast depend on the welding together of each individual turn by these smoothing

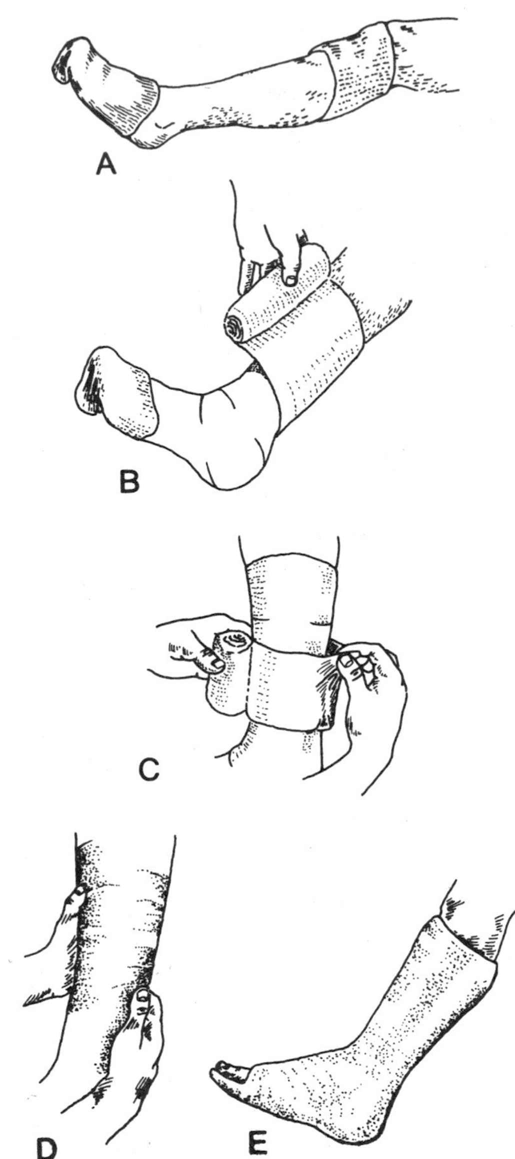

Figure 7.33. *A*: Apply stockinette to the locations of the ends of the cast. *B*: Apply cotton padding or Webril from the distal end of the limb proceeding proximally. See text for discussion. Roll a plaster bandage in the same direction as the padding, and overlap each turn over the preceding layer of plaster by half the width. *C*: As the limb tapers, make the bandages lie evenly by making small tucks with the index finger and thumb of the left hand as shown. *D*: Then smooth this down by the palms of the hands and the thenar eminences as shown. *E*: The final outcome is a well-molded, smooth, and strong cast.

movements of the left hand and the final smoothing out with both hands (Fig. 7.33*E*). Concentrate on making the two ends of the cast of adequate thickness; it is easy to make the center too thick, which provides no additional support at the fracture site (Fig. 7.34). A common problem is to use too many narrow bandages, which gives the cast a more lumpy appearance. Bandages of 4, 6, and 8 inches should be the most commonly used bandages for most casting. Another common mistake in bandaging is not applying the plaster tightly enough, especially over the proximal fleshy portion of the limb, where greater tension is needed than at the distal bony parts, resulting in a loose cast.

To reinforce the cast, as in an obese patient with a walking cast, add a fin to the front (Fig. 7.35), not posterior splints to the back which add no extra strength but add only weight to the cast. Use posterior slabs to add strength to the "sole of the foot" to prevent breakage there. Cast boots are available and are preferred to walking heels by most patients in the emergency center (Fig. 7.36). However, a walking heel

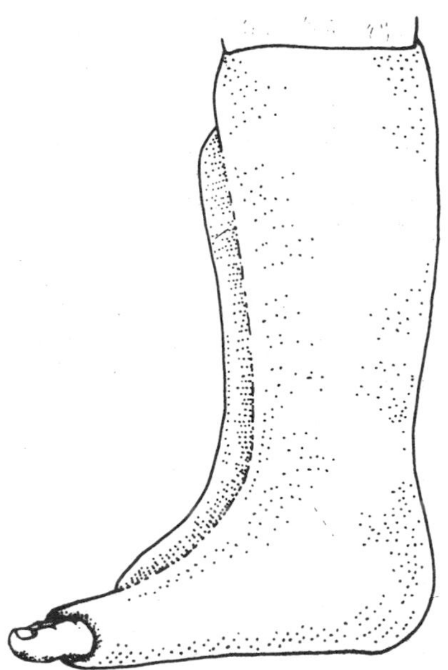

Figure 7.35. Apply a fin to the front of the cast to add strength to the cast at the ankle to prevent breakage there. Make the fin of two or three strips of 2-inch plaster slab applied over the anterior aspect of the cast. Cover this with a final roll of plaster, with the result being an anterior "fin."

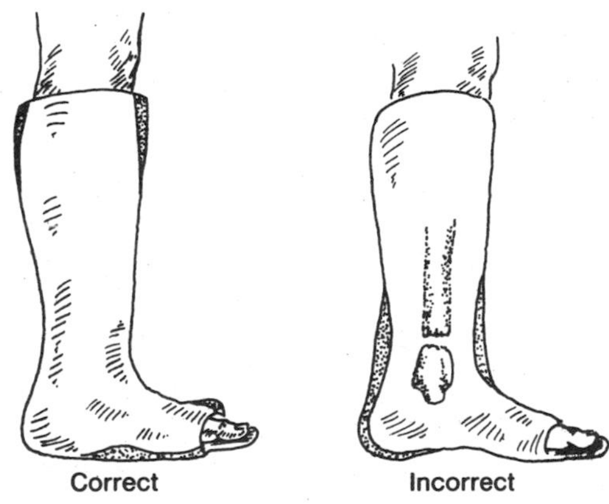

Figure 7.34. One of the most common mistakes is layering the plaster more thickly than is necessary around the fracture site by the physician who thinks this will increase the strength. Concentrate on making the two ends of the cast of adequate thickness, because this provides the most durable cast.

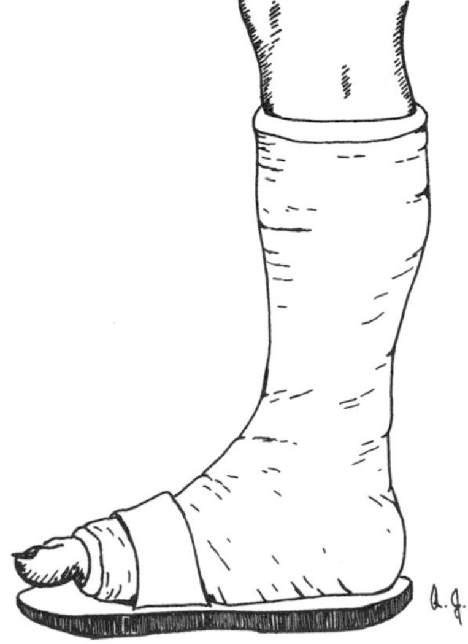

Figure 7.36. Walking shoe (boot). Use with a short-leg cast.

remains a commonly applied device for ambulation. The application of a walking heel should be under the center of the foot (Fig. 7.37).

When applying a cast to an upper extremity, leave the patient's hand free by stopping the cast at the metacarpal heads dorsally and the proximal flexor crease of the palm to permit normal finger motion (Fig. 7.38).

A window may be placed in a cast when a fracture is accompanied by a laceration or any skin lesions for care while treating the fracture. Windows are best made as shown in Fig. 7.39 by covering the wound with a bulky piece of sterile gauze and then applying the cast over the dressing in the normal manner (Fig. 7.39*B*). When casting is completed, cut the window in the cast over the "bulge" created by the gauze dressing (Fig. 7.39*C*). Always cover the defect with a dressing and, over the dressing, a piece of sponge rubber or felt held snugly in place with an Ace bandage

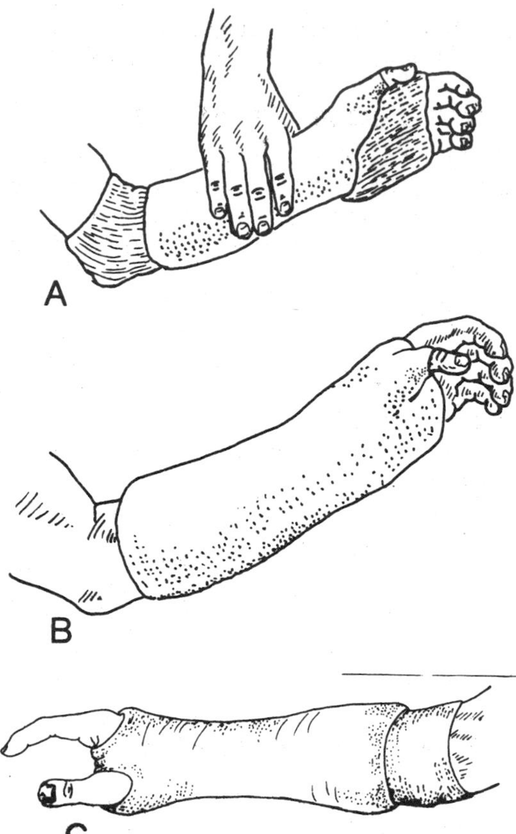

Figure 7.38. The fingers and the thumb should be free to move when a cast is applied to the forearm for fractures of the distal forearm.

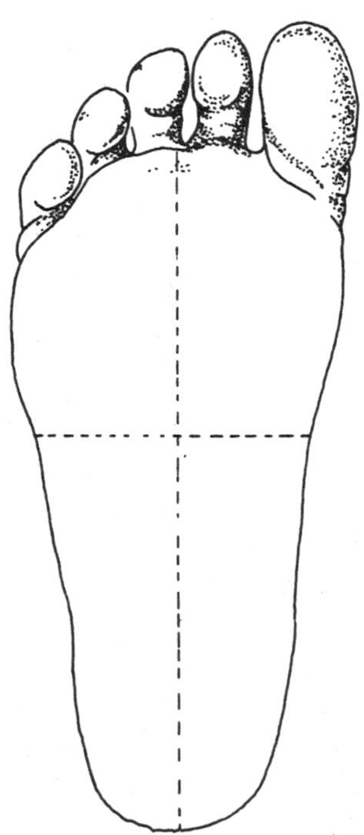

Figure 7.37. Apply walking heels under the center of the foot.

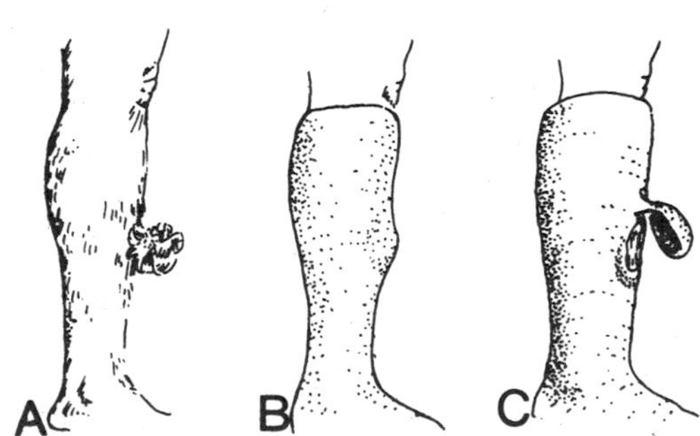

Figure 7.39. When a wound is present over the leg and the limb requires casting, cut a window out of the cast. *A*: Apply a wad of gauze over the wound after it is adequately dressed and/or sutured. *B*: Apply a cast over the wad of gauze. This creates a lump in the cast as shown. *C*: Then cut the "lump" out with a cast saw, which permits a window through which the wound may be managed.

so that herniation of the soft tissue and subsequent swelling around the window and ulceration of the skin from pressure at the sides of the defect does not occur.

There are many types of casts, such as spica casts, patellar tendon–bearing casts, and more recently, cast braces; however, these are not used by the emergency physician and are not discussed here. Recently fiberglass casts made of lightweight plastic have been introduced. These casts are durable and radiolucent and have the advantage of not being softened or damaged when they become wet. These have limited application to fresh fractures because they are more difficult to apply, and a snug fit is more difficult to achieve, but they are commonly used as a second or subsequent cast. They are especially useful for open fractures because the patient can use a whirlpool or other forms of "wet" therapy while in the cast.

Plaster sores are complications of plaster casts that can occur as a result of excessive pressure. Patients complain of a burning pain or discomfort. These can be avoided by eliminating sharp ends in the cast and by avoiding indented spots in the cast. Felt pads placed between the layers of padding in the cast tend to migrate, and pressure sores may result.

Splints also are commonly used to immobilize injuries. The most common splints used are the posterior splints to the lower extremity for ankle and foot injuries (Fig. 7.40); similar splints are used in the upper extremity. Splints offer the advantage of permitting soft tissue swelling without compromising the circulation. Ice packs can be applied to the site of injury along with elevation of the limb, because the splint will permit penetration of the cold to maximize its effect. These reasons, along with its ease of application, make splinting of upper and lower extremity fractures a commonly used method of immobilization in emergency management; later a more definitive cast is applied. The disadvantages of splinting are that it permits excessive motion and provides little stability for a fracture that has been reduced and must be maintained in a certain position.

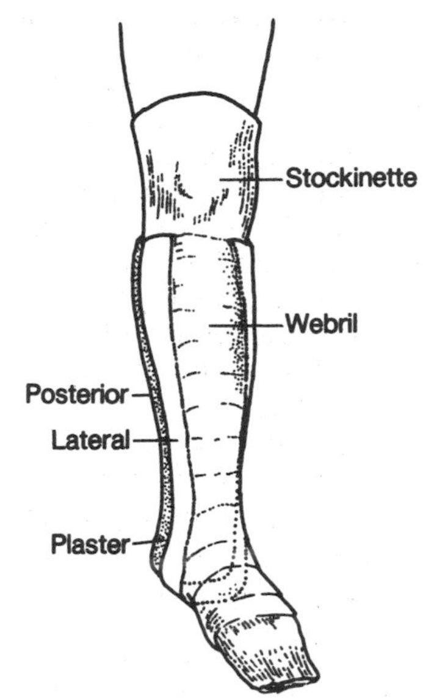

Figure 7.40. A posterior splint to the ankle. These splints offer the advantage of permitting soft tissue swelling without compromising circulation. Obtain added support by adding an additional piece to cover the medial and lateral sides to strengthen them. When Webril is applied under the plaster, incise it longitudinally to permit swelling to occur.

CHECKING CASTS

Accompany any circumferential cast with written instructions to the patient or family members about signs of the cast being too tight. *Increasing pain*, swelling, coolness, or change in skin color of the distal portions of the extremity are signs of a cast being too tight. Paresthesias, poor capillary refill, and pain on passive extension of the phalanges distal to the cast are important signs and symptoms of ischemia from a too-tight circumferential cast. Check the patient immediately, and make the patient aware of the dangers of ignoring such problems. As a general rule, we recommend that any circumferential cast be checked the following day for signs of circulatory compromise. Instruct the patient to elevate the limb for 24 hours after the application of a cast to avoid problems.

If the cast is too tight, remember to split not only the plaster casting but also the inner padding to reduce the pressure significantly. This was well demonstrated in a recent study that showed that there was no significant reduction in pressure when only the plaster was opened and that there was significant reduction when the padding also was incised (44).

ANESTHESIA FOR FRACTURES

Many forms of anesthesia can be used in fracture reduction. Many fractures require general anesthesia, particularly those in small children. Weigh the risk of general anesthesia against the advantages of regional blocks, which can be satisfactorily used in most of the common reductions performed in the emergency center. Injection of anesthetic into the fracture hematoma is commonly done but may not achieve adequate pain control.

Bier Block

A Bier block is an excellent form of anesthesia for leg, foot, forearm, and hand fractures. This type of anesthesia is discussed in detail in Chapter 3, Anesthesia and Regional Blocks; see that chapter for contraindications, complications, technique, etc.

Regional Block

This is another good form of anesthesia for upper extremity reductions. See Chapter 3 for complete information.

Special Considerations for Fracture Management: Open Fractures

Open fractures provide a significant challenge to the physician. Check the skin around the wound and note what contaminants may be in the wound. Do not attempt to explore the wound digitally in the emergency center, because little information will be provided, and an increased risk of infection will result. Local debridement is indicated in all cases. When a small wound is noted on the skin that overlies a fracture, and a question arises as to whether it communicates with the fracture, one can safely check the wound with a sterile blunt probe to see if bone is touched. If the question still remains, then prudent management mandates treatment as if it were an open fracture, with debridement of the wound in the operating room. Dress the wound with a sterile dressing, and splint the extremity. Some open fractures do not require meticulous debridement and have a good prognosis, including open fracture of the distal phalanx of the digits; this is the open fracture most commonly seen in the emergency center. The usual prudent therapy advocated for open fractures elsewhere is not necessary here, because the blood supply to the distal phalanx is excellent, and fractures clinically heal without osteomyelitis in this area. The treatment of open fractures of the distal phalanx includes cleansing the area, routinely treating the fracture and any open laceration, and monitoring the patient.

Gutter Splints

Gutter splints are used for the treatment of stable phalangeal and metacarpal fractures. The fractures that are most commonly treated by gutter splints are those that are simple with no rotational abnormality or significant displacement. In fractures involving the ring and little finger, immobilize the digit in a gutter splint as shown in Figure 7.41*A*. Form the splint by using plaster slabs cut to the proper size and then applied and molded into a U-shaped splint over the ring and little fingers, while holding the fingers in the position shown. The splint should extend from the fingertips to just below the elbow, permitting flexion and extension at the elbow joint. Approximately six to eight sheets of plaster provide an adequate thickness to give good support. Apply the plaster directly to the skin, as shown, with

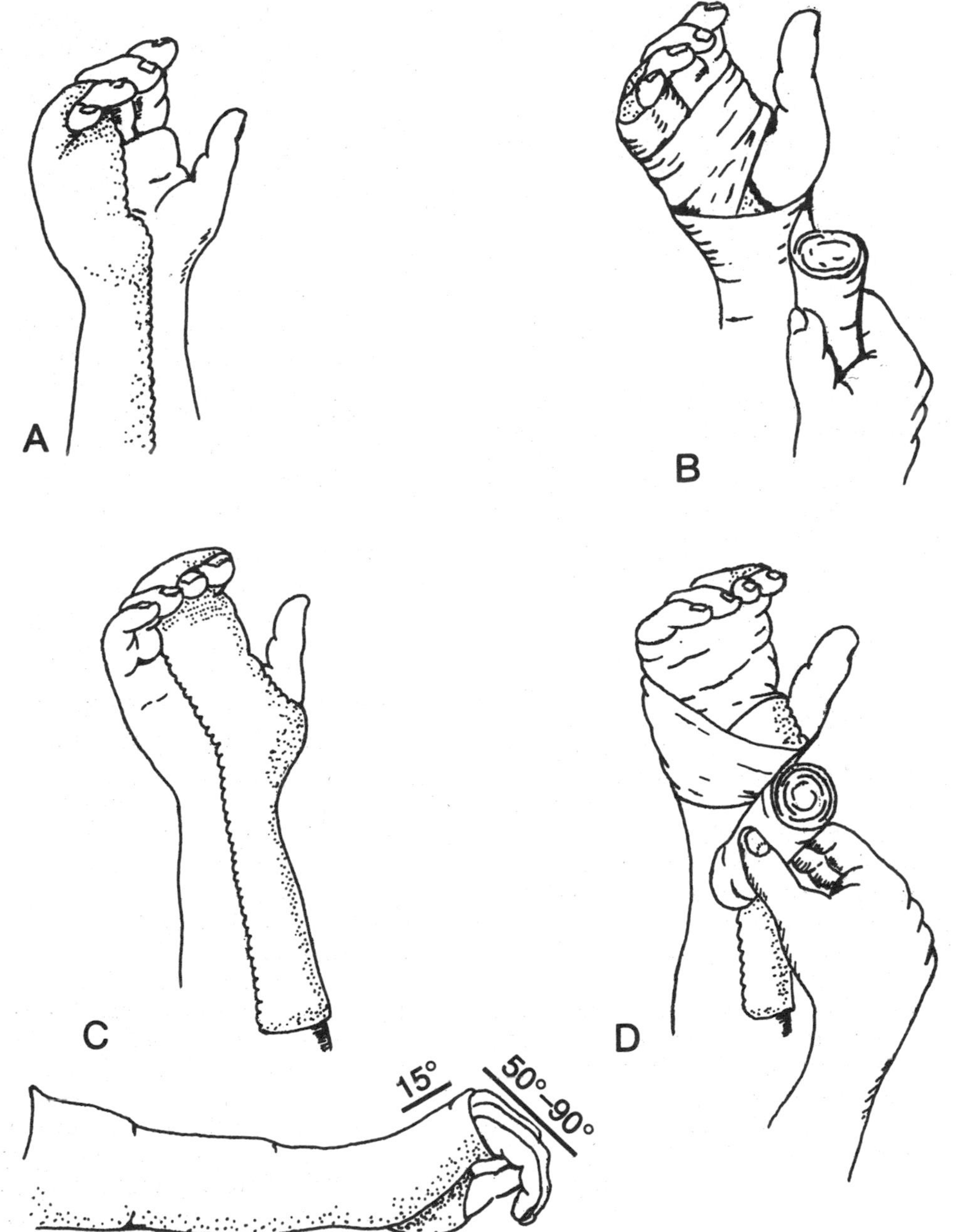

Figure 7.41. The technique for doing a gutter splint for phalangeal fractures and metacarpal fracture of the hand. Note that the wrist is splinted at 15 degrees of extension with the metacarpophalangeal joints at 50 to 90 degrees of flexion. See text.

the fingers held at approximately 50 to 90 degrees of flexion at the metacarpophalangeal joint and 15 to 20 degrees of flexion at the interphalangeal joints (Fig. 7.41*E*). With fractures involving the index and long fingers, use a similar splint, as shown in Fig. 7.41*C*. This splint has a piece cut out for the thumb. Hold the splints in place with an elastic bandage, as shown in Fig. 7.41*B* and *D*. Because of the light weight of these splints, the patient generally does not require a sling or support; however, advise the patient to elevate the hand continuously for the first 24 hours to prevent swelling, which is a common complication in fractures involving the hand and can lead to a significant loss of function.

Thumb Spica or Wrist Gauntlet Cast

The thumb spica is the most commonly used cast for management of scaphoid fractures of the wrist in the emergency center. It is made by applying a stockinette dressing to the arm and extending the stockinette from the hand to the midarm, or more proximally when a long-arm spica cast is desirable. The decision as to whether to use a short-arm or a long-arm cast must be individualized to the patient and is, in part, contingent on the philosophy of the treating physician. This is followed by the application of a cotton bandage (Webril), which is then followed by the application of plaster rolls (Fig. 7.42). The method for applying plaster rolls was discussed earlier in the chapter and is not repeated here. Before the application of the final roll, fold the stockinette back over the cast, and apply the final plaster roll, as shown in Fig. 7.43*B*, in which the distal end of the stockinette has been folded back. Maintain the position of the thumb as shown in Fig. 7.43*C* when applying this cast. Provide the optimal position for the thumb by asking the patient to imagine holding a glass. Although the interphalangeal joint may be incorporated in the cast we have described, there is controversy regarding the need to immobilize this joint in treating scaphoid fractures. Leave the fingers free so that there is full motion at the metacarpophalangeal joints. The position of the forearm shown here is the neutral position, midway between supination and pronation. In using this cast for scaphoid fractures, some authors advocate extending it above the elbow joint, thus making it a long-arm cast with the elbow flexed to 90 degrees; however, as mentioned earlier, this is controversial. Our preference is to use a short-arm cast in treating these fractures.

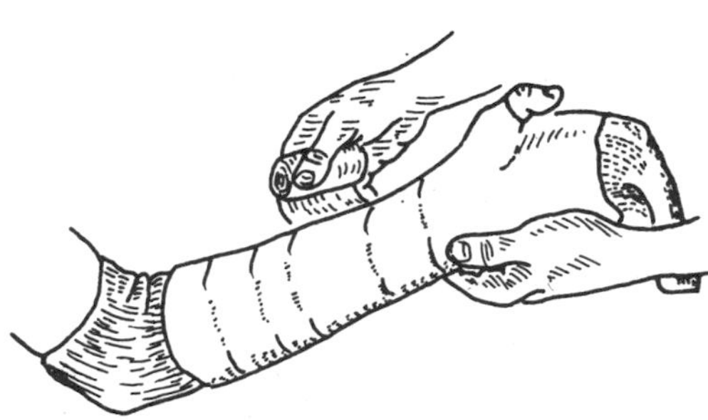

Figure 7.42. A thumb spica cast. See text for discussion.

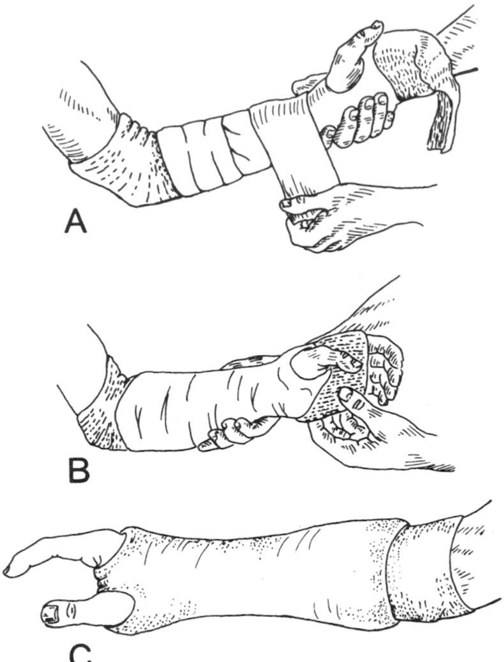

Figure 7.43. A short-arm cast. See text for discussion.

Short- and Long-Arm Casts

A short-arm cast is used in the emergency center for immobilization of a number of simple fractures involving the distal forearm and metacarpals. Make the cast by applying the stockinette from the fingers to above the elbow, as shown in Fig. 7.43*A*. Then apply a cotton bandage (Webril) over the stockinette with the thumb remaining free at the metacarpophalangeal joint and the fingers free at the same level. Apply two to three plaster rolls, maintaining the hand in the position shown in Fig. 7.43*B*. Fold the stockinette over this cast, and apply a final roll of plaster bandages (Fig. 7.43*C*). The patient should be able to use the fingers and thumb freely, without any impingement on normal motion after the cast is applied.

Produce a long-arm cast in a similar fashion, with the exception that it is extended above the elbow to approximately the midarm position, with the elbow flexed at 90 degrees. Use the long-arm cast in treating most fractures involving the forearm.

Dorsal Distal Phalanx Splint

Avulsion fractures involving the extensor tendon attachment to the distal phalanx can be treated in the emergency center with a dorsal extension splint applied over the dorsal surface of the distal interphalangeal joint (Fig. 7.44*B*). Either a dorsal or a volar splint is useful in treating avulsion fractures of the distal phalanx. We prefer the dorsal splint because it provides more support; there is less "padding" on the dorsal aspect of the finger, so the splint is in closer contact with the bone that it is to support. In using this splint, do not hyperextend the distal interphalangeal joint as was recommended in older textbooks. Full extension is the position of choice when applying the splint, and this position must be maintained for 6 weeks with the splint in place. Never remove the splint or flex the finger during this time. Position the splint so that it does not interfere with motion at the proximal interphalangeal joint. Most of these splints are made of flexible metal strips that are available in all emergency centers.

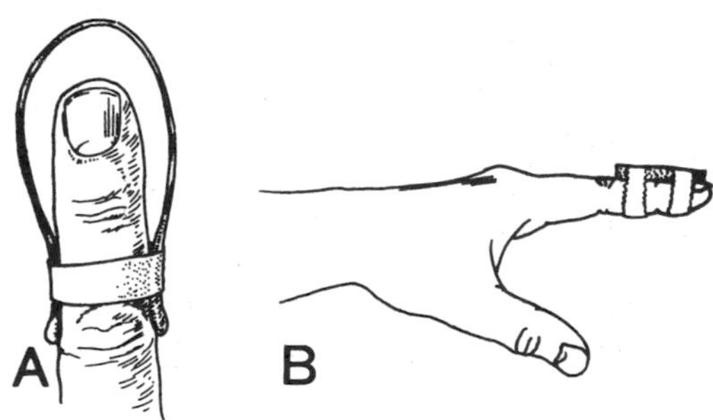

Figure 7.44. *A*: The hairpin splint is commonly used for comminuted fractures of the distal phalanx. *B*: Use a dorsal splint applied across the distal interphalangeal joint for treating ruptures of the central slip of the extensor tendon or mallet fractures.

Hairpin Splint

This splint is fashioned out of a thin metal strip or a large hairpin (Fig 7.44*A*) and provides excellent protection in fractures involving the distal phalanx of the fingers, which generally need no support but do need protection from external injuries, as in comminuted fractures. The hairpin splint provides this protection without allowing any contact between the splint and the skin surface, which might produce pain.

Dorsal and Volar Finger Splints

Dorsal and volar finger splints are used in the management of a variety of injuries, the most common being collateral ligament injuries involving the proximal or distal interphalangeal joint or the metacarpophalangeal joint. The splints are fashioned from commercially available metallic splints that have a sponge rubber padding on one side. Cut the splint to the proper size and shape as desired (Fig. 7.45). When the splint is to be applied for a prolonged period, position the metacarpophalangeal joint at 50 degrees of flexion and flex the interphalangeal joint to approximately 15 to 20 degrees. This position provides optimal stretch of the collateral ligaments of the metacarpophalangeal and interpha-

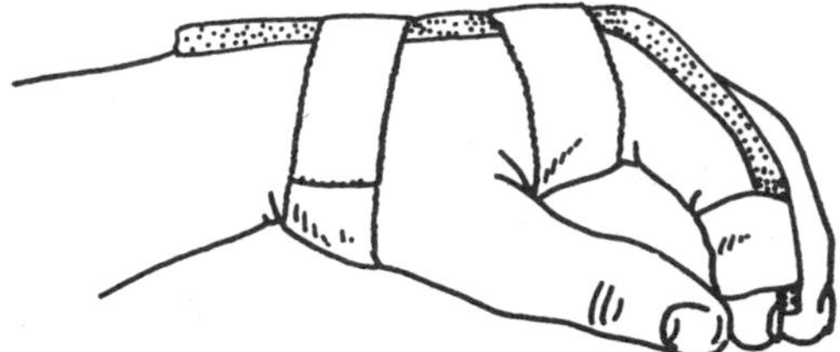

Figure 7.45. A dorsal finger splint. These splints provide support for sprains of the collateral ligaments of the digits; however, do not use them for fracture management. Flex the metacarpophalangeal joint to 50 degrees or greater, and flex the interphalangeal joint 15 to 20 degrees.

langeal joints and avoids the problem of contracture of these ligaments as healing progresses. One can test this on oneself by extending the long finger at the metacarpophalangeal joint and moving it from side to side. A wide range of motion is noted in doing this; with the finger flexed at 50 degrees at the metacarpophalangeal joint, side-to-side motion is markedly reduced because the collateral ligaments are taut in this position. When stress testing shows complete rupture of a collateral ligament, a gutter splint should be used.

Dynamic Finger Splinting

This form of splinting is used commonly in sprains involving the collateral ligaments of the interphalangeal joints of the hand. This type of splinting is used when there is minimal injury to the collateral ligament or after the collateral ligament has been treated with a splint and requires only moderate support. The most common joint injuries in which this type of splinting is used are stable first- and second-degree sprains of the proximal and distal interphalangeal joints. Splint the injured finger to the adjacent normal finger, which provides support for the injured digit while permitting motion primarily of the metacarpophalangeal joint and limited motion of the interphalangeal joint. Cut a piece of felt to the proper size and insert it between the fingers and the two digits, taped together as shown in Fig. 7.46. This method of splinting also is quite good for phalangeal fractures of the toe, for which alternative methods of splinting would be inconvenient.

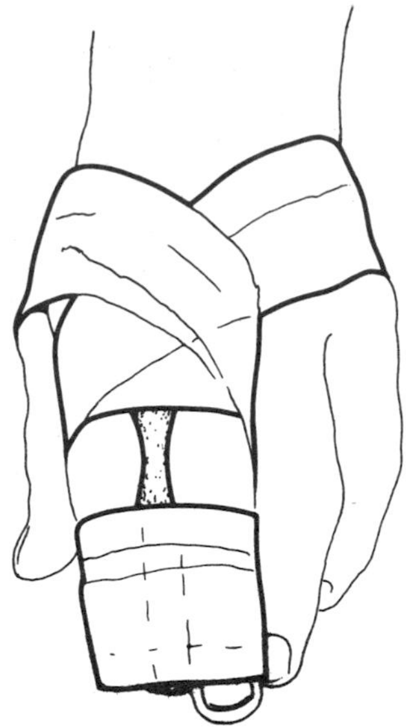

Figure 7.46. Dynamic finger splinting. Use this type of splinting when a collateral ligament is injured only minimally or after the collateral ligament has been initially treated with a splint and requires only moderate support.

Universal Hand Dressing

The universal hand dressing is used in a number of hand problems seen in the emergency center, including infections of the hand, serious lacerations, and some forms of tendonitis. The position in which the universal hand dressing immobilizes the hand provides optimal lymphatic drainage and a functionally resting position for all the joints to facilitate adequate healing. The optimal position in which to immobilize the hand for a hand infection or soft tissue injury is demonstrated in Fig. 7.47*A*. This position provides 15 degrees of extension at the wrist, 50 degrees of flexion at the metacarpophalangeal joint, and 20 to 30 degrees

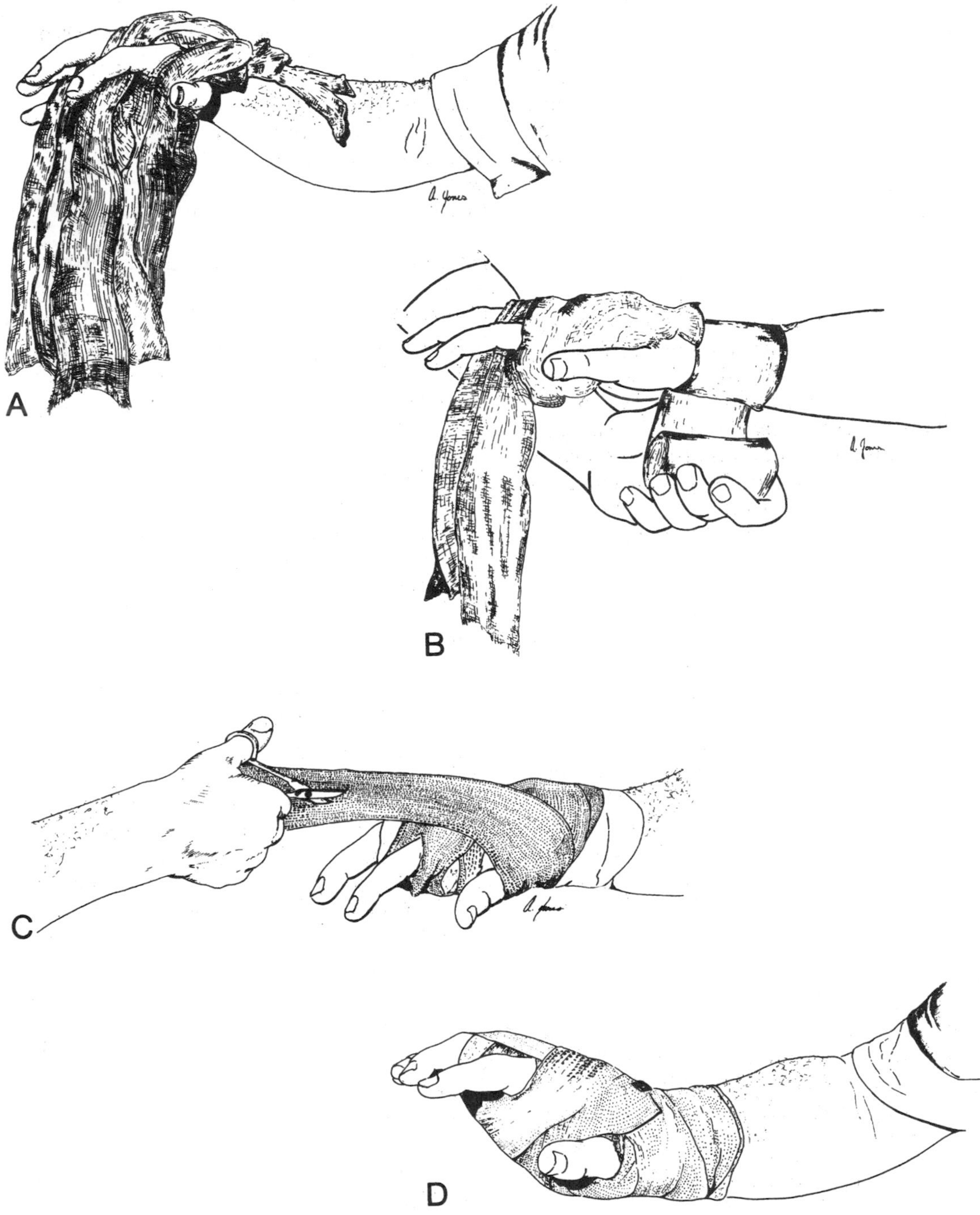

Figure 7.47. Universal hand dressing. *A*: Insert gauze fluffs between the fingers as shown. *B*: Then use a Kerlex gauze roll to wrap between the fingers. *C*: Apply an elastic bandage over the gauze as shown. Note that the elastic bandage is placed over the fingers with a hole cut into the bandage for the fingers to pass through. *D*: When applying the elastic wrap, be sure to prop up the wrist at 15 degrees of extension, allowing the metacarpophalangeal joint and interphalangeal joints to be placed in the position noted in the diagram (see text). This allows relaxation of the hand and maximal drainage. Extend the dressing to the distal interphalangeal joints whenever necessary.

of flexion at the interphalangeal joints with the thumb positioned as shown. This position permits optimal drainage for swelling, which occurs with virtually all serious hand problems and is a significant limiting factor for adequate healing. To maintain this position in a soft dressing, place fluffs between the fingers and thumb as shown in Fig. 7.47*A*. These fluff dressings should extend down to the midforearm. Follow this with the application of a gauze roll around the fluffs and between the fingers to secure them in place (Fig. 7.47*B*). Follow this with an Ace wrap with holes cut out for the fingers (Fig. 7.47*C*, *D*.) Finally, apply half-inch tape to hold the Ace wrap in position. Advise the patient to elevate the hand above the level of the heart to facilitate the drainage, especially with infections, for which the universal hand dressing has been applied.

Long-Arm Posterior Splints

A long-arm posterior splint is commonly used in the emergency center to immobilize a number of injuries involving the elbow and forearm. Produce the splint by wrapping a cotton bandage (Webril) around the forearm from the midpalmar region to the midarm. Then apply a plaster slab to the posterior aspect of the forearm, extending above the elbow with the elbow held in a position of 90 degrees of flexion, and the forearm maintained in a neutral position that is neither supinated nor pronated (Fig. 7.48). Apply a posterior plaster slab consisting of eight layers of plaster that are wide enough to provide a semicircular dressing around the circumference of the arm, as shown in Fig. 7.48. Cut this splint from rolls of plaster or make them from prefabricated slabs. Then apply an Ace wrap to hold the plaster slab in place. Use a sling after the splint has been applied. Commercially available splints incorporate the plaster slabs, cotton bandage, and a foam sponging that can be cut to the proper length and applied in a similar fashion.

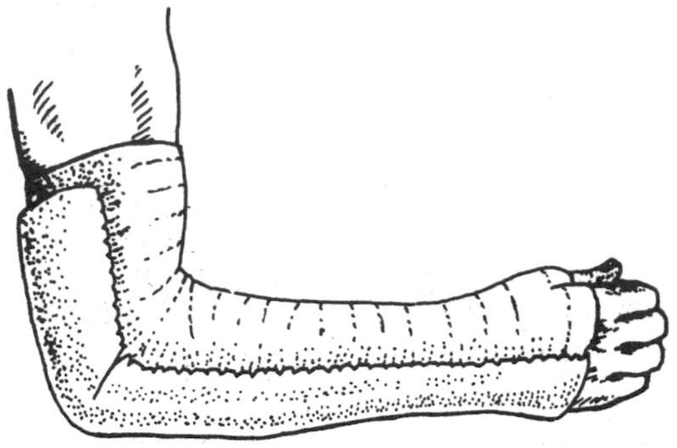

Figure 7.48. Apply a posterior plaster splint to the forearm. Extend the splint above the elbow, with the elbow flexed to 90 degrees. See text for discussion.

Anterior–Posterior Splints of the Forearm

Anterior and posterior molds are most often used for the initial management of fractures involving the forearm and wrist in which immobilization must be maintained in a more secure position than with a simple posterior splint and in which, because of anticipated swelling, a circular cast is not desirable. With these splints, the forearm can be maintained in any degree of flexion, supination, or pronation. Apply stockinette first over the forearm and the hand, and cut splints to the proper length from plaster slabs and apply them anteriorly and posteriorly to the forearm, as shown in Fig. 7.49*A*. With unstable fractures of the forearm, extend the splint above the elbow flexed at 90 degrees. Place the arm in a pronated or a supinated position to stabilize a fracture, depending on the site and position of the fracture being supported. Use a cotton bandage dressing (Webril) under the splint; however, if this is done, incise the bandage lengthwise to permit swelling of the limb. Use an elastic wrap to hold the splints in position (Fig. 7.49*B*). Use a sling to support the forearm after splinting.

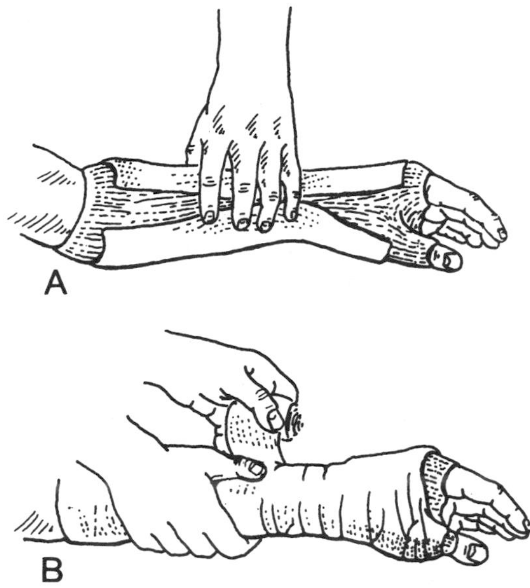

Figure 7.49. An anterior–posterior splint of the forearm. To make a long-arm anterior–posterior splint, extend the slabs to above the elbow. *A*: Apply stockinette over the forearm. After this, apply an anterior and a posterior plaster slab. *B*: Hold the anterior and posterior slabs in position with an Ace wrap.

Sugar-Tong Splint of the Forearm

The sugar-tong splint is commonly used to immobilize forearm fractures, particularly distal radius fractures at the wrist, in patients in whom it is desirable to maintain the forearm in some degree of supination or pronation. Place the forearm in a supinated or a pronated position during the application of the splint. First apply a cotton bandage (Webril) to the injured limb, followed by a single long plaster slab that extends from the distal palmar crease to the elbow, after which it courses around the elbow to the dorsum of the hand just proximal to the metacarpophalangeal joint, thus encircling the elbow joint (Fig. 7.50). The advantages of this splint are that it permits immobilization in a position of pronation or supination without applying a circumferential cast, with its attendant hazards, and is a very simple splint to apply. Use a sling after application of this splint.

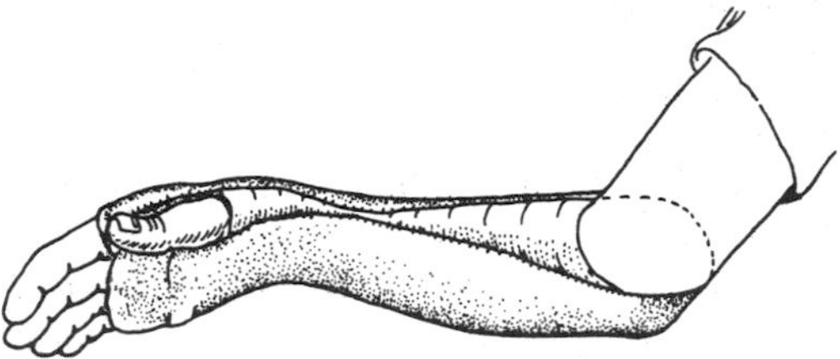

Figure 7.50. A sugar-tong splint. See text for discussion.

Sugar-Tong Splint of the Arm

A sugar-tong splint also can be used in the initial management of fractures of the humeral shaft. Humeral shaft fractures are often displaced and, after reduction, an assistant may have to maintain position of the fracture while the splint is being applied, as shown in Fig. 7.51*A*. The splint

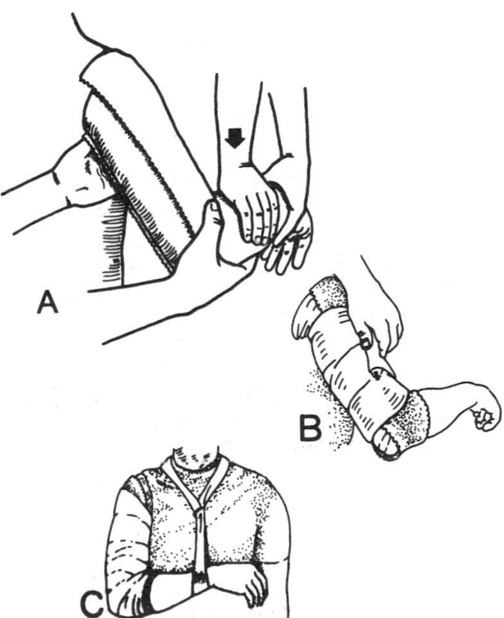

Figure 7.51. A sugar-tong splint of the arm or U-shaped coaptation splint. Apply Webril to the arm in a one-layer dressing. After this, apply a plaster slab, extending from the axilla to the deltoid region. *A*: During this application, an assistant holds the forearm at 90 degrees with compression as shown, to keep the ends of the fractured humerus separated and stabilized. *B*: An Ace wrap or an Esmarch's bandage holds the U-shaped splint in position. *C*: Then use a collar and cuff to maintain the elbow in the flexed position.

should extend from the axilla medially down the humerus, encircling the elbow joint, and up along the outer aspect of the humerus and over the acromion (Fig. 7.51*A*). Apply this over a cotton bandage as previously discussed under the section Sugar-Tong Splint of the Forearm. After this application, hold the splint in place with an Ace bandage, as shown in Fig. 7.51*B*, followed by the use of a collar and cuff (Fig. 7.51*C*).

Types of Slings

Three types of slings are commonly used within the emergency center: a common sling, a collar and cuff, and a stockinette valpeau. These are pictured in Fig. 7.52*A* through *C*, respectively. The common sling is most often used and is primarily used to support the arm in association with a number of injuries and disorders involving the upper extremity. The collar and cuff is an alternate method used to support the forearm and wrist in patients with humeral fractures treated with a coaptation splint (sugar-tong splint to arm) and in those patients in whom a stable humeral fracture requires only the application of a collar and cuff for support. A stockinette valpeau and swathe (the component that encircles the patient's waist) is used if there is an unstable fracture involving the proximal humerus, which has a tendency to displace because of contraction of the pectoralis major muscle. The position demonstrated in Fig. 7.52*C* relaxes the pectoralis major and prevents it from displacing fractures involving the proximal humeral shaft.

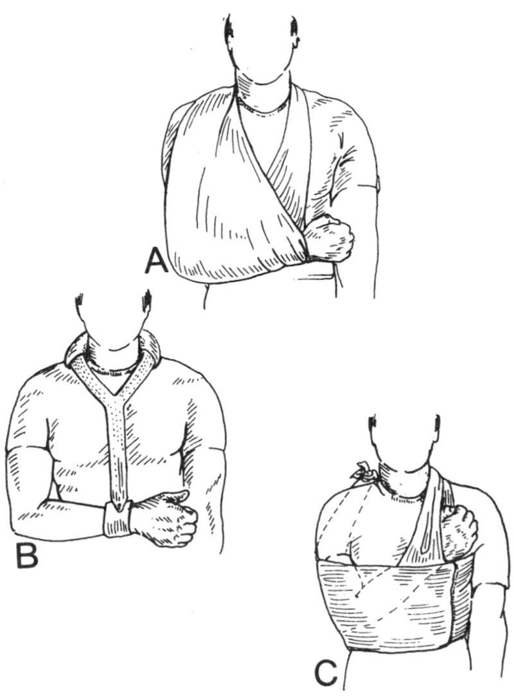

Figure 7.52. *A*: A common sling. *B*: A collar and cuff. *C*: Stockinette valpeau dressing.

Application of a Posterior Splint to the Ankle

This type of splint is commonly used in the emergency center for the initial management of complex ankle sprains and to immobilize fractures of the ankle, foot, and distal tibia until definitive care can be instituted or until swelling subsides. Posterior splints applied to the ankle allow the effective use of ice packs in the treatment of postinjury swelling while providing adequate immobilization of the injured extremity. Apply stockinette dressing over the leg to cover the area to which the plaster slabs are to be applied, and extend it well above the knee and below the toes, as shown in Fig. 7.53*A*. Apply a cotton bandage (Webril) over the stockinette (Fig. 7.53*A*), followed by the application of posterior slabs of plaster composed of eight to 10 sheets. The posterior splint should extend from the toes to below the knee, permitting comfortable flexion of the knee joint (Fig. 7.53*B*). With the splint properly applied, the patient should be able to flex the knee freely. Apply an additional splint medially to laterally, extending around the ankle held at 90 degrees. This provides additional support for the ankle joint. Then fold the stockinette over the plaster, and apply an elastic wrap that secures the plaster to the leg (Fig. 7.53*C*). When swelling is

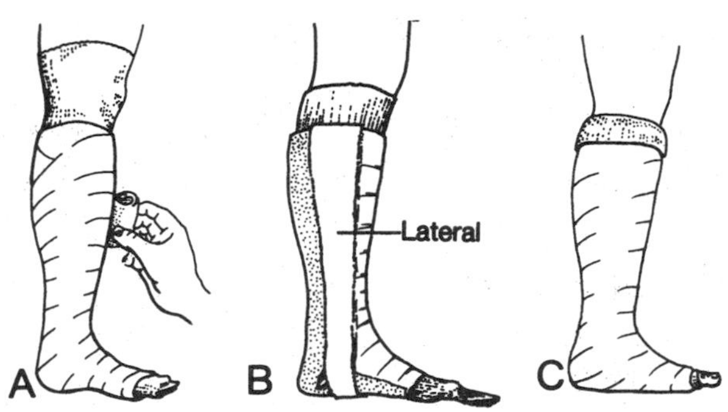

Figure 7.53. The application of a posterior splint to the ankle. See text for discussion. The posterior splint extends from the ball of the foot at the metatarsal heads to the posterior aspect of the knee just below the flexor crease. To add stability, extend a U-shaped lateral splint around the medial and lateral sides of the ankle. Commercial posterior splints are currently available for use in many emergency centers. Incise the Webril longitudinally to permit swelling to occur.

a significant concern (as with a fracture), incise the cotton bandage before the elastic wrap is applied because it may act as a compressive dressing. Posterior splints incorporating the cotton bandage, plaster slabs, and foam sponging are available commercially.

Jones Compression Dressing

A Jones compression dressing is commonly used for soft tissue injuries involving the knee joint. This dressing provides for immobilization of the limb and a compressive dressing for swelling while permitting some flexion and extension at the joint. Make the dressing by applying a layer of cotton bandage (Webril) that extends from the groin to just above the malleoli of the ankle. After this, apply an elastic wrap circumferentially from distal to proximal (Fig. 7.54). Then apply a second layer of Webril, followed by another elastic wrap. This additional layer provides added support, to maintain uniform compression when the first layer loses its elasticity.

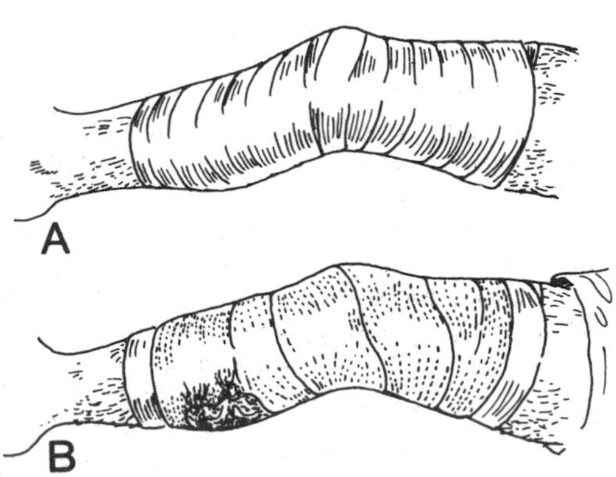

Figure 7.54. A Jones compression dressing.

REDUCTION OF SELECTED COMMON FRACTURES

Many of the fractures seen in the emergency center are splinted for immobilization and are referred for definitive care to an orthopedic surgeon. A detailed discussion of fracture management is beyond the scope of this text; however, a chapter on orthopedic procedures would not be complete without discussion of some of the common fractures managed by the emergency physician.

Clavicular Fractures (8, 31)

Clavicular fractures are the most common of all childhood fractures. Overall, clavicular fractures account for 5% of all fractures seen in all age groups. Eighty percent of all clavicular fractures seen in the emergency center occur in the middle one third of this bone. Childhood clavicular fractures generally require little treatment because rapid healing and full return of function is the usual outcome. Adult clavicular fractures may be associated with complications and, therefore, require a more accurate reduction and closer follow-up to ensure a full return to normal functioning. Adult fractures may be complicated by excessive callus formation and by neurovascular compromise secondary to compression against the first rib. With a clavicular fracture in the midportion, examine the patient for and document any neurovascular compromise distal to the injury in the upper extremity.

A figure-of-eight clavicular strap is often used in managing these fractures. Commercial devices are available and, when applied properly, they are quite useful in children older than 10 years. Instruct the family in the proper application and adjustment of this device (Fig. 7.55):

1. Pull both shoulders backward tightly, as if to stand in a military position.
2. Apply the commercial splint around both shoulders as if applying a backpack and tighten the posterior straps as shown in Fig. 7.55*A*.
3. Examine the patient for neurovascular compromise and educate the family as to the symptoms of this complication.
4. Instruct the family in the method of tightening the splint daily. The splint will require frequent tightening and should be worn until the patient can abduct the extremity without pain and there is evidence of clinical union. Children generally require 3 to 5 weeks of immobilization, whereas adults require 6 weeks or more.

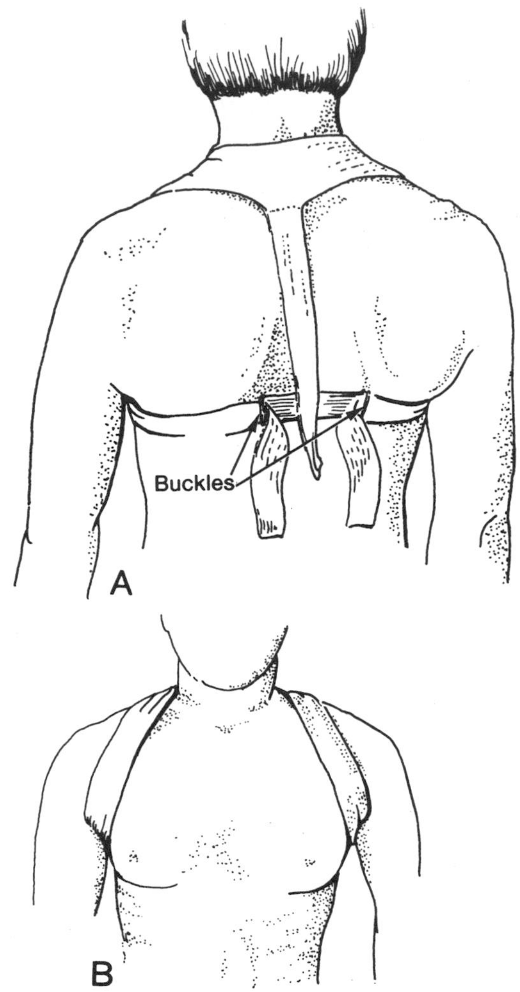

Figure 7.55. *A*: A figure-of-eight clavicular strap. Apply the straps around the shoulders, and adjust them by pulling on the two metal buckles. *B*: Instruct the patient to hold the shoulders back and the chest out, as if standing at attention, when the straps are tightened.

In children, a properly applied figure-of-eight clavicular strap that is adjusted frequently is the treatment of choice. See patients in follow-up to ensure proper reduction and maintenance of position. If the child or family is uncooperative and will not use the figure-of-eight splint properly, refer for consideration of a shoulder spica. Although a commercially available figure-of-eight splint can be used in the initial management in the emergency center for the reduction and maintenance of position of displaced clavicular fractures in the adult, if, after 1 week, the fracture is not adequately reduced, refer the patient to an orthopedic surgeon for a shoulder spica cast. If the patient is uncooperative initially and will not properly wear and maintain the figure-of-eight strap, referral for a shoulder spica is indicated.

Colles' Fracture (5, 6, 15, 16)

Only simple Colles' fractures can be managed by the emergency physician in the emergency center. Fractures of the distal radius and ulna with radiocarpal joint involvement and distal radial fractures with radioulnar joint involvement, in our opinion, should be referred because of the high incidence of associated complications, including secondary joint stiffness, postreduction swelling with secondary compartment syndromes, and cosmetic defects that may follow seriously displaced distal forearm fractures, as may malunion. Only those fractures that are extraarticular, involving the distal radius, or those involving the distal radius and ulna should be managed in the emergency center by the emergency physician. Colles' fractures, even when managed appropriately, frequently result in long-term complications. For this reason, treat only selected Colles' fractures. Splint all other distal forearm fractures and refer the patient for emergency treatment and follow-up.

The method of reduction of a Colles' fracture is demonstrated in Fig. 7.56.

1. The optimal method of anesthesia is a regional block, such as the Bier block (discussed in Chapter 3, Anesthesia and Regional Blocks). A less effective, but acceptable, method is to insert a needle into the fracture hematoma after adequate preparation, aspirate the hematoma surrounding the fracture, and inject 5 to 10 mL of lidocaine into the area. This form of anesthesia will

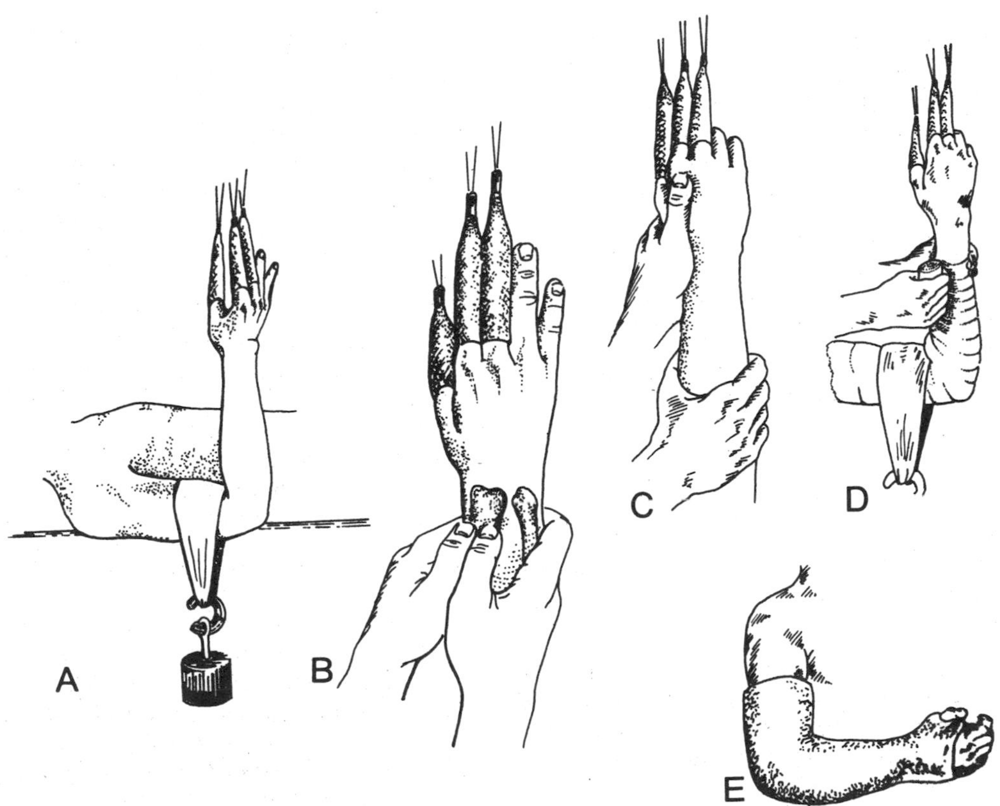

Figure 7.56. The reduction of a Colles' fracture. *A*: Fingers in a Chinese finger trap to disimpact the fracture fragments. *B*: Reduce the fracture by applying a reducing force with the thumbs directing the distal segment volarly, after reversing the mechanism of the fracture by dorsal angulation, until the ends of the fractured fragments come in contact. *C*: Correct ulnar and volar displacement. *D*: If the reduction is unstable, apply the initial portion of a plaster cast while the hand is in traction. *E*: Finished cast.

work in most patients; however, it is often incomplete.

2. The recommended method of reduction is with *traction* followed by *manipulation*. Place the fingers in a Chinese finger trap (Fig. 7.56*A*) and elevate the wrist with the elbow in 90 degrees of flexion. Eight to 10 pounds of weight is then suspended from the elbow for a period of 5 to 10 minutes or until the fragments disimpact.
3. After disimpaction and with continuing traction, apply dorsal pressure over the distal fragment(s) with the thumbs, and apply volar pressure over the proximal segments with the fingers (Fig. 7.56*B*). With the thenar eminence of the physician's hand applied over the fracture site, position the fragment in an ulnar and volar direction to achieve the proper positioning (Fig. 7.56*C*). When proper positioning has been achieved, remove the traction weight.
4. Immobilize the forearm in a position of slight supination or midposition with the wrist at 15 degrees of flexion and with 20 degrees of ulnar deviation. Some orthopedic surgeons prefer to immobilize the patient in pronation. The position of the forearm is controversial and, before treatment is undertaken, we recommend consultation with the orthopedic surgeon who is to monitor the patient.
5. Wrap the forearm in one layer of Webril, followed by the application of an anterior–posterior long-arm splint, sugar-tong splint to the forearm, or short-arm cast. Use short-arm splints under the following circumstances:
   a. Impacted fracture for which reduction is not necessary.
   b. Stable fracture in the elderly patient who needs to maintain mobility of the ipsilateral elbow, whether or not reduction of the Colles' fracture is needed.

NOTE

If reduction must be performed as indicated earlier, it is best to place the patient, especially children, in a long-arm cast.

Displaced Surgical Neck Fractures of the Humerus (1)

The emergency management of these fractures includes immobilization, ice, analgesics, and emergency referral. If emergency referral is not available in a situation of limb-threatening vascular compromise, perform reduction by the following method:

1. Adequate analgesia for this reduction is best provided under general anesthesia; however, intravenous narcotic analgesics or a high axillary nerve block may be used in the emergency center. With the patient lying supine, apply steady downward traction to the arm along the long axis of the humerus with the elbow flexed completely (Fig. 7.57*A*).

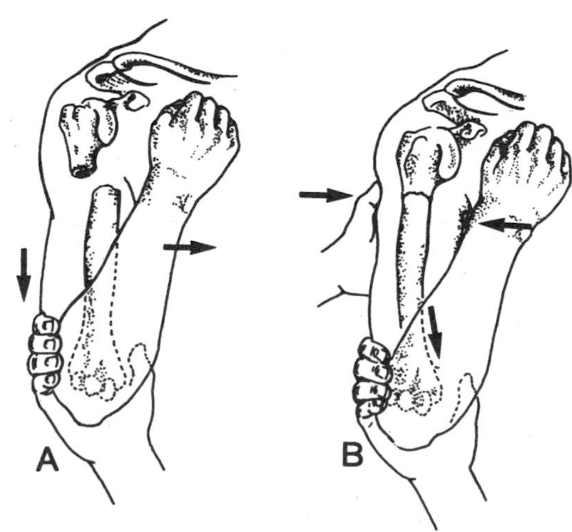

Figure 7.57. The reduction of a displaced surgical neck fracture of the humerus. See text for discussion.

2. While maintaining traction, abduct the arm across the anterior chest and slightly flex it.
3. While traction is maintained at the elbow, place the physician's other hand around the arm just distal to the fracture site along the medial border of the humerus, as shown in Fig. 7.57*B*. Manipulate the fragments manually back into position with lateral forces directed by the physician's fingers, and gradually release the traction.
4. Document a complete neurovascular examination before and after any attempt at a manipulative reduction. Then apply a sling and swathe dressing, or use a stockinette valpeau and swathe in situations in which there is an unstable fracture of the proximal humerus that has a tendency to displace because of contraction of the pectoralis major muscle. This position allows relaxation of the pectoralis major. Use a sugar-tong splint of the arm to aid in stabilization of the fracture in its proper position, and refer the patient to an orthopedic surgeon.

Supracondylar Fractures of the Distal Humerus (2, 3, 10, 11, 53, 61)

Supracondylar fractures of the distal humerus are seen often in children and less commonly in the adult. The acute problem in the initial management of these fractures is to ascertain if there is any impingement on the brachial artery from the displaced fracture fragments (Fig. 7.58). Assess the neurovascular status of the patient before any attempt at reduction. An experienced physician should be the one to attempt the reduction of these fractures especially when vascular compromise is in question. When vascular compromise is not a problem, give the patient a splint and have an orthopedic surgeon perform emergency reduction to avoid the delayed complications of ischemic contracture of the distal extremity. When reduction must be performed by the

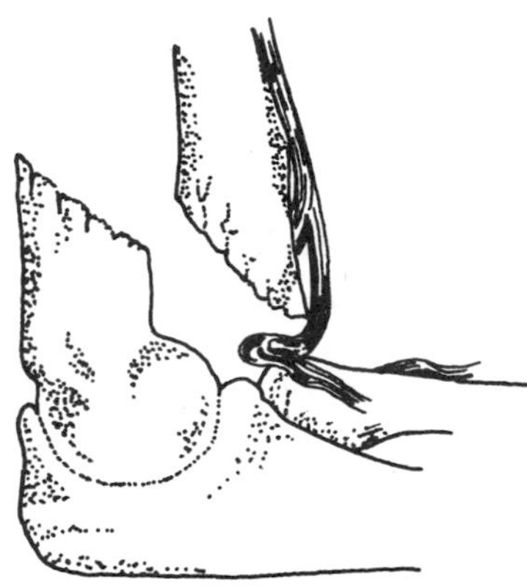

Figure 7.58. Supracondylar fracture of the distal humerus with brachial artery entrapment by the displaced fracture fragments.

emergency physician, the technique is as follows (the procedure must be performed in a two-stage maneuver, and these stages are described separately):

1. Use either an axillary nerve block or a regional Bier block to provide analgesia in reducing these fractures (described in Chapter 3, Anesthesia and Regional Blocks).
2. The initial maneuver in reducing these fractures involves extension of the elbow and distal traction on the wrist to disimpact the fracture fragments while an assistant applies proximal countertraction on the upper arm (Fig. 7.59*A*). After the fracture fragments are disimpacted, use the physician's opposite hand to mold the distal segment into its proper alignment with the proximal segment, as shown in Fig. 7.59*A*.
3. The second stage in reducing these fractures involves flexion of the elbow with forearm held in supination at the wrist and posteriorly applied pressure to the distal segment applied with the fingers of the opposite hand of the physician, as shown in Fig. 7.59*B*. This displaces the previously disimpacted distal fragment anteriorly into its proper position. Finally, with the thumb of the physician's opposite hand applying a medially directed

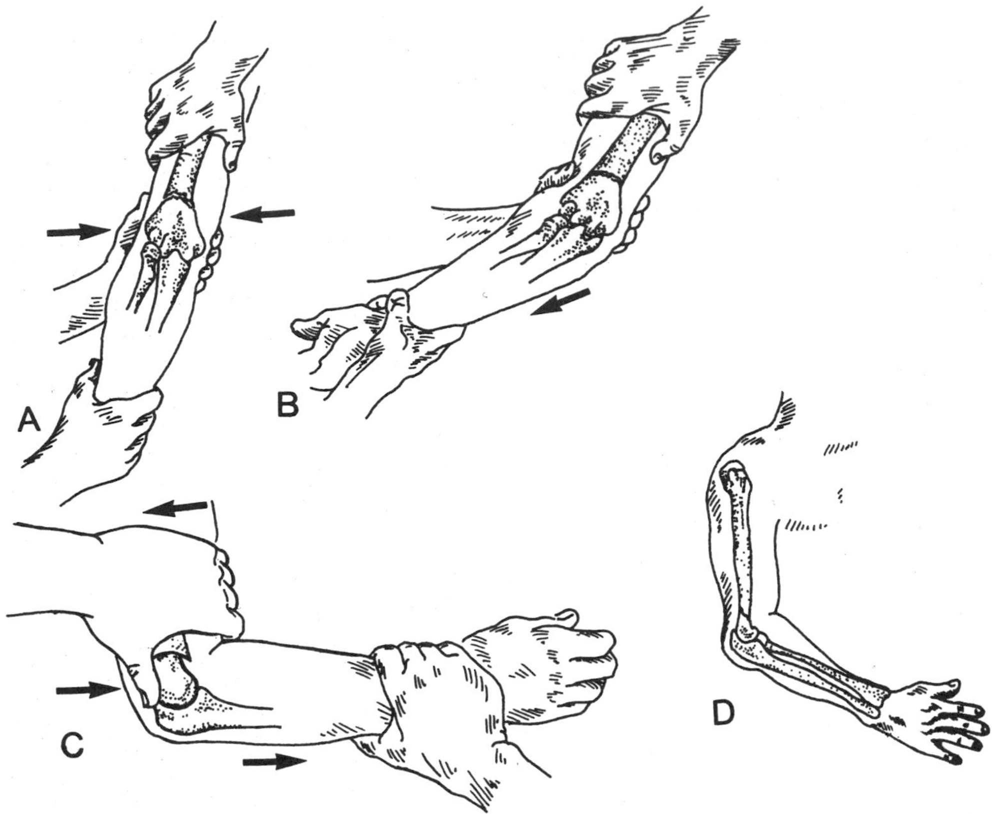

Figure 7.59. The reduction of a displaced supracondylar fracture of the humerus. See text for discussion.

force to the distal fragment of the humerus and the fingers wrapped around the proximal humerus (Fig. 7.59*C*), maneuver the distal fragment into its final position.

Place the patient in anterior and posterior long-arm splints. All these patients should be admitted to the hospital for observation for any evidence of delayed vascular complications.

REDUCTION OF SELECTED COMMON DISLOCATIONS

Anterior Dislocations of the Glenohumeral Joint (37, 49, 50)

An anterior shoulder dislocation is one of the most common problems in the emergency center and represents approximately 50% of all major joint dislocations seen by the emergency physician. The mechanism by which this injury occurs is usually abduction accompanied by external rotation of the arm, which disrupts the anterior capsule and the glenohumeral ligaments. A detailed description of this problem is beyond the scope of this chapter; however, emergency physicians always should examine the function of the axillary nerve before any attempt at reduction because this nerve is commonly injured in anterior dislocations (4). Assess this nerve by testing sensation to pinprick or two-point discrimination over the lateral aspect of the deltoid and comparing it with sensation on the uninjured side. In addition, evaluate the radial, ulnar, and brachial pulses as well as the integrity of the median, ulnar, and radial nerves.

There are many methods of reducing anterior dislocations of the shoulder, several of which are discussed. Administer intravenous narcotics and muscle relaxants before any attempt at reduction. Keep bag–mask, oral airway, and naloxone (0.4 mg), a narcotic antagonist, at the bedside of these patients so that any marked respiratory depression can be managed easily. Muscle relaxation is crucial in any attempt at reducing an anterior shoulder dislocation that cannot be reduced by the first technique described later. An alternate method of providing analgesia is by suprascapular nerve block; however, this is not commonly used. The techniques listed are in order of our preference. The least manipulative maneuvers are first attempted; if these are unsuccessful, go on to the other methods.

HENNEPIN TECHNIQUE (40)

This technique requires little manipulation and is safe. It has been studied and found to require no anesthetic and to have a high success rate (39, 40, 42). The technique requires gentle, steady external rotation of the shoulder. This is done over several minutes. Tell the patient to relax as you progressively externally rotate the shoulder with the elbow flexed. This brings the humeral head out from under the glenoid rim. After external rotation to 90 degrees, reduction is often achieved. If this does not occur, abduct the arm while it is held at 90 degrees of external rotation. During abduction, reduction is usually achieved (Fig. 7.60). This technique is preferred for reduction of anterior shoulder dislocations. The key point in using this technique is to be certain that the muscles are relaxed. It may be necessary to administer a sedative or analgesic intravenously while performing the maneuver. Often, the physician can talk to the patient and relax him or her. Remember not to force external rotation. This should be done slowly and gently, stopping intermittently whenever pain occurs. In performing the technique for shoulder reduction, follow the steps indicated in Fig. 7.60. Gently externally rotate the arm with the elbow at 90 degrees flexion while providing minimal traction in line with the humerus (Fig. 7.60*A*, *B*). The rotation must be done gradually, stopping whenever minimal pain occurs. This may take several minutes. Once the arm is rotated, so that the hand is in the same plane as the torso (Fig. 7.60*C*), continue traction on the elbow. Reduction will usually occur at this point. If reduction occurs, elevate the arm as shown in Fig. 7.60*D*. If it does not, use another technique described later.

STIMSON TECHNIQUE (59)

The Stimson technique is a safe procedure and an excellent choice in attempting to reduce an anterior dislocation of the shoulder. Place the patient in the prone position with the arm dependent and a pillow or folded sheet placed under the shoulder (Fig. 7.61). Apply a strap to the wrist or distal forearm and suspend weights (from 10 to 15 pounds) over a period of 20 to 30 minutes. This time period usually is sufficient for reduction to occur. Muscle relaxation is imperative, and the patient must be under constant observation for monitoring of the respiratory status and pulse. Twenty to 30 minutes is usually a sufficient amount of time for displacement of the humeral head, after which either a spontaneous reduction will occur or the examiner may rotate the humerus gently, externally and then internally, with mild traction; this usually reduces the dislocation.

TRACTION AND COUNTERTRACTION (47)

This method has been advocated for those anterior dislocations that are difficult to reduce by the Stimson technique. In this method, an assistant applies coun-

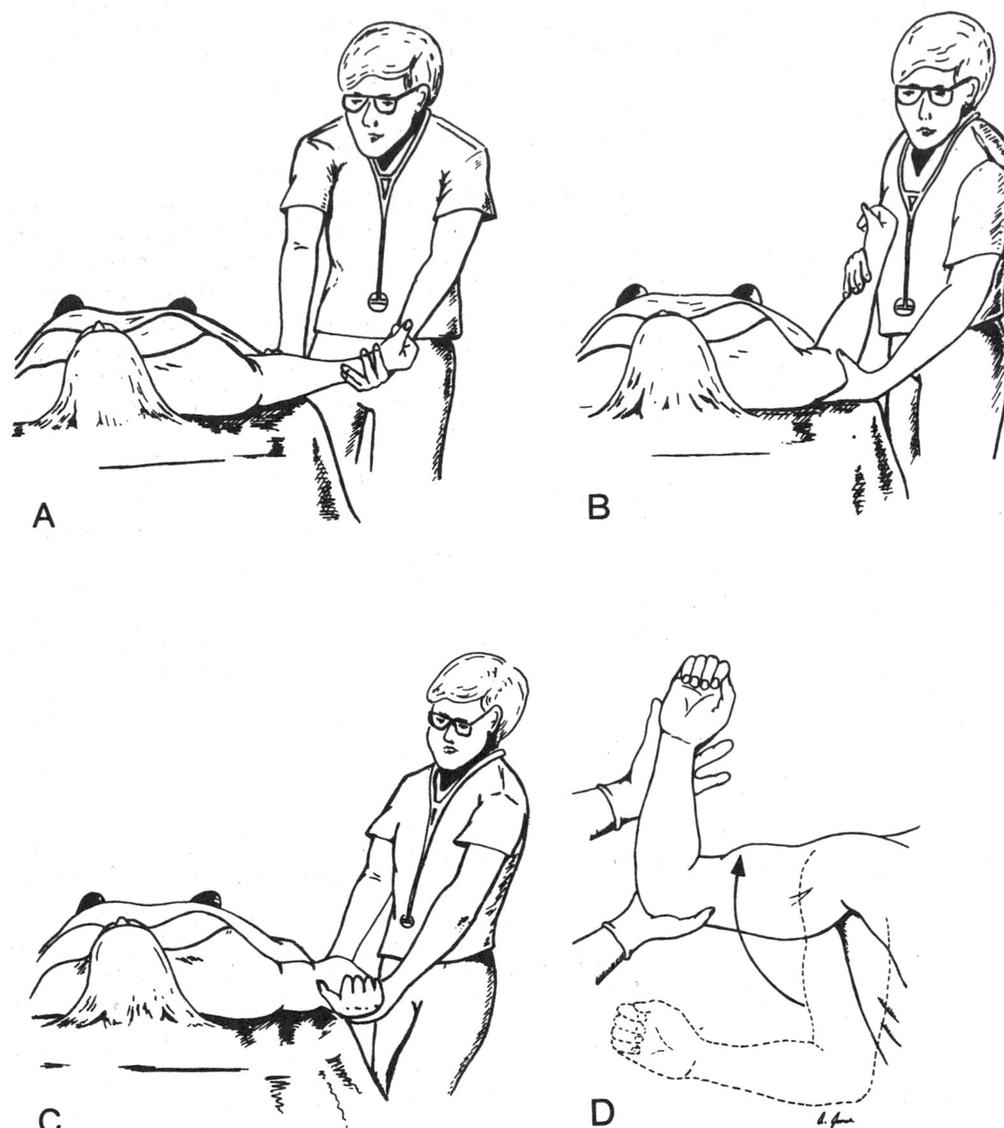

Figure 7.60. The Hennepin technique for reducing anterior shoulder dislocations. *A*: Place the patient supine with the elbow bent at 90 degrees; gently pull the elbow inferiorly. *B*: Gently rotate the arm outward (with the elbow bent) in small incremental stages, pausing whenever the patient experiences even minimal pain. Once the arm is at 90 degrees external rotation, the shoulder will usually reduce at this point *(C)*. If reduction occurs, elevate the arm as shown in *D*.

tertraction with a folded sheet wrapped around the upper chest, as shown in Fig. 7.62, and the examiner applies traction to the arm. This maneuver usually dislodges the humeral head, and slight lateral traction on the proximal humerus usually reduces the dislocation.

TRACTION WITH LATERAL TRACTION (47)

This maneuver is similar to the previous one; however, in addition to traction along the longitudinal axis of the humerus, lateral traction also is applied to the proximal humerus after disimpaction of the

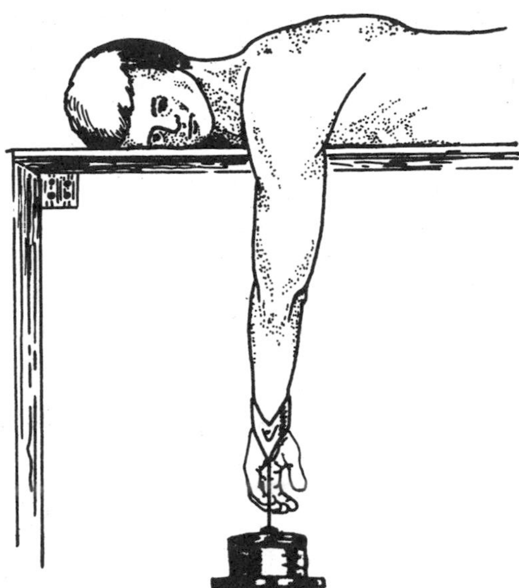

Figure 7.61. The Stimson technique for reduction an anterior shoulder dislocation.

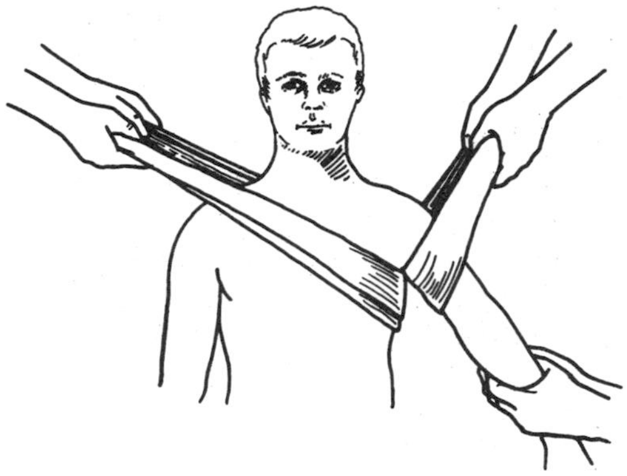

Figure 7.63. In reducing a difficult dislocation of the glenohumeral joint, apply traction on the forearm while an assistant applies countertraction by using a sheet that encircles the chest. This traction and countertraction disimpacts the humeral head from under the glenoid rim. Next, apply lateral traction by using a pillowcase around the upper portion of the arm as shown. Remember not to apply lateral traction until the humeral head is disengaged, which can be determined by slight elongation of the arm during traction and countertraction.

humeral head is achieved by the former procedure. The lateral traction is provided by an assistant with a pillowcase folded and wrapped around the proximal humerus as shown in Fig. 7.63. It is important that lateral traction not be applied until the humerus is disimpacted from under the glenoid. To prevent avulsion injuries during the reduction, the patient must have good muscle relaxation when this maneuver is used.

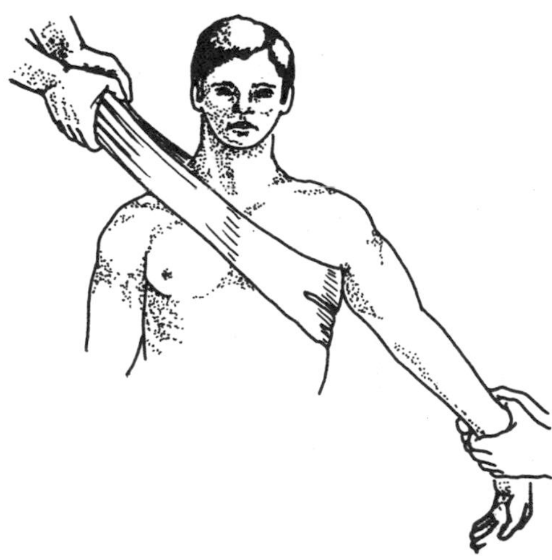

Figure 7.62. The traction and countertraction technique for reducing an anterior shoulder dislocation. This technique is preferred by many. It has the advantage of being quicker than the Stimson technique and is a safe procedure.

KOCHER MANEUVER (27, 32)

This maneuver is quite dangerous, is fraught with many complications, and should not be used by the emergency physician in reducing anterior dislocations of the shoulder. In our opinion, the Hippocratic technique (foot in axilla) also should not be used under any circumstances in reducing these dislocations. If the methods described earlier prove ineffectual in reducing the dislocation, then consider general anesthesia and reduction in the operating room. Irreducible dislocations are usually due to soft tissue interposition.

AFTERCARE

In patients younger than 40 years, we advocate the use of a sling and swathe or a shoulder immobilizer for a period of 3 weeks after reduction. In patients older than 40 years, we advocate the use of a sling and swathe for a period of 1 week with range-of-motion exercises (avoiding abduction and external rotation) to begin within 4 or 5 days after the injury. Once healing occurs, use an exercise program to strengthen the subscapularis muscle to prevent recurrences.

Luxatio Erecta (35, 55)

This is an unusual dislocation in which the humeral head is dislocated inferior to the glenoid. It occurs when the arm is abducted to 180 degrees. The patient presents with the arm raised directly over the head. Reduction is accomplished by applying traction to the arm in line with the deformity, followed by rotation through a 180-degree arc and bringing the arm back to the patient's side.

Sternoclavicular Dislocations (13, 51)

The sternoclavicular joint is stabilized by the sternoclavicular and the costoclavicular ligaments. Complete rupture of these two ligaments permits the clavicle to dislocate from its manubrial attachment. Dislocations at this joint are either anterior or posterior; by far the most common is the anterior dislocation. Posterior dislocations, although uncommon, may be life-threatening emergencies as a result of airway or vascular compromise from the posteriorly displaced clavicle impinging on the trachea. Patients with a posterior dislocation may have breathing difficulties secondary to tracheal compression or tracheal rupture. Posterior dislocations occur with serious vascular and pulmonary complications, including pneumothorax, laceration of the superior vena cava, and occlusion of the subclavian artery or vein. Approximately 25% of all posterior dislocations of the sternoclavicular joint are associated with tracheal, esophageal, or great vessel injury, which demonstrates the need for early reduction.

Dislocations are reduced as shown in Fig. 7.64. Place a folded sheet between the shoulders while the patient is in the supine position, which serves to separate the clavicle from the manubrium. Abduct the arm and apply traction by an assistant, as shown in Fig. 7.64*A*. To relocate an anterior dislocation, maintain traction on the ipsilateral arm and push the clavicle posteriorly into its normal position. In patients with a posterior dislocation, use the same maneuver; however, pull the clavicle forward while maintaining traction by

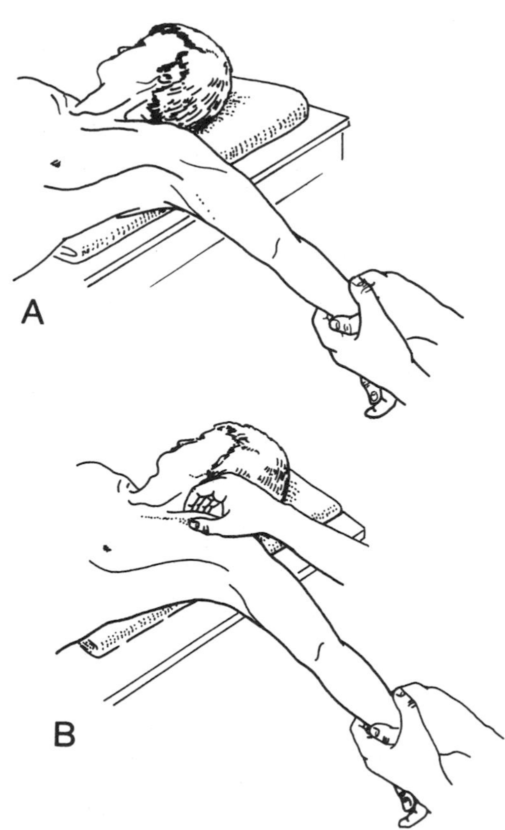

Figure 7.64. Reduction of a sternoclavicular joint dislocation. *A*: Place a folded sheet between the scapulae as shown. Then abduct the patient's arm, and apply traction. *B*: For posterior dislocation of the sternoclavicular joint, lift the clavicle back into its normal position. Use a towel clip if necessary to grab the clavicle and lift it anteriorly. For anterior dislocations, reduce the clavicle back into its normal position by applying posteriorly directed pressure over it.

grasping it as shown in Fig. 7.64*B*. In more difficult situations in which the clavicle may not be grasped with the examiner's fingers, use a towel clip to encircle the clavicle and apply traction in an anterior direction in a manner similar to that indicated earlier.

Dislocations of the Elbow (29, 30)

Elbow dislocations are among the most commonly seen dislocations of the body, second in frequency only to dislocations of the shoulder and the fingers. Posterior dislocations, in which the ulnar olecranon is displaced posteriorly in relation to the distal humerus, account for the majority of dislocations of the elbow. Anterior dislocations are far less common. With prolonged delays in reducing these injuries, the articular cartilage is damaged and swelling increases, which may cause circulatory compromise.

Accomplish reduction after administering an analgesic and a muscle relaxant. The best technique for reducing an elbow dislocation is a modified Stimson technique, as shown in Fig. 7.65. Place the patient in the prone position, always being careful that the airway and breathing are maintained after giving muscle relaxants and analgesics. Hang the elbow over the side of the bed with a folded sheet underneath the arm as shown. Weights (5 to 7 lb) are applied either by using a bucket strapped to the wrist or some other method, and reduction will ensue within 10 to 15 minutes. This technique is safe and requires minimal manipulation, so that hyperextension injuries do not occur, as with other techniques previously used. In addition, there is little risk of coronoid process fractures, which occur with more manipulative techniques.

Always assess the ulnar and radial collateral ligaments of the elbow for their integrity after reduction. These ligaments are commonly injured in dislocations and sprains of the elbow. Use a valgus and varus stress test of these ligaments to assess their integrity.

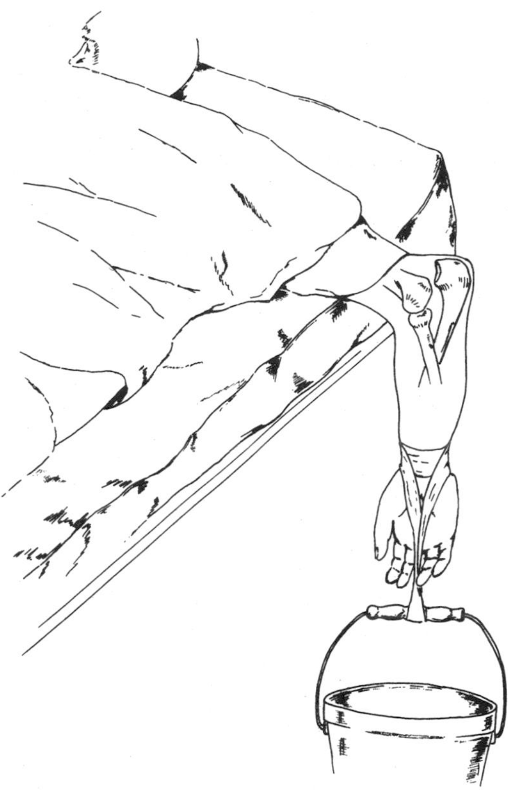

Figure 7.65. Reduce a posterior dislocation of the elbow best by a modified Stimson technique, in which the patient lies prone, with the arm hanging alongside the bed. Attach weights to the wrist as shown, and give the patient the appropriate muscle relaxants and analgesics. Over a period of 10 to 20 minutes, the posterior dislocation will reduce.

Subluxation of the Radial Head in Children

This is a common injury in children between the ages of 2 and 5 years. In children there is little structural support between the radius and the humerus; with sudden traction on the hand or forearm, such as occurs when a parent pulls a child up by the arm to prevent a fall, the annular ligament that attaches the radius to the humerus is pulled over the radial head and lies between it and the capitulum.

To reduce the subluxation, apply direct pressure with the thumb over the forearm in the region of the radial head and slowly supinate and extend the elbow, as shown

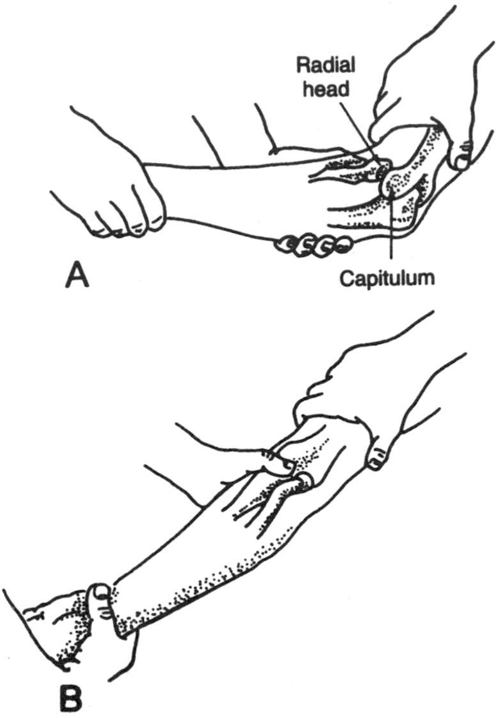

Figure 7.66. Reduction of a subluxation of the radial head in children. *A*: Apply direct pressure with the thumb over the displaced radial head. *B*: At the same time, distract and supinate the forearm with the right hand while extending the elbow. Usually a "pop" or a "snap" is palpable when the radial head reduces into its normal position.

in Fig. 7.66. A sudden release of resistance accompanied by a definite click signifies reduction. Take roentgenograms before any attempt at reduction. Then place older patients in a forearm sling for 1 week. Younger children are difficult to keep in a sling for any period, so do not apply slings in the young child.

Dislocations of the Interphalangeal Joints of the Hand

Dislocations of the proximal and distal interphalangeal joints of the hand are commonly seen in the emergency center and generally are easily reduced. Most dislocations of this joint are posterior dislocations, and the proximal interphalangeal joint is more commonly involved than the distal.

Provide analgesia by block of the metacarpal or digital nerve to the involved digit. After this, apply traction longitudinally in the line of the deformity to distract the articular surfaces of the involved joint. Then apply hyperextension to permit alignment of the articular surfaces, which is followed by flexion of the joint; this accomplishes reduction. After reduction, examine the collateral ligaments by stress tests to ascertain if there is complete rupture. Splint the involved digit in a volar or dorsal finger splint, and monitor the patient. However, if there is complete destruction of the ligaments with instability, use a gutter splint. Dislocations involving the thumb are often difficult to reduce because of entrapment of the volar plate or sesamoids, making this a complex dislocation that requires operative reduction. In attempting to reduce any interphalangeal or metacarpophalangeal joint dislocation involving the hand or foot and when failing after two attempts at reduction under good anesthesia, suspect a complex dislocation entrapping soft tissue in the joint.

Hip Dislocations (12, 60)

Hip dislocations require large forces and are frequently associated with acetabular fractures or ipsilateral extremity injuries. All hip dislocations must be regarded as true emergencies and must be reduced early to minimize the incidence of avascular necrosis of the femoral head. Posterior dislocations are far more common than are anterior dislocations. Anterior dislocations of the hip are best managed with early reduction under spinal or general anesthesia. Open reduction is indicated if attempts at closed reduction fail. We strongly recommend emergency referral for reduction. Manage posterior dislocations with immobilization and emergency referral for reduction. If the emergency referral is not available, attempt closed reduction with the following method:

1. Place the patient on a backboard and give intravenous muscle relaxants (diazepam; Valium) and narcotic analgesics for skeletal muscle relaxation and pain relief.
2. Lower the patient to the floor on the backboard, where an assistant immobilizes the pelvis as demonstrated in Fig. 7.67*A*.
3. Pull up on the distal calf to apply traction in line with the deformity and gently flex the knee to a position of 90 degrees (Fig. 7.67*B*).
4. At this point, gentle but firm pulling of the hip anteriorly by upward traction on the flexed calf with slight external rotation will result in reduction in most cases. If this is unsuccessful, perform reduction under general anesthesia. If reduction is successful, admit the patient for traction, strict non–weight bearing, and observation.

Stimson's method for reducing posterior hip dislocations (55) is shown in Fig. 7.68. This method also may be used; however, our experience indicates a lower success rate with this method than with the technique described earlier.

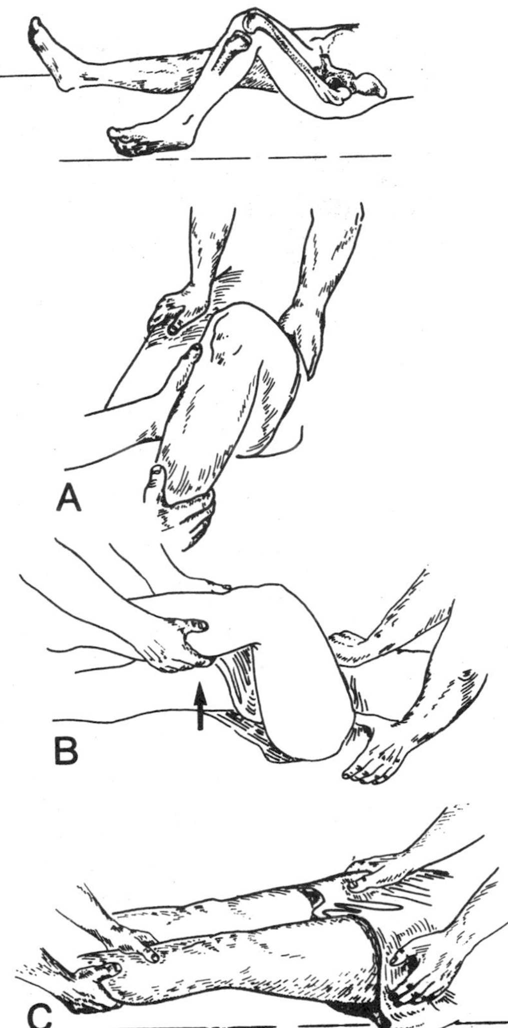

Figure 7.67. The reduction of a posterior hip dislocation. *A*: Lower the patient to the floor on a backboard while an assistant immobilizes the pelvis as shown. *B*: Then stabilize the patient's foot against the thigh and gently but steadily lift the flexed knee superiorly as shown with slight external rotation. *C*: After reduction, extend the hip into its normal position.

Dislocations of the Knee (25, 28, 52)

Dislocations of the knee are a true orthopedic emergency because a high incidence of popliteal artery compromise is associated with these injuries. Both anterior and posterior dislocations of the knee must be immediately reduced, and a follow-up arteriogram to examine the integrity of the popliteal artery must be performed. A neurovascular assessment should be done before any attempt is made to manipulate this injury. Posterior dislocations appear to be less common than are anterior dislocations.

In reducing these dislocations, apply traction longitudinally in the line of the deformity to the involved extended knee while an assistant applies countertraction above the knee, as shown in Fig. 7.69*A*. In posterior dislocations, after disengagement of the articular surfaces and with

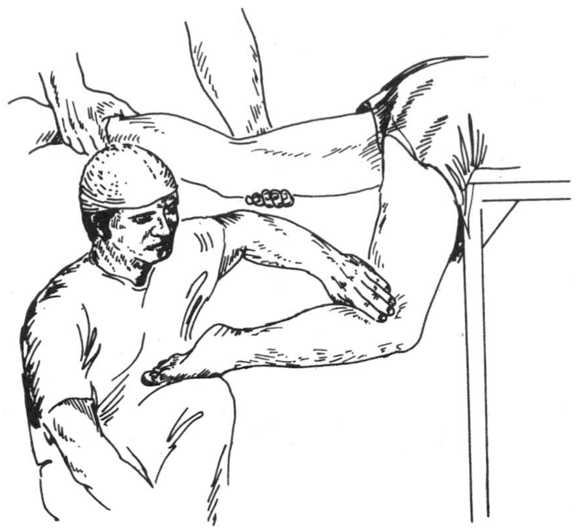

Figure 7.68. The Stimson method for reducing posterior hip dislocations. Place the patient in a prone position, and apply pressure to the flexed knee directly downward, with the foot held against the examiner's knee as shown. An assistant holds the opposite leg in extension.

traction maintained, rotate the hand to the undersurface of the tibia and displace it anteriorly into its normal position (Fig. 7.69*B*). Reduction of this fracture is generally performed without much difficulty; however, the incidence of associated complications due to the injury itself is extremely high.

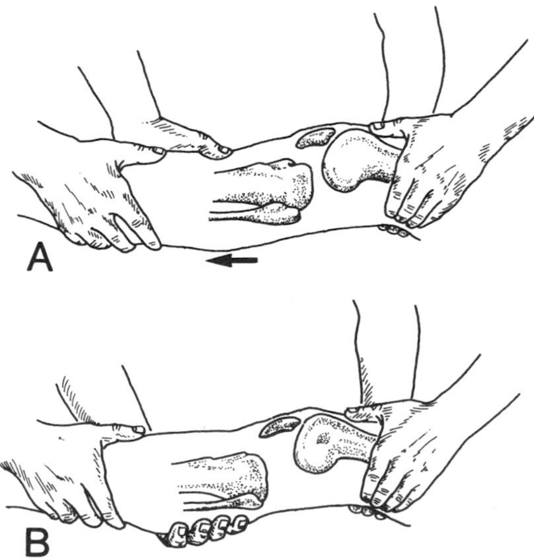

Figure 7.69. The reduction of a dislocation of the knee. *A*: Stabilize the femur proximally, and pull the leg inferiorly. *B*: After traction, lift the knee, which is posteriorly dislocated, back into its anatomic position.

Dislocations of the Ankle

There are four types of ankle dislocations: posterior, anterior, lateral, and superior (Fig. 7.70). The most common dislocation seen in the emergency department is the lateral dislocation. For all injuries, it is important to assess vascular integrity immediately, and obtain radiographs before attempting reduction. Once the dislocation is reduced, apply a posterior splint.

The posterior dislocation is commonly associated with a fracture of one or both malleoli. The mechanism of injury is a strong force applied to the posterior tibia in a posterior to anterior direction (9). The ankle is usually plantarflexed when the force is applied. On presentation, the foot is plantar flexed, and the leg is shortened. Achieve reduction by pulling the foot forward while maintaining the ankle plantarflexed (Fig. 7.71). Aftercare includes referral to an orthopedist for capsular tears, and fractures are often surgically repaired.

An anterior dislocation is almost always associated with a fracture of the anterior lip of the tibia. The mechanism causing this injury is usually a force that results in posterior displacement of the tibia on the fixed foot or forcible dorsiflexion of the foot (i.e., a fall on the heel with the foot dorsiflexed). The patient has the foot held

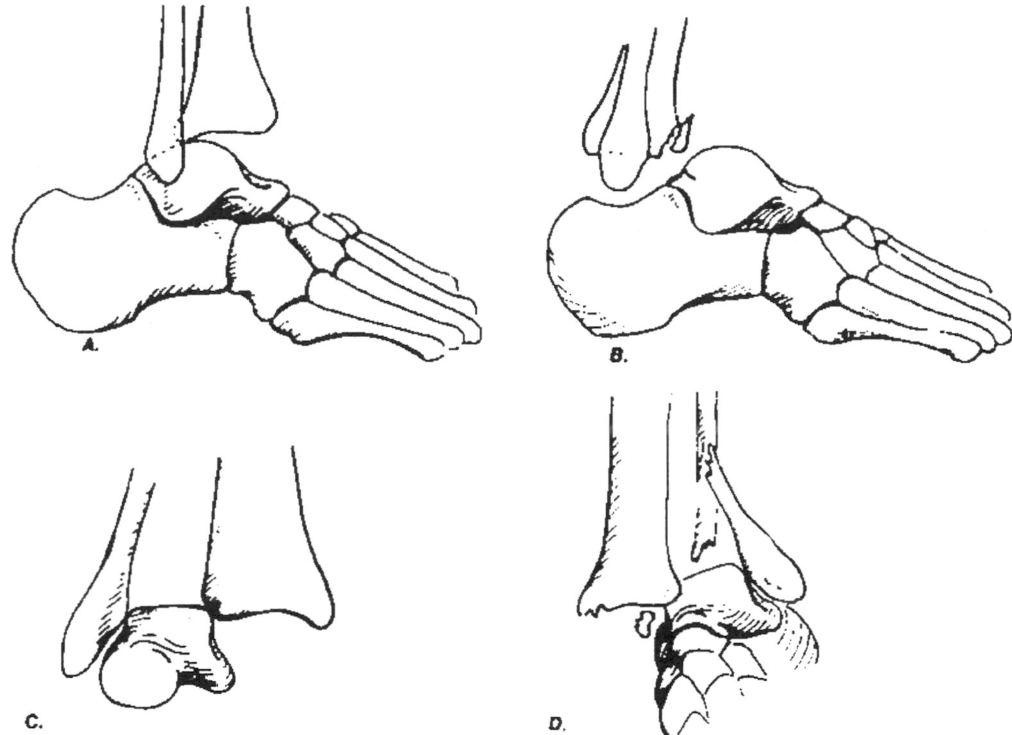

Figure 7.70. Four types of ankle dislocations. *A*: Posterior. *B*: Anterior. *C*: Superior ("diastasis"). *D*: Lateral. (From Simon RR, Koenigsknecht SJ: Emergency Orthopedics: The Extremities. New York: McGraw-Hill, 521, 2000, with permission.)

in dorsiflexion and lengthened. Moreover, the supporting ligaments and capsule are disrupted. A fracture of the malleoli also is commonly seen. Reduction is accomplished by dorsiflexing the foot slightly to disengage the talus and pushing the foot posteriorly back into position.

Superior dislocations (diastasis) are uncommon injuries but are often associated with articular damage. These cases require emergency consultation with an orthopedist.

The lateral dislocation is the most commonly seen in the emergency department and is always associated with fractures of the malleoli or distal fibula. On presentation, an obvious deformity is seen, with the foot being laterally displaced. In addition, the skin is taut over the medial aspect of the ankle. Associated injuries include a fracture of the medial malleolus or, less commonly, rupture of the deltoid ligament. Reduction of this dislocation is relatively simple but requires two people. One person applies longitudinal traction on the foot with one hand on the heel and the other hand on the dorsum of the foot, while another person applies countertraction to the leg. Gentle medial manipulation is required with the talus regaining normal position with little difficulty (Fig. 7.72).

Patellar Dislocations (18, 26, 44)

Patellar dislocations are commonly seen in the emergency center. The knee is at 20 to 30 degrees of flexion, and the patella usually is laterally displaced. The laterally dislocated patella is reduced by extending the knee while applying medially directed pressure over the patella to

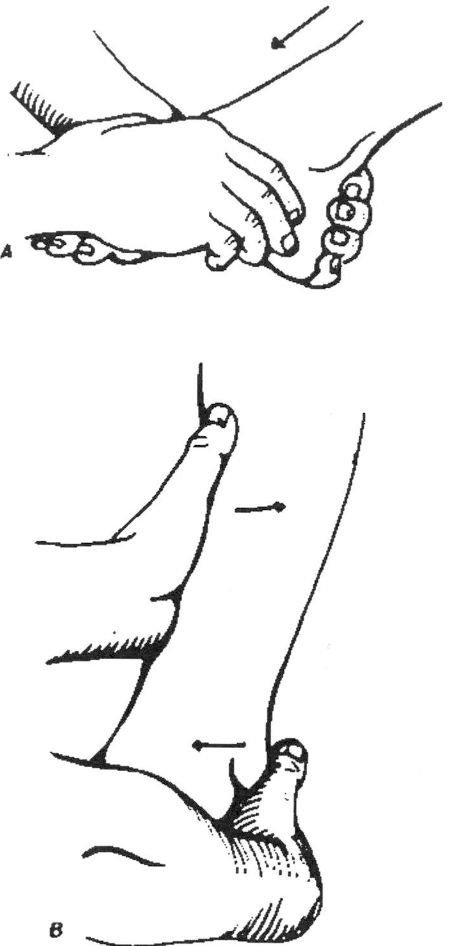

Figure 7.71. Reduction technique for a posterior dislocation. (From Simon RR, Koenigsknecht SJ: Emergency Orthopedics: The Extremities. New York: McGraw-Hill, 523, 2000, with permission.)

reposition it. This is done as a single maneuver. Patellar dislocations frequently relocate spontaneously before the patient arrives at the emergency center.

INJECTION AND ASPIRATION OF SELECTED SOFT TISSUE DISORDERS

De Quervain's Stenosing Tenosynovitis

This condition involves the abductor pollicis longus and extensor pollicis brevis tendons of the first dorsal wrist compartment. The pathognomic test, called "Finkelstein's test," which reproduces the pain, is performed by holding the patient's thumb in the palm with the remaining four digits covering it and having the patient make a fist with ulnar deviation of the wrist. Treat this form of tendonitis with the injection of steroids (triamcinolone, 10 mg) along the tendon sheath, as shown in Fig. 7.73. Place the needle along the tendon and not perpendicularly into the tendon. Install bupivacaine (Marcaine) and a steroid (triamcinolone, 10 mg) along the tendon sheath, which generally provides good relief. Surgical intervention may be required if the condition progresses.

Tennis Elbow

Tennis elbow is an undifferentiated term denoting radiohumeral bursitis or lateral epicondylitis of the humerus. The major feature of this syndrome is the localization of the tenderness over the prominence of the lateral epicondyle of the humerus (7). Certain severe cases of tennis elbow may require steroid injections. The landmark selected for this injection is the lateral epicondyle. Flex the patient's elbow when the steroid is injected (38). Perform the injection in the posterolateral direction and toward the lateral epicondyle. Insert the needle laterally along the condylar ridge of the humerus and direct it toward the lateral epicondyle. Inject the steroid at multiple sites at this point. Use a total of 20 mg of triamcinolone along with bupivacaine. Often multiple injections are necessary.

Olecranon Bursitis

The subcutaneous tissue superficial to the olecranon does not communicate with the elbow joint and presents no problems for arthrocentesis, because when it is distended, the entire extent of the bursa can be noted subcutaneously from the posterior aspect. Insert the needle from the posterior aspect perpendicularly through the skin and subcutaneous tissue and into the

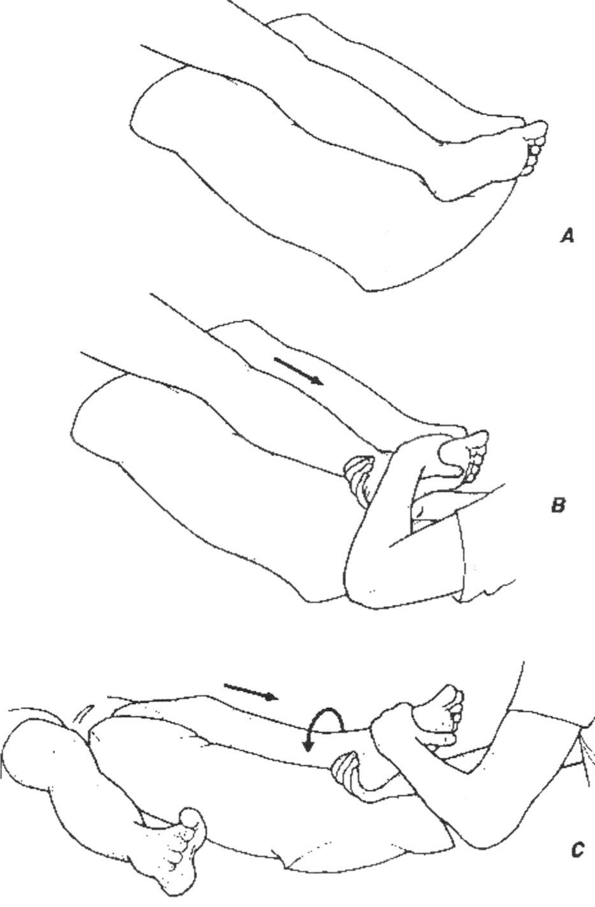

Figure 7.72. Lateral dislocation of the ankle. *A*: The typical position of a lateral ankle dislocation. *B*: The application of distal traction to the plantar-flexed foot. *C*: To reduce the dislocation, return the foot to its proper anatomic position while maintaining distal traction of the foot. This maneuver usually produces a palpable "thud." (From Simon RR, Koenigsknecht SJ: Emergency Orthopedics: The Extremities. New York: McGraw-Hill, 524, 2000, with permission.)

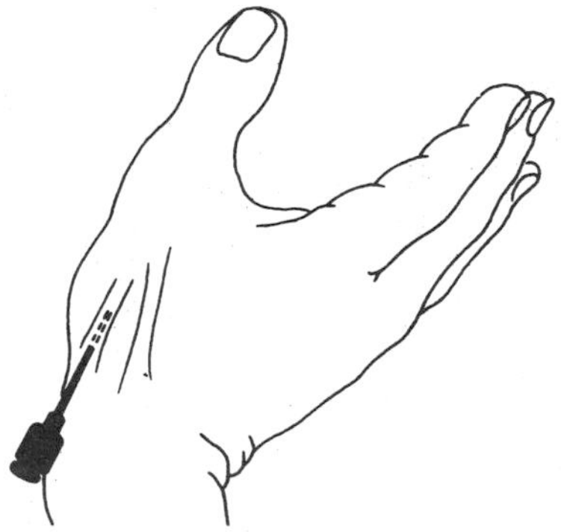

olecranon bursa. The indications for aspiration of the olecranon bursa are suspicion of septic bursitis and, in some cases, of chronic recurrent effusions within that bursa (38).

Figure 7.73. The injection into a tenosynovitis of the abductor pollicis tendon.

Subdeltoid Bursitis or Supraspinous Tendonitis

The optimal injection site for patients with subdeltoid bursitis or supraspinous tendonitis is at the point of maximal tenderness elicited on palpation beneath the acromial process (Fig. 7.74) (39). The anterior tip of the acromion is immediately adjacent to the subacromial bursa and is an ideal bony landmark that serves as a guide for injection or aspiration of this bursa. With the arm distracted downward

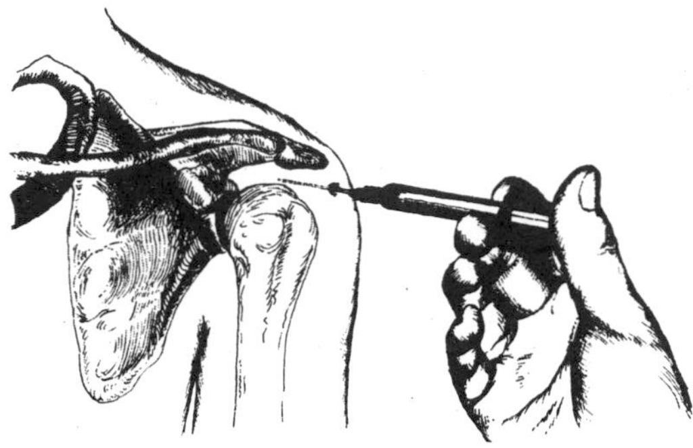

Figure 7.74. Injection into subdeltoid bursitis or supraspinatus tendonitis. The point of maximal tenderness is beneath the acromion and above the greater tuberosity. Perform the injection with multiple needle sticks into the bursa to release pressure.

to increase the separation between the bursa and the acromion of the shoulder joint, insert a needle just inferior to the acromion, and it usually enters the bursa. The lateral approach is preferred to the anterior approach to avoid the cephalic vein, as seen in Fig. 7.72 (38). Multiple needle punctures aid in relieving pressure from within the bursa. Then inject the steroid and anesthetic.

Stenosing Tenosynovitis

The flexor tendon sheath of the fingers or thumb is usually involved in this condition. The site of predilection in the sheaths is over the palmar aspect of the metacarpal heads. Localization is made easier if the patient slowly flexes the involved digit until a "snapping" of a trigger finger occurs. The site of injection for pain relief is slightly proximal to the point of tenderness. Ask the patient to gently flex and extend the finger, and then attempt to engage the injection site with the needle tip, and inject a small amount of steroid (58). Deposit the solution in the sheath and not in the tendon.

Bicipital Tendonitis

Bicipital tendonitis is a common condition in the emergency center and must be distinguished from pain in the shoulder secondary to subdeltoid bursitis or supraspinous tendonitis. In patients with bicipital tendonitis, the point of maximal tenderness is in the groove between the greater and lesser tuberosities of the humerus, which contains the tendon of the long head of the biceps. Inject bupivacaine into the biceps tendon sheath to differentiate this condition from other causes of pain in the shoulder. If the procedure relieves much of the pain, this can be followed by an injection of steroids.

Ask the patient to rotate the arm externally and abduct it approximately 15 to 20 degrees. Locate the point between the greater and lesser tuberosities of the humerus (just medial to the greater tuberosity). Insert the needle from an anteromedial approach, and direct the tip toward the tendon lying within the groove between the two tuberosities. Do not inject within the tendon but rather inject in a band-like fashion along the tendon sheath (Fig. 7.75). The injection is usually followed by significant relief of pain within 10 to 15 minutes.

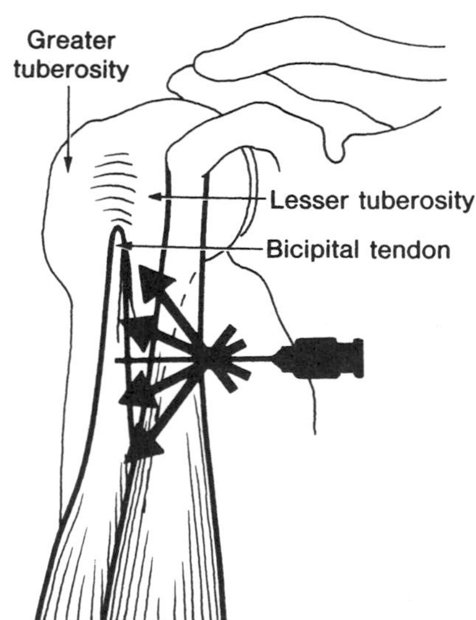

Figure 7.75. The injection into a bicipital tendonitis involves multiple needle sticks along the tendon sheath. Insert the needle at one point over the biceps tendon, and direct it along the tendon sheath.

Ingrown Nails

An ingrown nail is a common problem in the emergency center. The nail most commonly affected is that of the great toe. A number of techniques exist in dealing with this problem. Although many surgeons remove one third to one half of the involved nail, it has been our experience that this only delays healing and prolongs discomfort. Excise only the portion of the nail that is involved. Perform a digital block to provide anesthesia for the procedure (see Chapter 3, Anesthesia and Regional Blocks). A no. 11 scalpel and blade is used to make an initial incision along the nail, as shown in Fig. 7.76. Next, slide one jaw of a hemostat under the ingrown nail segment and grasp it firmly. Move this segment up and down to detach it from the nail bed and remove it (Fig. 7.76). Cauterize the underlying nail bed with phenol or use a rongeur on the nailbed and apply a dressing. Advise warm soaks if infection is present. The nail may not grow back for 9 to 12 months. With this technique, no suturing is necessary, and only a small dressing is needed.

When granulation tissue is the major problem, excise this as a wedge along with the distal corner of the nail (Fig. 7.77). A small spicule of nail is usually embedded in the granulation bed and is removed with this wedge resection of the distal corner. This prevents recurrences.

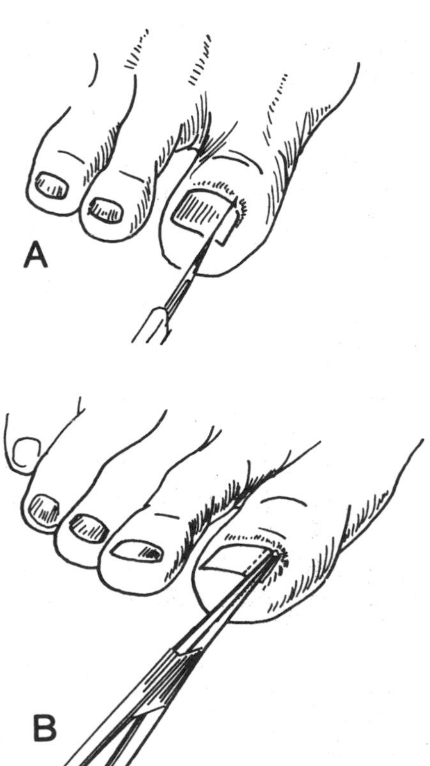

Figure 7.76. *A*: A no. 11 scalpel and blade is used to make an incision along the nail. *B*: After this, insert one jaw of a hemostat along the ingrown nail segment, and grasp the segment firmly. Then detach this segment from the base and the nail bed.

Drainage of the Paronychia and Eponychia

A paronychia is an inflammatory condition localized to the nail fold of a digit on either the ulnar or radial side. An eponychia, however, is localized to the basal

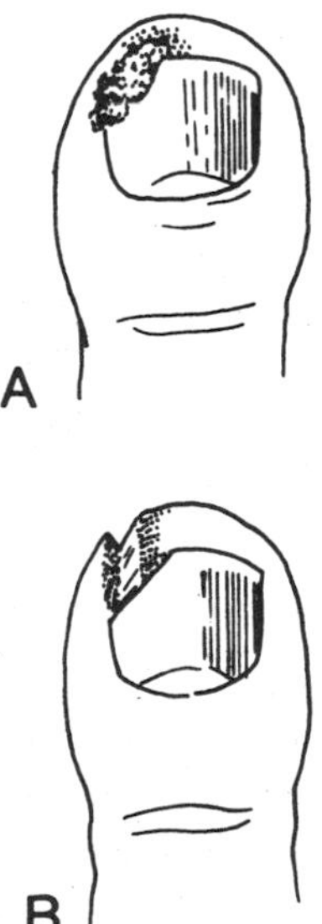

Figure 7.77. *A*: When granulation tissue covers the distal end of the nail over the ingrown segment, remove it. Beneath the granulation tissue is usually a spicule of nail that has grown into the distal nail fold. *B*: Excise a wedge from the distal segment containing the corner of the nail and granulation tissue.

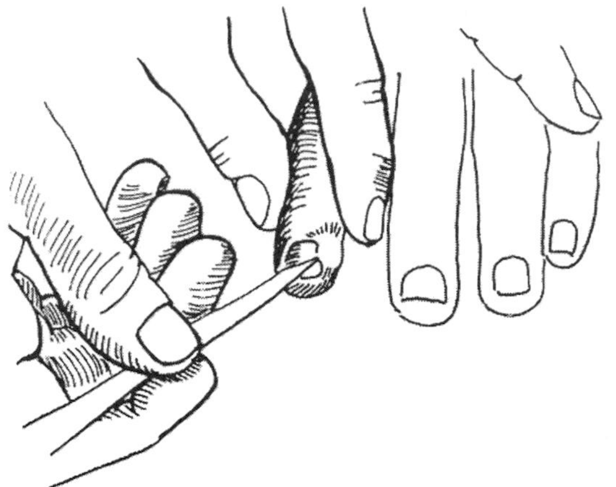

Figure 7.78. Drainage of the paronychia. (From Simon RR, Koenigsknecht SJ: Emergency Orthopedics: The Extremities. New York: McGraw-Hill, 190, 2000, with permission.)

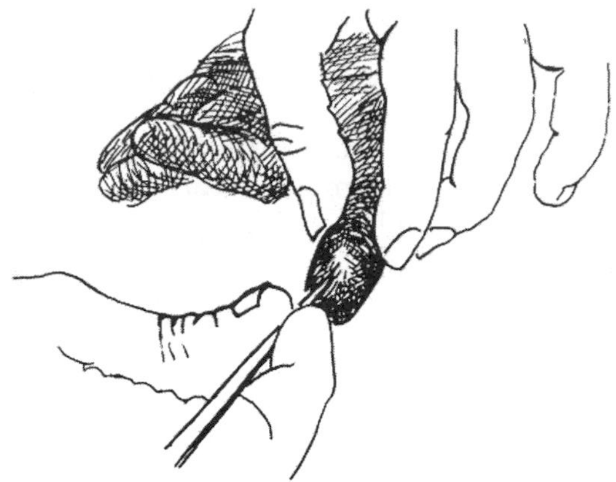

Figure 7.79. Drainage of the felon. (From Simon RR, Koenigsknecht SJ: Emergency Orthopedics: The Extremities. New York: McGraw-Hill, 191, 2000, with permission.)

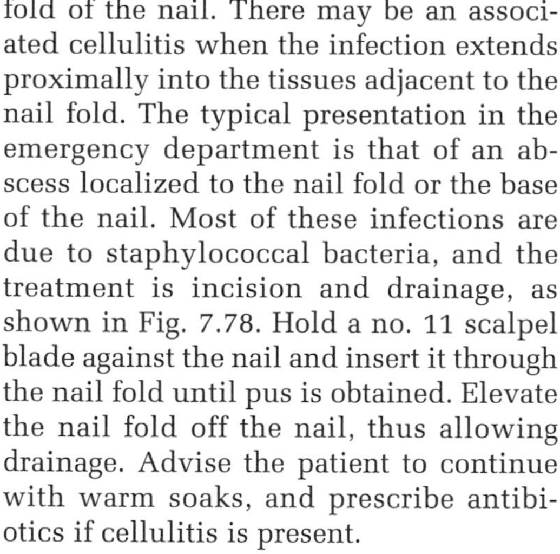

fold of the nail. There may be an associated cellulitis when the infection extends proximally into the tissues adjacent to the nail fold. The typical presentation in the emergency department is that of an abscess localized to the nail fold or the base of the nail. Most of these infections are due to staphylococcal bacteria, and the treatment is incision and drainage, as shown in Fig. 7.78. Hold a no. 11 scalpel blade against the nail and insert it through the nail fold until pus is obtained. Elevate the nail fold off the nail, thus allowing drainage. Advise the patient to continue with warm soaks, and prescribe antibiotics if cellulitis is present.

Drainage of the Felon

A felon is a pulp-space infection of the distal phalangeal region. The primary causative agent is a staphylococcus, and treatment is with incision and drainage. Insert a no. 11 blade at the point of maximal fluctuance, and extend a longitudinal midline incision, sparing the flexion crease (Fig. 7.79). This approach avoids injury to the vessels and nerves of the digit. Many other approaches have been advocated (i.e., fish-mouth, through-and-through, and lateral), but they invoke necrosis and ischemia and lead to anesthesia of the tip of the digit. Moreover, the resulting scar is less sensitive to pain after the midline incision. Prescribe systemic antibiotics in all cases.

COMPARTMENT SYNDROMES

Compartment syndromes are the result of increased pressure that develops within a closed-tissue space leading to tissue ischemia as a result of compromised blood flow. The development of a compartment syndrome is a potentially devastating problem in an emergency department. Early diagnosis and an understanding of the pathophysiology are critical for the emergency physician.

The development of a compartment syndrome is multifactorial, but the two most common causes are a decrease in compartment size or an increase in compartment contents (Table 7.5). The normal tissue pressure is approximately zero and never exceeds 10 mm Hg. Capillary blood flow is compromised within the compartment when the pressure is greater than 20 mm Hg. Ischemic necrosis of muscles and nerves can develop when compartment pressures exceed 30 to 40 mm Hg. Tissue ischemia leads to necrosis if the compartment pressure is not reduced promptly.

Table 7.5.
Factors Related to the Development of Compartment Syndrome

Decreased compartment size
Constrictive dressings and casts
Thermal injuries and frostbite
Application of excessive traction to a fractured limb
Localized external pressure
Increased compartment contents
Fractures
Soft tissue injury
Popliteal cyst
Bleeding secondary to vascular injury
Increased capillary permeability secondary to postischemic swelling
Intense use of muscles (i.e., exercise or seizures)
Severe contusions
Reduction and fixation of fractures
Snakebites
Vessel laceration
Prolonged immobilization with limb compression
Edema accumulation due to arterial injury

By the time the distal pulses are reduced, muscle necrosis has already occurred. Muscle ischemia is manifest by pain that is aggravated by both active muscle contraction and passive stretching.

The compartments clinically relevant to the emergency physician are those contained within the upper and lower extremities. In the upper extremity, the arm contains an anterior and posterior compartment; the anterior compartment contains the biceps brachialis muscle and the ulnar, median, and radial nerves. The posterior compartment contains the triceps muscle. In the forearm, there are volar and dorsal compartments (Fig. 7.80). The volar compartment contains the wrist and finger flexors, whereas the dorsal compartment contains the wrist and finger extensors. The interosseous muscles of the hand are contained within their own individual compartments.

In the lower extremities, there are three gluteal compartments in the buttock. One contains the tensor muscle of the fascia lata; another, the gluteus medius and minimus; and the third compartment contains the gluteus maximus. The thigh has an anterior compartment that contains the quadriceps group and a posterior compartment contains the hamstring group of muscles as well as the sciatic nerves. The leg contains four compartments: anterior, peroneal, posterior, and superficial posterior (Fig. 7.81). The anterior compartment contains the tibialis anterior muscle and the extensor muscles of the toes. This

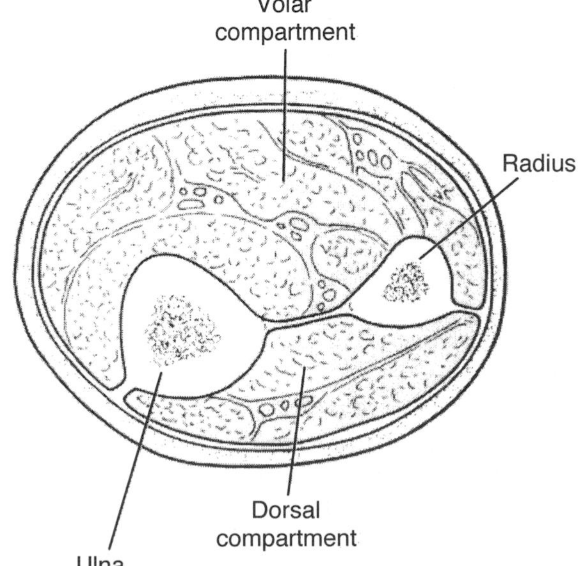

Figure 7.80. Compartments of the forearm. (From Simon RR, Koenigsknecht SJ: Emergency Orthopedics: The Extremities. New York: McGraw-Hill, 491, 2000, with permission.)

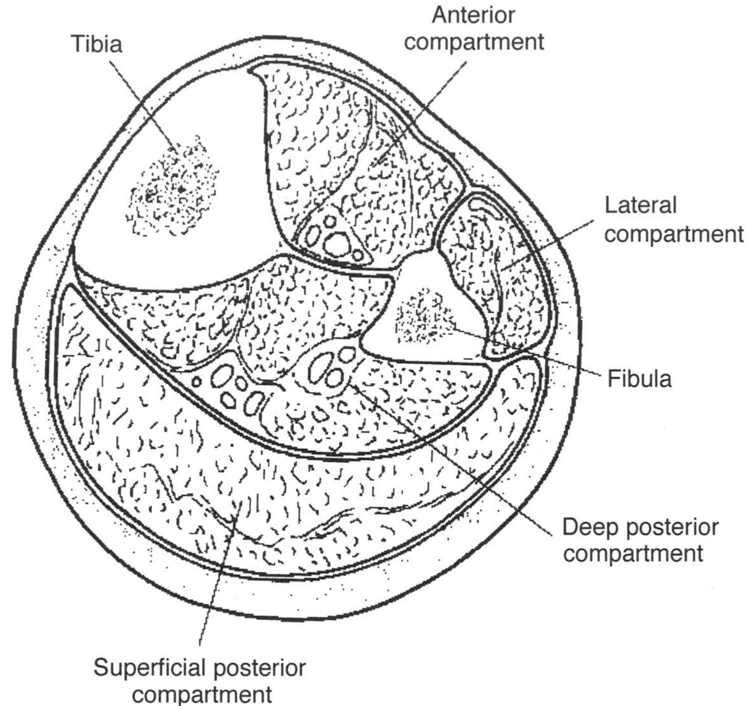

Figure 7.81. Compartments of the thigh. (From Simon RR, Koenigsknecht SJ: Emergency Orthopedics: The Extremities. New York: McGraw-Hill, 491, 2000, with permission.)

compartment is most commonly affected by this syndrome. The peroneal compartment contains the foot everters, peroneus longus and brevis, as well as the peroneal nerve. The deep posterior compartment contains the tibialis posterior muscle and the flexors of the toes. The superficial posterior compartment contains the gastrocnemius and soleus muscles as well as the sural nerve.

Anterior Thigh Compartment Syndrome

The anterior compartment syndrome typically results after tibial or fibular fractures. Other potential causes include thrombotic occlusion of the femoral artery, exercise, blunt trauma, or ischemia (48). The clinical presentation includes pain over the anterior tibia, weakness on dorsiflexion of the ankle and toes, and a variable degree of sensory loss along the deep peroneal nerve (47). The earliest and most reliable sign of a compartment syndrome is severe pain. The pain is not well localized and is out of proportion to the severity of the injury. Pain with passive stretch may be present and can be confused when there is a contusion. It is important to remember that paresis and paralysis are unreliable findings and occur late. The four signs of an anterior compartment syndrome are (a) pain on passive plantar flexion of the foot, (b) pain increased by dorsiflexion of the foot against resistance, (c) paresthesias in the space between the first and second toes, and (d) tenderness over the anterior compartment.

It is imperative to maintain a high index of suspicion to make this diagnosis. If one suspects the presence of a compartment syndrome, then measure compartment pressures. Compartment pressures can be measured quickly and easily by using a commercially available battery-powered monitor (Stryker STIC monitor), or they can be measured by using a device made up of items in the emergency department as shown later. For the method shown in Fig. 7.82, use the following supplies.

20-mL syringe
Two i.v. extension tubes
A four-way stopcock
A small bottle of sterile saline
A blood pressure manometer
An 18-gauge needle

Assemble these items as shown in the figure. Attach the 18-gauge needle to an i.v. extension tube and then to the stopcock. First insert the needle into the sterile saline and aspirate to approximately half the distance of the i.v. extension tubing. It is important to avoid getting any air into the tubing. Then attach the second i.v. extension tube to the four-way stopcock with the opposite end attached to the manometer (remove the black tubing from the manometer before this). Then place the needle into the compartment, and keep the apparatus at the level of the needle. Then turn the stopcock so that it is opened in all three directions. Slowly compress the syringe; when it is filled with air, the plunger causes air to move into both i.v. extension tubes. Watch the meniscus created by the saline in the extension tube attached to the 18-gauge needle for any movement. As soon as movement occurs in the fluid column, look at the blood pressure manometer: this is the compartment pressure.

Once the diagnosis is suspected, ice packs and elevation are essential to reduce compartment pressures. Once the compartment pressure exceeds 20 mm Hg, nerve and muscle damage can occur. This warrants surgical consultation as well as hospital admission. A compartment pressure between 30 and 40 mm Hg is typically an indication for an emergency fasciotomy in the operating room. Make a longitudinal incision in the skin over the compartment. Split the underlying fascia the length of the compartment, allowing the contained muscles to expand. Once muscle necrosis develops, the fibrous scar that develops is irreversible. A fasciotomy that is performed early (i.e., less than 12 hours from the onset of symptoms) results in the re-

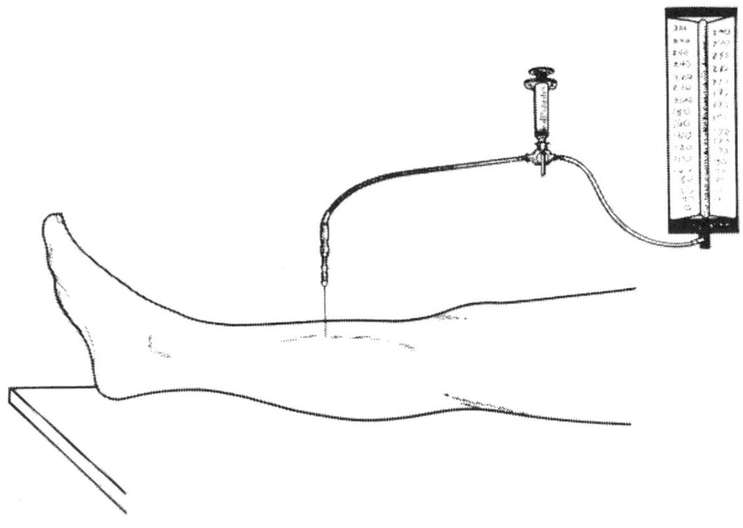

Figure 7.82. Schematic for a bedside compartment pressure measuring device. (From Simon RR, Koenigsknecht SJ: Emergency Orthopedics: The Extremities. New York: McGraw-Hill, 493, 2000, with permission.)

turn to normal function in 68% of cases, whereas only 8% of those with a fasciotomy performed after 12 hours had returned to completely normal function (53).

Deep Posterior Thigh Compartment Syndrome

The deep posterior compartment encloses the flexor digitorum longus, the tibialis posterior, and the flexor hallucis longus, as well as the posterior tibial artery and nerve. The clinical presentation is usually complicated by the involvement of other surrounding compartments. The most common cause of the syndrome is a fracture to the tibia or fibula in the middle or distal thirds (36). On initial presentation, there is a paucity of complaints. As the syndrome progresses, there is increased pain on passive extension of the toes and weakness on toe flexion. Hypesthesia over the distribution of the posterior tibial nerve (i.e., along the sole) is noted. The patient also has tenderness along the medial distal aspect of the leg, and this area will be tense. These signs may become evident from 2 hours to as long as 6 days after the inciting event.

Once the diagnosis is suspected, remove all circumferential dressings and completely examine the extremity. Once the syndrome is established, a fasciotomy is indicated. This is a more technically complex procedure than that required for an anterior compartment syndrome and has been described by Paranen (41).

REFERENCES

1. Adams JC: Outline of Fractures. Edinburgh: E & S Livingston, 1968.
2. Anderson L: Fractures. In: Campbell's Operative Orthopedics, 5th ed. St. Louis: CV Mosby, 1971.
3. Anderson R: Fractures of the humerus. Surg Gynecol Obstet 64:919, 1937.
4. Antal CS, Conforty B, Engelberg M, et al: Injuries to the axillary nerve due to anterior dislocation of the shoulder. J Trauma 13:564, 1973.
5. Carothers RG, Berning DD: Colles' fracture. Am J Surg 80:626, 1950.
6. Carothers RG, Boyd FJ: Thumb traction technique for reduction of Colles' fracture. Arch Surg 58:848, 1949.
7. Cave EF: Fractures and Other Injuries. Chicago: Yearbook Publishers, 1958.
8. Cronwell HE: Fractures of the clavicle. JAMA 90: 838, 1928.
9. Detenbeck LC, Kelly PJ: Total dislocation of the talus. J Bone Joint Surg Am 51:283, 1969.
10. Eastwood WJ: The T-shaped fracture of the lower end of the humerus. J Bone Joint Surg 19:364, 1937.
11. Edman P, Lohr G: Supracondylar fractures of the humerus. Acta Chir Scand 126:505, 1963.
12. Epstein HC: Traumatic dislocations of the hip. Clin Orthop 92:116, 1973.
13. Ferry A, Rook FW, Masterson JH: Retrosternal dislocation of the clavicle. J Bone Joint Surg Am 39:905, 1957.
14. Finder JC, Post M: Local injection therapy for rheumatic diseases: a practical guide. JAMA 172: 2021, 1960.
15. Fitzsimmons RA: Colles' fracture and chauffeur's fracture. Br Med J 2:357, 1938.
16. Furlong R: Injuries of the Hand. Boston: Little, Brown, 1957.
17. Geiderman JD, Dawson WJ: Arthrocentesis: Indications and method. Postgrad Med 66:141, 1979.
18. Gore DR: Horizontal dislocation of the patella. JAMA 214:119, 1970.
19. Henny FA: Intra-articular injection of hydrocortisone into temporomandibular joint. J Oral Surg 12:314, 1954.
20. Hollander JL: Intra-articular hydrocortisone in the treatment of arthritis. Ann Intern Med 39: 735, 1953.
21. Hollander JL: Technique of intra-articular injection with hydrocortisone acetate. Rahway, NJ: Merck & Co, 1953.
22. Hollander JL, ed: Arthritis and allied conditions: A textbook of rheumatology. Philadelphia: Lea & Febiger, 380–401, 1969.
23. Hollander JL, Brown EM Jr, Jessar RA: Intra-articular hydrocortisone in the management of rheumatic disease. Med Clin North Am 38:349, 1954.
24. Holzman RS, Bishko F: Osteomyelitis in heroin addicts. Ann Intern Med 75:693, 1971.
25. Hoover NW: Injuries of the popliteal artery associated with fractures and dislocations. Surg Clin North Am 41:1099, 1961.
26. Hughston JC: Subluxation of the patella. J Bone Joint Surg Am 50:1003, 1968.
27. Hussein KM: Kocher's method is 3,000 years old. J Bone Joint Surg Br 50:669, 1968.
28. Kennedy JC: Complete dislocation of knee joint. J Bone Joint Surg Am 45:889, 1963.
29. King OC: Fractures and dislocations about the elbow. Surg Clin North Am 20:1645, 1940.
30. Kini MG: Dislocation of the elbow and its complications. J Bone Joint Surg 22:107, 1940.
31. Kini MG: A simple method of ambulatory treatment of fractures of the clavicle. J Bone Joint Surg 23:795, 1941.
32. Kocher T: Eine neue Reductionsmethod fuer Schulterverrenkung. Berlin Klin 7:101, 1870.
33. Krause W, Kling DH: The synovial membrane and the synovial fluid with special reference to arthritis and injuries of the joints. Los Angeles: Medical Press, Chapter 24, 1938.

34. Landsmeer JMF, Koumans AKJ: Anatomical considerations in injection of the hip joint. Ann Rheum Dis 13:246, 1954.
35. Lynn FS: Erect dislocation of the shoulder. Surg Gynecol Obstet 39:51, 1925.
36. Matsen, FA, Clawson DK: The deep posterior compartmental syndrome of the leg. J Bone Joint Surg 57:34, 1975.
37. McLaughlin HL, MacLellan DI: Recurrent anterior dislocations of the shoulder. J Trauma 7:191, 1967.
38. Miller JA Jr: Joint paracentesis from an anatomic point of view, I: Shoulder, elbow, wrist, and hand. Surgery 40:993, 1956.
39. Miller JA Jr: Joint paracentesis from an anatomic point of view, II: Hip, knee, ankle and foot. Surgery 41:999, 1957.
40. Mirick MJ, Clinton JE, Ruiz E: External rotation method of shoulder dislocation reduction. JACEP 8:528, 1979.
41. Paranen J: The medial tibial syndrome. J Bone Joint Surg Br 56:712, 1974.
42. Parisien VM: Shoulder dislocations: an easier method for reduction. J Maine Med Assoc 70: 102, 1979.
43. Pels-Leusden. In: Kling DH, ed. The synovial membrane and the synovial fluid with special reference to arthritis and injuries of the joints. Los Angeles: Medical Press, 1938.
44. Percy EC: Acute dislocation of the patella. Can Med Assoc J 105:1176, 1971.
45. Roca R, Yoshikawa TT: Primary skeletal infections in heroin users. Clin Orthop 144:238, 1979.
46. Rockwood CA, Green DT: Fractures. Philadelphia: JB Lippincott, 1975.
47. Protzman RR, Griffis CG: Stress fractures in men and women undergoing military training. J Bone Joint Surg 59:825, 1977.
48. Rorabeck CHI, Macnab I: The pathophysiology of the anterior compartment syndrome. Clin Orthop 113:52, 1975.
49. Rowe CR: Anterior dislocations of the shoulder. Surg Clin North Am 43:1609, 1963.
50. Royle G: Treatment of acute anterior dislocations of the shoulder. Br J Clin Pract 27:403, 1973.
51. Salvatore J: Sternoclavicular joint dislocation. Clin Orthop 58:51, 1968.
52. Schmeiden. In: Kling DH, ed. The synovial membrane and the synovial fluid with special reference to arthritis and injuries of the joints. Los Angeles: Medical Press, 1938.
53. Sheridan GW, Matsen FA: Fasciotomy in the treatment of acute compartment syndrome. J Bone Joint Surg 58:112, 1976.
54. Shields L, Mital M, Cave EF: Complete dislocation of the knee: Experience at the MGH. J Trauma 9:192, 1969.
55. Simon R, Koenigsneckt K: Orthopedics in emergency medicine. New York: Appleton-Century-Crofts, 1982.
56. Spear HC, Jones JM: Rupture of the brachial artery accompanying dislocation of the elbow or supracondylar fracture. J Bone Joint Surg Am 33: 889, 1951.
57. Sperling IL: Hydrocortisone intra-articular use in rheumatic diseases. Mod Med 119:123, 1955.
58. Sternbach GL, Baker FJ: The emergency joint: Arthrocentesis and synovial fluid analysis. JACEP 5:787, 1976.
59. Stimson CA: An easy method of reducing dislocations of the shoulder and hip. Medical Research 57:356, 1958.
60. Thompson VP, Epstein HC: Traumatic dislocation of the hip. J Bone Joint Surg Am 33:746, 1951.
61. Wade FV, Batdorf J: Supracondylar fractures of humerus (a twelve year review with follow-up). J Trauma 1:269, 1961.
62. Wolf AW, Benson DR, Shoji H, et al: Current concepts in synovial fluid analysis. Clin Orthop 134: 262, 1978.
63. Yehia SA, Duncan H: Synovial fluid analysis. Clin Orthop 107:11, 1975.

8

Otolaryngologic and Ophthalmologic Procedures

EXAMINATION OF THE HEAD AND NECK

Physical Examination

As with all emergencies, attention to the airway, breathing, and circulation (ABCs) is paramount. Before proceeding with an evaluation of the patient with an otolaryngologic complaint, make sure that the airway is secure and can be protected. Afterward, a thorough examination of the head and neck is essential when evaluating the patient with an ophthalmologic or otolaryngologic complaint. This is often challenging because much of the area to be examined is not easily accessible to direct visualization. Specialized instruments and the skill to use those instruments are required to perform an adequate examination. The examination should begin with proper patient positioning, usually with the patient sitting in front of the examiner with the examiner either sitting or standing. Use a mask, eye protection, and gloves at a minimum to guard against blood or body fluid exposure. Proper illumination is essential for a thorough examination, and various options are available including a reflecting head mirror, headlight, otoscope, ophthalmoscope, slit lamp, and specialized equipment including fiberoptic instruments.

Indirect Laryngoscopy

One method for examining the larynx is the use of a headlight or head mirror and an angled laryngeal or dental mirror. Seat the patient upright with the legs uncrossed and the upper body leaning slightly forward, with the head in mild extension (the "sniffing" position). Pretreat the patient with a topical anesthetic such as benzocaine and tetracaine (Cetacaine) to help reduce the gag reflex. Use either a headlight or a head mirror for illumination, and either stand or sit. Reassure the patient and instruct to breathe slowly and continuously through the mouth and then protrude the tongue, which is grasped with a gauze sponge between the thumb and forefinger and pulled outward and downward (Fig. 8.1). Insert a warmed or defogged laryngeal mirror along the soft palate and uvula. Taken care not to contact the posterior tongue or the posterior pharyngeal wall, as contact with these areas usually elicits a gag reflex. Direct the light at the mirror and angle the mirror to visualize the larynx. Have the patient phonate to examine the anterior larynx and to assess vocal cord mobility. If the patient is having difficulty cooperating with the examination or if the examiner has difficulty visualizing the anatomy, use a right-angle laryngo-

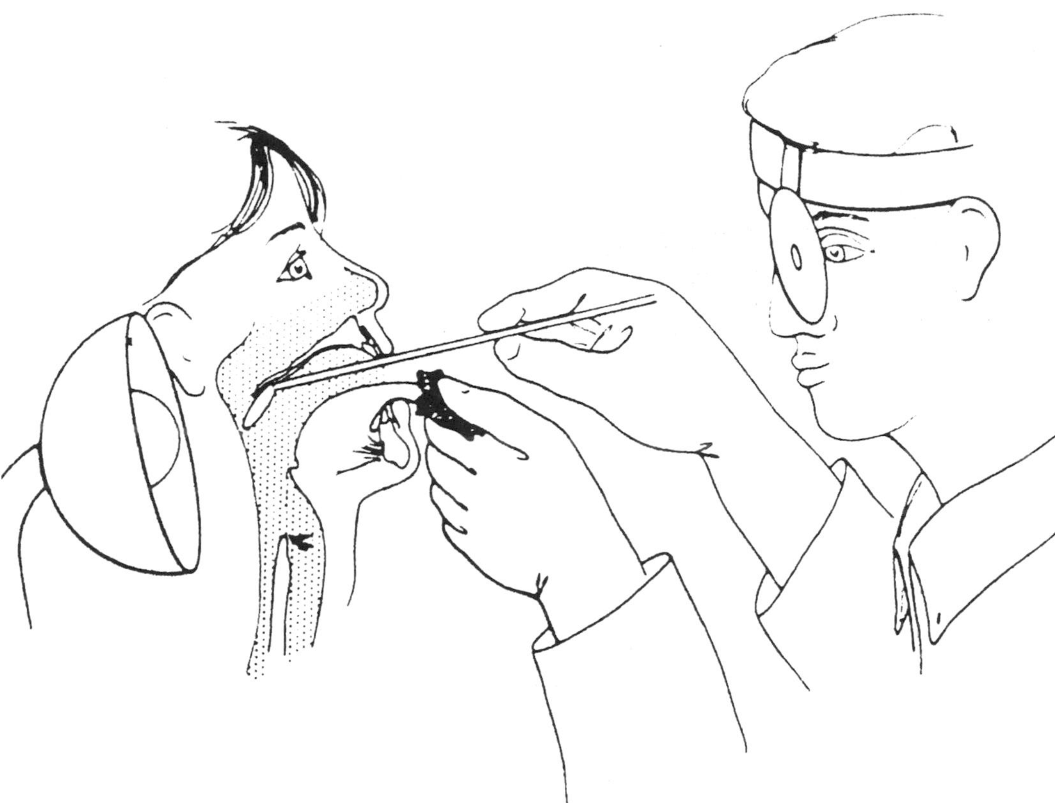

Figure 8.1. Examination of the larynx by using a lamp and head mirror (From Paparella MM, Shumrick DA: Otolaryngology, 3rd ed., Philadelphia: Saunders, 1991, with permission.)

scope. Position this patient in the same way as when using the angled mirror. Guide the laryngoscope so that the tip is just posterior to the tongue before placing the eye near the eyepiece, as in Fig. 8.2*A*.

Direct Laryngoscopy

Use direct laryngoscopy to examine or to remove foreign bodies (FBs) from the larynx or upper airway. The most commonly used approach is to position the patient supine with the head resting on a towel or a small pillow (the "sniffing" position). If the situation allows, apply topical anesthetic. Have a laryngoscope handle and the appropriate sized laryngoscope blade as well as a suction device and Magill forceps available at the bedside. Insert the laryngoscope blade slowly and carefully along the tongue with gentle traction along the handle. Take care not to "pry" with the blade, as this could cause damage to the teeth or other parts of the oral cavity. Insert the blade of the laryngoscope to the depth needed to visualize the larynx, as in Fig. 8.3. If an FB is present, attempt removal with the Magill forceps. For further information, see Chapter 2, Airway Procedures.

Fiberoptic Laryngoscopy

Fiberoptic laryngoscopy requires only a light source and a nasopharyngoscope, but the cost of this instrument often precludes its presence in the emergency department or generalist's office. It does provide an excellent tool to examine the patient who is unable to be examined by other methods. Pretreat the patient by applying a topical anesthetic and a vasoconstrictor medication to the nasal mucosa.

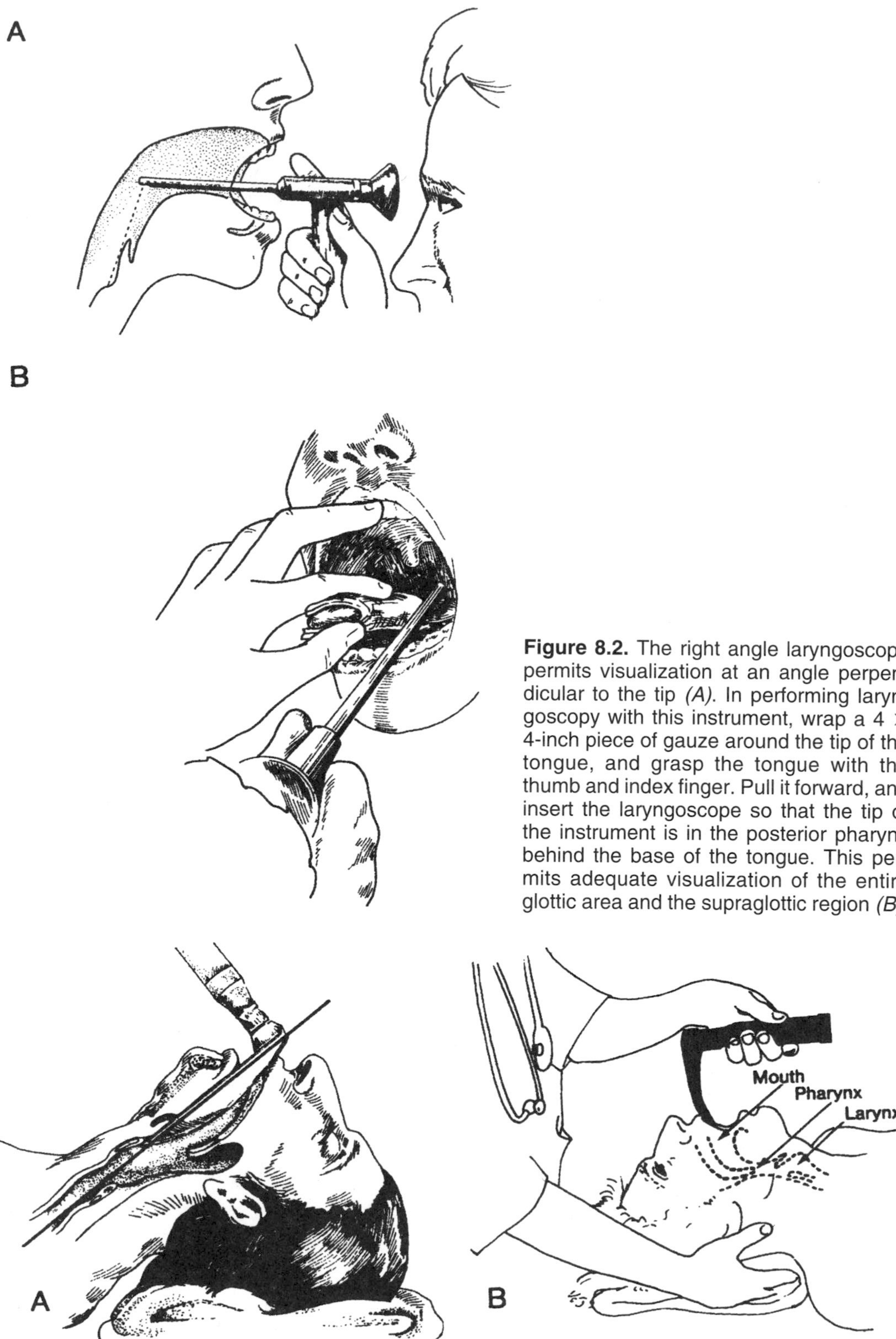

Figure 8.2. The right angle laryngoscope permits visualization at an angle perpendicular to the tip *(A)*. In performing laryngoscopy with this instrument, wrap a 4 × 4-inch piece of gauze around the tip of the tongue, and grasp the tongue with the thumb and index finger. Pull it forward, and insert the laryngoscope so that the tip of the instrument is in the posterior pharynx behind the base of the tongue. This permits adequate visualization of the entire glottic area and the supraglottic region *(B)*.

Figure 8.3. Direct laryngoscopy allows visualization of the posterior pharynx and the larynx.

Seat the patient with the head held in the sniffing position. Warm the scope to prevent fogging and place it into the nares. While looking through the eyepiece, advance the scope to visualize the structures of the nasopharynx, the pharynx, and the larynx, as in Fig. 8.4. Do not advance the scope beyond the tip of the epiglottis unless the larynx has been anesthetized. Having the patient swallow can usually clear a fogged scope.

AIRWAY AND ESOPHAGEAL FOREIGN BODIES

Upper Airway Foreign Bodies

Complete upper airway obstruction or partial obstruction with poor air exchange is a dire emergency and must be dealt with immediately. The details of management of acute upper airway obstruction are covered in Chapter 2, Airway Procedures.

Esophageal Foreign Bodies

Only one FB impaction in the esophagus is a true emergency: a large FB in the postcricoid area that causes either partial or complete airway obstruction. In complete obstruction or respiratory insufficiency, control of the airway with either endotracheal intubation or emergency cricothyroidotomy is indicated. All other FBs need emergency but not immediate removal.

The evaluation of the patient with a suspected esophageal FB should include a focused physical examination and radiologic evaluation. Posteroanterior (PA) and lateral radiographs of the neck, chest, and abdomen will identify the location of most FBs in the esophagus. Flat or irregular objects will align themselves in the esophagus such that on a PA radiograph, the object will appear side-on; flat objects in the trachea will usually align themselves end-

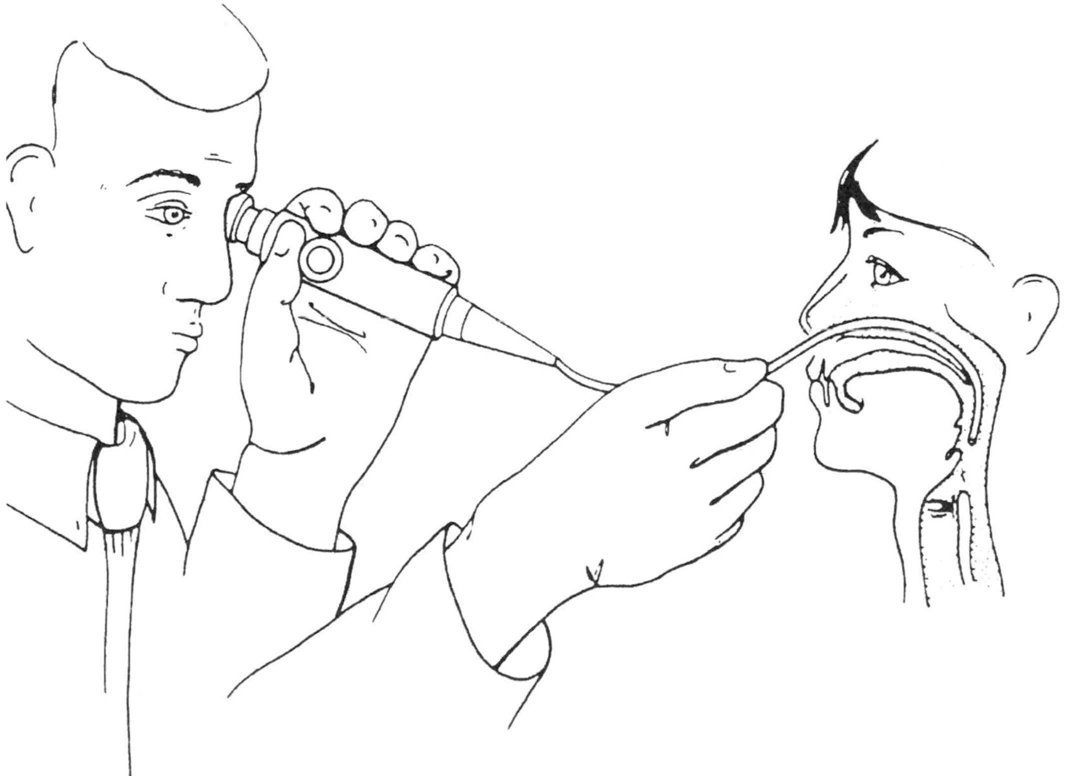

Figure 8.4. Examination of the larynx with a fiberoptic laryngoscope (From Paparella MM, Shumrick DA: Otolaryngology, 3rd ed., Philadelphia: Saunders, 1991, with permission.)

on on the PA radiograph (see Fig. 8.5). Perform a barium swallow in patients with a suspected FB but a negative radiograph to delineate the presence of a complete or partial obstruction. Having the patient swallow a barium-soaked cotton ball may help identify an irregularly shaped radiolucent object. Occasionally, a computed tomography (CT) scan may be required to identify esophageal FBs.

Removal of an esophageal FB can be divided into noninvasive and invasive methods. The noninvasive methods include the use of glucagon, nitroglycerin, nifedipine, gas-forming agents, and carbonated beverages (7, 19, 36, 43, 46). The use of proteolytic agents such as papain is *strongly discouraged* because of the possibility of esophageal erosion and perforation. Glucagon is most useful for meat impactions at the lower esophageal sphincter (LES) and is not effective for FBs in the upper or middle esophagus. Administer glucagon intravenously in a dose of 1 to 2 mg given over 1 to 2 minutes with the patient in the upright position. After administration, instruct the patient to drink a large glass or two of water to aid in moving the FB through the LES. If there are no results in 20 to 30 minutes, administer a repeated dose of glucagon. Glucagon is contraindicated in pediatric patients or patients with Zollinger–Ellison syndrome, insulinoma, pheochromocytoma, sharp FB, or an allergy to glucagon (47). Nitroglycerin can be used either alone or in conjunction with glucagon. Sublingual nitroglycerin decreases LES tone and is given in a dose of one or two 0.4-mg tablets sublingually, or 1 to 2 inches of nitroglycerin

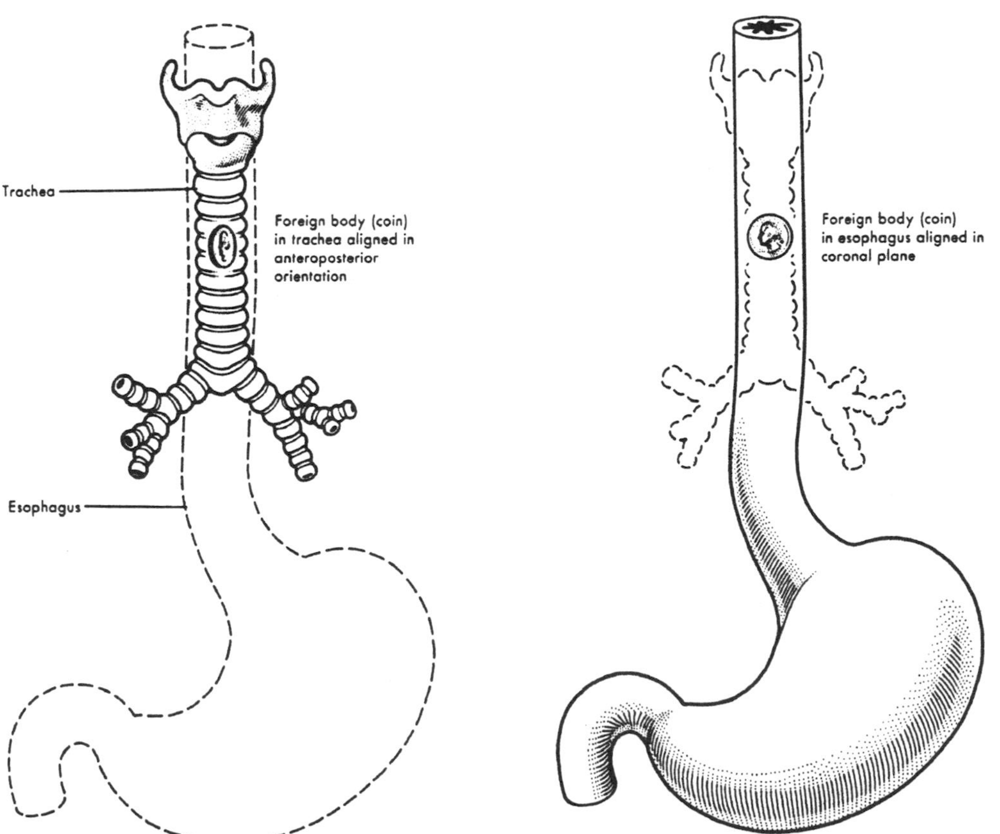

Figure 8.5. Orientation of a flat foreign body, such as a coin, in the trachea and esophagus. (From Rosen P, Barkin RM: Emergency Medicine: Concepts and Clinical Practice. 3rd ed., with permission.)

paste. Nifedipine also decreases LES tone and is given in a dose of 10 mg sublingually. Monitor patients that are given either nitroglycerin or nifedipine for signs of hypotension, especially if they are dehydrated. Another method of FB removal is by using gas-forming agents in the radiology suite under fluoroscopic guidance. A 15-mL aliquot of tartaric acid solution (18.7 mg/100 mL) is followed by 15 mL of sodium bicarbonate solution (10 g/100 mL), which is immediately followed by 60 mL of high-density barium. Additionally, give 100 mL of carbonated beverage followed by a mouthful of barium to a patient in an upright position. Movement of the FB into the stomach should be observed with fluoroscopy.

Invasive methods to remove esophageal FBs include Foley catheter extraction, nasogastric tube extraction, and esophagoscopy. Foley catheter extraction has been used by pediatricians, emergency physicians, family practitioners in the outpatient setting, and in the emergency department with good success (14, 20, 40). Patients need to be cooperative; pediatric patients can be restrained. Place the patient in an extreme head-down position, preferably prone, with the head turned to the side. Insert a 12- to 16-French Foley into the mouth, and pass it distal to the FB. Then gently inflate the balloon. If this procedure is performed in the radiology suite (preferred), instill a small amount of barium into the balloon to aid in visualization. Gently pull back the Foley catheter, with balloon inflated, until the FB is positioned in the oral cavity, as in Fig. 8.6. Perform another radiographic study to rule out the

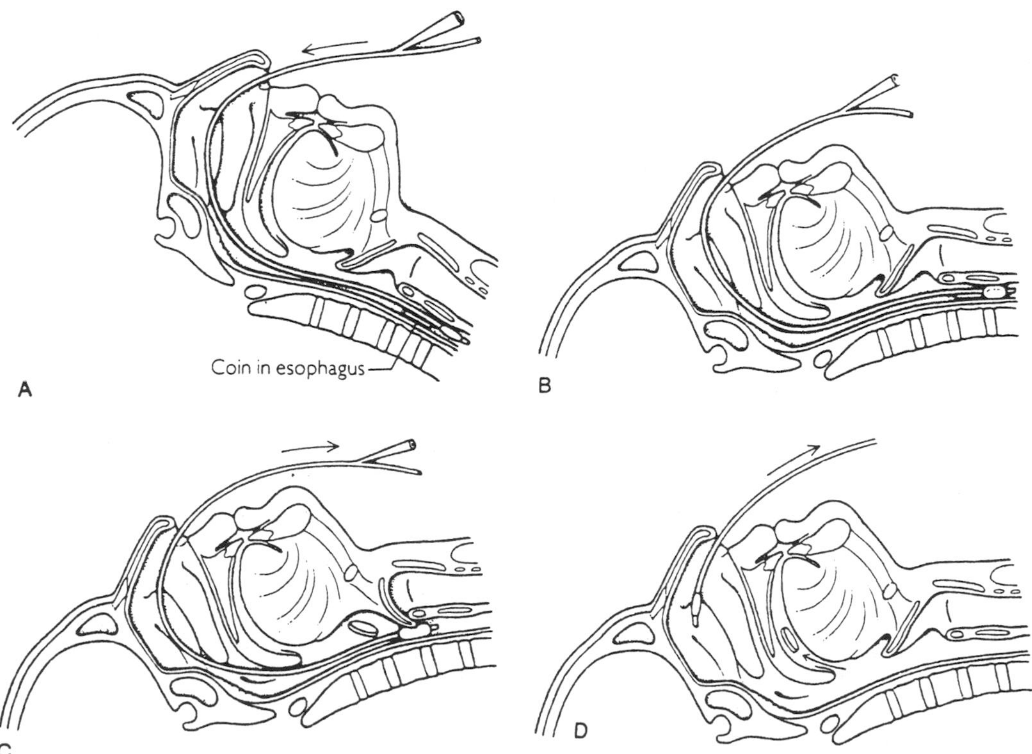

Figure 8.6. Removal of a foreign body with a Foley catheter. Position the patient prone with the head turned to one side. Introduce the catheter either through the nares or through the mouth. Advance the catheter past the foreign object *(A),* and then inflate the balloon *(B).* Slowly pull the foreign body out as the catheter is removed *(C).* Remove the foreign body from the oral cavity *(D).* This procedure may be more accurately done under fluoroscopy, with the catheter balloon filled with contrast material. (From McSwain N: Esophageal foreign body. Emerg Med 21:85, 1989, with permission.)

possibility of multiple FBs. Nasogastric tubes have been used to remove esophageal FBs. Cut off the tube at the most proximal side hole, and insert the tube until it abuts the impaction; then apply maximal suction to the tube, and gently extract the FB. Immediately refer patients with FBs that cannot be removed in this manner to a gastroenterologist or otolaryngologist for removal with endoscopy. Make special note of the patient who has ingested a button battery, often found in watches or hearing aids. These FBs have been found to cause esophageal injury secondary to leakage, electric current, and pressure necrosis, all of which may lead to esophageal erosion and perforation within a few hours of ingestion. Make every attempt to remove these batteries immediately by endoscopy or by use of a Foley catheter, as we do not recommend noninvasive methods.

Warn patients that undergo successful FB removal about the risk of delayed bleeding, recurrent impaction, and the probability of underlying pathology. Refer all adults with a history of esophageal FBs for follow-up endoscopy. Monitor FBs that pass into the stomach to make sure they pass in the stool. Either repeated radiographs of the abdomen or examination of the stool can confirm the passage of the FB.

EAR EMERGENCIES

Foreign Body Removal from the Ear

FBs in the external auditory canal (EAC) are a common problem, particularly in children. Presenting symptoms can include pain, drainage, bleeding, hearing loss, or observation that an FB was placed in the EAC. A wide variety of objects can be found, and the type of object should dictate the method of removal (11). Several methods of removal have been advocated and include suction, irrigation, super glue, direct removal, and use of a Fogarty catheter. Chemically immobilize animate objects, such as insects, before removal.

Animate objects, most commonly cockroaches and moths, usually cause the patient considerable discomfort and should be quickly immobilized before removal. Instillation of various substances including mineral oil, microscope immersion oil, lidocaine, isopropyl alcohol, hydrogen peroxide, antipyrine, benzocaine, and glycerin (Auralgan) and even succinylcholine have been studied. Recent in vitro studies showed that microscope immersion oil (a refined mineral oil) immobilized cockroaches quicker than the other substances listed previously (31). Viscous lidocaine 2% and lidocaine 2% also acted quickly to immobilize insects. When using immersion oil (mineral oil) or lidocaine, instill approximately 2 to 3 mL into the affected EAC, and in 30 to 45 seconds, attempt removal with direct visualization and the use of alligator forceps. Insects that fragment or are difficult to remove with forceps can often be irrigated out.

Irrigation of the EAC is often the first method of removal for many EAC FBs. Direct a pulsatile flow of body-temperature irrigation fluid against the superior wall of the EAC. Irrigate by using a Waterpik, a DeVillbiss irrigator (Sunrise Respiratory Products Division, Somerset, PA), a 20-mL syringe with either an 18-gauge Teflon intravenous catheter, or a butterfly infusion catheter with the metal needle and plastic butterfly cut off. Do not remove hygroscopic objects that will swell when exposed to water by this method, and do not irrigate when there is the possibility of a ruptured tympanic membrane.

If irrigation does not work, then remove under direct visualization with the use of alligator forceps, ear curette, right-angle hook, or Fogarty catheter (see Fig. 8.7). Adequate visualization of the EAC is a must in this circumstance and the use of a headlight and metal ear speculums, or an operating otoscope head will facilitate visualization. Patient cooperation is important and can be aided by topical, local, or general anesthesia. Topical anesthetics in-

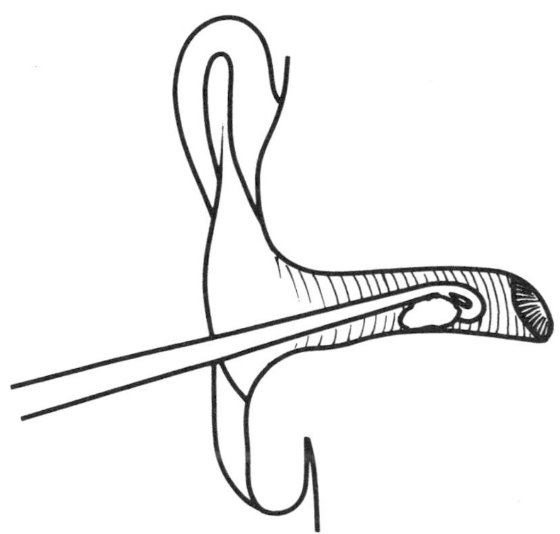

Figure 8.7. Removal of a foreign body of the ear with an ear curette. The first method that should be tried is irrigation, as explained in the text.

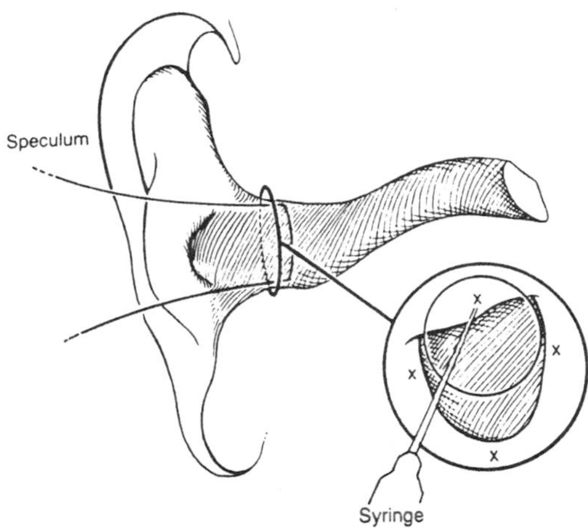

Figure 8.8 Local anesthetic in a four-quadrant block to the external auditory canal. Inject local anesthetic subcutaneously in small amounts (up to 0.5 mL) in each of the four quadrants. This block allows painless removal of most foreign bodies in the ear. (From Roberts JR, Hedges JR: Clinical Procedures in Emergency Medicine: 2nd ed.: Philadelphia, Saunders, 1991, with permission.)

clude Auralgan, tetracaine, and lidocaine. Accomplish local anesthesia by injecting 1% lidocaine with or without epinephrine into four quadrants to encircle the ear canal. Use a speculum to visualize the EAC, and inject less than 0.5 mL, or enough to raise a small wheal, in each quadrant, as depicted in Fig. 8.8. Within 2 to 3 minutes, attempt FB removal. The use of conscious sedation or general anesthesia may be required in more difficult cases; see Chapter 3 for details.

Smooth objects such as beads or pearls are difficult or impossible to grasp or irrigate out. With these objects, use a suction catheter with a soft, flexible "umbrella tip" (see Fig. 8.9). Additionally, apply a small drop of cyanoacrylate glue to the tip of an instrument and hold it lightly against the FB for approximately 1 minute, and then attempt removal. Take great care not to allow the instrument to adhere to the wall of the EAC. Styrofoam (polystyrene) also can be difficult to remove and is easily dissolved by filling a tuberculin syringe with an attached 22-gauge Teflon catheter with pure acetone (usually available in most hospital laboratories) and instilling 0.1 to 0.3 mL directly onto the styrofoam. The styrofoam will dissolve immediately; then irrigate the EAC with water to remove any residue (49).

After removal of EAC FBs, inspect the ear canal for any trauma or residual FB. Small lacerations or abrasion are com-

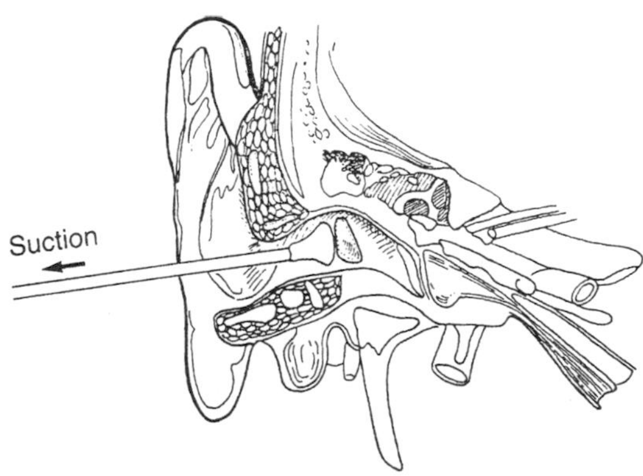

Figure 8.9. Use a suction catheter with a soft flexible tip to remove certain objects from the ear canal. (Courtesy of Richards Manufacturing Company.)

mon; treat them with a topical antibiotic solution. Significant lacerations, injury to the tympanic membrane, or the inability to remove a foreign object should prompt immediate referral to an otolaryngologist.

Cerumen Impaction

Cerumen impaction is a common problem that prevents visualization of the tympanic membrane. Soft cerumen can be removed by irrigation, as detailed earlier. Soften hard cerumen with either half-strength hydrogen peroxide, triethanolamine (Cerumenex), or preferably, docusate sodium (Colace) (44). Cerumen that cannot be removed with softening and irrigation can be removed under direct visualization with a cerumen spoon or curette.

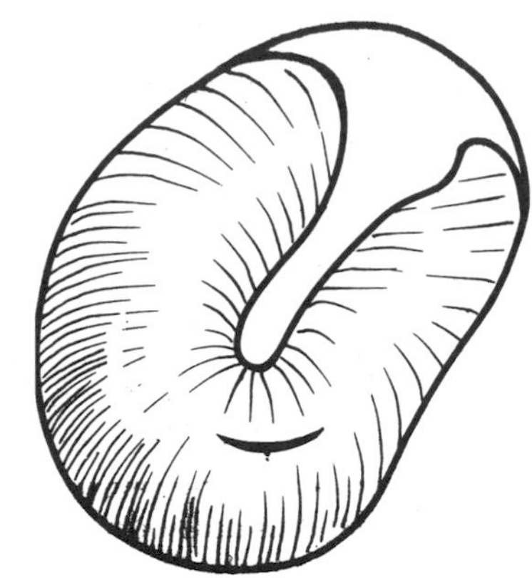

Figure 8.10. When performing a myringotomy or tympanocentesis, place the puncture site in the inferior aspect of the tympanic membrane to avoid damage to the ossicles.

Tympanocentesis and Myringotomy

Tympanocentesis and myringotomy are rarely performed in the emergency department and are better left to the expertise of an otolaryngologist. Indications for urgent myringotomy include severe pain from acute otitis media, septic neonate younger than 6 weeks with acute otitis media, and severe pain from barotitis media (1). Local anesthetic with topical or regional anesthesia, as described in the section on FB removal, is indicated. The patient must be cooperative or immobilized to prevent injury to the tympanic membrane and the ossicles. Make a small incision in the inferior aspect of the tympanic membrane with a myringotomy knife under direct visualization (see Figs. 8.10 and 8.11). If a myringotomy knife is not available, then use a 15-gauge spinal needle.

EYE EMERGENCIES

Intraocular Foreign Bodies

Most intraocular FBs are metallic shavings. The single most common cause of these is metallic particles struck off of a hammer or chisel. The longer the delay in the removal of an intraocular FB, the greater the likelihood of developing endophthalmitis. Use either a burr spud or 23-gauge needle to remove a superficial metal FB from the surface of the cornea with the aid of slit-lamp examination after adequate topical anesthesia (2).

Intraocular FBs may be difficult to visualize on plain radiographs. Metallic particles can often be visualized on plain radiographs; however, use a CT if an FB,

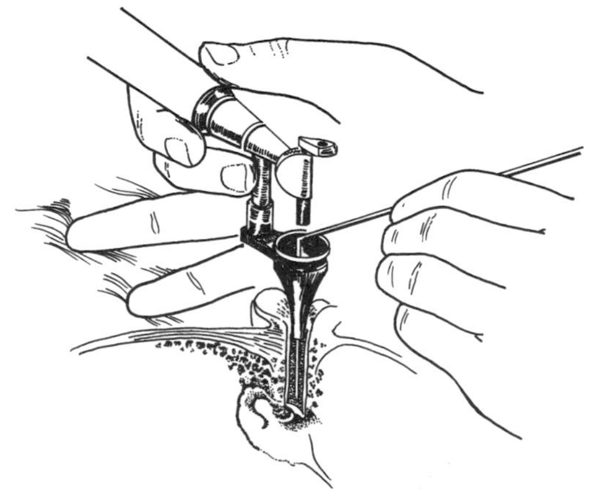

Figure 8.11. A myringotomy can be done as shown. Place the fingers against the scalp to aid in stabilizing the instruments.

metallic or nonmetallic, is highly suspected (12, 42).

Corneal Rust Stains

After the removal of metallic FBs from the surface of the cornea, there is often a rust ring around the site of the removed FB. Use a 22-gauge needle or a burr spud to remove the corneal rust ring. With either of these devices, gently lift a corneal rust stain off of the cornea by using the slit lamp for optimal visualization while using normal saline to irrigate the surface of the cornea. This procedure should be performed by someone experienced in corneal rust ring removal because of the risk of corneal scarring and inadvertent globe penetration. If the corneal rust is not easily removed, ophthalmologic referral is necessary (17).

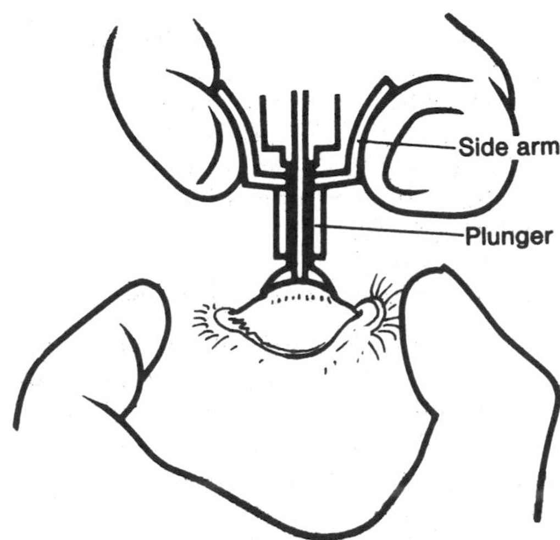

Figure 8.12. Use of a Schiotz tonometer. Before placement of the tonometer over the cornea, obtain adequate anesthesia by using topical anesthetics. The plunger of the tonometer will elevate and indicate the intraocular pressure.

Schiotz Tonometry

The Schiotz tonometer is used to measure intraocular pressures and to diagnose glaucoma. Accompanying the instrument is a series of weights (5.5, 7.5, 10.0, and 15 g) and a chart converting the units on the Schiotz tonometer to millimeters of mercury. The technique of tonometry is very simple and involves anesthetizing the eye with an appropriate topical anesthetic solution. Place the lowest weight (5.5 g) on the tonometer. Next, hold the tonometer with the left hand and rest it gently on the center of the cornea while the right hand retracts the lids, as shown in Fig. 8.12. Do not apply pressure on the orbit itself; rest the other fingers on the supraorbital and infraorbital ridges. Make sure the tonometer rests on the center of the limbus. Do not press the tonometer firmly against the limbus. Leave the side arm freely mobile; otherwise, erroneous readings will be obtained. Use a chart to translate the measurement of the pressure on the tonometer into millimeters of mercury. If the reading is too low for the chart, then apply a higher weight, and determine the value again. The lower the reading on the tonometer, the higher the intraocular pressure. If the pressure is elevated, then obtain a more accurate value by using applanation tonometry.

Applanation Tonometry

Perform applanation tonometry with the tonometer attached to the slit lamp. Topically anesthetize the eyes, and place fluorescein in each eye to be examined. Open the light beam to its widest setting, select the cobalt blue filter, and place the microscope on its lowest magnification with the light source set at the highest power. Set the light at an angle of approximately 45 degrees so that it shines near the applanation prism tip. Place the tonometer knob at 1 g, which is the equivalent of 10 mm Hg.

With the patient's eye wide open, move the prism anteriorly with the joystick while observing from the side. Place the prism on the center of the cornea with contact being confirmed by blue light filling the anterior chamber. As the examiner views through the microscope, two semicircles are visualized divided by a horizontal line. The semicircles should be equal in size, being approximately one tenth the diameter of the semicircle. Widened semicircles indicate excessive moisture, whereas narrow semicircles indicate lack of moisture. Remedy either situation by drying the surface of the prism as well as asking the patient to blink a few times.

Once contact has been made with the cornea, adjust the micrometer from the initial reading of 1 g until the inner borders of the two semicircles are approximated (Fig. 8.13). Then convert the micrometer reading into millimeters of mercury by multiplying the reading by a factor of 10. Any reading greater than 20 mm Hg warrants concern and, depending on the clinical scenario, the patient may need emergency ophthalmologic consultation if acute angle closure is suspected.

Slit-Lamp Examination

Gross visualization of the external eye may be adequate for obvious eye pathology. However, the slit lamp provides a microscope for viewing the detail of the cornea, anterior chamber, and iris. FBs, corneal abrasions, iritis, hyphema, and hypopyon may all be visualized with the aid of the slit lamp. FB removal can be facilitated with the use of the magnification of the slit lamp. Many slit lamps also have an applanation tonometer attached to allow intraocular pressure measurement.

GENERAL OUTLINE FOR SLIT-LAMP EXAMINATION

Position the patient comfortably with the chin in the chin rest and forehead pressed against the headrest by manipulating the patient's seat height as well as the height of the chin rest. Align the patient's eyes with the mark on the headrest support.

Turn on the slit lamp initially to the lowest power setting, and set the magnification to the lowest setting (see Fig. 8.14).

1. 45-Degree optic section illumination. Move the slit lamp's light source so that it shines at an angle of 45 degrees in a position lateral to the eye being examined. Grossly adjust the light source so that the light shines on the anterior chamber by

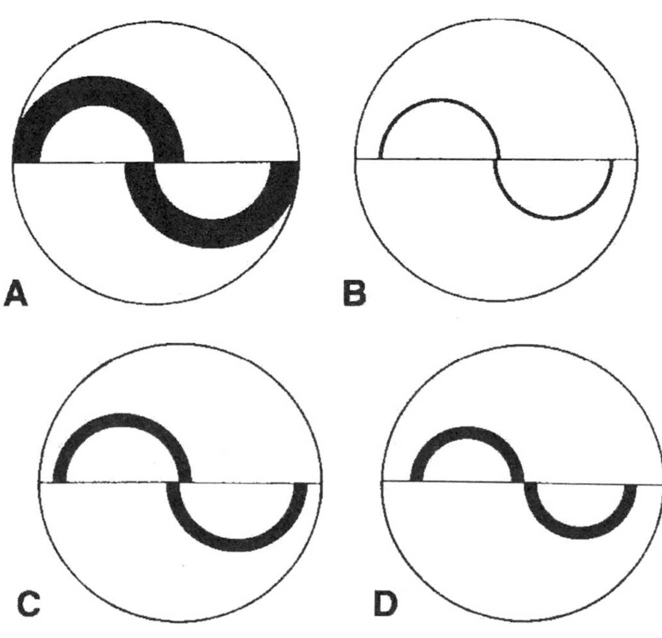

Figure 8.13. The semicircles of the Goldmann tonometer demonstrating the appropriate orientation of the inner borders of the semicircles for interpretation of the intraocular pressure *(C)*. *A*: Semicircles that are too wide, indicating excessive eye moisture. *B*: Semicircles that are too narrow, indicating corneal dryness. *D*: Semicircles that are improperly intersected. (Reprinted from Keeney AH: Ocular Examination, 2nd ed. St. Louis: CV Mosby, 1976, with permission.)

moving the slit-lamp assembly on its table. After looking into the binoculars, accomplish more detailed focusing by moving the joystick controlling the slit lamp toward and away from the patient. Examine the external eye for blepharitis, hordeolum, chalazion, ectropion, entropion, FBs, pterygia, and pinguecula. Limbal injection or redness may indicate iritis, whereas more diffuse injection throughout the conjunctiva may suggest conjunctivitis. Adjust the light beam so that it is as narrow and tall as the slit-lamp controls allow. Use the white light for this initial part of the examination. Then visualize the entire cornea by moving the slit-lamp base right and left while the light source remains at a constant 45 degrees. Note the smoothness of the cornea, the depth of its surface, the presence of debris or discharge. By moving the base of the slit lamp forward, visualize the entire anterior surface of the iris in a similar fashion as the cornea. Assess the depth of the anterior chamber in this manner. Examine the iris for elevated lesions, nevi, as well as new blood vessels, which may develop in states of retinal hypoxia. This setup also may be used to facilitate corneal FB removal.

2. Blue cobalt filter. With the light beam widened for more diffuse illumination, examine the cornea for injury with the aid of fluorescein stain. Place the fluorescein in the inferior cul-de-sac of the eye. The areas of corneal epithelial injury will become bright green with the staining of Bowman's membrane.

3. Conical section illumination. With the white light and the narrow beam shortened to approximately 3 mm, visualize the anterior chamber. Because of the small size of this light beam, a higher power is needed for adequate visualization. Use the joystick to focus the cone of light at a point midway between the cornea and anterior surface of the lens. Inspect the anterior chamber for flare, which represents an increase in protein in the anterior chamber that appears like a haze reflecting the light beam. Also visualize cells in the anterior chamber. Red blood cells appear yellowish, whereas white blood cells appear as white dots. These cells will move throughout the anterior chamber because of the fluid nature of the anterior chamber (8, 10, 39).

NASAL EMERGENCIES

Nasal Foreign Bodies

Nasal FBs are commonly seen in children and can present a special challenge. Edema and secondary infection can develop rapidly, making removal more difficult. Take special care to make sure that an FB in the nose is not dislodged into the pharynx, resulting in aspiration.

The initial method of removing an FB from the nose is to have the patient forcefully blow the nose with the unobstructed side pinched closed (35). In the uncooperative or young patient, two other methods are used to "blow" the object from the patient's nose. The first method is to have the parent blow a puff of air while the parent's mouth is sealed over the child's mouth. The other method is to use an Ambu bag and cover only the mouth, and then quickly to squeeze in a puff of air. In both of these methods, pinch the unobstructed nostril closed (9, 16).

If these methods do not work, then use a hooked probe or alligator forceps. Pass the hooked probe beyond the object and use it to pull the object forward. Alligator forceps work well to remove particulate matter and for objects that can be grasped easily. These methods work well for objects in the anterior part of the nasal cavity, but if the object is too far posterior, then the following techniques may aid in removal.

Balloon catheters, such as the Fogarty biliary balloon catheter in 5- or 6-French size, can be used to remove most FBs. Lubricate the catheter with 2% lidocaine jelly, advance it past the object, and inflate the balloon with 2 to 3 mL of air, and then pull the catheter forward. Additionally, use the inflated balloon to stabilize the FB,

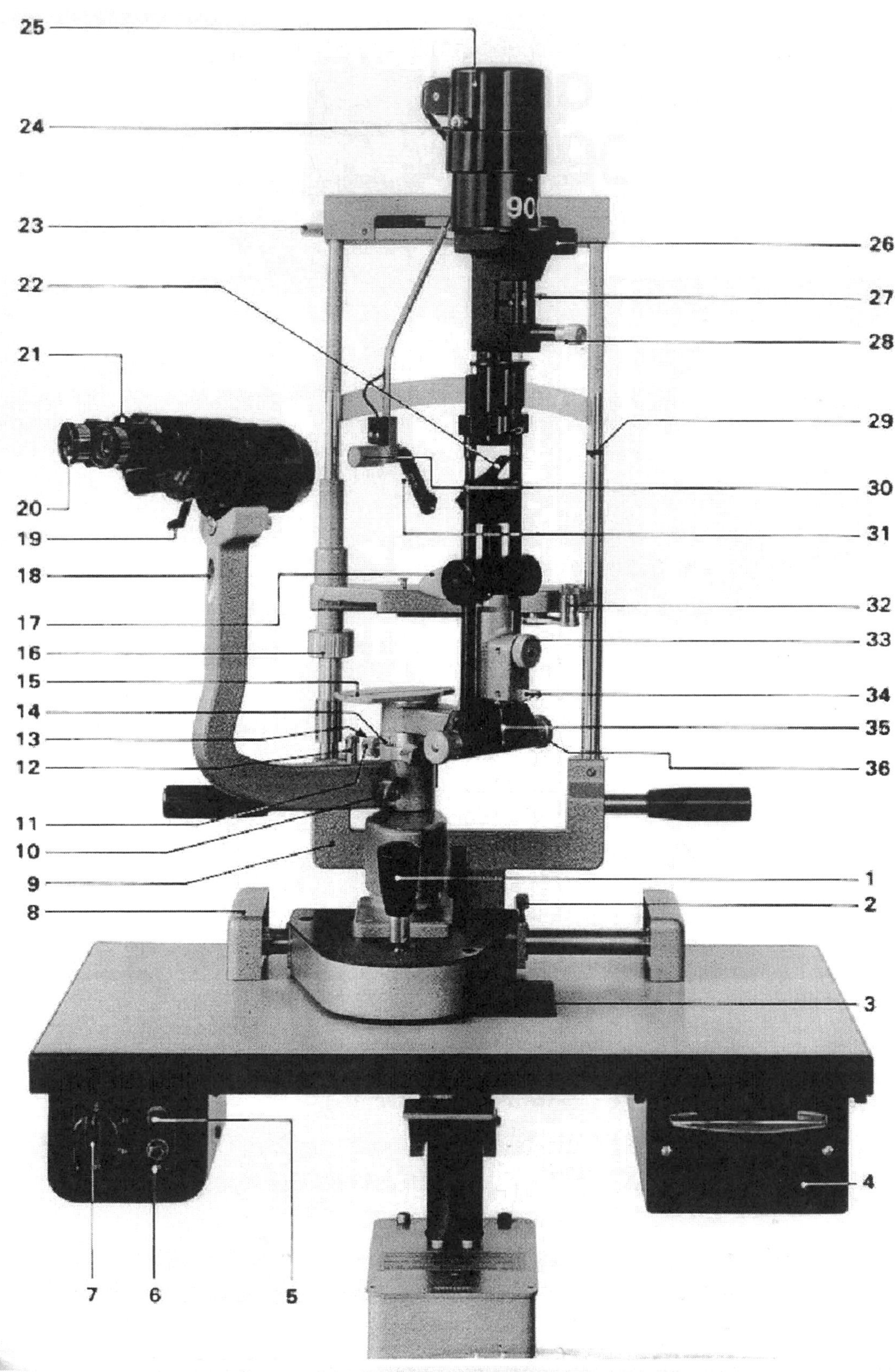
25
24
23
22
21
20
19
18
17
16
15
14
13
12
11
10
9
8
26
27
28
29
30
31
32
33
34
35
36
1
2
3
4
7
6
5
90

and use a wire loop or ear curette to remove it. Use suction to remove certain nasal FBs. Place a suction catheter with a plastic umbrella tip against the FB, and turn on the suction to 100 to 140 mm Hg. The object is removed as the catheter is removed from the nose (28). Cyanoacrylate glue also can be used to remove objects from the nose. Apply a drop of glue to the blunt end of a swab stick, and hold the stick in contact with the FB until the glue is dried, approximately 30 to 60 seconds, and then remove the object.

Nasal FB removal can be challenging, but most FBs can be removed with these procedures. Those that are unable to be removed or that develop complications should be immediately referred to an otolaryngologist.

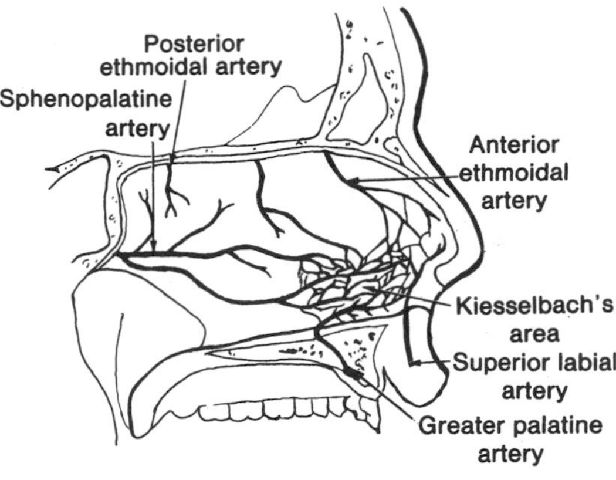

Figure 8.15. Nasal vessels supplying the septum. (From Laforce RF: Treatment of nasal hemorrhage. Surg Clin North Am 49:1306, 1969, with permission.)

EPISTAXIS

Epistaxis is a common problem in the emergency center. For the emergency physician to understand this disorder thoroughly, a basic understanding of the arteries and veins supplying the nose is mandatory.

The sphenopalatine artery, a terminal branch of the external carotid artery, courses through the sphenopalatine foramen to supply the nasal cavity. It divides into the medial and lateral branches. This artery supplies the majority of the posterior portion of the nose. The anterior and posterior ethmoidal arteries arise from the ophthalmic artery as it enters anteriorly along the crista galli just superior to the cribriform plate (Fig. 8.15). These arteries course downward and supply blood to the anterior superior portion of the nasal cavity. The arteries supplying the septum form a plexus of vessels anteriorly, called Kiesselbach's area (Little's area). This plexus, formed along the anterior portion of the nasal septum, is the most common site of epistaxis. Another common site for arterial bleeding is from the anterior superior portion of the nasal

Figure 8.14. Slit lamp and parts. *1.* Control lever for horizontal and vertical adjustment. *2.* Fixing screw for horizontal movements. *3.* Gliding plate. *4.* Accessory drawer. *5.* Pilot light. *6.* Fuse. *7.* Rotary switch. *8.* Rail covers. *9.* Headrest. *10.* Fixing screw for the microscope arm. *11.* Two knobs for coupling the microscope arm to the lamp arm. *12.* Roller for setting the angle between microscope and illumination. *13.* Index for reading angles. *14.* Scale for reading the angle between microscope and illumination. *15.* Guide plate for preset lens and applanation tonometer T 900.4.1. *16.* Level adjustment control for the chin rest. *17.* Chin rest. *18.* Fixing screw for the microscope. *18a.* Fixing screw for the microscope. *19.* Lever for changing the objectives. *19a.* Knob for changing the magnification. *20.* Interchangeable eyepieces. *20a.* Milled surface and thread for fixing the applanation tonometer. *21.* Knurled rings for setting the eyepieces. *22.* Interchangeable illumination mirror. *23.* Knurled knob for lateral adjustment of the fixation light. *24.* Clamping nuts for the lamp housing. *25.* Cover for lamp housing. *26.* Scale for slit diaphragms. *27.* Lever for three filters. *28.* Control for rotation of slit, for varying the slit length, and interposing the blue filter. *29.* Level marker. *30.* Fixation lamp. *31.* Handle for focusing the fixation target. *32.* Slide for preset lens. *33.* Centering screw. *34.* 5-degree stops. *35.* Latch for the angle of inclination. *36.* Controls (2) for setting the slit width. (Reprinted from Slit Lamp Systems 900: Instructions Use Maintenance. Haag-Streit AG, with permission.)

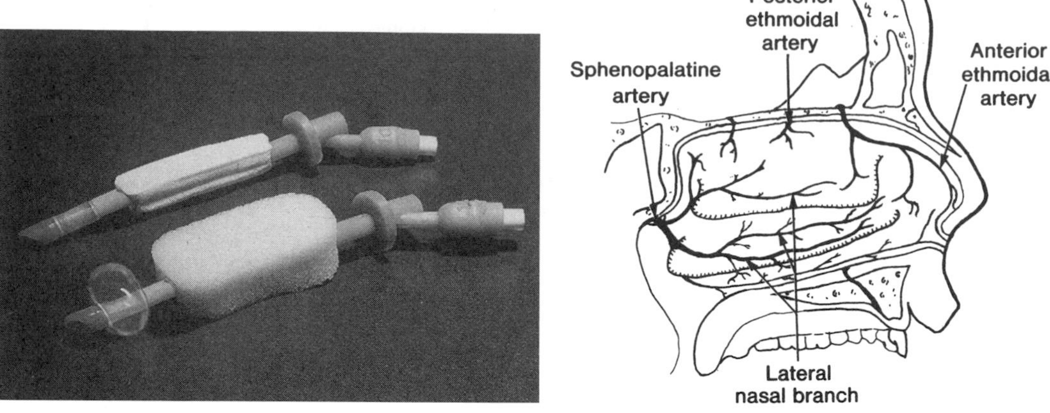

Figure 8.16. *A*: Nasal catheter. Epistat and Epistat II are manufactured by Medtronic Xomed (Courtesy of Medtronic Xomed, Jacksonville, Florida). *B*: Nasal vessels supplying the lateral nasal wall. (From Laforce RF: Treatment of nasal hemorrhage. Surg Clin North Am 49:1306, 1969, with permission.)

cavity supplied by the ethmoidal artery. A third site for arterial bleeding is from the sphenopalatine artery, and the patients usually have posterior nasal bleeding into the pharynx (Fig. 8.16) (21, 30, 41). The external carotid artery supplies the middle and inferior turbinates via the sphenopalatine artery, whereas the internal carotid supplies the superior and anterior portion of the nose via the ophthalmic arteries, which branch off to form the anterior and posterior ethmoidal arteries. The septum thus is supplied by both the external and internal carotid arteries; Kiesselbach's area can be thought of as the terminal branches of both the internal and external carotid system meeting on the cartilaginous nasal septum (15, 21, 22).

The venous system also may be the source of epistaxis. A common source of epistaxis is an area of dilated veins in the posterior end of the inferior turbinate called Woodruff's nasopharyngeal plexus. Bleeding from this source occurs particularly in older hypertensive patients and in patients with arteriosclerosis.

Always consider the etiologies in patients with epistaxis. Cardiovascular factors play a major role, not in the initiation of epistaxis, but in the continuation of bleeding (27). Our knowledge of the underlying cause of spontaneous nosebleeds remains sketchy. In one study involving 1,724 cases of epistaxis, 71% of the patients were found to be older than 50 years. Cardiovascular causes were implicated in 47% of the cases, and the cause was undetermined in approximately 30% (27). In the elderly, there seems to be a higher incidence of posterior sites of bleeding (13). Specific identifiable causes account for only 10% to 15% of all cases seen in the emergency center with epistaxis (45). In children with recurrent epistaxis, acute rhinitis or allergic problems may predispose to this difficulty. In the older age group, hypertension, arteriosclerosis, vascular anomalies, and coagulopathies are the leading causes of recurrent epistaxis (21).

When one sees a patient with epistaxis, ascertain whether the bleeding was associated with a traumatic etiology or was spontaneous. Trauma (including nose picking, auto accidents, falls, sneezing, etc.) accounted for only 13.5% of cases in one large study (22). Most of the bleeding associated with a traumatic etiology is in the anterior portion of the nasal cavity.

The causes of spontaneous bleeding are numerous; the most common are

1. **Acute and chronic infections** (15, 21, 22). Several severe cases of epistaxis occurred in patients with influenza (23). Acute and chronic nasal infections as well as systemic diseases including measles, chickenpox, or nasal congestion associated with an upper respiratory infection all have been documented as causes of spontaneous epistaxis, particularly in children (15, 21, 23).
2. **Vascular abnormalities.** Diseases of the vascular system account for a number of cases of epistaxis such as hereditary hemorrhagic telangiectasias (21, 22).
3. **Hypertension**, although an overdiagnosed etiology of spontaneous epistaxis, is, nevertheless, a known cause (22). Remember that all patients with epistaxis will be anxious, and many of them will have some degree of hypertension. Although this requires follow-up, it is uncommon for the hypertension to be the etiology of the epistaxis, particularly in the younger age group.
4. **High venous tensions**, as occur in emphysema, whooping cough, bronchitis, and tumors of the neck, account for some venous sources of epistaxis (22).
5. **Coagulation defects** account for a small percentage of patients with epistaxis.
6. **Neoplasms of the nose or sinus**, although uncommon causes, should be searched for.
7. **Other causes** include atherosclerosis, Cushing syndrome, uremia, and scurvy.

In patients suspected of having coagulation defects, obtain appropriate coagulation profiles. Suspect coagulopathies in a patient with a history of easy bruising, of recurrent nosebleeds without an obvious cause, or of bleeding from other sites and, finally, in patients with physical evidence of a coagulopathy or low platelet count, such as petechiae.

Anterior Epistaxis

The treatment of epistaxis basically includes the arrest of hemorrhage and the search for and treatment of underlying causes.

EQUIPMENT (30)

Headlight
Nasal speculum
Bayonet forceps
Epinephrine, 1:1,000 topical
Cotton balls or pledgets
Cotton-tipped applicators
Tongue blades
French Frazier angulated suction catheter
4 × 4-inch and 3 × 3-inch gauze
10-inch long umbilical tape, two pieces
Small rubber catheter, ½ inch wide
Vaseline-impregnated gauze strips
Antibiotic ointment
Epistat balloon
10- or 12-French Foley catheter

TECHNIQUE

1. Seat the patient upright with the head bent forward and ask the patient to hold the nose pinched for approximately 10 minutes (23). Both the patient and the physician should wear gowns, and the physician should wear a face mask and eye protection.
2. If bleeding continues, ask the patient to blow the nose to remove all clots.
3. With use of a nasal speculum and head mirror, suction all the remaining clots and bleeding.

NOTE

Many of these patients, particularly children, will be apprehensive. The use of morphine sulfate in a dosage of 10–15 mg intramuscularly or meperidine (Demerol) in a dosage of 100 mg for *adults* has been recommended by many authors (21, 33). In the child, administer a mild sedative hypnotic. When the bleeding is minimal, discover the source of bleeding before the administration of vasoconstrictors or topical anesthetics into the nose. When trauma is the etiology, look at Kiesselbach's area, particularly in patients with anterior bleeding. Not uncommonly, a small, bleeding septal vessel is noted in the anterior portion. When the anterior ethmoidal artery is the source of bleeding, notice bleeding coming from the anterior aspect of the middle turbinate. This bleeding often is intermittent, and the blood may "trickle" backward, making it seem like posterior bleeding. When the patient states that the bleeding occurred in the pharynx, first suspect the sphenopalatine artery as the source of posterior bleeding (23). When bleeding is brisk and the source cannot be identified, place multiple cotton strips soaked in 4% cocaine and a 1:1,000 solution of epinephrine along the floor of the nose. These should remain in place for 5 minutes (15, 18, 21, 23, 30). When the bleeding can be seen to be coming from one site, apply a cotton pledget soaked in cocaine and epinephrine to that site to decrease the amount of bleeding, thus permitting cauterization.

NOTE (20,21)

Silver nitrate sticks are commonly used to cauterize the bleeding point chemically. Persistent bleeding or high risk of recurrent bleeding may require electrocauterization. When silver nitrate is used, apply the applicator for at least 20 seconds (13). Vigorously bleeding vessels are commonly seen in hypertensives and in patients with arteriosclerotic disease; in these, electrocoagulation is necessary. Bipolar coagulation such as the Bantan Bovie unit is probably the best type to use (3, 13).

---

4. When a specific bleeding point cannot be identified, but the bleeding is ascertained to be coming from an anterior source, place an anterior pack.

   a. Squeeze antibacterial ointment into the plastic package containing the ½-inch wide Vaseline-impregnated gauze that is used for anterior packing.

NOTE

A number of authors advise the use of an antibacterial ointment on the pack, because, if it is left in for more than 24 hours, infection is commonly seen (3, 15). Bilateral anterior packs almost never should be used because of the increased risk of infection and septal damage and ulceration. Use them only when one cannot tell, by history or examination, which side the bleeding is coming from, which is most unusual. In addition to the antibacterial ointment, use oral broad-spectrum antibiotics for most patients with posterior packs; some authors advise them for patients with anterior packs as well.

---

   b. Place the gauze strips in rows, beginning in the floor of the nose along the posterior aspect, and layering the gauze stripping as shown in Fig. 8.17. Lay the gauze carefully and only after adequate shrinking of the congested nasal membranes and adequate anesthesia has been provided, as indicated earlier.

5. When anterior bleeding continues, take the following steps:

   a. A number of authors recommended the use of Surgigel or Oxygel as a packing agent (23). We do not recommend these because they often form a sticky, amorphous mess when left in place (13, 29).
   b. Remove the packing and place cotton strips soaked in cocaine and epinephrine solution; keep these strips in place until the bleeding decreases. Place a new anterior pack carefully, by following this procedure. If bleeding continues,

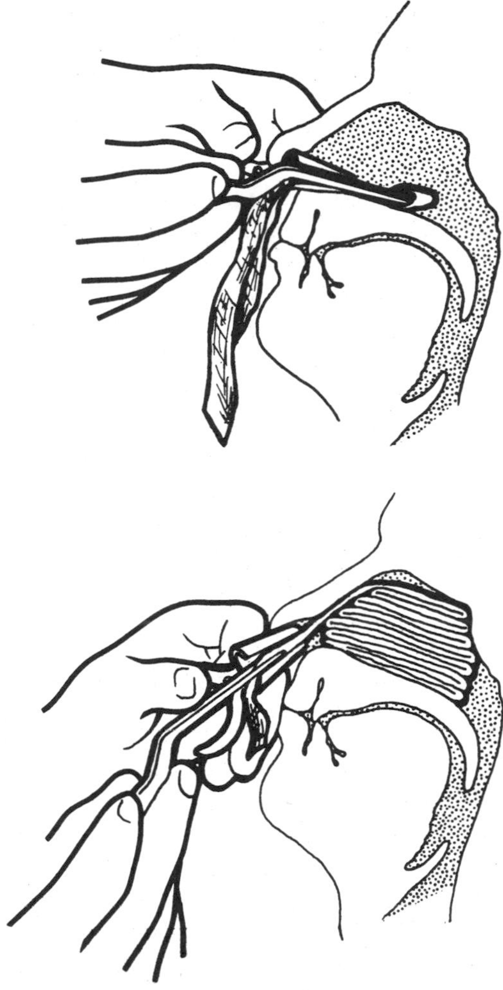

Figure 8.17. Place an anterior pack by layering ¼-inch gauze packing impregnated with antibacterial ointment along the floor of the nose. Add morc packing toward the superior aspect of the nasal cavity, and pack it down periodically to ensure a tight tamponading pack.

check these patients for a hemorrhagic diathesis. Try to ascertain whether the bleeding is coming from under the middle turbinates, suggesting an arterial cause, or from a superior site that an improperly placed pack may not adequately control (27).

c. Topical thrombin also may be quite useful in patients with coagulopathies (21).

d. The Epistat balloon (Merocel Corp., Mystic, CT) described later may be of benefit in unremitting anterior bleeds.

6. Leave the packing in place for 5 days, and then remove it.

NOTE

When bleeding occurs from both nostrils, this almost always is due to blood coming around the posterior portion of the nasal septum and across to the uninvolved side. Ascertain from which side of the nose the bleeding started first; examine this side for the site of bleeding (15, 30).

Posterior Epistaxis

Posterior bleeding, as indicated earlier, may be secondary to bleeding from Woodruff's plexus, in which case, hold a cotton pledget moistened with cocaine and epinephrine snugly below the inferior turbinate to decrease the bleeding (21). The sphenopalatine artery is another common site of posterior bleeding. Basically two methods have been described for the treatment of posterior bleeding: the placement of a posterior pack and balloon tamponade.

POSTERIOR PACK

Fold a 3 × 3-inch gauge bandage lengthwise (Fig. 8.18), roll it tightly until the thick end is less than ¾ inch in diameter, and bind it tightly around the middle by two pieces of umbilical tape, each measuring approximately 10 inches in length. Umbilical tape is superior to string because it does not cut into the palate (29). After this, insert a rubber catheter through the nose and pull it out through the mouth. Tie the umbilical tape to the catheter, and pull the pack back into the mouth and into the posterior choanae of the nose by pulling on the rubber catheter. The pack lodges securely in the posterior

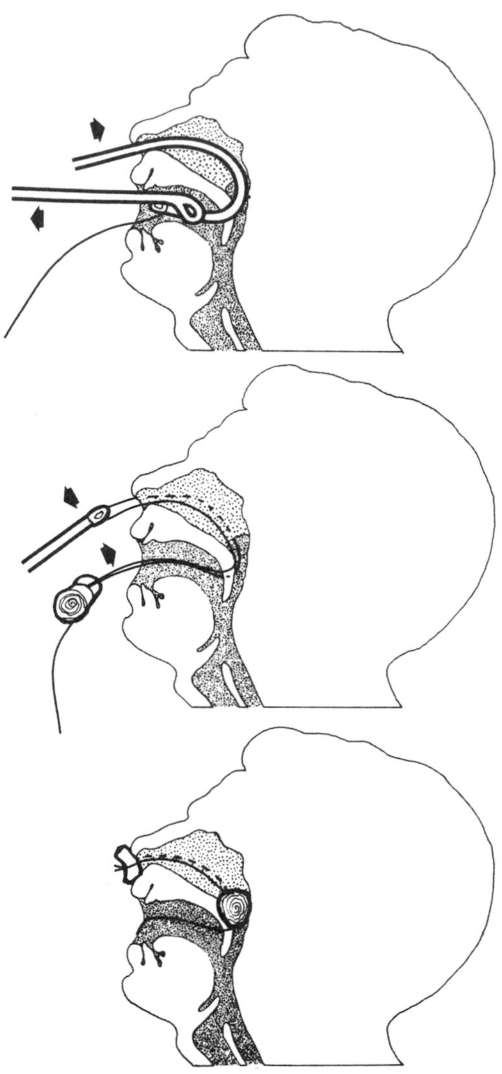

Figure 8.18. Technique for placing a posterior pack. See text for discussion.

choanae of the nose and tamponades bleeding at this point. Then secure the umbilical tape anteriorly by tying it around a piece of gauze to prevent posterior displacement of the pack. Apply an anterior pack on the same side on which the posterior pack was placed, because bleeding may resume at a later time just anterior to the posterior pack as a result of difficulties in maintaining constant pressure on the sphenopalatine artery. Most bleeding can be stopped with a properly placed posterior and anterior pack.

Complications

A number of complications have been described in association with posterior packs. If a string is used rather than umbilical tape, it may cut into the soft palate. Infections of the middle ear have been noted after posterior pack insertion. Osteomyelitis of the parasphenoid also has been described after pharyngeal infections from posterior packs (21). Abscesses in the pharynx may occur after posterior packs.

Give antibiotics to all patients with a posterior pack in place. Ventilation–perfusion abnormalities develop with a posterior pack, and arterial oxygen may decrease 20 to 30 mm Hg; admit all these patients to the hospital (21, 30).

BALLOON TAMPONADE

A number of authors have recommended balloon tamponade rather than a posterior pack because of poor patient tolerance and the complications associated with posterior packs (6, 27, 45, 48). Many nasal balloons have been developed and are currently commercially available. The Brighton and Eschman balloons function much like a Foley catheter and are held in place by an external balloon that, if accidentally deflated, could result in the entire device and pack slipping posteriorly and blocking the airway. The Noz-stop is a two-balloon device that is bulky and hard to place in the airway and also may block the airway if the outer balloon is deflated. Of all the balloons commercially available, the Epistat has been found by us and others to be the best-designed balloon on the market today (Fig. 8.19). This balloon is designed to act as an anterior and posterior pack. There is no need for an anterior pack with this balloon in place, because it occludes the area where the sphenopalatine artery exits, as well as all sites anterior to the artery.

Technique of Insertion

1. Inflate the balloons to ascertain that there are no leaks.

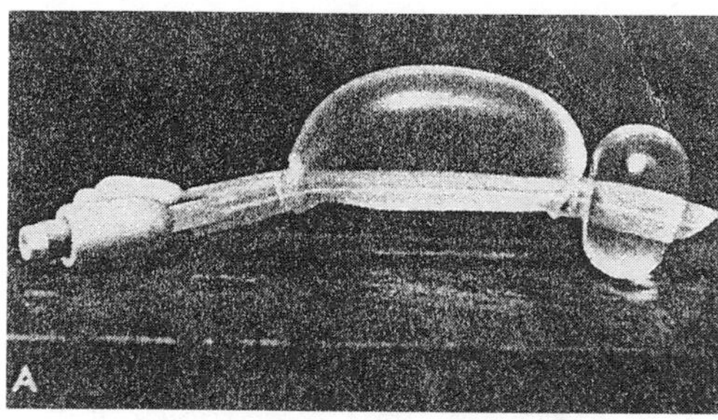

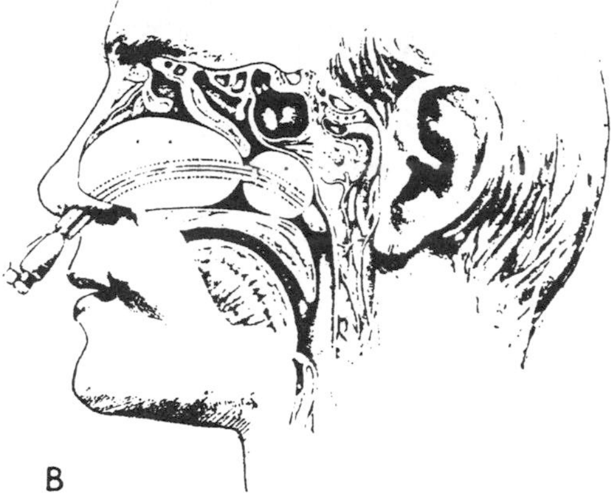

Figure 8.19. The Epistat balloon *(A)* and similar devices allow an easy method to provide control for either anterior or posterior epistaxis *(B)*. (Courtesy of Exomed Inc., Jacksonville, Florida.)

2. Lubricate the balloon with lidocaine (Xylocaine) jelly and introduce it along the floor of the nose.
3. Inflate the distal balloon first with air, injected very slowly to minimize the discomfort that may occur with rapid inflation, and then inflate the proximal balloon.
4. Inspect the oropharynx for evidence of continuing posterior bleeding. If posterior bleeding persists, slowly inject more air until either the posterior bleeding stops or the palate is seen to bulge inferiorly into the mouth. If the patient complains of a blocked feeling in the airway, the balloon may be overinflated and air should be withdrawn until the opposite airway is patent.
5. If no bleeding is noted posteriorly and the opposite airway is patent, withdraw and measure the air, and replace it with the same volume of water, because air will leak out over a short period.
6. Place a 2 × 2-inch strip of gauze between the nose and the bulb so as to prevent pressure necrosis. If anterior bleeding continues after the balloon is inflated, it is probably from the ethmoidal artery, so place an anterior packing superiorly in the nasal cavity. In some patients with a large nasal passage, or in patients with continuing ethmoidal bleeding, insert the balloon along the floor of the nose with an anterior pack applied over it, and then slowly inflate the balloon to stop the epistaxis.
7. Maintain balloon inflation for 48 hours. After this period, deflate the balloon, but leave it in place for an additional 12 to 24 hours. If no bleeding results at this time, remove the balloon.

NOTE

When an Epistat or other balloon device is not available, use a 12- or 14-French Foley catheter. Insert the Foley catheter along the floor of the nose until it reaches the nasopharynx. Then inflate the balloon with approximately 7 mL of water and draw it forward until it lodges in the posterior portion of the nose (Fig. 8.20). If bleeding does not stop, add an additional 15 mL of water. Then place an anterior pack anteriorly against the balloon for the same reasons as indicated earlier for the posterior pack. This combination has been used successfully to control posterior bleeding (7, 45, 48).

INJECTION BLOCK OF THE SPHENOPALATINE ARTERY

In the patient who has unremitting posterior nasal hemorrhage, a method has been described for controlling the hemorrhage by blocking the sphenopalatine artery as well as the descending palatine

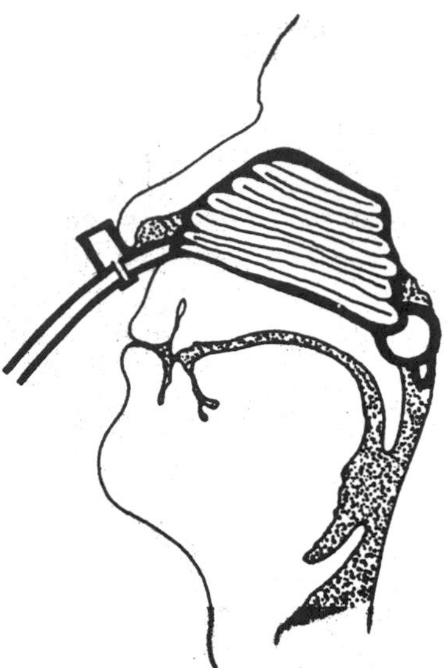

Figure 8.20. For posterior nasal bleeding, place a Foley catheter in the nasopharyngeal area and add an anterior pack. Then inflate the Foley catheter and pull it to form a tight seal at the site of the sphenopalatine artery. This method will stop most posterior nose bleeds that may be resistant to other methods.

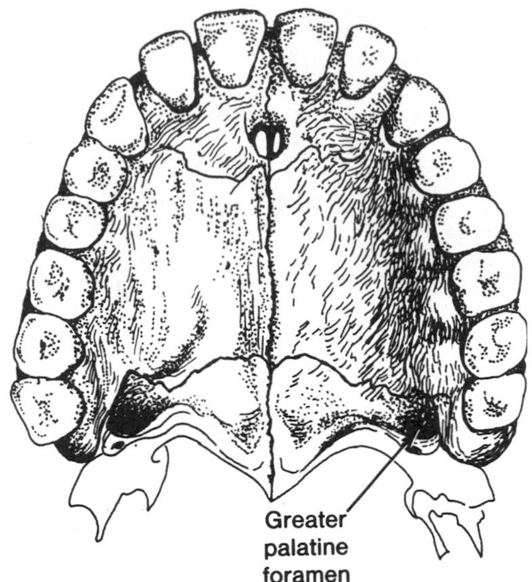

Figure 8.21. Greater palatine foramen. The technique of blocking the sphenopalatine artery is discussed in the text.

arteries. Place the patient in a supine position with the mouth opened, and palpate the greater palatine foramen (Fig. 8.21). Be accurate in locating the foramen because the needle must pass through it to obtain a good block. It is located in the hard palate just anterior to the junction with the soft palate. Palpate a slight depression under the palatal mucosa just distal to the third molar, or locate it with a needle probe. With a 22- or 23-gauge spinal needle on a 5-mL syringe, inject 3 mL of 2% lidocaine with 1:100,000 epinephrine through the greater palatine foramen into the pterygopalatine fossa via the pterygopalatine canal. When properly placed, injection here blocks the sphenopalatine artery and also the descending palatine artery. The ideal depth of injection is 28 mm (41); insert the needle to this depth once within the foramen. The active agent reducing bleeding is epinephrine; lidocaine merely reduces the pain of injection, because the sphenopalatine nerve courses with the artery in the pterygopalatine canal. In one study using this procedure, posterior bleeding was controlled or stopped in 10 of 11 patients within 3 minutes after the block was instilled (41). Authors using this technique advocated that it should be attempted before insertion of any posterior pack, because when bleeding is controlled by this means, the difficulty of inserting a pack and the discomfort of a balloon in place for a prolonged period are avoided (30, 41).

Arterial ligation is indicated only when packing or a balloon tamponade have failed and should be left to the expertise of an otolaryngologist.

Summary

Figure 8.22 presents a useful guide for management of patients seen in the emergency center with epistaxis.

NASAL FRACTURES

Nasal fractures are very commonly seen in the emergency center. The physician

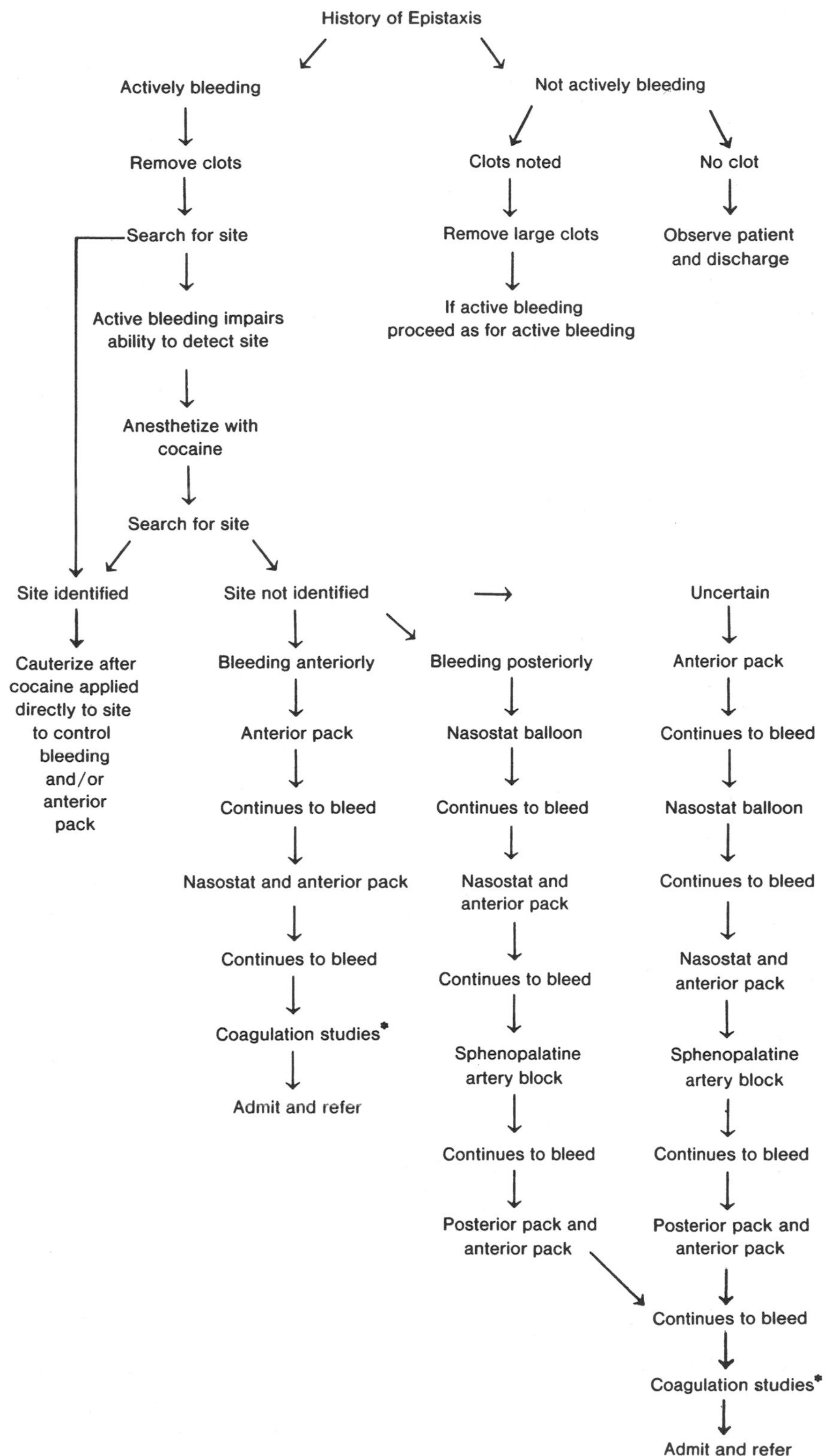

Figure 8.22. A guide for the management of and approach to a patient with epistaxis. In the patient with an anterior nose bleed and a suspected coagulopathy, try topical thrombin early in the course of therapy.

first seeing the patient must make an early diagnosis before the development of edema, which may impair the ability to diagnose a displaced fracture. In children, edema develops very early, whereas, in adults, it develops much later. Although nasal bones heal by bony union without scar contracture, nasal cartilage does not. Cartilage heals by deposition of scar tissue with contracture that may cause curling and buckling around an organized inflammatory exudate and a chondritis formed during healing. One has a grace period, during which time a reduction of nasal fractures can be done by the emergency physician in the emergency center. This grace period is before swelling occurs. If the patient comes in after swelling is significant, then reduction should be delayed, and the patient referred to an otolaryngologist. Reduction of a nasal fracture can be done 7 to 10 days after the swelling has subsided, by using a closed technique after the injury. In children, bony fusion may occur earlier, and therefore reduction should be done at an earlier time. If there is any doubt about the ability to perform an adequate reduction, refer the patient to a specialist.

We recommend the following protocol in diagnosing fractures of the nose:

1. Look for any deformity or depression of the nasal bone.
2. Palpate the bridge of the nose for any crepitus. Be cautious not to palpate too vigorously. Fractures may be present in this area without any obvious crepitation.
3. Examine the inside of the nose after applying 4% cocaine to shrink the nasal membranes. Look for submucosal hemorrhage or hematoma formation, particularly along the septum, and for mucosal tears or deviation of the septum or lateral nasal wall. A hematoma of the septum has normal mucosal coloring and is not ecchymotic, making it difficult to identify. Identify a septal hematoma; missing this diagnosis may lead to the formation of a septal abscess or devitalization of the cartilage and saddle deformity of the nose. Palpate the septum to feel a fluctuation over a hematoma. When a septal hematoma is identified, incise and drain it as discussed in Chapter 10, Plastic Surgery Principles and Techniques. The technique for drainage through an L-shaped incision is shown in Fig. 10.77. Find lateral swelling resulting from buckling of the lateral cartilage or submucosal hemorrhage.

   All of these conditions will be seen with inability to shrink the mucous membrane with cocaine. If the membranes do shrink with the application of cocaine, search for mucosal membrane tears. When a mucosal membrane tear is large and accessible, repair it with plain catgut suture. When one is unable to repair a large defect of the membrane, pack the area to prevent hematoma formation.
4. As a final step, obtain radiographs. It is reported that only 50% of fractures of the nose are seen on routine radiographs (4, 25).

Nasal fractures can be classified into three categories:

1. *Greenstick fractures.* In this situation, there is bending of the nasal bones or septum but no complete fracture line is visualized.
2. *Linear fractures.* A linear fracture may be displaced or undisplaced. When the patient has an undisplaced fracture in good position, the treatment is ice to decrease swelling and analgesia. If there is a linear fracture with either lateral displacement or depression present, the treatment consists of blunt elevation with splinting and/or intranasal Vaseline-impregnated gauze packing.
3. *Comminuted fractures.* Comminuted fractures of the nasal bones are often open, with mucosal tears exposing the

bone. The treatment of these injuries is similar to that of displaced and depressed lateral fractures.

The most common fracture seen in the adult is one with lateral displacement or depression of the nasal bone.

An analysis of nasal fractures indicates that patients with greenstick fractures and linear fractures without displacement or depression have a 100% good outcome. Linear fractures with displacement have a 40% good outcome and a 25% poor outcome, and depressed fractures have a 20% good outcome and a 45% poor outcome. In patients with comminuted fractures, only 10% have good results, and 70% have poor results (26). These figures are despite the usual therapy for the fracture.

EQUIPMENT

Asch forceps
Vaseline-impregnated gauze, ½-inch wide, for nasal packing
Bayonet forceps
Anesthetic prep
1% lidocaine with epinephrine
5-mL syringe
25-gauge, 1.5-inch needle
18-gauge needle
4% cocaine
Cotton balls
Cotton-tipped applicators
Head light
Prefabricated metal splint, or casting material cut to appropriate shape and size
¼ inch adhesive tape
Tincture of benzoin
Periosteal elevator
Salinger elevator

Technique of Reduction

The physician must have a clear understanding of the anatomy of the nose before attempting reduction of a nasal fracture (Fig. 8.23). The nasal part of the frontal bone is posterior and inferior to the nasal bones and adds strength and support to the bony arch of the nose. Therefore fractures involving the nasal portion of the frontal bone require more uplift and support to prevent postreduction depression of the bridge of the nose. After reduction, splint the fractures and pack properly. Lateral cartilaginous plates also extend upward on the inner surface of the nasal bones and intimately fuse with them, so trauma to the nasal bones often injures these cartilages as well.

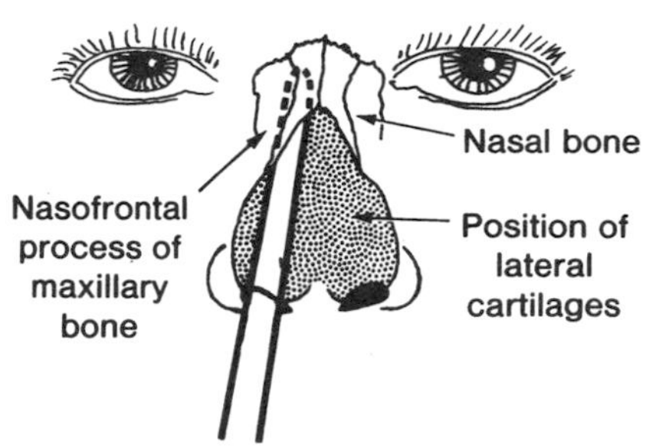

Figure 8.23. Note the anatomy of the nose and the placement of the cartilages.

Use the following principles in reduction of nasal fractures:

1. Provide anesthesia by the technique discussed in Chapter 3, Anesthesia and Regional Blocks.
2. Evacuate any hematomas or effusions and examine carefully for any cartilaginous damage.
3. Reduce the displaced fracture fragments. The bridge of the nose may have to be separated from the nasal part of the frontal bone, as shown in Fig. 8.23. This is done by inserting the Asch forceps into the appropriate nostril and elevating the nasal bone fragments into proper position by applying outward pressure with the forceps (Fig. 8.24*E*). Place the finger on the outside of the nose to aid in properly aligning the nasal bone (Fig. 8.24*B* and *E*). A Salinger forceps is our preferred tool for reducing depressed nasal fractures (see Fig. 8.24*D* for description). Adequate anesthesia is essential for this procedure. With an Asch forceps, rotate outward the na-

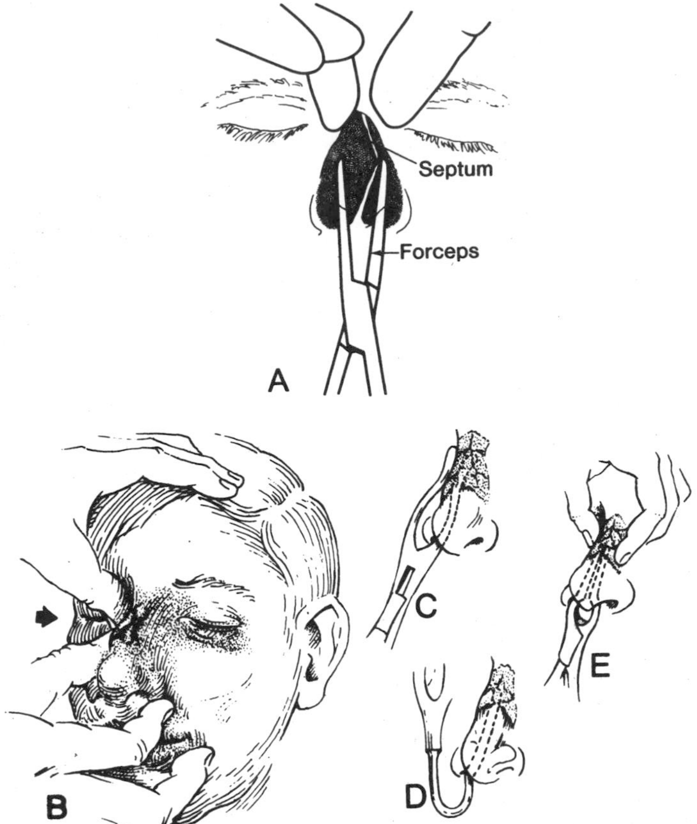

Figure 8.24. Use an Asch forceps to correct a deviated septum, and use a Salinger elevator or the handle of a scalpel to elevate a depressed nasal fracture. Use the opposite side of the nose for a comparison, and palpate to reduce these fractures adequately. Manual reduction of laterally angulated nasal fractures often can be done immediately after injury and with only momentary discomfort. *A*: An Asch forceps correcting a deviated nasal septum. *B*: A finger placed on the outside of the nose can manipulate a displaced fragment back into position. *C*: A Salinger or Walsham forceps may be used to correct a laterally depressed fracture. *D*: A Salinger elevator (preferred method) can be used to reposition a depressed fragment. *E*: A forceps inserted inside the nose can anatomically reposition these fragments. (From Schultz RC: Nasal fractures. J Trauma 15:321, 1975, with permission.)

sofrontal process of the maxillary bone if it is depressed, for the nasal bones to be properly aligned with it. Do this with the Asch forceps by applying outward pressure against these processes (Fig. 8.24*C*). By applying inward pressure with a digit over the laterally displaced segment and with the Asch forceps inserted inside the nose to provide adequate counterpressure, reduce laterally displaced segments.

4. Reduce a deviated septum by replacing it in the groove of the vomer with the Asch forceps, as shown in Fig. 8.24*A* (see legend to figure for a more detailed description).
5. After reduction of the nose and septum, pack the nose internally on both sides with ½-inch Vaseline-impregnated gauze to provide internal stabilization of the reduced segments. Provide external stabilization by splints that are made of either dental compound or casting material or by a specially made metal splint that is commercially available (Fig. 8.25). Leave

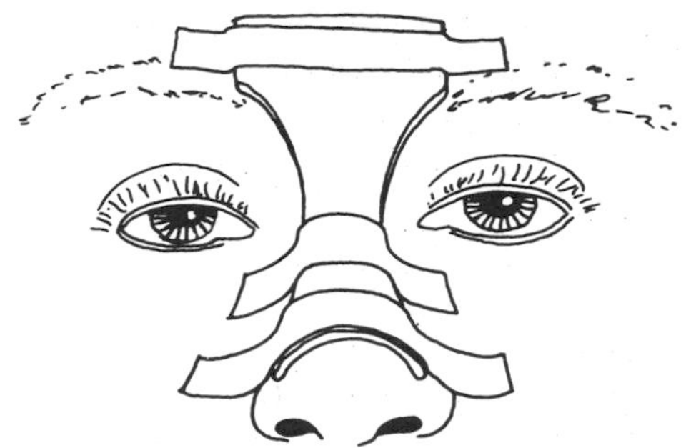

Figure 8.25. A prefabricated nasal splint used for external support of a reduced fracture. This does not provide a great deal of support, but cautions the patient against further trauma to the site of the nasal fracture.

the splint in place over the dorsum of the bony arch and cartilage to maintain position for 10 days. Continue internal splinting for 5 to 7 days.

When a splint is formed from casting material, cut out the splint from several sheets of casting material in a shape similar to that of the metal splint shown in Fig. 8.25. To secure the plaster splint to the nose, paint tincture of benzoin on the nose and apply a strip of adhesive tape ("sticky side up") to the area where the cast will lie. Then form the cast and place it in the proper position over the adhesive tape, which aids in keeping it in its proper location. Place ¼-inch adhesive strips over the casting material in a fashion similar to that shown in Fig. 8.25 for the metal splint. Remember that with complex nasal fractures, open reduction may be required if one cannot place the fragments together properly. Again, if there is any doubt about your ability to perform an adequate reduction, refer the patient to a specialist, especially with comminuted fractures.

NOTE

In children, because there is less ossification, there is a higher incidence of greenstick fractures, and crepitation may not be palpable even with significant displacement. Less force is required to fracture the cartilaginous structures of the nose, and there is a tendency to form more scar tissue, with deformity increasing as the child grows. If the child has edema, and the history suggests a fractured nose, arrange for adequate follow-up, even if the radiographs are normal. For children with depressed fractures, the treatment is basically similar to that for the adult, with the exception that one must shrink the nasal membranes with cotton strips saturated with cocaine before any procedure. Wrap the cotton around a periosteal elevator, dipped in cocaine and Vaseline, and use it to elevate the depressed nasal arch. Maintain the position with lateral splints.

HEAD AND NECK ABSCESSES

Although abscesses of the head and neck are a relatively commonly seen problem in the emergency center, only a few can be drained on an outpatient basis. Small superficial abscesses in the anterior triangle (the area anterior to the sternocleidomastoid muscle) may be drained, but any deep abscesses in a patient who has torticollis or trismus should be drained in the operating room, with the exception of peritonsillar abscesses. There are various potential spaces within the neck that are beyond the scope of discussion in this text. Abscesses may drain or may extend into the carotid sheath or paratracheal region, requiring extensive incisions to promote adequate drainage.

Preparatory Steps in Treating Intraoral Abscesses

It is helpful to rinse the mouth with bicarbonate solution to dissolve excess mucus when dealing with intraoral abscesses, particularly those in the peritonsillar region. After the mucosa is sprayed with a topical anesthetic, such as Cetacaine, rub the site of the proposed incision with a

10% cocaine stick until blanching occurs. Then perform the incision with the patient in the sitting position and leaning forward whenever possible to avoid pulmonary aspiration of purulent material.

Peritonsillar Abscesses

Muller (38) stated that although incision and drainage are often done for these abscesses, when compared with immediate tonsillectomy in 186 cases, no problems were encountered with this procedure, and a faster return to normal activity was noted. Many authors recommend immediate tonsillectomy as the treatment of choice for peritonsillar abscesses (4, 34, 46). Other authors also noted that it is often hard to obtain adequate drainage of an abscess in the peritonsillar area with a simple stab incision (38). Evidence of loculated nondraining purulent material may be slow resolution of the abscess, trismus, and persistence of pain in patients treated with incision alone. Immediate tonsillectomy assures total evacuation of the purulent matter, and the patient is spared a later admission for an interval tonsillectomy. In view of these data, the emergency physician should review the criteria for immediate tonsillectomy with the referring otolaryngologist. When interval tonsillectomy is elected, drain the peritonsillar abscesses in the emergency center. If no trismus or torticollis is present, one can safely assume that there is no extension into the neck. If these are present and are severe, consider drainage of the abscess in the operating room.

TECHNIQUE FOR DRAINAGE

1. We advise, before incision and drainage, aspiration with a 20-gauge spinal needle and syringe at the point of maximal bulge in the soft palate. Make a safety stop by removing the needle guard and cutting off the distal 1 cm and carefully placing the guard back on the needle. This will leave only 1 cm of the needle exposed and will help prevent overpenetration by the needle.

NOTE

Internal carotid artery aneurysms seen as acute peritonsillar abscesses have been reported, and, therefore, we advise confirmatory needle aspiration in every patient with a peritonsillar abscess (24). Bloody return or pulsatile nature of the lesion should make one suspicious of this diagnosis.

---

2. Make an incision superolaterally to the tonsil at the point of maximal bulge in the soft palate and extend it slightly laterally. The length of the incision should be approximately 1 to 1.5 cm and should be horizontal. We recommend a no. 11 blade for the incision, and hold a Frazier suction tip at the tip of the blade and guide it in front of the blade to prevent any aspiration of purulent material. The suction should be continuous, high-flow wall suction (Fig. 8.26).

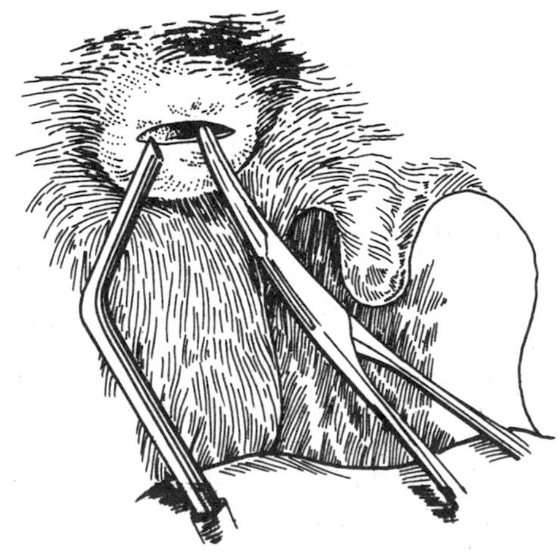

Figure 8.26. When draining a peritonsillar abscess, hold a suction tip at the tip of the abscess while the hemostat spreads apart the abscess. This allows the pus to be suctioned from the oral cavity and prevents possible aspiration of the purulent material.

3. Packing generally is not indicated and bleeding is usually minimal. Advise the patient to rest prone or in the lateral decubitus position with the side of the abscess down. Whenever possible, we advocate that a peritonsillar abscess not be drained late in the evening before bedtime, particularly in the debilitated patient. Aspiration of purulent material as the patient rolls over into the supine position during sleep may result in a severe infection of the lungs.

NOTE

Approximately 78% of the pathogens found in peritonsillar abscesses are streptococci (38). In one large series, only one patient had *Bacteroides* and two patients had *Haemophilus parainfluenzae* and *Enterobacter* cloacae, both of which were sensitive to penicillin. Therefore, the treatment of choice for these abscesses, once drained, is penicillin.

Retropharyngeal Abscesses

Retropharyngeal abscesses can be due to FBs in the pharynx, extension of infections from the ear, or infections in the posterior pharyngeal wall. Although drainage has been performed on an outpatient basis under local anesthesia for small high-lying abscesses, we recommend admission and drainage in the operating room (31). These infections may extend to produce a severe mediastinitis with a high mortality.

Sublingual Abscesses

The sublingual space is localized along the floor of the mouth above the mylohyoid muscle. Intraoral drainage of abscesses occurring in this area is sometimes possible. Be careful to avoid incision in the posterior lateral region of the floor of the mouth because this contains the lingual artery, vein, and nerve (32).

TECHNIQUE FOR DRAINAGE

Anesthetize the roof of the abscess with 1% lidocaine with epinephrine. Open the abscess cavity with a horizontal incision, using a no. 11 blade under local anesthesia. Insert a Kelly clamp into the abscess cavity and open it to separate any loculations and promote drainage. These patients usually require some type of sedation or intramuscular analgesia before the procedure. Drains generally are not inserted into the abscess cavity. Give the patient broad-spectrum antibiotics and advise to use mouthwashes with hydrogen peroxide 3 times daily.

Abscesses of the Parotid Duct

Parotid duct abscesses are seen in patients who have calculi obstructing the orifice of the duct or who have strictures causing stenosis and proximal dilatation. These abscesses should not be drained by probing the external orifice of the duct; achieve drainage by direct incision intraorally over the point of maximal bulge of the abscess. After drainage, pack the abscess cavity with fine strips of gauze, and refer the patient to an otolaryngologist for follow-up care.

Aftercare of Intraoral Abscesses

After drainage of the abscesses in the oral cavity, encourage the patient to use mouthwashes with half-strength hydrogen peroxide 5 times daily until the cavity is healed. The hydrogen peroxide solution aids in breaking up the purulent matter, and the foaming action permits cleansing and debridement of the abscess cavity.

References

1. American Academy of Otolaryngology-Head and Neck Surgery, Inc.: Clinical indicators: Myringotomy and tympanostomy tubes: Clinical indicators for otolaryngology. Head Neck Surg OTO-HNS web page, 2000.

2. Applebaum A: Simplest instrument for removal of foreign body from cornea. Arch Ophthalmol 30:262, 1943.
3. Barelli PA: The management of epistaxis in children. Otolaryngol Clin North Am 10:91, 1977.
4. Becker OJ: Nasal fracture: analysis of 100 cases. Arch Otolaryngol 48:344, 1948.
5. Beeden AG, Evans JN: Quinsy tonsillectomy: A further report. J Laryngol Otolaryngol 84:443, 1970.
6. Bell AF, Eibling DE: Nifedipine in the treatment of esophageal food impaction [Letter]. Arch Otolaryngol Head Neck Surg 114:682, 1988.
7. Bell M, Hawke M, Jahn A: New device for the management of postnasal epistaxis by balloon tamponade. Arch Otolaryngol 99:372, 1974.
8. Berliner ML: Biomicroscopy of the Eye, Vols. 1 and 2. New York: Hoeber, 1949.
9. Botma M, Bader R, Kubba H: "A parent's kiss": Evaluating an unusual method for removing nasal foreign bodies in children. J Larynol Otol 114:598–600, 2000.
10. Braneth RH: Clinical Slit Lamp Biomicroscopy. San Leandro, CA: Blaco Printers, 1978.
11. Bressler K, Shelton C: Ear foreign body removal: A review of 98 consecutive cases. Laryngoscope 103:367–370, 1993.
12. Bronson NR: Nonmagnetic foreign body localization and extraction. Am J Ophthalmol 58:133, 1964.
13. Call WH: Control of epistaxis. Surg Clin North Am 49:1235, 1969.
14. Campbell J, Foley C: A safe alternative to endoscopic removal of blunt esophageal foreign bodies. Arch Otolaryngol 109:323, 1983.
15. El Bitar H: The etiology and management of epistaxis: A review of 300 cases. Practitioner 207: 800, 1971.
16. Finkelstein JA: Oral Ambu-bag insufflation to remove unilateral nasal foreign bodies. Am J Emerg Med 14:57–58, 1996.
17. Galin MA, Harris LS, Paperiello GJ: Nonsurgical removal of corneal rust stains. Arch Ophthalmol 74:674, 1965.
18. Giammanco P, Binns PM: Temporary blindness and ophthalmoplegia from nasal packing. J Laryngol 84:631, 1970.
19. Gibson MS: Nitroglycerin use in esophageal disorders [Letter]. Ann Emerg Med 9:280, 1980.
20. Ginaldi S: Removal of esophageal foreign bodies using a Foley catheter in adults. Am J Emerg Med 3:64, 1985.
21. Hallberg OE: Severe nosebleed and its treatment. JAMA 148:355, 1952.
22. Hara HJ: Severe epistaxis. Arch Otolaryngol 75: 84, 1962.
23. Harpman JA: Management of epistaxis other than from Little's area. Arch Otolaryngol 75:254, 1962.
24. Henry RC: Aneurysm of the internal carotid artery presenting as a peritonsillar abscess. J Laryngol Otolaryngol 88:379, 1974.
25. Hersh JH: Management of fracture of nasal bony vault. Ann Otolaryngol 54:534, 1945.
26. Hurst A: The importance of nasal fractures. Laryngoscope 70:68, 1969.
27. Juselius H: Epistaxis: A clinical study of 1,724 patients. J Laryngol Otolaryngol 88:317, 1974.
28. Kadish HA, Corneli HM: Removal of nasal foreign bodies in the pediatric population. Am J Emerg Med 15:54–56, 1997.
29. Kamer FM, Parkes ML: An absorbent, non-adherent nasal pack. Laryngoscope 85:384, 1975.
30. LaForce RF: Treatment of nasal hemorrhage. Surg Clin North Am 49:1305, 1969.
31. Leffler S, Cheney P, Tandberg D: Chemical immobilization and killing of intraural cockroaches: An in vitro comparative study. Ann Emerg Med 22:1795–1798, 1993.
32. Levitt GW: The surgical treatment of deep neck infections. Laryngoscope 80:403, 1970.
33. Lynch MG: Minor surgery of the ear, nose and throat. Surg Clin North Am 31:1315, 1951.
34. McCurty JA: Peritonsillar abscess. Arch Otolaryngol 103:414, 1977.
35. McMaster WC: Removal of foreign body from the nose. JAMA 213:1905, 1970.
36. Mohammed SH, Hegedus V: Dislodgment of impacted esophageal foreign bodies with carbonated beverages. Clin Radiol 37:589–592, 1986.
37. Moses RA: Adler's physiology of the eye, 6th ed. St. Louis: CV Mosby, 1975.
38. Muller SP: Peritonsillar abscess: A prospective study of pathogens, treatment and morbidity. Ear Nose Throat J 57:46, 1978.
39. Nemeth SC: Basic slit lamp techniques. J Ophthalmic Nursing Tech 15:134, 1996.
40. Nixon G: Foley catheter method of esophageal foreign body removal: Extension of applications. AJR Am J Roentgenol 132:441, 1979.
41. Padrnos RE: A method for control of posterior nasal hemorrhage. Arch Otolaryngol 87:85, 1968.
42. Percival SPB: A decade of intraocular foreign bodies. Br J Ophthalmol 56:454, 1972.
43. Rice BR, Spiegel PK, Dombrowski PJ: Acute esophageal food impaction treated by gas forming agents. Radiology 146:299–301, 1983.
44. Singer AJ, Sauris E, Viccellio AW: Ceruminolytic effects of ducosylate sodium: A randomized, controlled trial. Ann Emerg Med 36:228–232, 2000.
45. Stell PM: Epistaxis. Clin Otolaryngol 2:263, 1977.
46. Templer JW, Hollinger LD, Wood RP II, et al: Immediate tonsillectomy for the treatment of peritonsillar abscess. Am J Surg 134:596, 1977.
47. Trenker SW, Maglinte DDT, Lehman GA, et al.: Esophageal food impaction: Treatment with glucagon. Radiology 149:401–403, 1983.
48. Wadsworth P: Method of controlling epistaxis [Letter]. Br Med J 1:506, 1971.
49. White SJ, Broner S: Use of acetone to dissolve styrofoam impaction of the ear. Ann Emerg Med 23:580–582, 1994.

9

Common Dental Emergencies

LOCAL ANESTHESIA (2)

EQUIPMENT

1% lidocaine (Xylocaine)
5-mL syringe
18-gauge needle
23-gauge, 1.5-inch needle

Local dental anesthesia is a valuable procedure needed for many of the dental emergencies discussed in this chapter. In conjunction with oral analgesics, the techniques described herein provide comfort to the patient throughout the night, until a dentist can be seen the next morning. Local anesthetics also can be used as a diagnostic tool to determine if the pain is of dental or nondental origin.

Intraoral injections should be performed with a 25-gauge, 1.5-inch needle and topical anesthetic, which, when applied to the oral mucosa, will reduce the pain of injection.

Posterior–Superior Alveolar Nerve Block

The maxilla is very porous and highly vascular. Thus anesthesia of the maxillary teeth can be accomplished by using one or a combination of three types of injections:

1. A posterior–superior alveolar nerve block.
2. Buccal infiltration over the root apices.
3. Palatal infiltration over the root apices.

The advantage of the posterior–superior alveolar nerve block over the other two techniques is that one can anesthetize several molars and the buccal soft tissue with one injection (Fig. 9.1). The maxillary first molar is often innervated by the middle superior alveolar nerve, which exits from the infraorbital foramen, and the palatal roots of this tooth are supplied by the palatal nerves. Thus adequate anesthesia for the maxillary molars may require both buccal and palatal infiltrations in addition to a posterior–superior alveolar block.

To perform the posterior–superior alveolar block, retract the upper cheek with a finger until *the most posterior and superior depth of the mucobuccal fold* is seen. The coronoid process sometimes makes it difficult to "visualize" the posterior maxilla. This visualization can be made easier if the patient shifts his mandible toward the injection side. Align the needle at approximately 45 degrees to the sagittal, frontal, and horizontal planes (Fig. 9.1). Advancing slowly along the mucobuccal fold, deposit 2 to 3 mL of anesthetic, being sure to aspirate before injecting (3).

Apical Nerve Blocks

Buccal infiltration of anesthetic solution over the root apices of teeth is quite effective because the bone is so porous. Remember that the root apices of teeth are

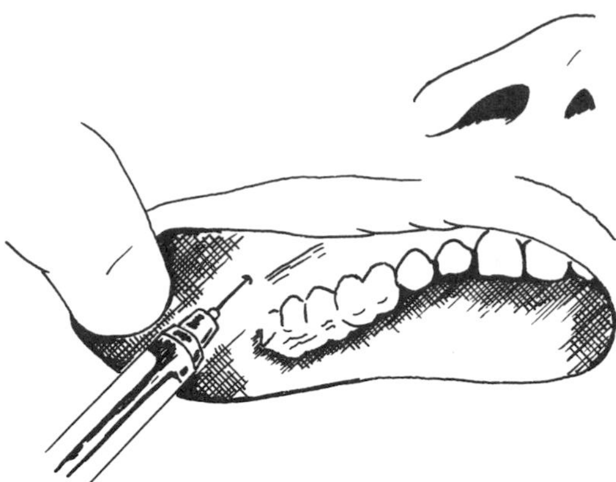

Figure 9.1. The posterior–superior alveolar nerve block. See text for discussion.

high in the maxilla. To perform this technique, retract the lip to visualize the superior aspect of the mucobuccal fold over the tooth to be anesthetized. Align and insert the needle along the long axis of the tooth (Fig. 9.2). Deposit approximately 2 mL of anesthetic. One may have to do palatal infiltration because anesthetic solution administered by buccal infiltration may fail to diffuse to the palatal root.

Palatal Infiltration

If palatal infiltration must be done, insert the needle into the palatal gingiva over the approximate root apex and deposit 5 mL of anesthetic (Fig. 9.3). This injection may be somewhat painful (1).

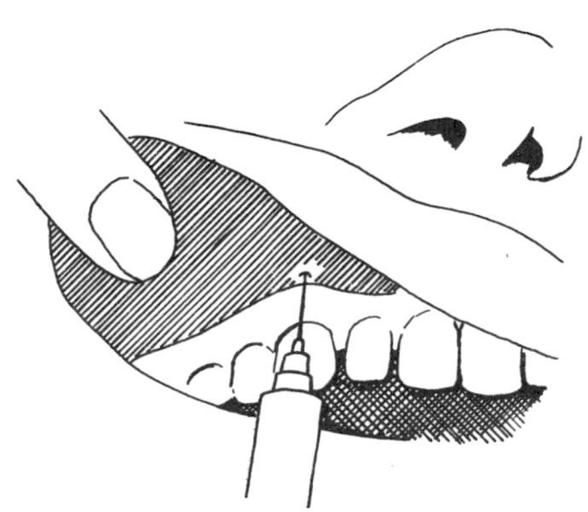

Figure 9.2. An apical nerve block.

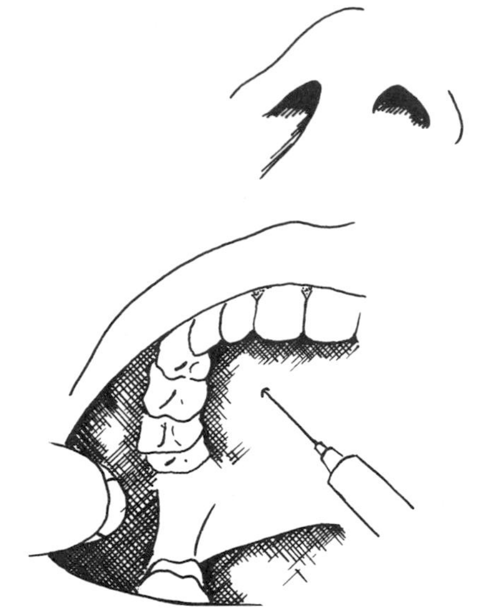

Figure 9.3. Nerve block of the molars along the palatal area.

Inferior Alveolar Nerve Block

The teeth in the mandible are surrounded by dense cortical bone, which prevents the anesthetic from diffusing through. Thus it is necessary to deposit the anesthetic over the mandibular nerve trunk at a site before the trunk enters the mandible. This can be done by anesthetizing the inferior alveolar nerve, thus causing anesthesia of all the mandibular teeth on one side of the midline and the buccal soft tissues anterior to the bicuspid. Half of the tongue is also anesthetized because the lingular branch of this nerve is blocked also.

The inferior alveolar nerve block is difficult to master, because the area to be entered is small and located deep under soft tissues. With the patient's mouth open, locate the anterior and posterior aspects of the ramus with a thumb intraorally, posterior to the last mandibular molar, and an index finger extraorally (Fig. 9.4). This allows you to imagine visualizing the mandibular foramen, located between the index finger and thumb. The foramen is typically found slightly above the level of the mandibular molars and midway be-

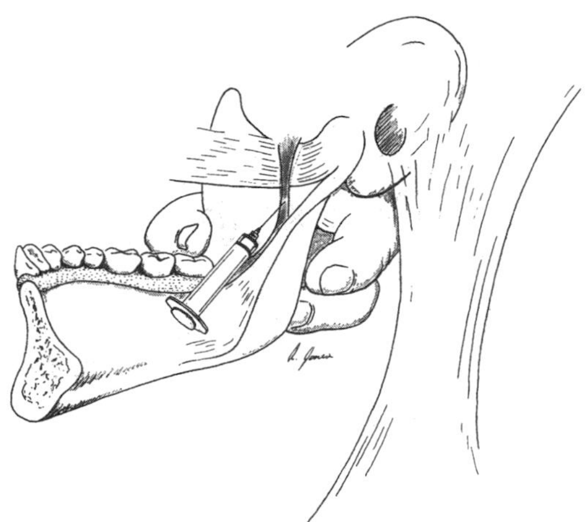

Figure 9.4. The inferior alveolar nerve block. The inferior alveolar nerve is located midway between the thumb and index finger, which have been placed on either side of the ramus of the mandible. See text for discussion.

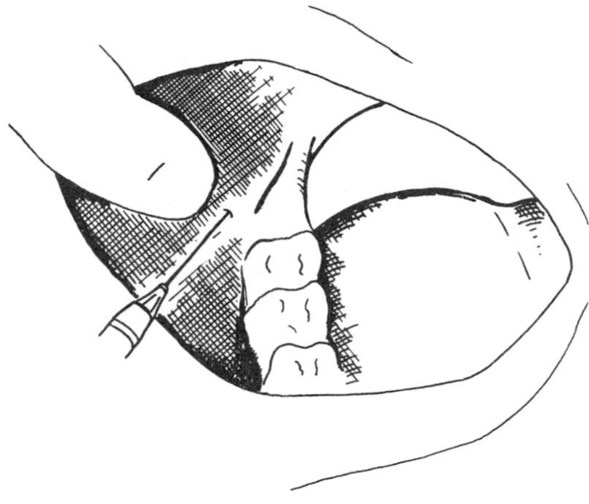

Figure 9.5. Buccal nerve block for a third molar.

tween the anterior and posterior border of the mandibular ramus. Insert the needle into the soft tissues of the ramus from the lateral side (as shown in Fig. 9.4), through the pterygomandibular triangle at a level that bisects the physician's thumbnail. Advance the needle until it makes contact with the bone. This advance should be between 1 and 2 cm. If contact occurs before 1 cm of penetration, then the inferior oblique ridge of the mandible has obstructed the track. In such a situation, redirect the needle more posteriorly, and advance the needle again. After aspirating, inject 2 to 4 mL of anesthetic solution (3).

Anesthetize the buccal nerve by infiltrating 0.5 mL of anesthetic in the sulcus between the mucosa and the mandibular third molar. After stretching the mucosa with the finger, insert the needle until bone is contacted (Fig. 9.5).

FRACTURED TEETH

A tooth may fracture at several points. Although the emergency physician will generally refer patients with fractured teeth to a dentist, he or she should be aware of the basic treatment rendered for such injuries. Seven types of tooth fractures are identified, which include dislocations of teeth (7). The degree of tooth damage will both determine the prognosis and indicate the appropriate treatment in the emergency center (Fig. 9.6). Emergency treatment of only a few of the more pertinent injuries is discussed here.

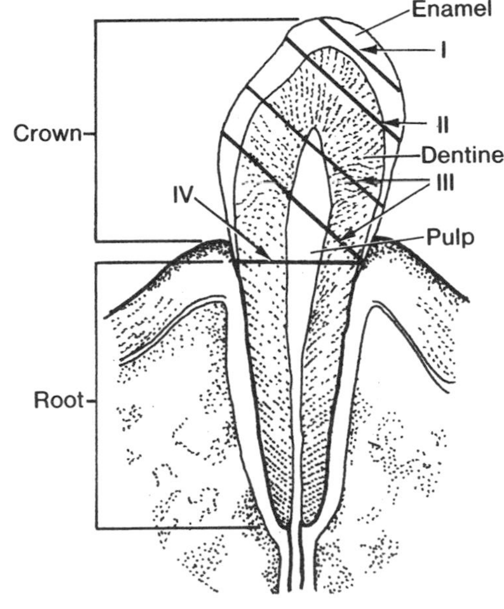

Figure 9.6. Various levels of fracture of a tooth. See text for complete discussion.

When intraoral radiographs are not available, a Panorex view is useful. One must do a careful, oral soft tissue examination so as not to overlook tooth fragments that are buried in a lip or tongue. Any tooth after trauma, regardless of how minimal the damage, may undergo devitalization. Movement at the apex of the tooth or inflammation may disrupt blood flow to the pulp, causing death of the tooth. Chronic endodontic infections can result after even the slightest fracture. Such infections can remain undetected for years, leading eventually to loss of the tooth. Thus early detection and treatment are essential (1). All patients who have fractures of their teeth should be advised to seek follow-up care from a dentist.

Crown Fractures

Crown fractures are incomplete fractures of the teeth, without true separation of fragments. They may occur due to occlusive forces. These fractures are usually of no consequence. However, if symptoms of sharp pain occur with biting or cold stimuli, this usually indicates a deeper fracture requiring further evaluation and treatment. Advise these patients to use a mild analgesic and seek dental consultation (3).

Type I Fractures (4)

This is a fracture that involves only the enamel; the physician primarily notices a chip off of the white portion of the tooth. Symptoms may or may not occur. The most common complaint is increased sensitivity to temperature changes. Furthermore, the sharp edges of the tooth may result in irritation to surrounding soft tissues. Treatment of these injuries is relatively straightforward: file the sharp edges with an emery board. Refer to a dentist for further care.

Type II Fractures

These dental fractures involving the dentin are very sensitive to cold and to touch. The dentin appears yellow and contains microtubules with nerve processes. Bacteria may directly invade the pulp. Carefully examine the exposed tooth surface for evidence of pulp exposure, which indicates a type III fracture.

When the type II fracture has a large cavity defect (particularly in the molars), place a Dentalone-soaked cotton pellet into the crater. On top of this, apply Cavit G and mold it over the tooth. Instruct the patient to bite down for 15 minutes to allow this to seal. Arrange follow-up with a dentist for permanent restoration.

With type II fractures of the anterior teeth, the defect is too small to allow placement of a cotton pellet. Therefore, simply apply a Dentalone-soaked cotton pellet over the dentin to provide some anesthesia. If the pain is significant, a dental block may also be required. Apply the Dentalone for approximately 5 minutes. Afterward, remove the cotton pellet and apply Cavit G to the defect and the adjacent teeth, and instruct the patient to bite down for 10 to 15 minutes. It is important to apply Cavit G over the affected and adjacent teeth, for there is no retentive area over the anterior teeth after a type II fracture. Refer these patients to a dentist for follow-up care.

EQUIPMENT NEEDED FOR DENTAL FRACTURES AND PULP CAPPING

Mouth mirror
Periodontal probe
2 × 2-cm gauze pads
Emery board
Cotton pliers
Dentalone
CaOH paste (Dycal)
Cavit G
Cotton pellets
Absorbable sponge (Gelfoam)
Dental explorer (Fig. 9.7)

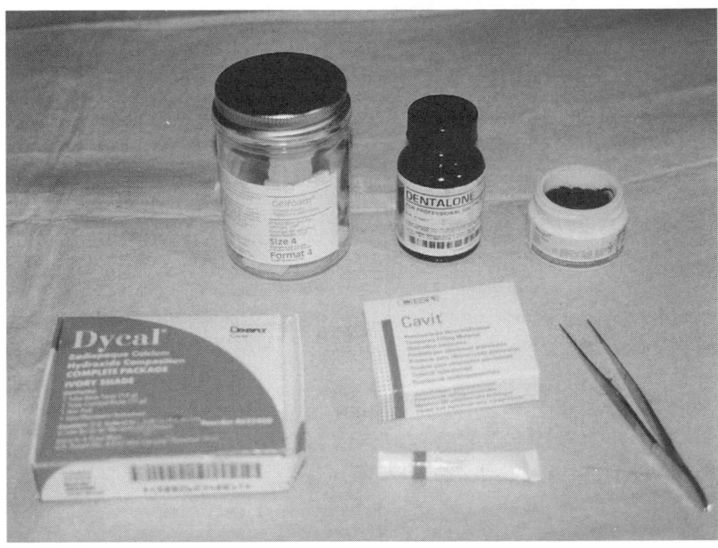

Figure 9.7. The items commonly used in an emergency department for all of the dental procedures covered in the text. They include absorbable gelatin sponge (Gelfoam), Dentalone, dry socket paste, Dycal, and cavit G.

Type III Fractures

Type III fractures involve the pulp. One will see an area of hemorrhage in the middle of the tooth if the pulp is exposed. This type of injury results in pain and allows contamination by bacteria from the oral cavity (5).

Treatment involves controlling the bleeding by applying a saline-moistened cotton pledget over the hemorrhagic area. Apply direct pressure for at least 5 minutes until the clot forms and bleeding stops (Fig. 9.8). It is important to use a moistened cotton pledget when doing this. Once the tooth is dry, apply CaOH paste over this area. Dycal is mixed on a paper pad using the catalyst and base. Then apply one pea-sized portion of the catalyst with one pea-sized portion of the base onto a paper pad, and mix them together until a uniform color is achieved. Apply this over the exposed pulp and dentin. Cover this area with a 3 × 3-inch piece of gauze and hold it for approximately 3 minutes until the Dycal has dried. Once the Dycal has hardened, apply Cavit G over the area, and have the patient bite down for approximately 5 to 10 minutes to allow the Cavit G to harden. A more rapid hardening of Cavit G may be accomplished when the patient is difficult to manage by applying a moistened cotton ball over the Cavit G after it is applied on to the tooth (8). With anterior teeth, one may need to smooth the Cavit G over adjacent teeth so

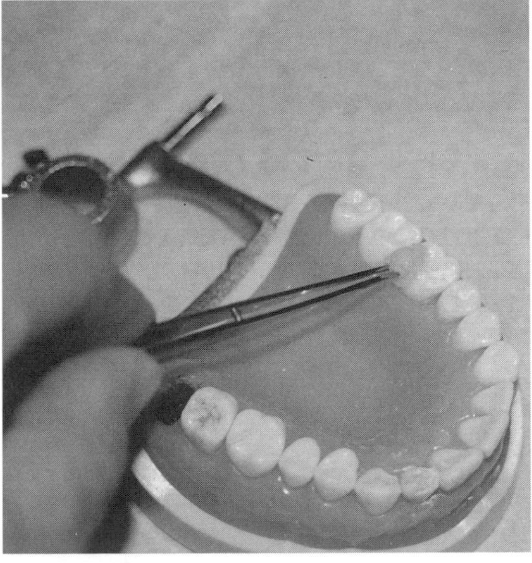

Figure 9.8. Hold a Dentalone-saturated cotton pledget against the type III tooth fracture involving the pulp until the bleeding stops.

that it will hold. Instruct the patient not to bite down on the temporary restoration and to maintain a soft diet until seen by their dentist. In addition, discharge the patient with penicillin because of the possibility of pulpitis evolving after the exposure to oral microbes. In the penicillin-allergic patient, clindamycin or clarithromycin are alternatives.

Type IV Fractures

Type IV fractures are uncommon and are usually vertical fractures. These injuries often require radiographic evaluation to make the diagnosis (14). Furthermore, computed tomography (CT) scans have been shown to be superior to conventional radiography for diagnostic purposes (C). These injuries usually involve crown fractures that extend below the gingival margin and have a resulting mobile fragment. If a mobile fragment is present, it is best to anesthetize the affected tooth by using blocks described in a previous chapter. Once adequate analgesia has been obtained, the mobile fragment can be removed with a hemostat. Afterward, treat these injuries as if they were type III fractures, if the fracture involves the nerve. Otherwise, prescribe antibiotics and refer to a dentist within 24 to 48 hours for definitive care.

DISPLACEMENT INJURIES OF THE TEETH

Complete avulsions are common in the emergency center. These teeth should be repositioned as soon as possible, to increase the success of treatment. Primary teeth should not be replanted or repositioned, to avoid damaging any permanent teeth below. Sometimes a local anesthetic is necessary to relieve the pain before manipulation.

There are many types of displacement injuries. In a concussion injury, the supporting structures are not involved, and there is no mobility of the tooth. A *subluxation* injury results in minor tooth mobility, but there is no displacement from the original position in the alveolus. No emergency treatment is necessary for these two types of injuries, other than mild analgesics and follow-up with a dentist (6).

A *luxation* injury results in physical displacement of the tooth. Teeth with minor luxations may need minimal repositioning, with or without splinting, depending on the degree of tooth mobility, stability, and position. However, teeth with major luxations need splinting. With major luxations, the dental neurovascular supply and periodontal structures sustain significant injury. Vitality tests are unpredictable.

Avulsion, the total dislocation of the tooth from its normal position in the socket is a major injury. Replantation remains controversial. The average life span of a replanted tooth is 5 to 10 years, and success of replantation diminishes inversely with the time out of the socket. Good success is achieved if the tooth is replanted within 30 minutes. One can anticipate reasonable success rates as long as the tooth is replanted within two hours after the avulsion, although significant root absorption occurs beyond 30 minutes. Therefore, if the patient calls an emergency department stating that the tooth has been dislodged from socket, advise that person to put the tooth back into socket and come to the emergency department immediately. If immediate replantation is impossible, normal saline is the ideal transport medium. However, if this is not available, milk at room temperature is an excellent substitute. Alternatively, place the avulsed tooth under the patient's tongue, bathed in saliva. However, this is the least desired option, for the saliva is relatively hypotonic, and there is an increased risk of bacterial contamination (1, 3, 6).

No simple technique can be easily mastered by the emergency physician to stabilize an avulsed tooth. Initially, it is best to pull down slightly on the avulsed tooth and clean out any debris. After this, push the tooth back into socket. Have the patient close the mouth so that the teeth are clenched together. Then, with the patient's finger, press on the outer lip (upper or lower lip depending on which tooth is involved) so that it pushes against the avulsed tooth. In essence, the pressure of the tongue on the lingular side and the lip on the buccal side will guide the tooth into position and hold it in place. This position should be maintained for at least 15 minutes to allow for some stabilization within the socket. Instruct the patient to keep the mouth closed as much as possible, and stay on a very soft diet. Avoid chewing until seen by a dentist.

POST EXTRACTION BLEEDING

Postextraction bleeding is a common problem in the emergency department. This usually occurs as a result of suction applied to where the molar has been extracted. First, apply a piece of gauze or cotton into the affected socket and have the patient bite down for approximately 5 minutes. This usually stops the bleeding or reduces the flow. If the source of bleeding is identified to be from a gingival laceration, repair this. If not, pack the socket with Gelfoam. Work the Gelfoam so that it resembles the shape of the socket. Insert the Gelfoam into the socket until a solid mass of Gelfoam is achieved, usually with two to three pieces. After this, apply a 3 × 3-inch piece of gauze over the socket, and instruct the patient to bite down for approximately 30 minutes. This will usually stop the bleeding. If the bleeding continues and is found to come from inside the socket, apply bone wax. However, if bone wax is to be used, refer the patient, because this may delay the healing of the affected tooth.

PAIN: POST-EXTRACTION PAIN AND DRY SOCKET

EQUIPMENT

Mouth mirror
2 × 2-cm gauze pad
Scissors
Cotton pliers
Cotton rolls
Irrigating syringe
Dry socket paste (eucalyptole and balsa wood)

Sudden onset of severe pain within 72 hours after dental extraction may indicate the development of alveolar osteitis (dry socket). A dry socket typically occurs after removal of a molar, and the cause remains uncertain. Treatment is directed toward providing patient comfort until healing occurs. If necessary, perform a dental block. Usually this is not necessary if one can irrigate the debris from the socket, which will result in some pain relief. Once this is done, apply dry socket paste into the socket (Fig. 9.9). Attempt to maximally fill the socket with the dry socket paste; the patient should report almost instantaneous relief. Apply Gelfoam on top of this, and compress this into the socket. Apply a piece of cotton gauze over this, and instruct the patient to bite down for as long as possible. Pain will return if the medicinal packing is disrupted. Prescribe appropriate pain medicine and an antibiotic if there is evidence of a secondary infection. Refer the patient to a dentist for follow-up within 24 to 48 hours. The medicated dressing may need to be changed daily to provide continuing pain relief.

DENTAL CARIES

Frequently dental emergencies are the result of caries that have undermined enamel and/or dental restorations; these problems may arise from high mastication forces and cause tooth sensitivity. Provide relief in the emergency department with a temporary restoration to cover the exposed pulp.

The treatment of a carious tooth depends on the presence or absence of a crater. If there is no crater, the treatment of choice is antibiotics. The first-line agent is penicillin, whereas clindamycin or clarithromycin are reserved for the pa-

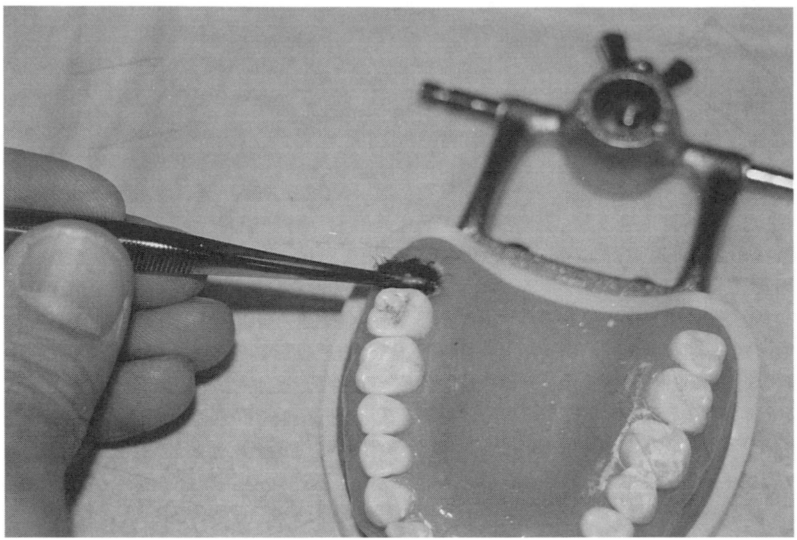

Figure 9.9. Insert dry socket paste into the cavity where the molar has been extracted.

tient allergic to penicillin. Prescribe antibiotics and analgesics for 7 to 10 days. If a crater defect is causing pain, the treatment of choice is to take a small cotton pellet dipped in Dentalone and apply it into the crater (Figs. 9.10 and 9.11). On top of this Dentalone-soaked pellet, apply Cavit G. Be sure to press the Cavit G firmly into the socket and then smooth it over the tooth (Fig. 9.12). Ask the patient to bite down firmly for 10 to 15 minutes, which will allow the Cavit G to harden and thereby reduce pain. Refer these patients to a dentist.

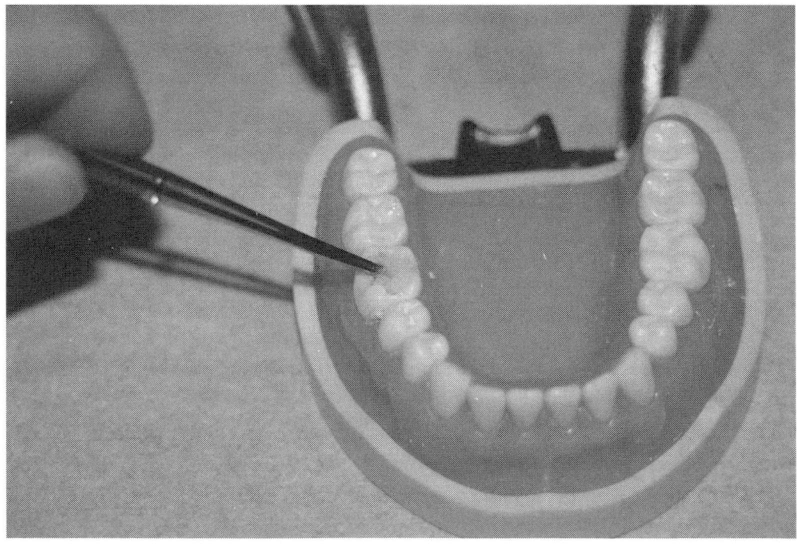

Figure 9.10. In a patient with a severe carious cavity, particularly in a molar, insert a Dentalone-soaked cotton pledget into the cavity.

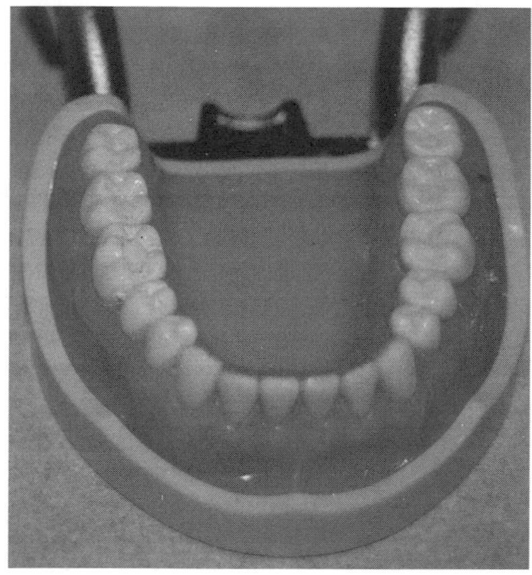

Figure 9.11. Pack the pledget into the cavity and leave it there.

PERIODONTAL ABSCESS

A periodontal abscess can produce gingival inflammation and enlargement. An acute periodontal abscess is typically accompanied by throbbing, radiating pain, and exquisite tenderness to palpation. Tooth mobility, lymphadenitis, systemic fever, leukocytosis, and malaise may accompany an acute abscess. An abscess may be associated with periodontal disease, endodontic disease, or both. A periodontal probe helps determine the diagnosis. Continuity between the gingival sulcus and abscess indicates periodontal involvement (Fig. 9.13).

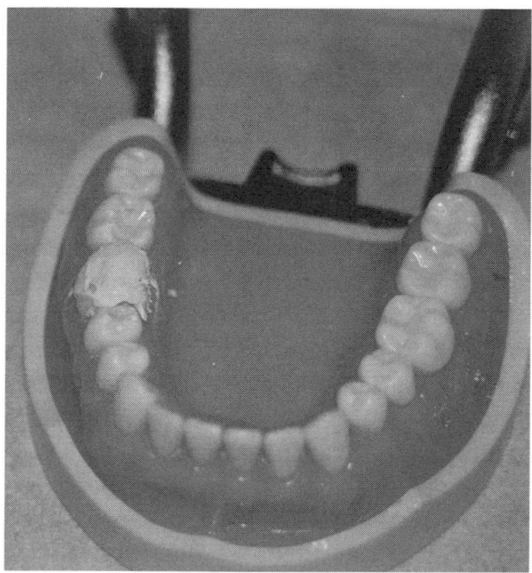

Figure 9.12. After the insertion of the Dentalone-soaked cotton pallet, cover the area with cavit G.

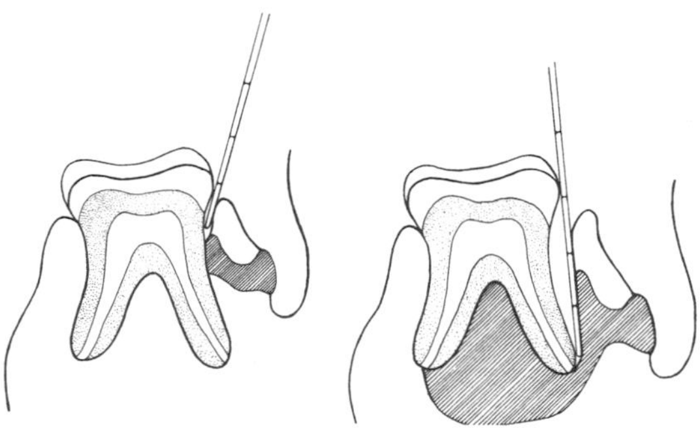

Figure 9.13. With a periodontal probe, determine whether there is communication with an apical abscess.

Application of gentle digital pressure to the most fluctuant area will express a purulent exudate from the gingival sulcus. If this is not successful, incise and drain the abscess to provide immediate relief. Periodontal abscesses are usually seen along the border of the premolars and molars. Drain these abscesses with an incision that parallels the gingival border over the point of maximal fluctuance (Fig. 9.14).

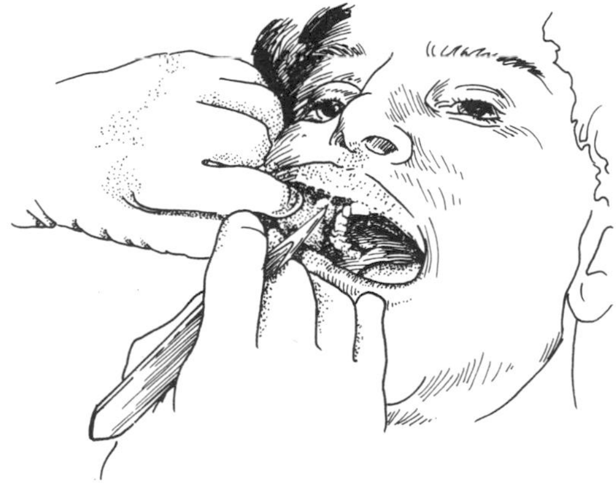

Figure 9.14. Drain a periodontal abscess by an incision made in the sulcus of the mouth where the gingiva meets the buccal mucosa. Make the incision over the point of maximal fluctuance.

Local nerve block will relieve the discomfort. If the patient has cellulitis, fever, or lymphadenopathy, prescribe antibiotics. Refer the patient to a dentist for follow-up whether or not incision and drainage of the abscess was performed.

References

1. American Dental Association. Accepted Dental Therapeutics. 40th ed. Chicago: American Dental Association, 1984.
2. Allen GD: Dental Anesthesia and Analgesia. 3rd ed. Baltimore: Williams & Wilkins, 1984.
3. Berry HM: Emergency Physician's Guide to Dental Care. Philadelphia: University of Pennsylvania Press, 1983.
4. Buonocore MG: A simple method for increasing adhesion of acrylic resin filling materials to enamel. J Dent Res 34:849, 1955.
5. Cooper JR: Dental Problems in Medical Practice. London: Heinemann Medical, 1976.
6. Grossman LI, Shipp II: Survival rate of replanted teeth. Oral Surg 29:899, 1970.
7. Heiman GR, Biren GM, Kahn H, et al: Temporary splinting using an adhesive system. Oral Surg 31:819, 1971.
8. Horn HR: Symposium on composite resins in dentistry. Dent Clin North Am, 25:2, 1981.
9. Johnson WT, Goodrich JL, James GA: Replantation of avulsed teeth with immature root development. Oral Surg 60:420, 1985.
10. Matusow RJ: Clinical observations regarding the treatment of traumatically avulsed mature teeth: Part 1. Oral Surg 60:94, 1985.
11. Matusow RJ: Clinical observations regarding the treatment of traumatically avulsed mature teeth: Part 2. Oral Surg 60:428, 1985.
12. Medford HM: Temporary stabilization of avulsed or luxated teeth. Ann Emerg Med 11: 490, 1982.
13. Vilkins BM: Treatment guidelines for the avulsed tooth. Endodont Rep Fall/Winter:16, 1986.
14. Youssefzadeh S, Gahleitner A, Dorffner R, et al. Dental vertical root fractures: Value of CT in detection. Radiology 210:2, 1999.

10

Plastic Surgery Principles and Techniques

INTRODUCTION

The evaluation and treatment of lacerations is an essential skill for the practice of emergency medicine. In 1996, approximately 11 million wounds were treated in emergency departments throughout the United States (83). The principles of wound care remain grounded in a sound understanding of the anatomy and physiology of human skin and the proper use of proven tools and techniques in its repair. Scar formation is a natural result of the healing process; all wounds leave some scar. Patients as a rule are usually concerned about the appearance of the healed wound; therefore the conscientious physician works to achieve the least noticeable and hence most aesthetically pleasing healed wound. The goals of wound care remain remarkably simple—achieve a well-healed, functional scar that is cosmetically acceptable to the patient and, at the same time, avoid complications such as wound infection, dehiscence, hypertrophic scar, etc., which may compromise the outcome. Meeting these goals requires an understanding of the principles and techniques of wound care, which have evolved as a result of sound scientific research. Thus the study of wound healing, anesthesia, techniques to remove wound contaminants, principles of debridement of devitalized tissue, handling of tissue during repair, choice of suture or alternative materials used for wound closure, use of the various techniques for suturing or closure of wounds, and postrepair wound care is essential to the physician who cares for the patient with a laceration.

SKIN ANATOMY AND FUNCTION

SKIN STRUCTURE

The skin is composed of an epidermal and a dermal layer, the thicknesses of which vary in different parts of the body. The epidermis of the palms and soles is quite thick, measuring 0.4 to 0.6 mm. The skin in the remainder of the body ranges in thickness from 0.075 to 0.15 mm. The dermis consists of fibroelastic connective tissue, containing both collagen for strength and elastic fibers for stretch and flexibility. The thickness of the dermis varies from 1 to 4 mm and is greatest in the back, followed by the thigh, abdomen, forehead, wrist, and scalp, and is least in the eyelid. Dermal thickness varies inversely with the age of the patient.

The color of normal human skin is related to the number, size, type, and distribution of melanocytes. The clinical applicability of this fact is discussed later in this chapter.

NORMAL REPAIR (40, 61, 57, 106)

Classically wound healing has been divided into three phases: inflammation, tissue formation, and remodeling. Advances in our understanding of wound healing on a cellular level have shown this to be a much more complex overlapping process than was originally perceived. It is now known to be a continuous and dynamic process mediated not only by skin and blood cells, blood vessels, and collagen fibers, but also by a complex "soup" of various chemical factors elaborated by the cells in the wound. These chemical factors influence the interactions between the cells and extracellular matrix, which develop in the wound and play a crucial role in the regulation of the entire healing process from injury onset to final remodeling. Indeed malfunction in the timing or amounts of these factors may play a key role in wound healing gone awry, such as with hypertrophic scars, keloid formation, or failure to heal. The current knowledge of these cellular level processes is far from perfect, but we hope that the ongoing research will further expand the science of wound healing and may offer some therapeutic adjuncts to augment or replace traditional wound treatment methods. For the present, however, it is sufficient to put this knowledge of the cell-level biochemical processes into the overall framework of the steps that take place during normal wound healing [at present, synthesized recombinant growth factors are not yet approved by the Food and Drug Administration (FDA) for use in laceration repair].

Laceration of the tissue causes disruption of blood vessels along with extravasation of blood into the wound. Formation of blood clot along with constriction and thrombosis of the injured vessels at the wound site achieve local hemostasis. Uninjured blood vessels adjacent to the injured tissue dilate and become more permeable, permitting the migration of additional platelets and white blood cells, which are chemotactically attracted to the wound by the various chemical signals released by the damaged parenchymal cells in the wound and/or the activated complement and coagulation pathways. Within a few hours of injury, the tissue is infiltrated by granulocytes and macrophages. During the first 24 hours, neutrophils and lymphocytes begin to remove debris, bacteria, and devitalized tissue from the wound. Platelets at the wound site produce transforming growth factor (TGF) in α and β forms, which stimulate fibroblasts and vascular endothelial cells to migrate into the wound. In addition, these factors enhance epithelial migration and neovascularization into the wound. Platelets also produce platelet-derived growth factor (PDGF), a small dipeptide that attracts fibroblasts and smooth muscle cells to the injured area. PDGF enhances the formation of procollagen and collagen fibrils, increasing wound tensile strength. TGF-β stimulates the production of other growth factors and retards wound hydrogen peroxide synthesis, which, if left unchecked, would destroy fibroblasts. Epithelial cells in the wound margins detach themselves from their underlying basement membrane, multiply, and migrate into the epidermal defect, eventually forming a bridge across the wound. By day 2, this growth factor–mediated epithelial bridging of the wound is well under way, and the wound usually becomes essentially watertight within 48 to 72 hours. This epithelial covering also acts as a barrier preventing bacterial penetration into the wound from adjacent skin and skin appendages (e.g., hair). The time for completion of this epithelial bridge is directly affected by the technique of closure used to repair lacerations. *Eversion* of the skin edges permits epithelial bridging of the laceration to occur within 18 to 24 hours, whereas *end-to-end approximation* of the wound edges may cause an additional 12-hour delay. If the wound edges are *inverted*, this bridging of new epithelium across the wound can take up to 72 hours.

AXIOM

Inversion of the wound edges results in a threefold increase *in the time it takes for epithelial bridging of a repaired laceration.*

Downward growth of the epithelial cells occurs not only at the laceration site but also at any interruption of the skin, including any suture tracks. This invasive epithelium begins to regress by day 10 to 15 and leaves behind a small keratinized epithelial "spur," commonly known as a **suture puncture mark**. If percutaneous sutures are removed *before the eighth day*, invasive spurs of epithelium regress, leaving no discernible mark. Sutures that are removed more than 8 days after repair result in a permanent scar with a cross-hatched or "railroad track" appearance. The severity of suture puncture-mark scarring is affected by the region of the body at which the laceration occurs. Skin of the eyelids, soles, and palms seldom shows such scars, but they are common on the back, chest, upper arms, and lower extremities. The size of the sewing needle and suture used play a relatively insignificant role in the development of these scars.

The process of **neovascularization** begins early. Angiograms have shown that within 10 hours after a laceration, there is relatively sparse vasculature, and the wound edges appear no different from the rest of the surrounding skin (86). By the third day, ingrowth of new vessels is under way, and some local vasodilatation at the wound periphery persists. New blood vessels may be seen bridging the wound space of primary wounds, and in open wounds, a rose-colored hue can be noted where the first few vessels appear. A number of chemical mediators play a role in this angiogenesis, including TGF-α, TGF-β, vascular endothelial growth factor, angiogenin, angiotropin, angiopoietin 1, and thrombospondin. Tissue hypoxia and local lactic acid production also may stimulate new blood vessel growth. Many of these chemical factors stimulate the production of basic fibroblast growth factor and vascular endothelial growth factor by macrophages and endothelial cells. These various angiogenesis factors are immediately released from macrophages and local epidermal cells after injury. Proteolytic enzymes are released into the connective tissue matrix and begin the degradation of extracellular matrix proteins such as collagen. In addition, fragments of these matrix proteins attract additional peripheral blood monocytes to the injured tissue, where they become activated macrophages and in turn release chemical factors to facilitate new blood vessel growth. Some of these factors activate plasmin and collagenase enzymes, which digest local basement membranes. This allows stimulated endothelial cells to migrate and form new blood vessels into the injured tissue. Thus by day 5, an occasional new blood vessel can be seen crossing the width of the wound, and by day 7, there is a marked increase in the number of vessels in the wound. The healthy wound bed is filled with moist, beefy red, friable granulation tissue—new blood vessels, fibroblasts, some early collagen, and so on. Once the wound is filled with new granulation tissue, this neovascularization ceases, and many of the new blood vessels gradually dissipate, again probably under the influence of local chemical signals. However, when most patients return for suture removal (7 to 8 days), often an increased vascular hue around the wound edges is still present, which is often so intense as to give the false impression of an infection. By day 21, the wound vascularity has returned to a grossly normal appearance, yet capillary vessels within the scar continue to decrease over a period of 6 months (hence scar color may continue to fade during this period).

Evaluation of the various suture materials used to repair wounds and their effect on local vascularity reveals that there is no difference between wounds closed with nylon, chromic catgut, plain catgut, or even tape (86). However, the effects of *tightly tied sutures* is striking. By the third day, wounds tightly tied show an absence of blood vessels. After 7 days, completely avascular areas up to 3 mm in size may be noted around tightly tied sutures. (86). Histologic sections reveal microinfarction and necrosis in the wound produced by tight suturing. Mattress sutures are much more likely to devascularize the wound than are simple or continuous sutures, unless extreme care is taken to tie the suture loosely. Remember that because of the injury response, wounds will develop local edema during the first few days, and sutures that are tightened too much during the repair may become much tighter during the first few days. The goal of suture repair is to approximate the wound edges while doing the least harm to the damaged tissue. Because the process of neovascularization and growth of granulation tissue in a wound depends on the influx of blood cells and the chemical factors that they elaborate, care must always be taken not to strangulate a wound with sutures that are too tight.

AXIOM

Sutures that are tied too tightly result in strangulation of tissue in the wound edges and result in impairment of wound healing, an increased risk of wound breakdown and dehiscence, and may thus potentiate wound infection.

Within a few days of injury, activated macrophages produce a host of growth factors (PDGF, TGF-α, TGF-β, fibroblast growth factor, macrophage-derived growth factor, and interleukin-2) that stimulate and recruit fibroblasts. The fibroblasts in turn lay down a significant amount of procollagen by day 5. Procollagen is subsequently converted to collagen fibrils that can contract with the aid of smooth muscle cells. Smooth muscle cells are similarly stimulated to contract by PDGF and macrophage-derived growth factor. Newly formed collagen appears in the wound by as early as the second day, reaching its peak synthesis by day 5 to 7. During the second week, fibroblasts in the wound transform into myofibroblasts with large bundles of actin containing microfilaments laid out along the faces of their cytoplasmic membranes. The microfilaments link cell to cell and the cells to the extracellular matrix elements (i.e., collagen) and begin the process of contracting the wound edges together and compacting the wound. **Wound contraction** will continue until the force generated by the open wound is equalized by the tension of the surrounding skin. This occurs because of the movement of full-thickness skin toward the center of the skin defect by the drawing in of surrounding normal skin. Wounds therefore become smaller if permitted to contract. In some areas, such as the face, contraction may pull and distort normal skin, resulting in a noticeable change in the skin contour of the area and a more noticeable scar. In wounds that require skin grafting for coverage, a full-thickness skin graft greatly diminishes the force of the resulting wound contraction. The initial orientation of collagen fibers is disorganized and must be remodeled. Thus collagen synthesis, breakdown, and remodeling begins and continues for 6 months to 1 year. Proper collagen remodeling is dependent on continued synthesis and breakdown of collagen at a low rate and is controlled by several proteolytic enzymes, the matrix metalloproteinases, which are produced by macrophages, epidermal and endothelial cells, and fibroblasts. Dysregulation of this process may result in malformation of healing, leading to hypertrophic or keloid scars. The most rapid rate of increase in the **tensile**

strength of the wound occurs by the *third week* (indeed the wound may only have about 20% of normal tensile strength at this time), and the wound has its greatest mass. Paradoxically, although the tensile or breaking strength of the wound is increasing during the first 7 to 10 days, because of its still low tensile strength, dehiscence is more likely to occur at this early time rather than at 3 weeks or after (Fig. 10.1).

Factors Affecting Normal Repair (40, 106)

Many factors have a significant effect on normal wound repair that the emergency physician must be aware of both for therapy and for prognostic purposes.

DRUGS

When administered within 3 days after injury, **steroids** can cause problems in repair and are able to suppress the inflammatory response necessary for proper wound healing (61). Polymorphonuclear leukocytes and macrophages fail to enter the wound, and fibroplasia is suppressed. However, steroids alone rarely halt repair unless given in large doses. In open wounds, the effect of steroids is much worse than in closed wounds, because open wounds require more tissue healing than do primarily closed wounds. Contraction and epithelialization of open wounds take longer with steroids. Antiinflammatory steroids begun after injury inhibit repair considerably less than do steroids started just after wounding.

Vitamin A can be administered therapeutically in selected individuals to stimulate healing when steroid suppression of wound healing is a factor. Vitamin A facilitates the migration of macrophages into a wound, which is important for the initiation of wound healing and is inhibited by glucocorticoids. In addition, poor vascular regeneration in steroid-treated patients is reversed by vitamin A. The dose of vitamin A is 25,000 U/day and is safe and effective over a period of weeks. Topical vitamin A (1,000 U/g) is used with good results when applied 3 times per day

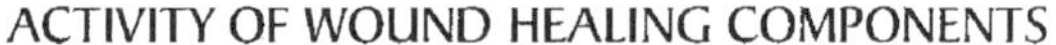

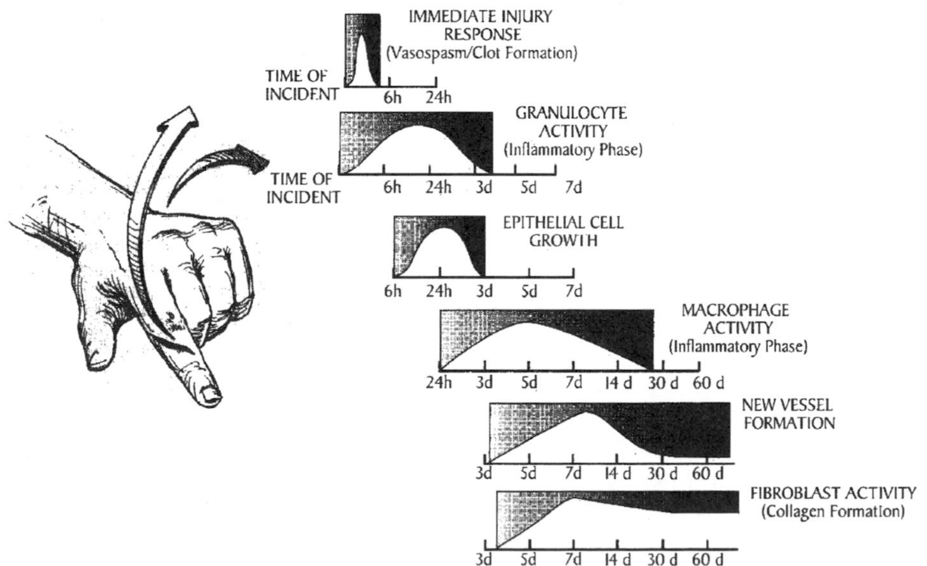

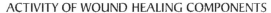

Figure 10.1. The chronology of early wound healing (From Trott A: Wounds and Lacerations: Emergency Care and Closure. St. Louis: Mosby-Year Book, 16, 1991, with permission).

in patients with nonhealing wounds, particularly steroid ulcers. If topical or systemic vitamin A is given, the effects of steroids can be partially overcome.

Wound repair also is inhibited by **sex hormones**. *Estrogen* depresses collagen synthesis and thereby mildly decreases the tensile strength of wounds. *Progesterone* increases neovascularization and oxygen supply to the wound and increases inflammation, but inhibits collagen synthesis. When estrogen is added to progesterone, neovascularization is reduced to normal, and thus the total effect is a marked decrease in wound repair. Therefore, progesterone depresses collagen synthesis markedly, and a combination of progesterone and estrogen depresses collagen synthesis even more markedly. Most women, however, have no problem with repair during pregnancy or while ingesting oral contraceptives.

Aspirin, phenylbutazone, and **vitamin E** inhibit inflammation, and this effect is reduced by vitamin A. Vitamin E has been dispensed in over-the-counter preparations advertised as an agent that decreases scar formation when applied topically over a wound. Vitamin E appears to decrease scar contracture; however, this has not been adequately proven.

Vitamin C is essential in the synthesis of collagen, and deficiencies in this vitamin impair wound healing. **Colchicine** interferes with microtubule function and slows collagen transport from the cell to the extracellular space.

ASSOCIATED CONDITIONS

Diabetics heal poorly. The function of white cells is impaired during episodes of hyperglycemia, and minor infections (even those that are remote from the wound site) may cause poor blood sugar control in diabetics, leading to impaired healing. Diabetics have impaired leukocyte migration and macrophage function. The loss of microvasculature and development of sensory neuropathy that ensue during diabetes may lead to the formation of cutaneous ulcers from relatively minor skin trauma coupled with a lack of awareness by the patient of skin pressure or injury. In addition they have an impaired ability to grow new vessels in a wound. Thus diabetics may have both dysfunctional white blood cells and a paucity of local blood vessels in their wounds, both of which are crucial defects for proper wound healing. Major infections also occur more readily in diabetic patients. For these reasons, it is important to avoid anemia, hypoxia, and hypovolemia during the process of repair in the diabetic with wounds. It should be obvious then that the injured tissue in the wound must be handled with the utmost care during the repair of a laceration in a diabetic patient. Similarly, any other patient with impaired peripheral vascular circulation or peripheral tissue hypoxia due to heart failure, atherosclerosis, chronic obstructive pulmonary disease, septicemia, or severe anemia may have impaired wound healing and must be treated with care.

Other factors that may adversely affect healing include those things that decrease collagen synthesis such as infection, associated major traumatic injuries, hypoxia, uremia, advanced age, and circulatory impairment. Any illness or disease (including nutritional deficits) that leads to an overall catabolic state may lead to poor healing. Cancer patients may be at risk for poor healing not only because of the possibility of being in a catabolic state, but also because some of the chemotherapeutic or radiation treatments that they take may impair normal local wound-repair processes.

REGION

Certain areas of the body heal better than others, depending on skin thickness, pigmentation, and location. Thick skin heals more poorly than thin skin. Wounds over the back, chest, and shoulders tend to heal with more scarring than do wounds of the eyelids (58). Darker skin tends to heal more poorly than light skin because melanin deposition may occur at the wound site. In addition, hypertrophic scars and keloids occur more with thick and dark skin. Oily skin has a greater tendency for scar formation. Certain regions heal with a much thicker scar regardless of meticulous care. This is particularly true for lacerations over the sternum and lower extremities. Patients with skin disorders obviously will heal more poorly than will those with normal skin.

Abnormal Repair (40, 60)

KELOIDS

A keloid is a large, firm mass of scarlike tissue composed of homogeneous, eosinophilic bands of collagen mixed with fibers and fibroblasts. Keloids can originate from a wound or skin lesion such as acne. The hypertrophic tissue extends beyond the original wound margins, and the epithelium tends to be *darker* than the normal skin. Keloids tend to occur over areas of increased skin pigmentation and are more common in wounds over the ears, waist, arms, elbows, shoulders, and especially the sternum. Certain individuals are predisposed to keloid formation, and such a patient can often give a history of prior keloid formation. Keloids are more common in patients of African descent.

A number of theories exist as to the etiology of keloids. Some authors believe they are due to excess melanocyte-stimulating hormone (MSH) (66), which is corroborated by the observation that dark-skinned patients are more prone to form keloids, that keloids are rare on the palms and soles (where melanocytes are rare), and that keloid development is enhanced during puberty and pregnancy when MSH levels are higher. Other authors believe that keloids are due to increased tension on the wound edges (66). More recent work suggests that keloids result from a dysregulation of the healing process at the cellular level, with abnormalities in cell migration and proliferation, inflammation, collagen synthesis, cytokines, and wound remodeling.

To decrease keloid formation, we advocate a closure that provides the *least tension possible* on the wound edges and a pressure dressing over the wound. All patients who are prone to form keloids should be followed up closely—when the wound is in a conspicuous region, refer these patients to a plastic surgeon as early as possible in the course of their care. Intradermal corticosteroid injections have been used to suppress MSH secretion and may even cure small keloids by accelerating collagen lysis. These injections are placed in the upper dermis, and a pressure dressing is applied. Larger lesions can be excised and the wound grafted and irradiated during the first 24 hours of excision and resuturing. Another alternative is to inject the wound edges with a corticosteroid at the first sign of keloid formation and, as an adjunct, apply firm pressure dressing during the healing period.

HYPERTROPHIC SCARS

Hypertrophic scars are bulky scars that remain within the boundaries of the wound. They occur more often around joints and areas of motion or tension. Keloids rarely resolve spontaneously, whereas hypertrophic scars tend to develop a peak size and often regress over a period of months to years.

There are two theories for the pathogenesis of a hypertrophic scar. One is that a continuous inflammatory response occurs as a result of infection, which causes more connective tissue formation. Another theory states that these scars are due to tension on the wound edges. Incisions that cross flexion creases often become hypertrophic; be particularly careful in dealing with these wounds.

In patients with a tendency to form hypertrophic scars, the application of a pressure dressing and splinting may be preventive. A firm pressure dressing at the level of capillary pressure (2 mm Hg) causes diminution of the mass of collagen and probably retards the synthesis of collagen by diminishing circulation. It often takes months of splinting and pressure to aid in the prevention of hypertrophic scars. Small scars may be treated with antiinflammatory steroids; radiation also has been used.

MECHANISM OF WOUND INJURY (40, 54)

Wounds may occur as a result of three types of forces: shearing, tension, and compression. A wound from a sharp-edged object such as a knife or piece of glass results in a classic example of a **shear injury**. This type of wound often does not have associated soft tissue damage around the laceration. The surface area of the tissue contacted by the wounding instrument is relatively small, and tissue failure occurs with a resulting small amount of energy imparted to the area. **Tension** wounds occur as a result of a blunt or flat object striking and stretching the skin, until it fails. An example would be a flat object such as a spatula striking the tissue that overlies a bony prominence or a fall at low speed from a standing position against a flat surface such as a piece of furniture. With this type of wound, there is usually some contusion injury to the tissue surrounding and/or underneath the laceration. **Compression** injuries result when two equal forces are oriented toward each other and result in a *stellate-type laceration*. An example of compression injury is the wound caused when a hard round object (e.g., rock) strikes a bony prominence (e.g., skull). The energy required (and hence transferred to the tissues) for a compression force wound is greater than that for a shear or tension laceration. Damage occurs to the wound edges with an associated reduction in blood flow and *100-fold increased* susceptibility to infection. There may be significant injury to the adjacent and underlying tissues with any compression-type wound.

AXIOM

Wounds that are due to compressive forces (e.g., stellate lacerations) are associated with a 100-fold increased susceptibility to infection as compared with those due to shear forces (e.g., a knife).

One recent wound registry project by Hollander et al. (54) found that most lacerations occur in young adults between ages 19 and 35 years, with men predominating over women. More than 50% of all lacerations were caused by blunt injury or a sharp object such as metal, glass, or wood that produced a shear force–type injury. Only a small minority (5%) of wounds were caused by bites. Most wounds were located on the head (37% face, 14% scalp) or on an upper extremity (34%), predominantly the hand or fingers (28%).

SUTURE MATERIAL AND ADJUNCTS FOR WOUND CLOSURE

SKIN TAPE

Skin tape may be used to close superficial wounds or deeper wounds once the subcutaneous dermal layers have been approximated by absorbable suture material. Skin tape should not be used in widely separated wound edges. The tensile strength of the surgical tape must be sufficient to maintain wound approximation during healing. Weak tapes will not resist pull at the wound edges and will tear, permitting the wound to separate. Adding reinforcing rayon filaments to the backing of the tape may increase tensile strength fourfold (22). Skin tapes come in many sizes: 1/8-, 1/4-, and 1/2-inch wide strips, that are approximately 2 to 3 inches in length. Before skin tape is used, cleanse the skin with acetone or alcohol to remove all oils and particles that may cause the tape to form a poor contact with the skin, even though the skin has been scrubbed with an iodophor.

Contaminated wounds whose edges were approximated by suture material had a higher infection rate than did contaminated wounds whose edges were not opposed (21). Irritation of the skin by tape can be correlated in part with the degree of tape occlusivity, which leads to accumulation of fluid underneath the tape, promoting tissue maceration and bacterial growth. The microporous tapes that are now used have interstices that permit moisture to be absorbed, and a dry skin surface is maintained below the tape. Tape closure will not work well in some areas, such as the skin of the axilla, palms, and soles. In addition, tape closures should not be used in areas where there is much moisture, such as over flexor surfaces of joints. Tape closure should not be used on crush-induced injuries in which there is a laceration. The optimal lacerations that can be closed with skin tape are wounds that are caused by sharp instruments.

Ideally skin tape should be applied for 2 to 3 weeks. In patients with oily skin, the tape may loosen in 7 to 9 days rather than the usual 2 to 3 weeks, or the tape may cause sebaceous duct inflammation (25, 80).

The *advantages* of skin tape are

1. No anesthetic is needed.
2. No suture marks are left when the tape is removed.
3. No skin reactivity occurs.
4. Tape can be left in place for a long time beneath casts.
5. Tape saves time in both application and removal.

The *disadvantages* of skin tape are

1. Tape does not adhere well to oily skin.
2. Tape does not provide for eversion of the wound edges and can actually produce inversion when used in wounds that are deeper than the dermis.
3. A child may remove the tape prematurely.
4. Tape cannot be applied to skin over joint surfaces or wounds that are under significant tension when closed.

When To Use Skin Tape for Closure

Skin tape can be used in lacerations that extend only partially through the dermis. These wounds are not widely separated and can be easily approximated with the use of skin tape. Skin tape also can be used in the closure of full-thickness lacerations that are small and are oriented such that they are parallel to skin tension lines, resulting in very little separation of the wound edges. Do not use skin tape in closing lacerations that are in regions of the body where there is excessive motion, such as over joints, eyelids, and fingers. Skin tape is especially useful in those wounds in which the edges are cleanly incised and "come together" naturally without tension.

With the advent of newer and better cyanoacrylate-based tissue adhesives, many wounds that are amenable to tape closure (i.e., superficial wounds that can be approximated easily under no tension and are not over a joint or area of excessive motion) may be more easily managed with tissue glue (Figs. 10.2–10.5).

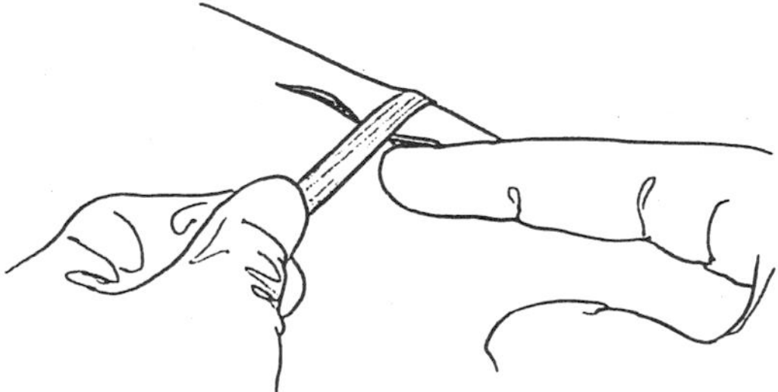

Figure 10.2. Bring tape over the wound as the wound is apposed with the finger of the opposite hand. (From Trott A: Wounds and Lacerations: Emergency Care and Closure. St. Louis: Mosby-Year Book, 252–253, 1997, with permission.)

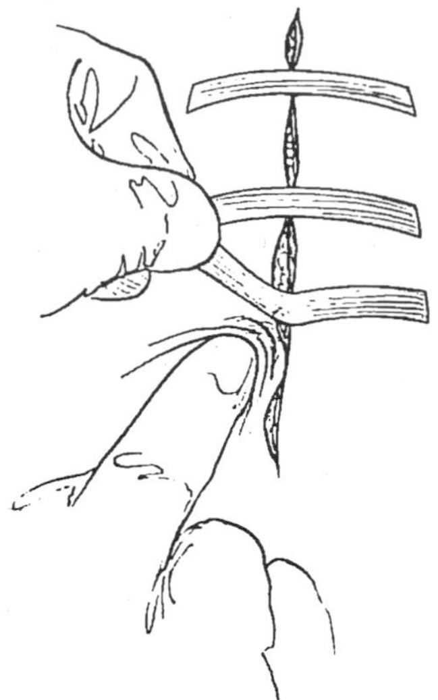

Figure 10.3. Place further tapes in a similar manner. (From Trott A: Wounds and Lacerations: Emergency Care and Closure. St. Louis: Mosby-Year Book, 252–253, 1997, with permission.)

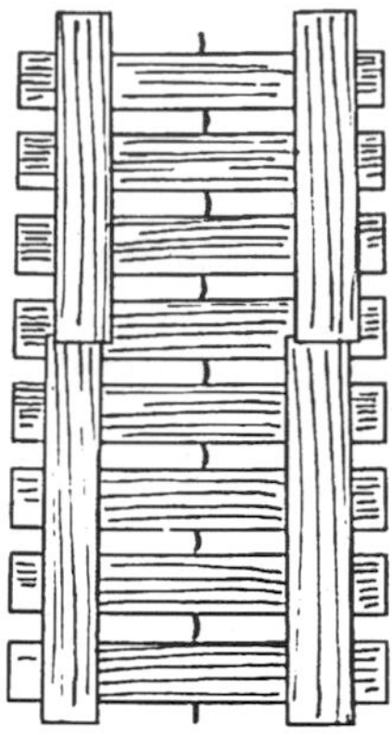

Figure 10.5. Cross stays are placed over the tape ends to prevent skin blistering and premature removal. (From Trott A: Wounds and Lacerations: Emergency Care and Closure. St. Louis: Mosby-Year Book, 252–253, 1997, with permission.)

SKIN CLIPS AND STAPLES

Skin clips are no longer in use and have been replaced by skin staples. The staples provide a good approximation of the wound edges. When used properly, they do not penetrate the skin surface and hence do not leave suture mark scars when removed. If there is tension on the wound, then the skin clips or staples may leave suture mark–type scars. The steel used is inert, and thus causes less tissue reaction than do most sutures and is associated with a low incidence of wound infection in contaminated wounds (40). The staples, however, seem to have a damaging effect on local tissue defenses. Stapled wounds seem to be more susceptible to infection than are taped wounds. This increased susceptibility to infection argues against the use of staples in superficial wounds that are contaminated, which are the most common type seen by the emergency physician (37). When using skin staples, close the subcutaneous tissue if involved, first with a deeper layer of absorbable suture. Staplers on the market today come as disposable units, with about 35 staples in each unit. In their favor, some studies on their use in the emergency department setting would seem to indicate that stapling is less costly than suturing, that this advantage appears to increase as laceration length increases, and when used in properly selected wounds may achieve adequate healing with acceptable cosmesis (16, 89). The *advantages* of staples are

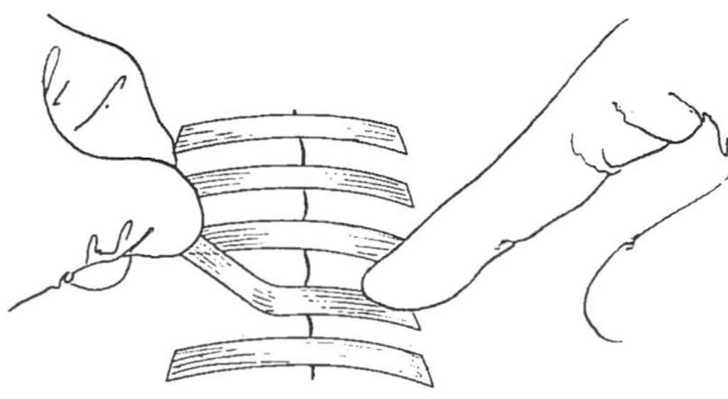

Figure 10.4. Enough tapes are placed so that wound gapping does not occur. Usually there is a space of 2 to 3 mm between tapes. (From Trott A: Wounds and Lacerations: Emergency Care and Closure. St. Louis: Mosby-Year Book, 252–253, 1997, with permission.)

1. A wound can be closed more rapidly with staples than it can with sutures.
2. Staples are easier to place than are sutures.

3. Placement of staples requires less skill than the placement of sutures.
4. In terms of time saved, they may be more cost effective than suturing, particularly with multiple or long lacerations.

The *disadvantages* of staples are

1. Staples can be more expensive than sutures, particularly for short or small lacerations.
2. Wounds closed with staples are more susceptible to infection.
3. Staples do not permit eversion of the wound edges, particularly in irregular lacerations.

Staples are best used in clean linear wounds located in areas that are not easily contaminated, such as the back, arms, and thighs. Despite their drawbacks, they have grown in popularity in many emergency departments. The decision to use staples versus other methods of closure, particularly sutures, must be made on a case-by-case basis, with all of these factors weighed carefully in the clinician's decision (Fig. 10.6).

WOUND-TISSUE ADHESIVES

Large strides have been made in recent years in the development of adhesives suitable for use in laceration repair. Cyanoacrylates were first manufactured in 1949 but were not tested for clinical use until the late 1950s by Coover et al. (27). Cyanoacrylate adhesives are formed by the combination of cyanoacetate and formaldehyde in a heat vacuum along with a base, resulting in the formation of a liquid monomer. If the monomer is exposed to water (moisture on the skin surface), it rapidly changes chemically to form a solid polymer (that binds to the top layer of epidermis). This exothermic reaction releases some local heat, which is occasionally noted by patients as a mild

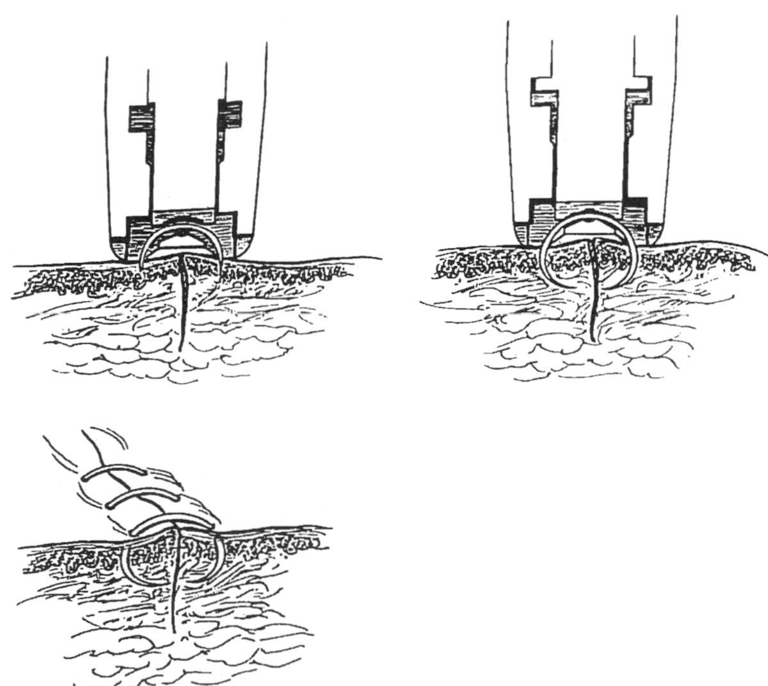

Figure 10.6. During triggering, the staple is reconfigured to approximate wound edges. (From Trott A: Wounds and Lacerations: Emergency Care and Closure. St. Louis: Mosby-Year Book, 258, 1997, with permission.)

burning sensation. Early derivatives used in wound repair included methyl-2- and ethyl-2-cyanoacrylates ("Crazy Glue" is an ethylcyanoacrylate), which, although provides acceptable closure, resulted in significant complications. These short alkyl-chain forms were found to degrade rapidly into cyanoacetate and formaldehyde, which produced histotoxicity and both acute and chronic inflammation (112). Eventually cyanoacrylates with longer alkyl chains were found to have much less tissue toxicity. The longer alkyl side chain retards breakdown significantly, thereby reducing the accumulation of toxic byproducts in the tissues. *N*-butyl-2-cyanoacrylate (Histoacryl Blue), developed in the 1970s, is the cyanoacrylate adhesive that has enjoyed wide use outside of the United States and indeed has been successfully used for wound repair worldwide for more than 20 years (95). Studies have shown it to provide cosmetic results comparable to those of suture repair with complications such as infection occurring at a rate no higher than those with traditional wound-repair techniques. Unfortunately Histoacryl Blue does retain some histotoxic properties, has a tendency to fracture if stressed by movement, and a 1985 study using rat peritoneum demonstrated a propensity to induce sarcomas. The development of human malignancies related to Histoacryl Blue use has not thus far been reported. Histoacryl Blue has not been approved for use in the United States by the Food and Drug Administration (FDA) (112).

2-Octylcyanoacrylate (Dermabond, Ethicon Inc. Summerville, NJ) is a newer-generation medical-grade tissue adhesive approved for use in topical wound closure in the United States by the FDA in 1998. It is a clear purple fluid packaged in single-use sterile 0.5-mL glass cylinders encased in plastic with a round cotton-like fiber tip to serve as the applicator. At the time of this writing, the cost to the hospital for a single-application vial is in the $20 to $25 range, but actual charge to the patient per vial varies among facilities. Most simple lacerations amenable to closure with Dermabond can be repaired with one or two vials. Suture material by comparison generally costs $3 to $5 per suture. If consideration is given to the added costs of suture instruments and the additional physician time required for suture repair versus adhesive, it is possible to see a potential cost savings with adhesive wound repair.

Dermabond has been formulated using a longer alkyl-chain cyanoacrylate in combination with some added plasticizers, which on polymerization, produces a strong yet flexible polymer that binds readily to the epidermis. Dermabond has been shown to have less tissue toxicity, reaches maximal bonding strength in about 2.5 minutes (equivalent to that of healed tissue at 7 days after repair), and has almost 4 times the bonding strength of *N*-butyl-2-cyanoacrylate (Histoacryl Blue) (18). When used for wound closure, it holds the epidermal edges of the wound together and permits normal wound healing underneath, eventually being shed in the natural process of exfoliation of the outer epidermal layer. Dermabond has been marketed as an alternative to sutures that are 5-0 or smaller in diameter. Proper use of Dermabond requires the clinician to understand its limitations. The use of Dermabond may permit wound repair without the use of local anesthesia in selected cases, but this feature must not persuade the clinician to forego sound wound-management principles, especially adequate wound cleansing and debridement. Failure to adhere to such principles may lead to a higher than expected infection rate. Despite its increased flexibility, Dermabond is often not adequate by itself to hold a wound under tension together. Subcutaneous sutures may need to be placed to draw the wound margins together adequately, so that the epidermal layer is well apposed under no tension, at which point Dermabond may be an effective alternative to skin sutures. Adequate hemostasis in the wound must be achieved before using Dermabond; otherwise, the blood accumulating at the wound margins may prevent the adhesive from binding adequately with the epidermis. Dermabond should *never* be placed in a wound, as it will polymerize rapidly when it contacts the moisture and blood within, resulting in a wound that is actually held *open* by the adhesive. If it enters the wound accidentally, sponge it out immediately with gauze; should this fail, it may require complete removal by careful debridement and/or excision to allow subsequent reclosure with adhesive or sutures. Polymerized glue allowed to remain inside the wound may lead to foreign-body reactions and serves a potential nidus for infection (119). Dermabond also will bind unwanted items such as latex glove fingertips and instruments such as forceps to the wound margins if the glue is allowed to contact them, necessitating their careful removal. Dermabond is a thin runny liquid, so take care to position the patient in such a way as to prevent inadvertent adhesive from running off into unwanted areas such as mucous membranes or the eyes. The placement of moistened gauze adjacent to the wound to prevent run off of the glue toward unwanted areas may help to prevent such complications (moistened rather than dry gauze is less likely to be glued to the skin) (119).

Always exercise good judgment when choosing which wounds to close with a tissue adhesive. Use Dermabond only with the intention of closing the epidermal layer of a wound, in lieu of other alternatives such as sutures, staples, or tape. Properly selected superficial wounds on the face, extremities, and torso may be safely closed with Dermabond. Extremity and torso wounds, particularly those that extend into the subcutaneous tissue, tend to heal better when subcuticular sutures are placed first. Despite its increased flexibility over older tissue glues, Dermabond should probably not be used for wounds in areas under high tension or with high mobility such as joints (unless the area will be immobilized by splinting). Exercise caution in choosing to use tissue glue to close a wound on the hand or foot because of the tension generated on the skin in such areas with normal movement. It is also probably best to avoid its use for bite and other heavily contaminated wounds, ulcers, puncture wounds, jagged or stellate lacerations, and mucous membranes (including mucocutaneous junctions). It is probably wise to avoid tissue adhesive use on patients who are prone to keloids, because a pressure dressing cannot be applied on top of the repair to discourage keloid formation. Scalp wounds may be closed with Dermabond, but use care to prevent excessive adhesive from binding adjacent hair; keep the wound dry for at least 5 days. Areas prone to excessive moisture such as the groin or axillae are probably best avoided for they are more prone to adhesive failure (19). A number of recent studies have demonstrated that wounds closed with Dermabond can heal with cosmetic results equivalent to those of suture repair, that wound repair with Dermabond is faster than with sutures and hence may be more cost efficient, that patients (and especially parents of children) are comfortable with this technique, and that physicians with proper training can rapidly become proficient in the technique of wound repair with Dermabond (18, 53, 82, 93, 94).

The *advantages* of tissue adhesives are

1. No anesthetic may be needed.
2. No suture mark scars are formed as the wound heals.
3. The epidermal layer of the wound can be closed more rapidly with adhesive than with sutures, saving time and perhaps reducing cost.
4. The adhesive forms a waterproof barrier over the wound, which may prevent bacterial encroachment and hence infection.
5. The patient may shower with the wound uncovered so long as pro-

longed immersion into water is avoided.

6. Wounds closed with adhesives require no additional dressing.
7. Return visits for suture removal are not required, as the adhesive is shed naturally from the skin during normal sloughing after a week or so.

The *disadvantages* of tissue adhesives are

1. They cannot be used as the sole method of wound approximation for lacerations into the subcutaneous tissues that are under tension.
2. Adhesive may fail under conditions in which the wound is placed under repeated tension or stress as a result of normal movement (e.g., over joints, on the feet, hands, and digits).
3. Adhesive may be picked off before adequate healing by curious children who cannot comprehend why they should not do so.
4. Tissue adhesives may not retain their adherence to the wound edges long enough to prevent dehiscence in patients with delayed healing (such as diabetics), in which longer than usual retention of wound approximation may be preferable (i.e., with sutures or staples).
5. Excessive exposure to water (such as prolonged immersion in a bath) may lead to adhesive failure before completed healing.
6. The bond between adhesive and the skin may be accidentally broken by inadvertent exposure to acetone or other petroleum-based products (including gasoline and antibiotic ointments), leading to dehiscence before the wound is fully healed.
7. Clinicians may be tempted to use adhesive because of the advantage of being able to forego local anesthesia before wound closure, and in so doing, not provide adequate wound cleansing and debridement before repair, thereby increasing the risk of infection.

Technique for Dermabond Closure of Lacerations (19, 119)

1. Inspect the laceration carefully to determine if there may be contaminants or foreign bodies present, determine the depth of the wound (and hence whether a layer of subcutaneous suture is needed), and then examine the patient for associated injuries to deeper or adjacent structures such as tendons and nerves.
2. Determine if the wound edges can be adequately approximated under little or no tension and hence whether use of a tissue adhesive for closure of the superficial layer of the laceration is appropriate (taking into account also the location of the wound itself).
3. Determine if topical and/or local infiltrative anesthesia, or regional anesthesia will be needed for the wound repair, keeping in mind that adequate cleansing and adequate exploration of the laceration may require the use of anesthetic (anesthesia will of course be needed if subcutaneous sutures are needed to achieve wound approximation without tension).
4. Prepare and drape the wound in the same manner used for traditional suturing.
5. Anesthetize the laceration if necessary, allowing time for adequate onset of anesthesia (see section on anesthesia of wounds later in this chapter).
6. Perform adequate cleansing of the wound with sterile saline irrigation (or appropriate antiseptic) and debride/remove devitalized tissue and contaminants thoroughly (if the wound is found to be heavily contaminated, reconsider the choice of tissue adhesive versus suture).
7. Close the subcutaneous layer if necessary with absorbable suture, and then reassess the approximation of the epidermal layer to make sure that the wound edges can be easily approximated with little or no tension; if not, consider using suture rather than Der-

mabond to close the skin. (TIP: Do not apply Dermabond over skin sutures or near to adjacent skin sutures because it may spread out to encompass and adhere to nearby sutures, making them very difficult to remove until the glue has broken down).

8. Be certain that adequate hemostasis has been achieved along the wound margins (a small amount of topical 1:10,000 epinephrine solution or the use of a local anesthetic agent with epinephrine may be helpful); the wound edges must be dry!
9. Position the patient in such a way as to try to ensure that excess Dermabond will not inadvertently run off downhill into sensitive adjacent structures such as the eyes or mouth. Use of some moistened (damp but not dripping) sterile gauze placed several centimeters away from the wound margins may help prevent accidental runoff of the adhesive into unwanted areas. An application of an ointment such as triple antibiotic or petroleum jelly to adjacent sensitive areas (around the orbit or mouth) may prevent unwanted glue attachment if the Dermabond should run onto them. If any glue manages to run onto adjacent areas of skin, quickly wipe it up with gauze before it hardens (acetone on a cotton swab may be used to remove unwanted glue from the skin if the glue dries before it can be removed; do not use acetone near the mouth or near the eyes).
10. Wear vinyl gloves if possible during the actual closure of the wound with Dermabond (it is much less adherent to vinyl than to latex). Squeeze the plastic casing of the Dermabond capsule, thereby crushing the glass ampule inside, and immediately invert the container with the applicator tip toward the floor so that the adhesive begins to flow into the applicator. (Be careful when doing this, and do not hold the applicator over the patient until you are ready to apply the adhesive, to avoid accidentally dripping or splashing adhesive onto the patient.)
11. Once the applicator becomes moist with adhesive, approximate the edges of the wound by using gentle manipulation with gloved fingers or alternatively metal smooth-tipped forceps or one of the plastic skin-approximation devices now available for use with tissue adhesives. (It is generally not easy or altogether not possible to achieve eversion of the wound edges with this technique, but always avoid inversion of the edges.) We also have had success with a wound-approximation technique using gentle pressure along opposite sides of the laceration with the long wooden sticks of two sterile cotton-tipped swabs to approximate the wound margins.
12. Then apply the adhesive longitudinally along the wound edges with gentle brushing motions (at no time should the applicator tip be allowed to penetrate into the wound; a light touch with no pressure on the wound is the key), and then hold the edges together for at least 30 seconds before releasing the wound. It may be necessary to recoat the wound one or two additional times before releasing, and apply more adhesive in an oval pattern around the wound edges for 0.5 to 1 cm to encompass additional skin surface area for the glue (this adds greater overall strength to the laceration repair). In general, apply at least three light coats of glue (allowing some time between coats for partial polymerization of the previous coat) to ensure optimal strength, but avoid creating an excessively thick patch. Fanning or blowing on the wound will *not* speed up the polymerization of the glue. Try to avoid touching the glue with the gloved fingertips, forceps, or other tools to prevent inadvertent adhesion to the wound margins. (If this does occur, gently remove

the glove or forceps from the skin, perhaps with the assistance of an acetone-dampened cotton swab, taking care not to pull so hard as to break the glue and reopen the wound, and avoiding contact of the acetone with the glue on the wound if possible.)

13. Do not touch the laceration until adhesive has thoroughly dried (generally waiting at least 5 to 7 minutes would be best, although it may be dry in less than 3 minutes). Inspect the wound for adequacy of closure and initial cosmetic appearance. If the wound has been inadequately closed or has an unacceptable initial cosmetic appearance, consider removal of the glue and reclosure of the wound. Apply bacitracin, triple antibiotic ointment, or petroleum jelly to the glue to loosen and facilitate its removal, but this may take some time (30 minutes or more) and in some cases, careful manual removal of some of the glue may also be required.
14. No additional dressing on top of the wound is necessary and *do not* apply antibiotic ointment to the repair, as it may loosen the glue from the skin. Once the glue has thoroughly dried, gently clean blood, prep solution, and so on from areas adjacent to the wound with water/soap and towels, but take care not to scrub the wound or to immerse it in water.

Aftercare of Dermabond Wound Repair (19, 119)

Instruct patients to leave the wound uncovered (the glue acts as a water-resistant bandage) and explicitly tell them *not* to apply topical antibiotic ointment or any other ointment or lotion to the wound (as this may loosen the glue prematurely). Similarly they should avoid inadvertent contact of the wound with other petroleum products such as gasoline or mineral spirits, which may similarly loosen the bond of the glue. Patients may shower normally, avoiding any scrubbing of the wound, and gently dab the wound area dry with a towel. Avoid baths; prolonged immersion of the wound into water may loosen the bond between the glue and skin. Advise patients to avoid picking at the glue to prevent its premature loosening and wound dehiscence (especially important for children and their parents). For particularly active children, apply a gauze bandage to the wound site to discourage them from picking at the glue. Dermabond will usually spontaneously peel off of the skin in 5 to 10 days, making a repeated visit to remove it generally unnecessary. Instruct patients to monitor the wound for typical signs of infection including increased pain or tenderness, local warmth or systemic fever, excessive redness, seeping of drainage from underneath the glue, and premature breakdown or loosening of the glue. Suspected infection of the wound below the adhesive without significant local swelling or fluctuance and without loosening of the glue, *may* respond well to a course of oral antibiotics. (Reported rates of wound infection after tissue adhesive repair have thus far been comparable to those of sutured wounds.) Purulent material from a true infection generally lifts the dried glue polymer away from the skin. In such cases, remove the glue and initiate standard wound-care measures for infection (cleaning, debridement, antibiotics, etc.), and allow the laceration to heal by secondary intention. Avoid reapplication of Dermabond for delayed closure in these cases. In rare cases, the adhesive may persist on the skin longer than is typically needed for adequate wound healing (generally 5 to 10 days). Instruct patients to return to the emergency center if the Dermabond has failed to slough off after 8 to 10 days (prolonged adherence to the skin may lead to infection between the adhesive and overlying glue). If the wound appears to be adequately healed, apply petroleum jelly or ointment to the glue and allowed it to sit for 30 minutes to facilitate its loosening and gentle removal (Figs. 10.7–10.9).

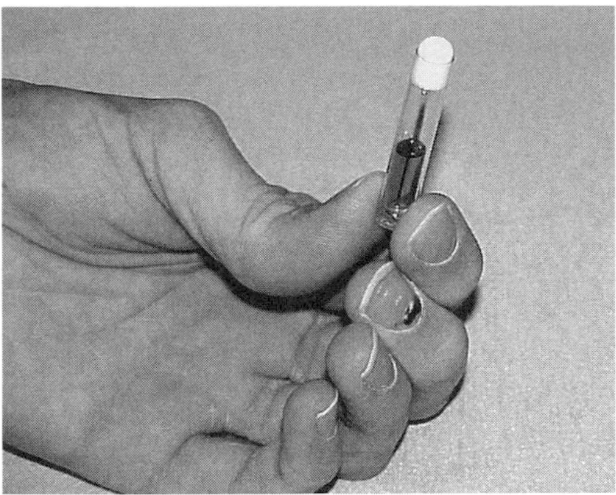

Figure 10.7 Invert the Dermabond adhesive capsule, and then gently squeeze to crush the glass ampule inside. [From the product sheet for Dermabond, demonstrating the activation of the vial and its application (Figs. 2–4), with permission.]

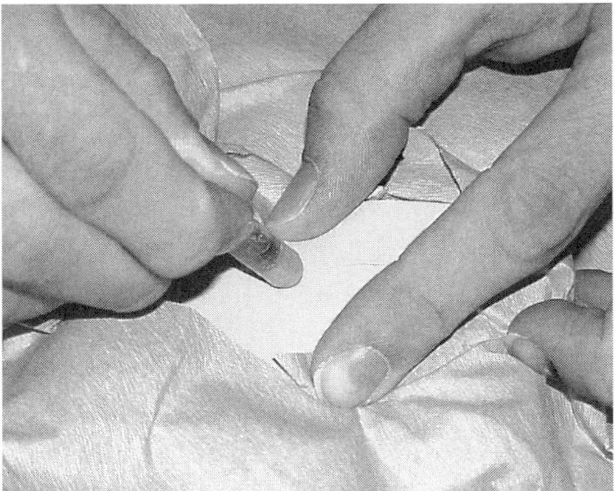

Figure 10.9. Apply Dermabond adhesive to the top of the wound with the wound edges held in apposition. Three to four "light" layers of adhesive are usually sufficient. [From the product sheet for Dermabond, demonstrating the activation of the vial and its application (Figs. 2–4), with permission.]

SUTURE MATERIAL

Absorbable Sutures

The absorbable suture materials available for use in the emergency department include plain gut, chromic gut, polyglycolic acid (Dexon; PGA), polyglactin 910 (Vicryl), polydioxanone (PDS II), and poliglecaprone 25 (Monocryl). Most of these absorbable sutures in size 4-0 or smaller are completely absorbed in 3 to 6 weeks, but the newer synthetics, particularly Monocryl and PDS II, may persist for several more weeks (70). Suture material that is larger than 4-0 size may last even longer, even up to 4 months. The absorption process involves an inflammatory reaction produced around the suture material, in a way similar to the typical reaction of tissues to a foreign antigenic body. All absorbable sutures produce some tissue reaction, so in general, the ideal absorbable material would produce the least amount of tissue reaction. In addition, the rate of absorption and subsequent loss in tensile strength of the suture material varies somewhat from one tissue type to another (mucous membranes absorb faster than fascia or muscle) and is dramatically increased by the presence of an infection. The infection magnifies the inflammatory response at the wound site, thus speeding the dissolution of the suture material and speeding the loss of wound tensile strength.

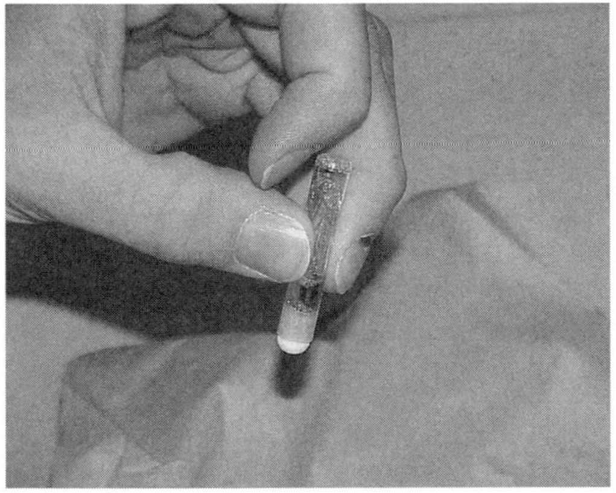

Figure 10.8. Invert the Dermabond applicator to start the flow of adhesive into the applicator pad. Be careful to avoid drips into unwanted areas of the patient. [From the product sheet for Dermabond, demonstrating the activation of the vial and its application (Figs. 2–4), with permission.]

Catgut was at one time one of the most commonly used suture materials, and although it is still used in certain circumstances, in the emergency center, it has been superseded by the newer synthetic absorbables Vicryl, Dexon, PDS II, and Monocryl. Catgut is made of collagen harvested from the submucosal layer of the small intestine of sheep and the serosal layer of cattle small intestine. The smaller the caliber or diameter of the catgut, the more rapidly it is absorbed. Catgut is digested by collagenase in the tissues, usually within about 10 days, leading to a significant tissue reaction and hence should not be used for skin closures.

Chromic catgut is soaked in chromic acid salts, similar to the chemicals used to tan leather, which permits the suture to retain its tensile strength for 2 to 3 weeks (117) with about 90% absorbed in 30 days and with complete absorption by 50 days (40). Chromic catgut offers the advantage over catgut of prolonged retention in the wound; however, it also eventually incites an even greater inflammatory response. The degree of inflammation caused by chromic catgut can lead to significant foreign-body reaction, localized abscess formation, and increased local tissue fluid. Both chromic catgut and catgut are packaged wet because drying damages them and causes the suture to become friable. Compared with the newer synthetic absorbable sutures, both catgut and chromic catgut have considerably lower initial tensile strength and greater inflammatory response with shorter duration of retention in the wound. Both should be generally avoided for closure of the skin, but are still useful in some instances, such as for mucosal wounds.

Dexon, Vicryl, and Monocryl are synthetic absorbable suture materials that retain their strength in wounds for at least 3 to 4 weeks (Table 10.1) (40, 70). Dexon is a polymer of polyglycolic acid introduced in the early 1970s. It is absorbable, braided, and relatively stiff, has a higher tensile strength than catgut, and contains no collagen, protein, antigens, or pyrogens. Dexon produces minimal tissue reaction and has an infection rate lower than that seen with either catgut or chromic catgut. Vicryl, a polymer of polyglactic, was introduced in 1971. Like Dexon, Vicryl is a braided synthetic that is also relatively stiff. Its tensile strength is less than that of Dexon but still greater than catgut or chromic catgut. Vicryl can induce bacterial growth and is contraindicated for use on the skin. Vicryl is supplied as a clear or violet suture. Both Vicryl and Dexon, by virtue of their stiffness, are more difficult to tie than catgut or chromic catgut. Attempts were made to produce both Vicryl and Dexon as monofilaments, but these were simply too stiff to be practical. PDS II or polydioxanone is an absorbable monofilament developed to address the concerns of braided sutures (increased infection). It has a very long duration of absorption (up to 6 months) and an extremely high tensile strength (50% remains at 28 days compared with 20% to 30% for Monocryl at 14 days and 30% for Vicryl at 21 days) (70). However, PDS II is stiff and difficult to handle and knot. It does have relatively low tissue reactivity and will maintain its integrity even in the presence of bacteria. It is supplied in undyed and violet forms.

Table 10.1
Absorbable Suture Material

Plain gut
Chromic gut
Dexon (PGA; polyglycolic acid)
Vicryl (polyglactin 910, Ethicon)
PDS II (polydioxanone, Ethicon)
Monocryl (poliglecaprone 25, Ethicon)

Monocryl (poliglecaprone 25) is a newer synthetic absorbable, undyed monofilament suture material introduced in 1993. It is the most pliable of the monofilament absorbable sutures. This lack of stiffness provides excellent handling properties, facilitates easy knot tying and retention, and eliminates the memory that some of the other absorbable sutures have for their shape while in the package (70). Monocryl retains approximately 20% to 30% of its strength after 2 weeks *in vivo*, and absorption is complete by 91 to 119 days (see

Table 10.2
Time of Absorption of Absorbable Sutures

Plain gut	7–14 days
Chromic gut	20–40 days
Coated Vicryl	60–90 days
Monocryl	91–119 days
PDS II	90–180 days

Table 10.2 for comparisons). Monocryl incites minimal tissue reaction, is not genotoxic, cytotoxic, pyrogenic, irritating, or antigenic. Monocryl is produced as an undyed clear monofilament, which takes on the color of the tissue in which it is placed; it is less noticeable under the skin than in dyed suture material. It is comparable in cost to plain and chromic catgut and generally a bit less expensive than Vicryl or Dexon (70). Monocryl has been reported to have superior tactile handling qualities compared with chromic, Vicryl, and Dexon when used in various surgical procedures on the head and neck by surgeons. In one series of 80 cases, it was found to produce excellent wound repair with no cases of stitch abscess or excessive wound inflammation (70). In this same series, Monocryl also was used in some cases for skin closure without any noticeable skin inflammation, microabscess formation, or sinus tract formation, and in the mucosal oral and nasal closures for which it was used, no tissue reaction was observed (70). The prudent emergency physician will become familiar with the various available absorbable sutures and guide the choice of absorbable suture used based on the known qualities of the material, the desired duration of persistence of the suture, and personal experience in the handling and knot tying of the various sutures.

Needles

There are two types of needles, tapered and cutting. A needle is classified according to its shape, its cross section, its point, and whether it has an eye. In emergency practice, there is virtually no need for an eye needle, which produces large cutaneous holes. A swaged needle does not produce a larger hole than is necessary. In this needle, the thread is attached directly to the needle without a hole, and the needle is the same diameter as the thread. This is the needle type that is used in an emergency center. There are two shapes of needles: straight and curved. The straight needles are placed in tissue with the hand, and the curved needles are used with a needle holder. The curved needles most commonly used are the 3/8-circle needle and the half-circle needle, which is the most commonly used needle in general surgical practice. Cutting needles at one time were made with the "cutting edge" placed along the line of stress (the line of pull of the suture material) into the tissue, and the cutting edge on the inside diameter of the curved needle. This placement caused the hole to enlarge as the two opposing edges of the tissue were brought together. Cutting needles now are of the reverse cutting type (Fig. 10.10). This type of needle does not place a "cut" along the direction of the suture's line of stress and does not produce an enlarging hole in the wound; the cutting edge also is on the outside diameter of the curved needle. Cutting needles are used to go through tough tissue such as skin and fascia. The taper needle has a round cross section that does not cut tissue; it is used in vascular work and fine mucosal closures (Fig. 10.10). Packages of suture material will state "cutting needle," even though it is a reverse cutting needle; their use is so common that the word "reverse" has been dropped in labeling.

A number of different needle types and sizes are used in the emergency center. The emergency physician should be familiar with some basic information to select intelligently the proper needle and size. Two basic varieties of needles are cuticular and plastic. Cuticular needles are honed (sharpened) 12 times. Plastic needles are designed for cosmetic closures and are honed 24 additional times to cause less trauma when penetrating the tissue. Cutic-

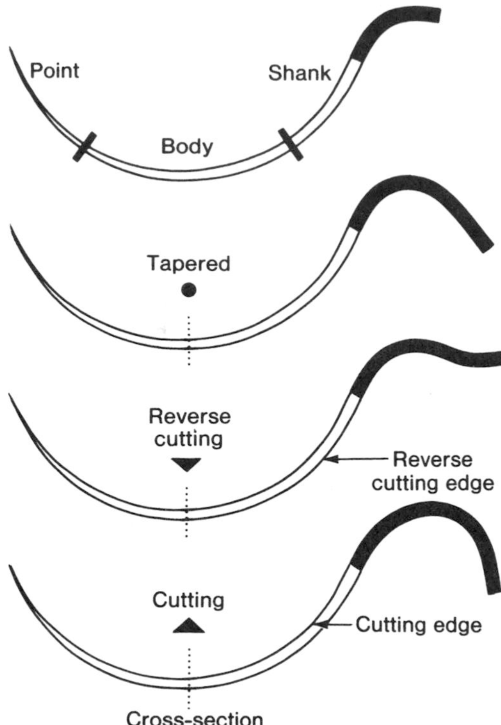

Figure 10.10. Needles used in suturing. See text for discussion. Note that, with the reverse cutting needle, the "base of the triangle" is in line of suture pull as it passes through tissue, thus avoiding enlargement of the hole as suture tension and wound edema ensue.

ular needles come in various series: C (cuticular) and FS (for skin). Plastic needles also have a letter designating the series: P (premium or plastic) and PS (plastic surgery). Within the series of a particular brand of sutures, a number coming after the letter indicates the needle size *within that series*. They are not cross-related; thus a PS-6 needle is not necessarily the same size as an FS-6. The larger the number, the smaller is the needle size within a series. Thus a PS-1 is larger than a PS-3.

Suture Materials and Risk of Infection

The chemical composition of the suture material is an important determinant of early infection. The greatest incidence of infection encountered in tissues is with cotton or silk sutures (39). Nylon and polypropylene sutures have a lower infection rate than any other nonabsorbable suture. Of the absorbable sutures, PGA has produced the least inflammatory response in contaminated tissues (39). Plain gut elicits less infection in contaminated tissues than does chromic gut in the same tissue. When one looks at other nonabsorbables, nylon and polypropylene have been found to elicit the least infection rate in contaminated tissue, and the infection rate is actually lower than that with metallic sutures (4). The infection rate in contaminated tissues containing either nylon or polypropylene does not differ.

Interesting differences exist between monofilament with multifilament sutures. It requires 10^6 *Staphylococcus pyogenes* per gram to elicit purulence and to form clinically significant infection when monofilament sutures are placed in a contaminated wound (40). With braided silk sutures, however, the number required is reduced to 100 staphylococci (40). Silk sutures potentiate infection 10,000-fold when compared with nonbraided nylon (41). The infection rate of contaminated tissue containing braided nylon is lower than that with any other multifilament, nonabsorbable suture. In general, tissues with knotted multifilament sutures have a higher infection rate than do monofilament sutures. When an inert material is used to cover a filament of Dacron, it is found to play no part in altering the rate of infection. Because silk and cotton have higher rates of infection than any other nonabsorbable sutures, never use silk in a contaminated wound. Regarding the lower infection rate with nylon and PGA sutures, the degradation products of both of these materials are potent antibacterial agents (40).

The Wound and Suture Material

Wounds that are parallel to the natural lines of the face and parallel to the flexion or extension lines above the joints heal better and with decreased scarring. Whenever possible, make surgical incisions parallel to these lines. Studies have shown that there is little difference in suture marks between absorbable and nonabsorbable sutures; the method of closure determines the **suture mark** (76). Suture marks are largely preventable by early removal of the sutures and by following the principles and techniques outlined later in this chapter. As a general rule, 5-0 Vicryl is used for subcutaneous closure and 6-0 nylon for skin (72, 107, 115). Some authors have recommended 6-0 chromic gut for the closure of skin in small children to avoid suture removal (115). When using this material, keep the suture moist (e.g., with bacitracin ointment or Vaseline-impregnated gauze) for early dissolution of sutures to occur. Approximate divided muscle with 4-0 chromic gut (74, 107). Special types of wounds are discussed later in this chapter.

TOOLS FOR SUTURING

A few necessary tools for optimal closure of wounds include the Webster needle holder with jaws designed to hold 6-0 suture material, two skin hooks, and no. 11 and 15 Bard–Parker scalpel blades. Two types of scissors are necessary: an Iris scissors for use on the skin and a suture scissors (Fig. 10.11) (115).

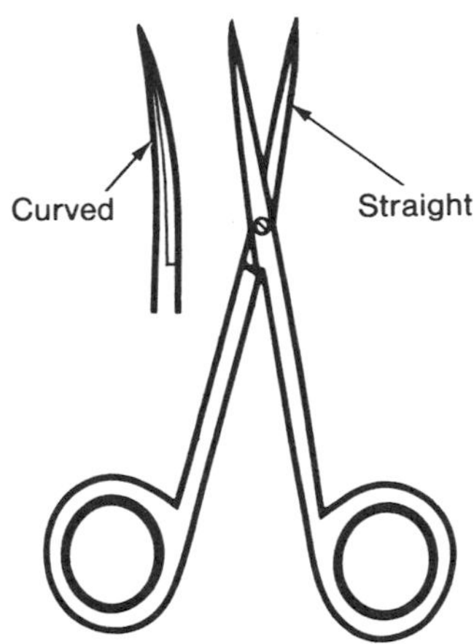

Figure 10.11. Iris scissors.

Instrument Holder

For ideal eversion of wound margins, the needle of a suture should enter the skin at a 90-degree angle or more. This angle is difficult to achieve if the instrument holder is grasped by the thumb and third finger. Hold the needle holder in the palm, providing greater flexibility in the angle of entry into the skin.

Forceps

Toothed forceps are used in subcutaneous fascia and thick muscle fascia. An Adson forceps is a fine-toothed, atraumatic forceps used for skin. A smooth forceps has no teeth and is used for grasping gauze sponges or tissue that may be perforated, and is not used for skin (Fig. 10.12).

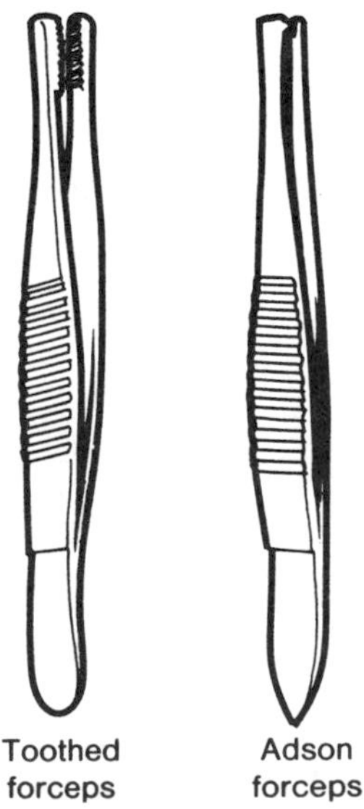

Figure 10.12. A toothed forceps and Adson forceps.

Scalpel Blade

The configuration of the cutting edge of a scalpel blade (Fig. 10.13) is designed to accomplish specific tasks. Three types of

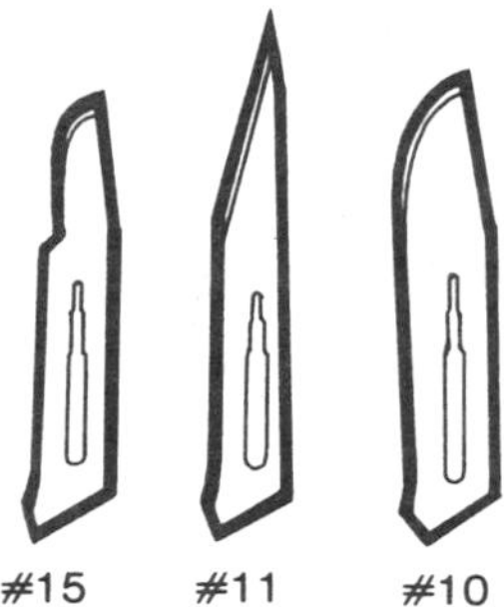

Figure 10.13. Various blades. A no. 15 blade is used for fine precision work, a no. 10 for larger incisions, and no. 11 for stab incisions.

blades are in current use in the emergency center. These include a no. 10 blade, which is predominantly straight except for its curved distal end. Hold the scalpel handle with this blade as you hold a violin bow so the long straight cutting edge of the blade contacts the skin. One sweep of the blade results in a deep straight incision. Holding a no. 15 blade in the same manner prevents the cutting edge from contacting the skin. Hold a no. 15 scalpel and blade as you hold a pencil (Fig. 10.14). Use this blade for precise, short incisions that often must follow an irregular anatomic landmark. When using these blades, learn to cut to the desired depth

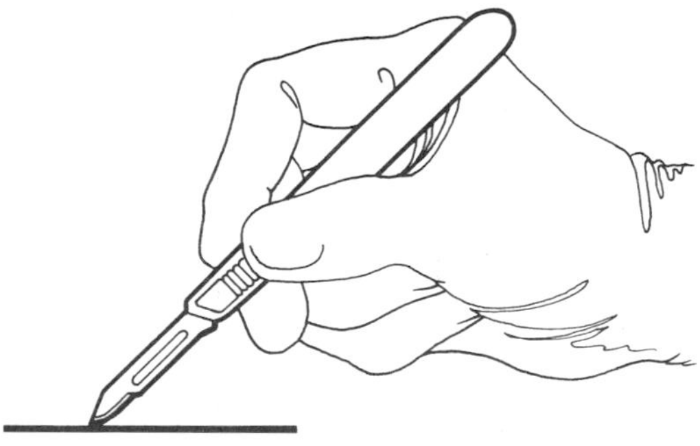

Figure 10.14. Hold a no.15 scalpel and blade like a pencil, with the point directed downward as shown. When the no. 15 blade is held like the no. 10 blade, then the belly of the blade rather than the sharpened point (which is the cutting edge of this blade) is in contact with the skin edge to be incised.

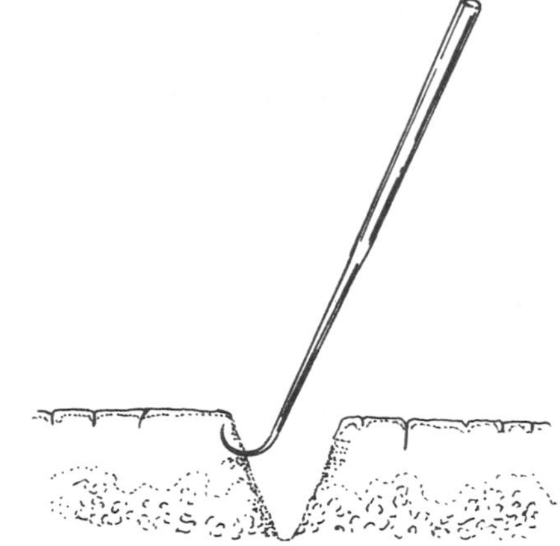

Figure 10.15. A skin hook is preferred over a forceps, because it causes no trauma to the wound edge. It takes practice to become skilled in handling a skin hook.

with one sweep of the blade, which will result in a wound that is more resistant to the development of infection. Use a no. 11 blade in emergency medicine for a stab incision, such as incision of an abscess or cricothyrotomy.

Skin Hooks

Skin hooks are ideal for picking up wound edges. They can be used, with experience, with greater ease and produce less trauma to the tissue than does a forceps. A skin hook is a needle-pointed instrument that enters the wound edge from its undersurface, thus producing a very small puncture rather than compressing the wound edge, as one would do with a forceps (Fig. 10.15).

TRAUMATIC WOUNDS (GENERAL PRINCIPLES)

Contaminated Wounds: Preparation

INFECTION-POTENTIATING FRACTIONS IN SOIL

Soil has four major components; inorganic materials, organic matter, water, and air. The major component is inorganic minerals. The organic content of soil ranges from 1% to 7% and is restricted primarily to topsoils. In swamps, bogs, and marshes, there is an increase in the organic content (98%). The organic component is chemically very reactive.

Fractions of soil with large particle sizes have small surface areas and low levels of chemical reactivity. Silt particles are smaller than sand, with a surface area and chemical reactivity 3 to 4 times greater than those of sand. The inorganic component of soil with the smallest particle size is clay. Clay-containing minerals have a large surface area, associated with high levels of chemical reactivity.

Sterilized samples of topsoil and subsoil consist mainly of inorganic matter that impairs the ability of a wound to resist infection. Wounds contaminated by 5 mg of sterile soil require only 100 bacteria to elicit purulence (40). When the soil is fractionated, the fractions found to potentiate infections reside predominantly in the clay and organic components. These "infection-potentiating" fractions (IPFs) in soil have a number of effects. These fractions inhibit leukocytes from ingesting bacteria. The surface of clay and other organic particles is anionic and surrounded by cations. Soil IPFs have considerable impact on nonspecific humoral factors, and exposure of fresh serum to IPFs eliminates bacteriocidal activity. All therapeutic measures should be directed at physically removing the IPFs of soil from the wound.

BACTERIAL CONTAMINANTS AND INFECTION

The skin has varied numbers of bacteria in different areas of the body. In most regions, the bacterial colonization is limited to the outermost layer of the skin, which is composed of a sloughing mass of dead cells. Beneath this layer is the stratum corneum, which is composed of tightly packed cells, providing an effective barrier against bacterial invasion.

Over most body surfaces, the density of the bacterial population is low, measuring only a few thousand or fewer organisms per square centimeter. The number of organisms on the palms and dorsum of the hand is sparse, numbering only in the hundreds per square centimeter. Most of these organisms on the hands reside beneath the distal end of the nail plate or adjacent proximal or lateral nail folds (37).

The type of bacteria contaminating a wound is less important than the number of bacteria in the development of infections. The infective dose of aerobic bacteria in wounds in healthy tissue has been determined to be 10^6/g or greater. When the bacterial counts are below this level, the wounds will heal without infection except in the presence of sutures, when small numbers of bacteria (10^4/g) can produce infection (39, 40, 62). The critical number of anaerobes that will elicit soft-tissue infections has not been documented.

Covering the surface of the skin with an *occlusive cover* promotes skin hydration, which encourages bacterial growth. A dramatic increase in bacteria is encountered with such occlusive dressings. Wounds to be covered with dressings should have an ointment such as Vaseline-impregnated gauze or bacitracin over the wound to preclude hydration of the skin but still prevent desiccation of the wound margin.

SHAVING OF HAIR AROUND WOUNDS

The shaving of hair around wounds in areas where there is much hair growth has been advocated as beneficial in decreasing the source of bacterial contamination. Studies by Seropian and Reynolds (105) demonstrated that the infection rate of surgical patients after razor preparation was 5.6% compared with a rate of 0.6% after use of a depilatory agent, because of the trauma inflicted by the razor. It also was shown that skin shaved with a recessed blade was more resistant to bacterial contamination. We recommended that hair removal be performed only when hair will interfere with wound closure and then only by either scissors or shaving with a recessed blade (30, 105). Never shave the eyebrows.

ANTISEPTICS AND WOUND PREPARATION (15)

Many types of antiseptic solutions are commercially available for use on the skin around lacerations. The ideal agent must be safe and fast acting, with a broad antibacterial spectrum with little damage to tissue (Table 10.3). This ideal antiseptic should be capable of reducing the number of organisms in intact skin after a single application.

The **iodophors** are now the best-known agents for providing good antimicrobial activity and cleansing with little tissue toxicity or damage. These agents are complexes of iodine that possess a broad spectrum of activity against fungi, viruses, and gram-positive and gram-negative bacteria. Three general categories of iodophors are in clinical use: solubilized inorganic elemental iodine, as tincture of iodine; iodine complexed with various surfactant compounds; and iodine complex. Iodine compounds are very stable, do not stain, have no odor, and are less irritating to the tissues than is tincture of iodine. After contact with wounds, these complexes release iodine slowly, resulting in prolonged activity. These complexes are basically composed of iodine plus an organic molecule. The forms most commonly used in the emergency center are a solution or a soap [e.g., povidone–iodine (Betadine)].

Table 10.3
Antiseptic Solutions and Tissue Damage

Antiseptic solution	Cellular damage resulting when no saline irrigation is performed later (%)[a]	Cellular damage after subsequent saline irrigation (%)
Alcohol	100	100
Hydrogen peroxide	100	90
Ordinary soap	90	25
pHisoHex	25	5
Distilled water	5	0
Polyvinylpyrrolidone iodine (1%)	5	0
Saline solution	0	0

[a] Some antiseptic solutions cause a great deal of tissue damage, some of which can be avoided by subsequent irrigation.

Mercury compounds have been commercially available for a long time; however, these agents are unacceptable for use in the emergency center. Organic mercury (Merthiolate) penetrates the skin very little, is bacteriostatic, and is not effective against spores. In addition, these agents may sensitize the skin.

pHisoHex, a soap, has been shown to cause central nervous system damage in neonates, and its use in the emergency center in wound preparation is discouraged.

Alcohol cleans the skin surface of dirt and oils; however, it is not an effective antiseptic. Alcohol has been widely used as a skin disinfectant because of its ability to remove lipids from the skin surface and its bacteriocidal action. The action of alcohol as a disinfectant, however, is restricted because of its inability to kill spores at normal temperatures, and for this reason, alcohol is not reliable as a skin disinfectant. Alcohol is active against gram-positive and gram-negative organisms. Ethanol is most effective at concentrations of 50% to 70%. Isopropyl alcohol is significantly more active than ethanol, is less volatile, and is more commonly used for skin disinfection.

Hydrogen peroxide in a 3% solution is a very weak disinfectant whose primary use is in the cleansing and debridement of wounds. When hydrogen peroxide is applied to tissues, oxygen is rapidly released by tissue catalases, and the germicidal action is brief. It also is toxic to tissue in open wounds.

Quaternary ammonium salts are dilute solutions of cationic surface-active agents with organically substituted ammonium compounds. Gram-positive organisms seem more susceptible than gram-negative ones to these salts. Gram-negative *Pseudomonas* are resistant to quaternary ammonium compounds and actually may grow in these solutions. These agents are not safe for use in surgical wounds. They contain toxic anionic detergents that damage the tissue defenses and potentiate the development of infection. Contaminated wounds subjected to topical treatment with these agents develop more infection than do contaminated wounds subjected to 0.9% saline (40). Benzalkonium chloride (Zephiran) is a quaternary ammonium salt that is a fast-acting bacteriocidal agent with good penetration into wounds. It is antagonized by soap and tissue fluids; during its use, benzalkonium chloride forms a film, and bacteria remain intact under this protective film. The bacteriocidal action of these agents is slower than that of the iodine preparations.

Pluronic F-68 (Shurclens) is a surfactant that has little or no local or systemic toxicity. This agent meets many of the criteria of an ideal agent wound cleanser. Experimental studies (99) show that this agent prevents the development of infection and, when used around the wound as well as in the wound, did not result in any significant damage to cellular components of the blood, wound healing, or resistance to infection. In a clinical trial involving 1,000 patients, it was decided that this was the agent of choice, when compared with iodinated solutions and normal saline. The cellular damage produced by various antiseptic solutions is shown in Table 10.3.

DEBRIDEMENT

Debridement is an essential part of preparing a traumatic wound for closure. It removes bacteria and tissue heavily contaminated by IPFs in soil and protects the patient from invasive infections. It removes permanently devitalized tissues that impair the ability of the wound to resist infections. All devitalized tissue left in a wound impairs wound healing and potentiates infection (56). There are three mechanisms by which devitalized soft tissue enhances infection. The devitalized tissue acts as a culture medium, promoting bacterial growth. This tissue also inhibits leukocyte phagocytosis and provides an anaerobic environment within the wound that also acts to limit leukocyte function.

In ascertaining the margin of devitalized tissue, one often must use clinical judgment. Within 24 hours after injury, there is a sharp demarcation, often apparent, between the devitalized skin and the viable skin. The margin to excise on a wound is based on the region of the body and the appearance of the tissue, as well as on the degree of maceration and contamination. Facial wounds require little debridement as compared with wounds of the lower extremity, because of the high vascularity of the region. Nonviable tissue must be debrided, and the configuration of the debridement depends on the location of the wound. When a wound is in a nondemonstrative area and is parallel to natural wrinkle lines, then an elliptical excision of the wound is preferred (Fig. 10.16*C*). To conserve tissue, use a curvilinear excision, as indicated in Fig. 10.16*B*. When tissue must be preserved over critical sites without excess tissue, such as the nose or forehead, then perform a jigsaw excision (Fig. 10.16*A*). To preform a jigsaw excision properly requires a good deal of expertise. A technique that has been used to demarcate the area for debridement in a devitalized wound is to apply a fluorescein dye to a gauze pack and pack the wound. Complete excision of the stained (devitalized) wound margins will minimize debridement of uninjured tissue. Alternatively, excise a wound until active bleeding is noted, indicating viable skin. The best debridement includes high-pressure irrigation followed by limited excision of any loose bone or edges of tissue that clearly are not viable (Fig. 10.17). Periosteum and other specialized tissue such as tendons should be saved unless

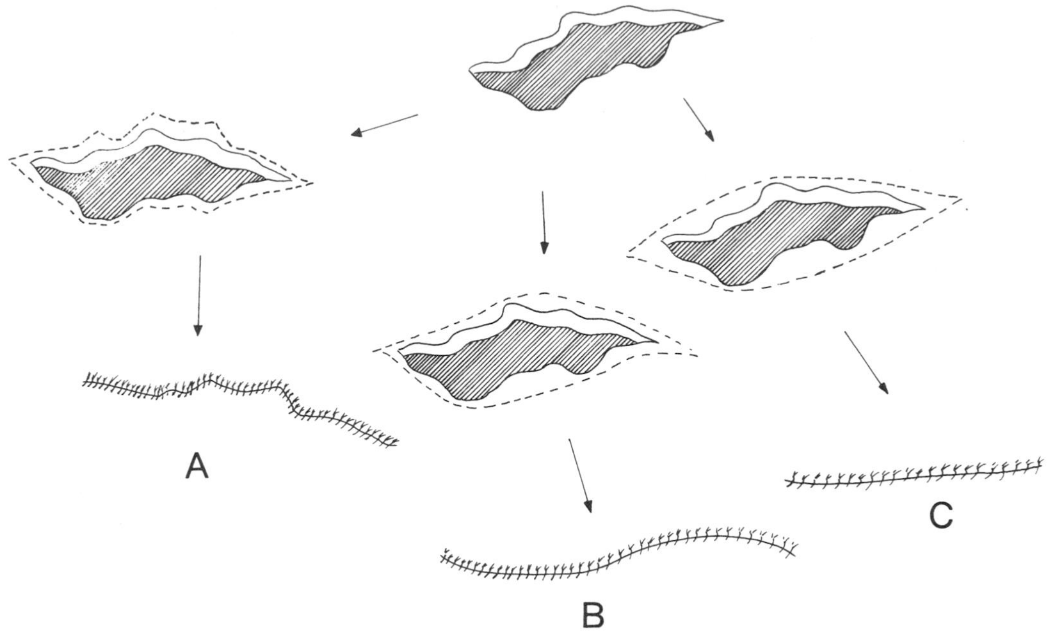

Figure 10.16. Techniques for debriding a wound. See text for discussion.

severely contaminated (56). Debridement of a wound should be done after stabilizing the skin edges with skin hooks (Fig. 10.18). With the fingers, pull the skin being debrided perpendicular to the direction of the laceration. Then excise the tissue to be debrided. This technique prevents "rolling in." The scalpel (no. 11 or 15) should be held angulated away from the wound, so that eversion is achieved when approximating the edges (Fig. 10.18). Debride subcutaneous tissue by using an iris scissors.

The decision whether to close a wound primarily or secondarily is to a large extent based on the adequacy of initial debridement and the location of the wound. If there is any question about the adequacy of debridement of a badly contaminated wound, it is best to do a delayed primary closure, rather than risk the chance of infection. Almost always close facial wounds primarily after initial wound care. This debridement is aided by irrigation with copious amounts of isotonic sodium chloride.

In **abrasions**, deep "ground-in" particles of dirt may be embedded in the wound after accidents such as falls on dirt roads. If these particles are left in place, they lead to what is called a traumatic tattoo. A **traumatic tattoo** represents particles of dirt that have remained embedded in an abrasion and have epithelialized. Most of the particles are superficial, and immediate removal is the procedure of choice. Removal may be aided by a surgical scrub brush or a sterile toothbrush after adequate field block or regional nerve block anesthesia (Fig. 10.19) (1). Lidocaine (Xylocaine) gel, 5%, applied for 5 to 10 minutes over an abrasion can work extremely well in providing adequate anesthesia for this procedure. Alternatively, use tetracaine, adrenaline, and cocaine (TAC; see "Anesthesia for Wounds," later). The point of a no.11 scalpel blade will aid in removing deeply seated particles from the abrasion. A sterile, hard, natural-bristle toothbrush can be used with either sterile saline or surgical soap. Rinse and blot the area fre-

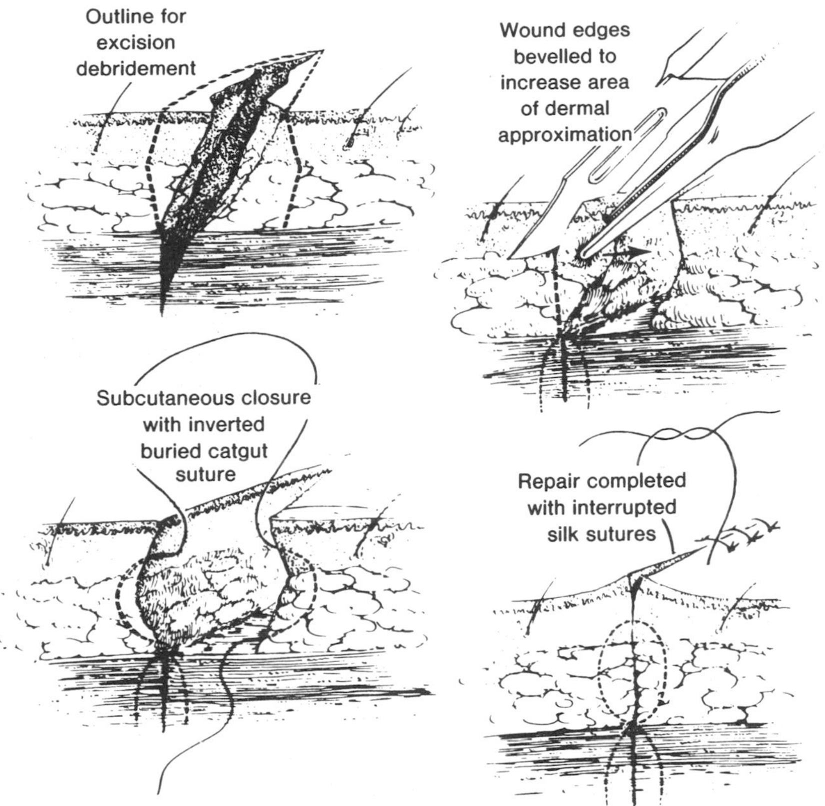

Figure 10.17. Excision of the macerated edges of a traumatic wound. Angulating the blade bevels the wound edges so that a subcutaneous closure will result in eversion of the edges, permitting no tension on the epidermis and dermis. (From Straith RE, Lawson JM, Hipps CJ: The subcuticular suture. Postgrad Med 29:164, 1961, with permission.)

quently until all pigment has been removed. Remove tar embedded in wounds easily with the use of Vaseline or polymyxin B, neomycin, and bacitracin (Neosporin) ointment, mayonnaise, or, as a last resort, acetone (32).

Leave the abraded areas open, and cleanse the involved area with a mild detergent 4 times per day. Use a topical antibiotic ointment (1), and the lesion usually heals in 2 to 3 weeks. Alternatively, use an antibacterial-impregnated gauze dressing (Xeroform) over the wound. Traumatic tattoos of the explosive type (as opposed to the abrasive type discussed earlier) leave the pigment deposited deeply in the central focus of the abrasion (1) and may require dermabrasion.

MECHANICAL CLEANSING (IRRIGATION)

Irrigation of a contaminated wound is an excellent means of removing soil and bacterial contaminants; perform it routinely on all traumatic lacerations with the exception of those that are caused by a sterile instrument. The force of the irrigating solution must exceed the adhesive forces of the contaminants; therefore provide enough force in the irrigating stream to dislodge the particles.

The amount of hydraulic force needed to dislodge a particle is decreased as the velocity of the irrigation stream is increased. Large volumes for extended times are required when small syringes are used. Irrigation has been studied, and the data,

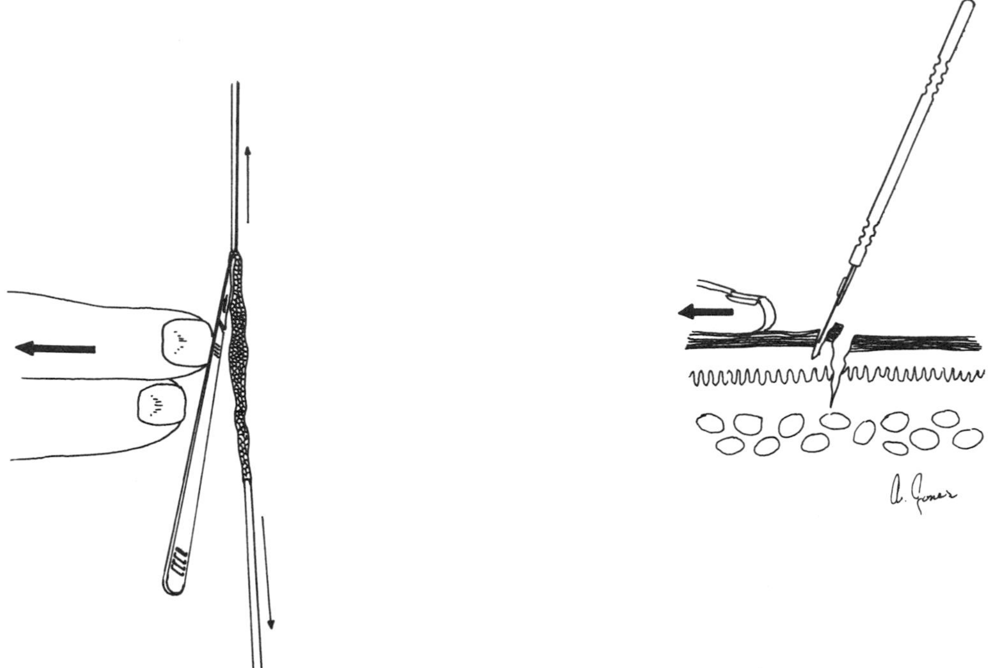

Figure 10.18. Debridement of a wound with a scalpel. Use skin hooks to retract a wound at both ends, while a finger pulls loose skin perpendicular to the length of the wound to allow easy debridement. Note the angle at which the scalpel blade debrides the wound. See text for discussion.

in the our opinion, show that the preferred method of irrigation causing the least tissue injury from too high an irrigating pressure and the maximal particle dislodgment is obtained by using a 35-mm syringe with a large-bore needle or plastic cannula, such as a 16 or 18 gauge (81, 100). This technique provides approximately 8 pounds of pressure per square inch. Pressure below this level is considered low-pressure irrigation, and that above it is referred to as high-pressure irrigation (Fig. 10.20). The concern that high-pressure irrigation would result in increased tissue injury is true. Weigh the effect of contaminated particles remaining in the wound against the risk of tissue injury. Concern that high-pressure irrigation forces particles deeper into wounds is not true. Low-pressure irrigation is most effective in dislodging relatively large particles from wounds. Direct scrubbing of a wound with a gauze sponge soaked with saline does not decrease the incidence of infection and does not impair the ability of the wound to resist infection.

CONTAMINATED WOUNDS, DELAYED CLOSURE, AND ANTIBIOTICS

The optimal time in which to repair a traumatic laceration without an increased risk of infection generally is regarded as less than 6 hours (7, 56, 79). With oral antibiotic coverage, the time for primary closure can be extended to 14 to 16 hours (7, 79). Proper cleansing of the wound and debridement include removal of all foreign bodies and nonviable tissue. Mechanical debridement and irrigation are the best means of ensuring a clean wound with the least tissue destruction (36, 79). Hemostasis, closure of the dead space, and approximation of the wound edges without tension are vital. For an excellent repair, adequate wound immobilization

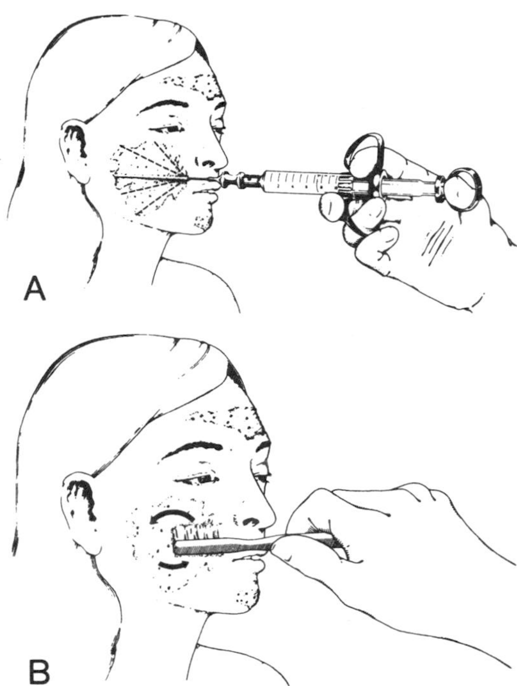

Figure 10.19. *A:* Technique for anesthetizing a traumatic abrasion with embedded particles. *B:* Removal of the particles with either an ordinary toothbrush or a bristle brush used for scrubbing hands. The tip of a no. 11 blade can be used to remove deeply embedded or larger particles. (From Agris J: Traumatic tattooing. J Trauma 16:799, 1976, with permission.)

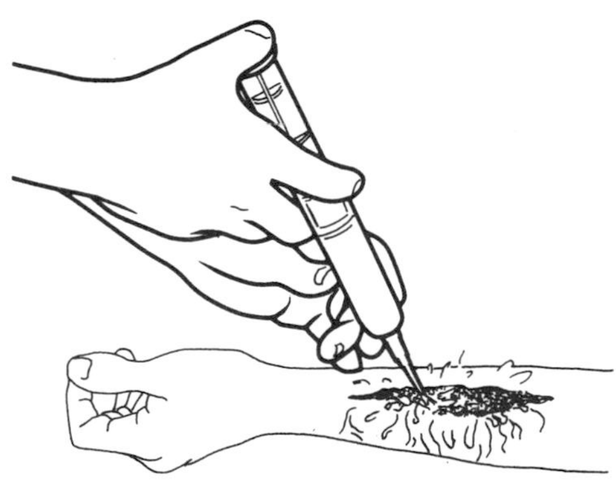

Figure 10.20. Irrigation of a traumatic wound decreases the bacterial content significantly and dislodges particulate matter from the wound. A 16- or 18-gauge needle or plastic cannula attached to a 35-mL syringe is ideal for providing proper irrigation pressures. See text for discussion.

with a properly applied pressure dressing is essential (7). Keep strong antiseptics away from the injured tissues. Substandard results are due mostly to a failure to remove foreign material and to a failure to excise irregular devitalized edges (80).

Indications for antibiotic therapy after wound closure remain controversial. The length of time a wound has been open and the level of contamination play important roles in the decision-making process. The effect of topical antibiotics is limited by the fibrinous coagulant that surrounds the bacteria and prevents contact with a topical antibiotic. Indications for antibiotics are affected by the mechanism of injury. Shear forces secondary to glass or a knife are responsible for most lacerations, and these wounds are highly resistant to infections, requiring 10^6 organisms per gram of tissue to produce infection (101), whereas compression injuries resulting in stellate lacerations weaken the local tissue defenses and increase the susceptibility to infection (101). When the risk of infection is high, we advocate oral antibiotic therapy for the first 3 to 5 days after suturing (47).

The earliest sign of infection is tenderness at the wound edges (7, 79). Remember that erythema may occur with normal healing. Later, lymphangitis and swollen, tender regional lymph nodes develop, followed, in severe cases, by systemic signs of infection. If suppuration develops, some or all of the sutures should be removed. In less cosmetically important areas, such as the trunk or extremities, a more conservative approach for heavily contaminated wounds is to leave the wound open for drainage, simply covering it or packing it with saline gauze dressings, changing them every 6 hours for the first 2 or 3 days, and then performing a *delayed closure* to decrease the risk of infection (7). When dressing a wound that will be subjected to delayed closure, pack the wound with sterile fine-mesh gauze and then cover it with 4 × 4-cm gauze pads and a gauze roll (Kling) (Fig. 10.21). It has

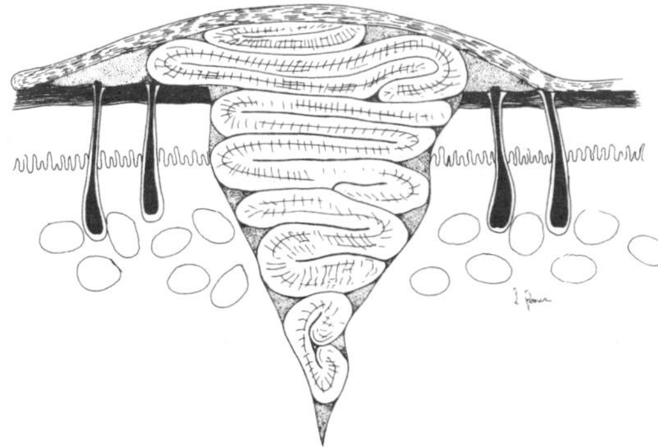

Figure 10.21. Gauze packing of a wound. See text for discussion.

been shown that the optimal time to suture a contaminated wound by a delayed closure is the fourth day (97). It is at this time that the tissue reaches peak resistance to infection.

ANESTHESIA FOR WOUNDS

Three anesthetic agents are in current use for providing local anesthesia: procaine (Novocain), bupivacaine (Marcaine), and lidocaine (Xylocaine). Of these, the agent that is by far the most commonly used is lidocaine with or without epinephrine, 1:100,000. Anesthesia by local infiltration is the method most commonly used in most emergency centers today. Regional nerve block or field block anesthesia is the optimal method to use when one is dealing with anything other than a small laceration. This method provides less tissue damage at the laceration site and avoids the inadvertent introduction of more contaminants into the injured tissue. Cleansing the wound of bacteria, soil contaminants, and debris, as well as surgical debridement of infected wounds cannot be effectively accomplished without anesthesia.

Lidocaine is the most commonly used local anesthetic agent. Loss of sensation occurs within 5 minutes and lasts an average of 97 to 156 minutes (2). Lidocaine does not exhibit antimicrobial activity and does not damage the local wound defenses. The addition of epinephrine, a potent vasoconstrictor, overcomes the vasodilating effects of lidocaine. The reduction of blood flow induced by epinephrine limits the clearance of the anesthetic agent from the tissue and prolongs the duration of anesthesia by up to 50%, permitting an increased dosage of lidocaine without toxicity. The toxic dose of lidocaine containing epinephrine (1:100,000) is 7 mg/kg; do not exceed 500 mg total or 50 mL of 1% lidocaine. When using lidocaine without epinephrine, 4.5 mg/kg is the toxic dose; do not exceed 300 mg or 30 mL of 1% lidocaine. Epinephrine does impair tissue defenses, which militates against its use in heavily contaminated wounds (2, 28). This must be tempered by the fact that epinephrine reduces bleeding and therefore decreases the chance of hematoma formation. Hematoma formation increases the chance of infection. Epinephrine is a strong vasoconstrictor and decreases bleeding; however, it should never be used in lacerations of terminal structures such as the fingers or toes.

In the usual circumstance, inject a 1% or 2% solution of lidocaine through a 27-gauge needle. Some fibrous tissues, such as scalp or scar tissue, require a 22-gauge needle for infiltration and may require longer periods for anesthesia than do other tissues (106). Although one can inject the wound from within, the optimal method is a field block or a regional block (79). Infiltrating the wound edges swells the edges and makes a cosmetic closure more difficult. As mentioned earlier, regional block anesthesia is the preferred technique because it is removed from the wound site and thus avoids contamination of the wound.

Patients with an overdose from an inadvertent intravenous injection of lidocaine will develop nausea, vomiting, headaches, transitory excitement, apprehensiveness, and/or convulsions. Secondary signs are an irregular pulse (which may be rapid or slow), hypotension, and a decrease in tidal volume. Patients allergic to lidocaine will

Table 10.4
Onset of Action and Duration of Various Anesthetic Agents

Drug	Concentration (%)	Approximate relative potency	Onset time (min)	Reappearance of pain sensation (min)
Procaine	1	2	7 = 1	60–90
Mepivacaine	1	4	4 = 1	120–240
Prilocaine	1	4	3 = 0.6	120–240
Lidocaine	1	4	5 = 1	90–200
Tetracaine	0.25	16	7 = 2.5	180–600
Bupivacaine	0.25	16	8 = 3.2	180–600

tolerate procaine (see Chapter 3: "Anesthesia and Regional Blocks").

Procaine has an onset of action of 3 to 10 minutes, as well as a duration of less than 1 hour, and a maximal dose of 700 mg or 10 mg/kg. Bupivacaine also has an onset of 3 to 10 minutes, with a duration of action of 4 to 12 hours, making it useful where prolonged anesthesia is desirable.

Table 10.4 summarizes the various agents used and indicates the onset of action as well as the duration of anesthesia. A topical local anesthetic agent has been tested in minor lacerations; this is a combination of tetracaine 0.5%, adrenaline 1:2,000 solution, and cocaine 10% (TAC). This composition of TAC yields an average dose of cocaine of 590 mg/5 mL and an average dose of tetracaine of 25 mg/5 mL. This agent was not tested in lacerations of the pinna or other end organs such as parts of the ear, the penis, or the digits, because of the possibility of compromising their vascularity. Mucosal lacerations were not anesthetized with this agent because of the increased vascularity of the mucosa, which accelerates the absorption of these anesthetics and increases the risk of toxic side effects. This agent was studied in 158 patients and compared with lidocaine with epinephrine (91). Most of the patients who were tested were children with small lacerations. The time required for surgical repair for patients matched for age and length of lacerations was essentially identical for older children. For children younger than 5 years, the time required for repair of lacerations using TAC was significantly shorter than that for the lidocaine-with-epinephrine group. The anesthetic agent (TAC) was applied topically after completion of wound preparation with a saturated sterile 2 × 2-inch gauze pad with firm pressure for a minimum of 10 minutes. Five milliliters of TAC was applied to all wounds less than 3 cm in length, and an additional 5 mL was applied for each increase in length of 3 cm (91). Our experience with this agent has shown it to be useful, particularly in children and in cleansing abrasions. Topical anesthesia can be used to anesthetize a large wound by soaking a gauze dressing soaked with 4% lidocaine over the wound (Fig. 10.22). This gauze dressing, applied over the wound, should be wrapped firmly with Kerlix gauze and left in place for approximately 10 minutes. If additional anesthesia is needed after this time, it can be applied again topically, and the wound rewrapped for an additional 10 minutes. This is a highly useful procedure for abrasions and larger cutaneous wounds.

HEMORRHAGE AND HEMOSTASIS

A wound hematoma almost always is associated with controllable bleeding that has been inadequately controlled. In a patient with a bleeding wound, **direct pressure** with a 4 × 4-inch gauze pad should be applied over a broad area. If bleeding continues to be uncontrolled, pressure over a proximal artery may be used. A blood pressure cuff can be inflated above

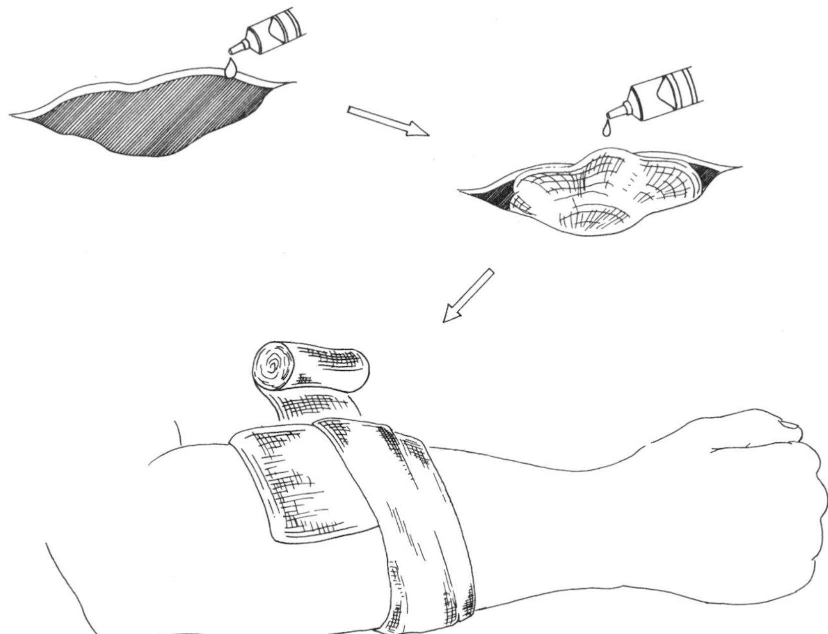

Figure 10.22. Topical anesthetic applied to a wound. See text for discussion.

systolic pressure when bleeding is a problem. Diffuse oozing from a wound often accompanies coagulation defects. Bleeding also may be a particular problem in patients with excessive ingestion of aspirin or other anticoagulants.

When a single vessel is found to be the cause of bleeding, use **ligation** with a small hemostat (7). Proximal control of a bleeding site in an extremity can be achieved with the use of a blood pressure cuff inflated to above systolic pressure, or, if the bleeding is from a digit, use a small rubber Penrose drain, secured with a hemostat, proximal to the bleeding site (Fig. 10.23). Maintain pressure for 15 to 20 minutes.

BASIC PRINCIPLES IN WOUND CLOSURE

Linear Scars and Skin-tension Lines

A number of skin-tension lines have been described (Figs. 10.24 and 10.25), some of which are relevant to the emergency physician in considering the repair of lacerations, in determining the cosmetic outcome of a scar, and in planning the revision of a laceration. Skin lines are divided into static and dynamic skin-tension lines. The natural **static skin-tension lines** are dependent partly on the natural characteristics of dermal fibers and partly on the pattern in which they are woven. Clinical evidence of these tension lines in the skin is the retraction of skin edges

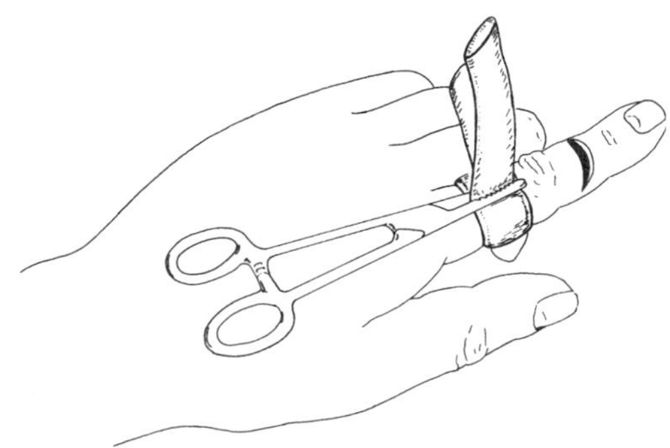

Figure 10.23. A Penrose drain, with a hemostat clamped over it, functions nicely to prevent bleeding from a finger wound. See text for discussion.

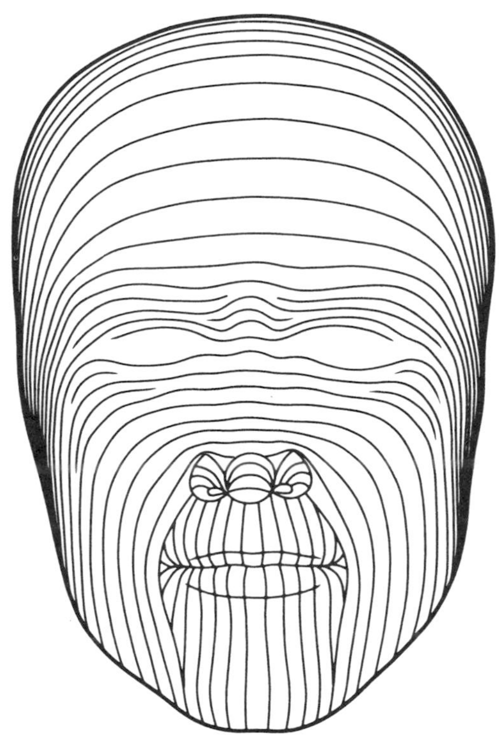

Figure 10.24. Lines of skin tension on the face. Perform elective incisions or modifications of existing wounds along these lines. See text for discussion.

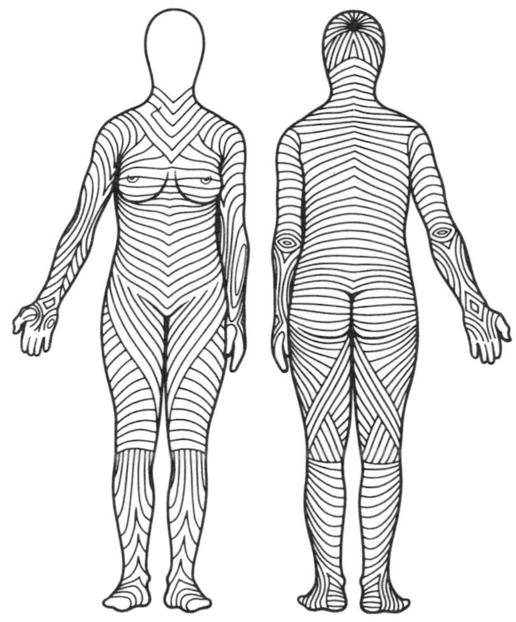

Figure 10.25. Skin-tension lines. In the male patient, the semicircular lines over the deltoid region extend down over the breasts, producing curved radial lines, as opposed to the horizontal lines demonstrated above in the female patient. Authors vary in their descriptions of the posterior skin-tension lines. Kraissl (62) stated that the skin-tension lines meet in the scapulae and that the latissimus dorsi and trapezius produce a vertically oriented semicircular pattern rather than the more horizontal pattern over the posterior shoulder and thoracic region. Kraissl also believed that the skin-tension lines are transversely oriented along the entire lower extremity from the hip to the foot, similar to those shown above in the calf region.

noted around a laceration when the laceration is perpendicular, as opposed to parallel to these lines of tension. Wounds that result in a wide scar occur from strong opposing static skin tensions. When there is minimal separation of the wound edges, repair occurs with a fine scar.

Wrinkle lines or **dynamic skin-tension lines** result from the contraction of the muscles underlying the skin (12, 102). These lines cross at right angles to the long axis of the muscles and are caused by contraction of these muscles (12, 13, 102, 109). The skin is attached to the underlying muscles by fascia, causing the skin to be thrown into accordion-like folds or lines at right angles to the direction of the muscle (102). Scars become adherent to the underlying tissue, so they least interfere with skin dynamics if placed transversely across muscles and joints and in the same lines as wrinkles (69). Optimally, the scar then becomes an exaggeration of the normal skin-tension lines (69). In the face, the wrinkle lines are called lines of facial expression; more recently, the term *relaxed skin tension lines* has been used in discussing elective incisions and the prognosis of wound healing (12). These are similar to wrinkle lines in most instances, but not in all cases. Wrinkle lines are primarily influenced by muscle pull, whereas other factors enter into relaxed skin-tension lines. On the forehead, vertical contraction of the frontalis demonstrates the relaxed skin-tension lines. In the elbow, transverse relaxed skin-tension lines are noted on the anterior and posterior aspect (12). References to Langer's lines in standard texts are inaccurate; these lines have little practical use because they do not consider the effect of dynamic skin tension on a healing scar (12, 13, 69, 102).

When possible, incise skin parallel, never perpendicular, to the normal tension lines and relaxed skin-tension lines to produce the most inconspicuous scars. Revisions can often be done in a laceration by the use of "Z-plasty" as early as 2 months after injury (13), but 6 months is preferable.

Tension and Layer-by-layer Closure

Close each layer separately: periosteum, fascia of muscles, and subcutaneous fascia (Fig. 10.26). Layered repair should be carried out with sutures that are snug but do not strangulate the tissue (74). When muscle is divided, use a two-layer closure to approximate it (74).

Before considering special situations, several axioms can be derived from the principles discussed earlier.

AXIOM

Use the smallest suture needed to approximate the edges of a wound.

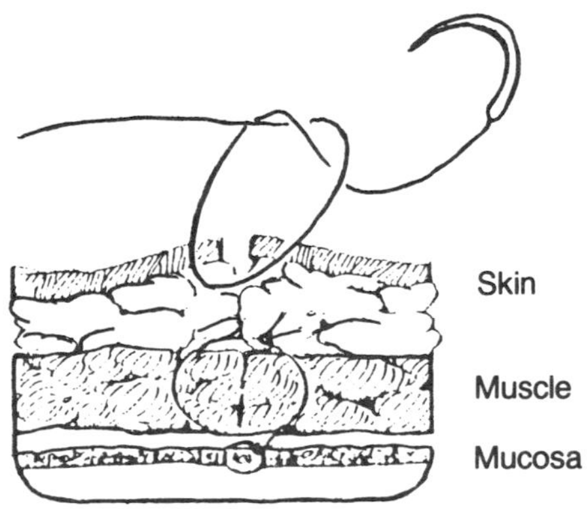

Figure 10.26. A layer-by-layer closure. Note that the subcutaneous suture that incorporates the muscle fascia does not have to be buried, and that it is far enough away from the wound edge that it will not irritate the edge.

AXIOM

Use small sutures placed closer together rather than larger sutures placed farther apart.

AXIOM

Edema occurs after closure, so only approximate the edges; do not strangulate the tissue.

AXIOM

Use forceps as little as possible; skin hooks, when one learns to handle them properly, offer the best means of handling a wound edge.

In general, an irregular wound should be perceived as a "jigsaw puzzle"; that is, if the most complicated section is closed first, then the remainder is closed more simply. If the laceration is jagged, the margins can be excised and removed, resulting in a linear laceration that can then be closed more easily.

RELATION OF SUTURE TO THE WOUND EDGE

When placing a skin suture, pass the needle perpendicular to the wound edges, as shown in Fig. 10.27. If the needle passes tangential to the surface of the skin, more tissue will be encompassed by the suture loop near the surface than will be encompassed deeper down, resulting in inversion of the wound edges. When the wound edges are difficult to evert, then pass the needle at an angle greater than 90 degrees to the skin. When the suture loop thus formed is closed, the tissue at the bottom of the loop comes together first (because more tissue is enclosed within the bottom of the suture loop by this technique), resulting in the pushing of the more superficial tissue upward and eversion of the wound edges.

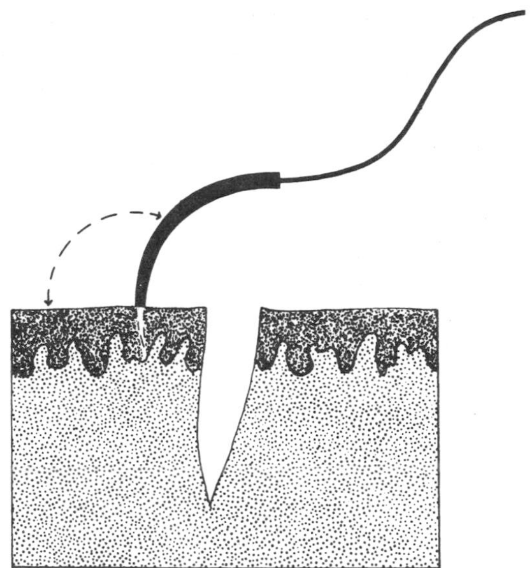

Figure 10.27. The needle passes perpendicular to the skin.

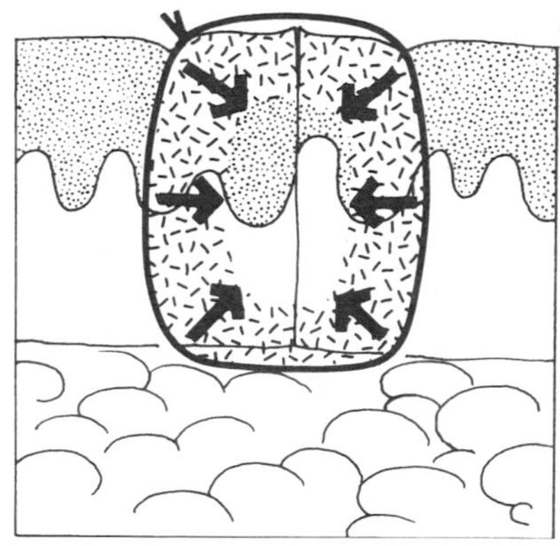

Figure 10.28. Intrinsic tension within the wound produced by a suture loop. See text for discussion.

Place sutures close to the wound edges. The farther from the skin edges a suture is placed, the greater the force needed to approximate the edges and the greater the tension within the tissue enclosed by the loop of suture. Edema develops in a wound during the first 48 hours after injury and tightens the sutures further (58). Tension in a wound is divided into intrinsic and extrinsic (29). *Intrinsic tension* within a suture loop is produced by an "inward" constricting tension within the wound (Fig. 10.28). *Extrinsic tension* on a wound is the pulling tension or the outward force that maintains the wound edges separated. Subcutaneous sutures tend to decrease the extrinsic tension from the skin sutures and permit early removal of the latter, leaving little or no scarring (29). In certain wounds, place tension sutures to remove the extrinsic tension from the wound edge and prevent scar spread (31).

Large "bites" result in large suture marks because of the constricting effect of the suture (intrinsic tension) on tissue vascularity (Fig. 10.29). Use the least number of sutures necessary to bring the skin edges together without causing increased

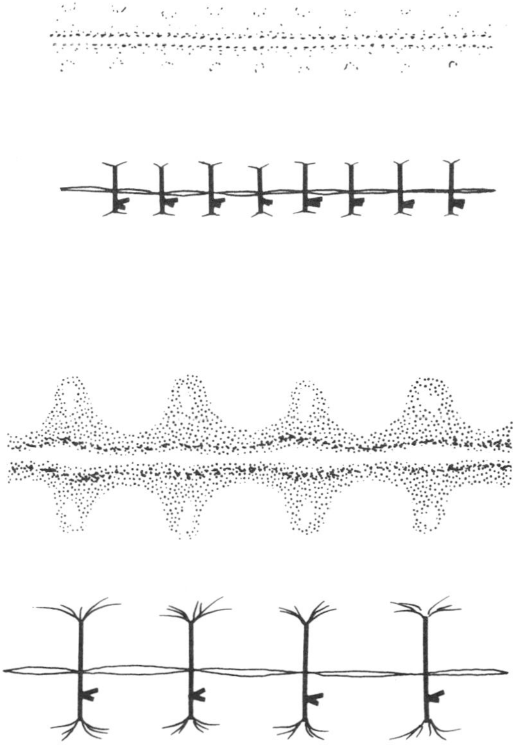

Figure 10.29. Place sutures closer together, taking smaller "bites." Large suture bites result in larger, thicker suture marks because of the constricting effect, which causes increased intrinsic pressure within the suture loop.

tension at the wound edges. The distance between sutures should be approximately the same as the depth of the sutures (Fig. 10.30). Sutures should enter 2 to 3 mm from the edge of the wound, roughly equal to the skin thickness (7). Place the sutures about 3 to 5 mm apart. In the face, even more meticulous care is needed for ideal healing. Never encompass more than 2 to 3 mm of tissue on either side of wounds on the face. The maximal amount of tissue encompassed by a single suture on the face, as a general rule of thumb, should be 4 mm between the entrance and exit sites on the two sides of the wound (74).

Horizontal and vertical forces act on wound edges, causing them to flatten gradually (115). Eversion of the wound edges helps in overcoming these forces. Eversion of the wound edges is most important in areas where the laceration lies perpendicular to the relaxed skin-tension lines, because of the greater tendency for "spread" of the scar with these lacerations. In addition, slight eversion of the skin edges compensates for contracture of the scar that always follows any wound healing (7). If the edges persist in being inverted, the result will be an unaesthetic, depressed scar.

The methods of everting the edges include the following:

1. With thick skin, incise the edges so the surface of the wound overhangs the perpendicular (Figs. 10.17, 10.18, and 10.31). Thus when the suture is placed, the top of the skin will come together before the bottom, causing eversion.
2. Reflect the wound edge when placing the suture to aid in incorporating more tissue in the lower half of the suture loop than in the top, which will cause eversion of the edges when closed (Fig. 10.32).
3. Place buried sutures in the manner shown in Fig. 10.31, which incorporate the lower part of the dermis within the loop, to aid in providing eversion of the edges.

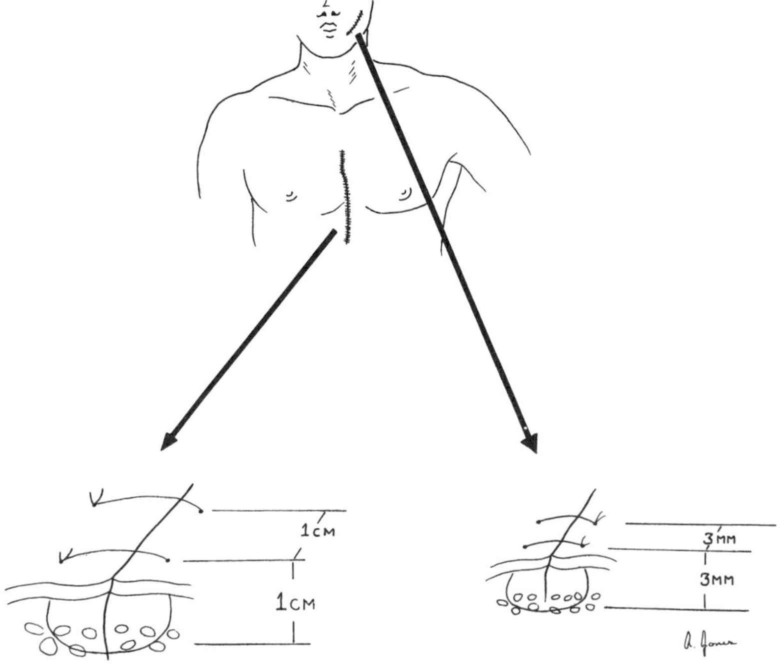

Figure 10.30. Separate sutures in the face and neck by approximately 3 mm. Separate those in the chest, arm, or back by approximately 1 cm. See text for discussion.

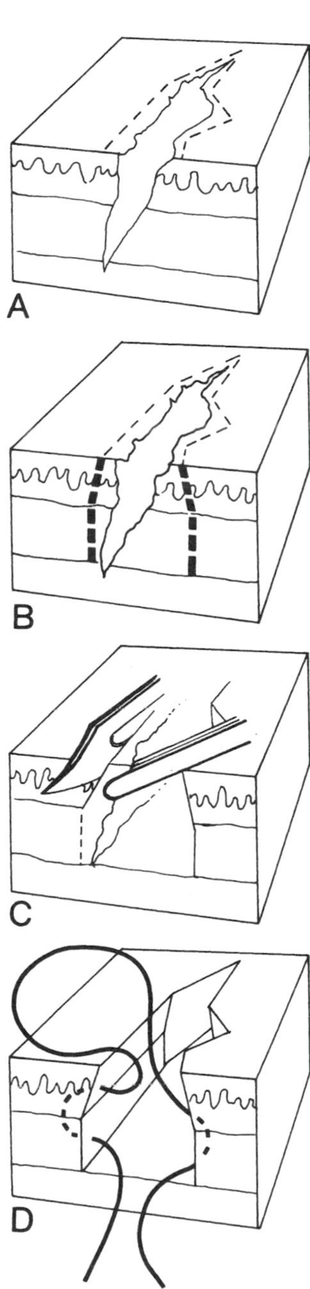

Figure 10.31. *A:* Excision of the macerated edges of a traumatic wound. *B:* Incise the edges so that the surface of the wound overhangs the perpendicular. This permits approximation of the top of the surface of the wound before the base of the wound and allows eversion of the wound edges. *C:* This is best done with a no. 15 or no. 11 blade. *D:* A buried suture going through the deep dermal layer.

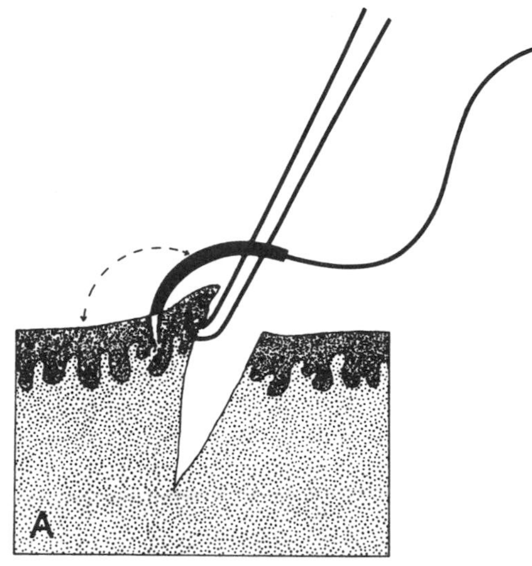

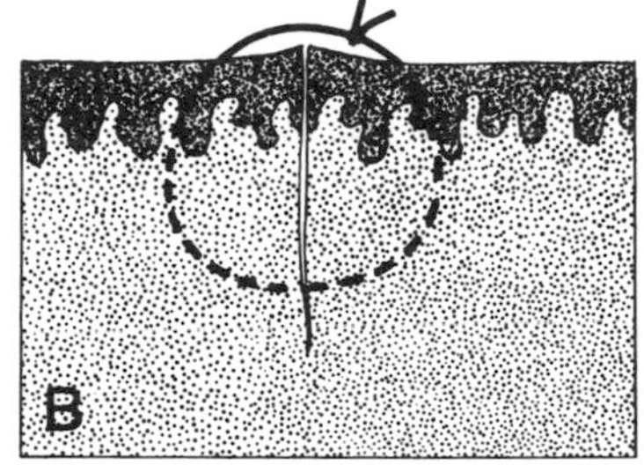

Figure 10.32. *A:* Reflection of the wound edge permits passage of the needle so that it incorporates more tissue at the base of the suture loop than at the top and aids in eversion of the wound edge. This is especially useful in thin skin over wrinkle lines or creases, which tend to invert. In this figure, the skin hook is shown reflecting the wound edge. *B:* This technique incorporates more tissue in the lower half of the suture loop than in the top and permits eversion of the wound edges when the suture loop is tied.

4. Adequate undermining is essential for eversion and is described in the next section.
5. In those wounds in which the edges persist in inverting after a simple closure, use a vertical mattress suture (7).

Timing of Closure

The timing of a closure is vitally important and was discussed in the section entitled Contaminated Wounds, Delayed Closure, and Antibiotics, earlier. *Primary closure* is generally performed in a wound less than 6 to 8 hours old, the exception being in the face, in which, if the wound is clean, closure can be safely performed up to 24 hours later (40). If the wound is clean, and the patient happens to be ingesting oral antibiotics at the time of injury, then the wound may be repaired primarily within the first 24 hours. Continue the antibiotics for 3 days after the suturing. For *delayed closure*, debride the area, and apply a dressing of fine-mesh saline absorbent gauze. Administer antibiotics and close the wound when it is clean. In the delayed repair, use few subcutaneous sutures because there is an increased risk of infection with sutures. Always do a delayed repair rather than risk a chance of infection in severely contaminated wounds, particularly in wounds caused by compressive forces (see the section, Contaminated Wounds, Delayed Closures, and Antibiotics, earlier).

Four days after injury is the ideal time for delayed wound closure (97). When packing a wound for a delayed closure, use loose mesh gauze to pack the wound open and apply a Kerlix wrap (Fig. 10.33). Maximal neovascularization and monocyte infiltration will occur in approximately 4 days. The wound can be closed by the third or fourth day after debridement of the edges and irrigation.

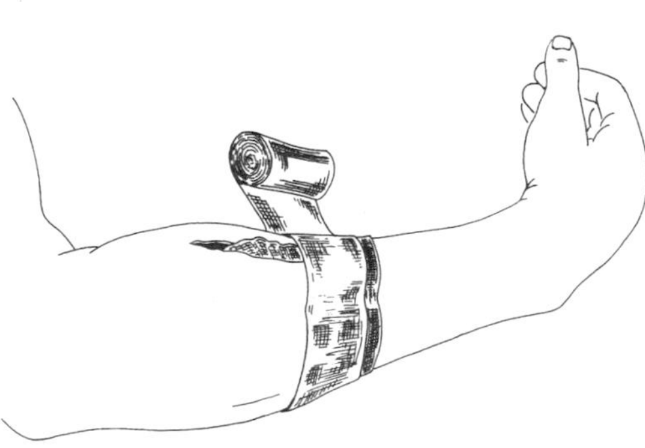

Figure 10.33. Packing a wound for a delayed closure. Insert fine-mesh gauze into a wound, followed by a gauze wrap. See text for discussion.

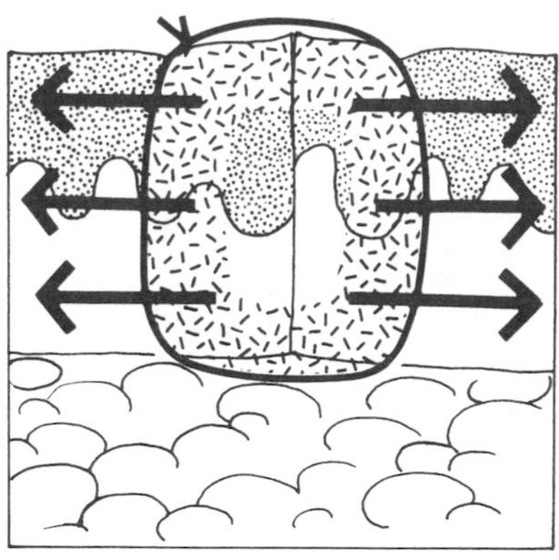

Figure 10.34. Extrinsic tension caused by elastic fibers in tissue will separate wound edges and increase pressure in the suture loop.

Undermining

The extrinsic tension on a wound is the "pulling" tension of a wound outward to maintain separated edges (Fig. 10.34). This tension varies with the direction of the laceration in relation to the skin-tension lines. Undermining involves the separation of the skin and attached superficial subcutaneous tissue from deeper subcutaneous tissue and fascia (Fig. 10.35). Undermining is important because it relieves extrinsic tension. Do not perform undermining in all wounds: wounds

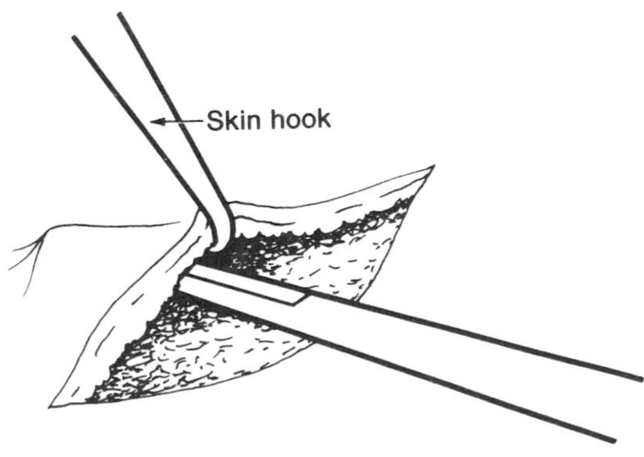

Figure 10.35. Undermining involves the separation of the skin and attached subcutaneous tissue from the deeper subcutaneous tissue and fascia. This is done in a natural tissue plane to relieve some of the extrinsic tension on the wound edge.

that are on the palm of the hand or the sole of the foot should not be undermined. In addition, do not undermine wounds of the fingertips. Undermining may lead to additional scar formation and should be performed only when release of extrinsic tension allows closure of the wound. The amount of undermining necessary to close a laceration is approximately double the width of the gap of the laceration at its widest point (115).

AXIOM

The amount of undermining necessary to close a laceration has been determined to be approximately double the width of the laceration at its widest point.

This gap is largely determined by the orientation of the laceration to the skin-tension lines. For example, undermine a 1-cm wide laceration 1 cm on both sides of the wound. Undermining also is important in allowing the eversion of the skin edges as well as in relieving the extrinsic tension from the skin sutures, thus aiding in obtaining a small scar (see discussion on eversion in the section on Relation of Suture to the Wound Edge, earlier).

The techniques of undermining are as follows:

1. Undermining may be performed by the use of blunt Iris scissors. The scissors should dissect in a normal fascial or areolar plane when possible. When this is not possible, dissect in the depth of the wound beneath the subdermal subcutaneous tissue (115), as shown in Fig. 10.35.
2. Undermining could be performed with the no. 11 blade by using multiple connecting stab incisions (115).

Closure of Dead Space

Condie and Ferguson (22) demonstrated that obliteration of the dead space by the use of subcutaneous sutures reduces the rate of infection in clean wounds. In heavily contaminated wounds, avoid suture closure of the dead space whenever possible. Place only a minimum number of sutures in the subcutaneous layer because the infection rate increases progressively in these wounds with more sutures. Perform closure of the dead space with "buried" sutures (Fig. 10.36), and use a minimal number of sutures (80).

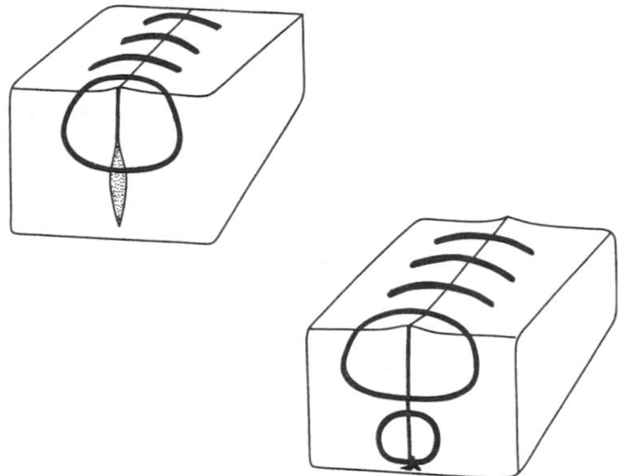

Figure 10.36. Closure of the dead space with buried sutures. Use the least number of sutures necessary to close a subcutaneous space.

Absorbable buried sutures are best in wounds that are not clean. Permanent deep sutures placed in contaminated wounds are frequently "spit out" weeks or months later.

AXIOM

Closure of the dead space will relieve surface tension and, thus, decrease scar spreading, particularly when the laceration is perpendicular to the skin-tension lines or the orientation of the muscles.

Closure of the dead space is best done with the least number of sutures and with just enough tension to approximate the tissue. The greater the number of sutures used, the greater is the infection rate.

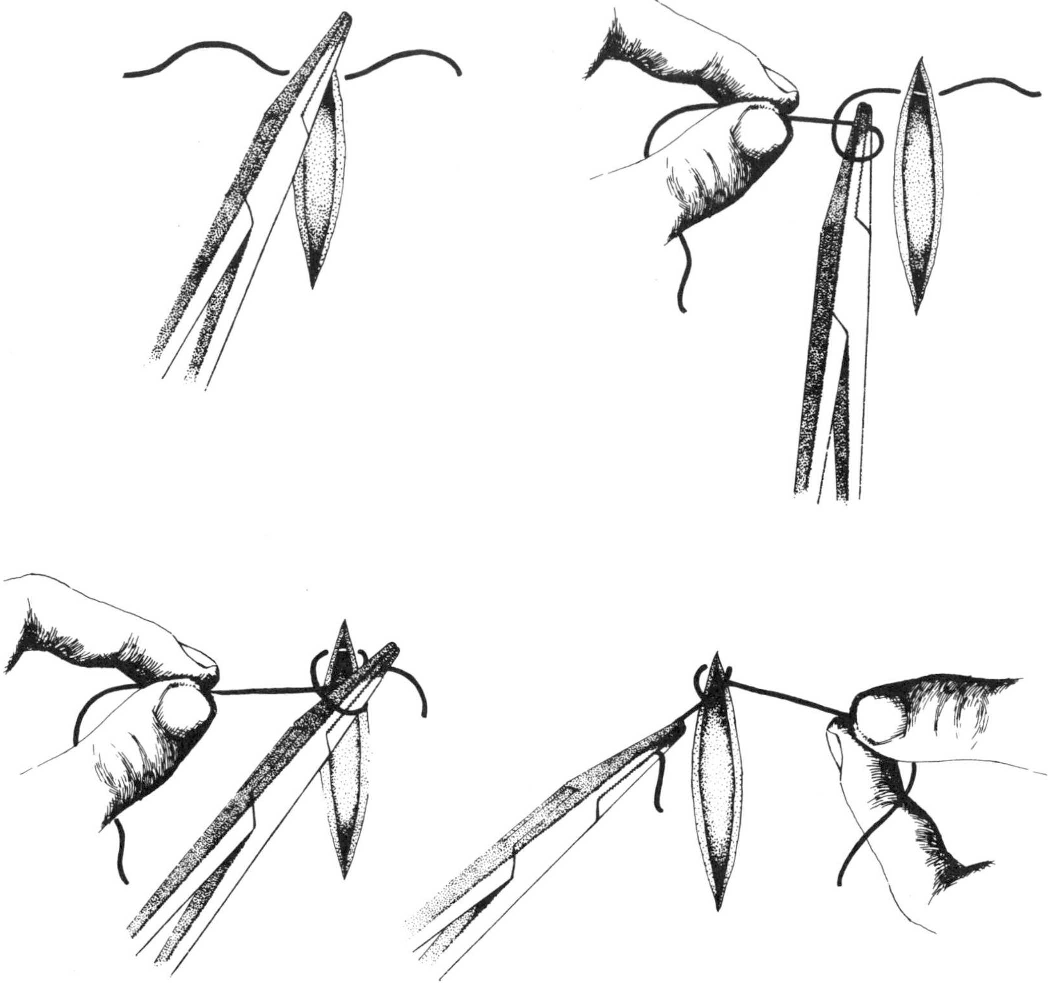

Figure 10.37. The instrument tie. Wrap two loops of suture around the distal portion of the needle holder, and then grasp the free end of the suture and pull it through the loop thus formed. Wrap a third suture loop around the needle holder in the opposite direction, and pull it in a direction opposite to the first tie to form a square knot.

BASIC SUTURING TECHNIQUES

Instrument Tie

Only the instrument tie is discussed here (Fig. 10.37). This tie is the most commonly used in the emergency center for simple closures. For this discussion, the suture is divided into two parts, the end close to the needle, termed the "needle end," and the end far from the needle, termed the "free end." Wrap two loops, or a "double-throw,"[1] of suture from the needle end (one loop shown in diagram for simplicity) around the distal portion of the needle holder, and grasp the free end of the suture and pull it through the loop thus formed. (Note that two loops are used to fix this half-knot in place to resist the

[1]Two loops are used to fix this half-knot in place and resist the extrinsic tension of the wound in the interim, before the square knot is finished. Occasionally, three loops may be needed with nylon.

extrinsic tension of the wound in the interim, before the square knot is finished. Occasionally, three loops may be needed with nylon.) Keep the free end short before pulling through the loops to form the first knot; otherwise too much suture material will be discarded with each instrument tie. Wrap the next suture loop around the needle holder in the opposite direction, and pull it in a direction opposite to the first tie to form a square knot. After all the knots are placed squarely, shift the mass of knots out of the center of the wound and to one side to decrease tissue reaction of the wound.

Simple Closures

SIMPLE INTERRUPTED

Simple interrupted sutures are the most commonly used sutures in the emergency center. The proper technique for this suture to provide eversion and good apposition of the wound edges is quite difficult to master. To assure the best results in placing simple interrupted sutures:

1. Take equal volumes of subcutaneous tissue from both sides. In wounds in which there is unequal thickness on one side, bring over the subcutaneous tissue from the thicker to the thinner side before approximation of the skin, as discussed in the general section.
2. Insert the needle into the skin edge at an angle of 90 degrees or greater (see Fig. 10.27), with the angle of exit ideally the same as the angle of entrance.

AXIOM

The closer the needle to the wound edge, the greater the control on the ultimate position of that edge.

---

3. When eversion of the edges is difficult to achieve in a wound, obtain it by passing the needle at a more acute angle than perpendicular to the skin, thereby taking a wider bite of subcutaneous tissue from the base of the wound than from near the skin edge (see Fig. 10.32). When the stitch is tied, the tissue at the base of the suture loop will come together before the tissue at the surface, thereby uplifting and everting the wound edges. In addition, before tying the first knot, lift up on the stitch ends, more accurately to appose the wound edges. When nylon is used, place at least four knots to be certain that unraveling does not occur. With polypropylene (Prolene), Vicryl, or silk, use three knots to secure the suture in place.
4. Hold the needle by the needle holder about halfway along the length of the needle. If held too near the end where the suture attaches to the needle, the needle may bend when passed. Always follow the curve of the needle. Do not pass the needle at a more acute angle by bending or pushing on the needle, but rather by lifting the edge of the skin with the forceps or skin hooks and/or by entering the skin at a greater angle. If a more acute passage is needed (in the intertriginous space between the fingers or toes), use a half-circle needle. When making the first throw of the simple interrupted suture, lift up on the wound edges and bring them together within the suture loop. When making the second throw, as the loop is being formed just before cinching the second throw (Fig. 10.38), swiftly pull the stitch to one side and close the loop. It is important that this be done with a rapid movement to prevent deforming the approximation of the wound edges created by the first throw.

OPEN-LOOP SIMPLE INTERRUPTED

This tie is a modification of the simple interrupted in which the same basic technique is used, with the exception of tying

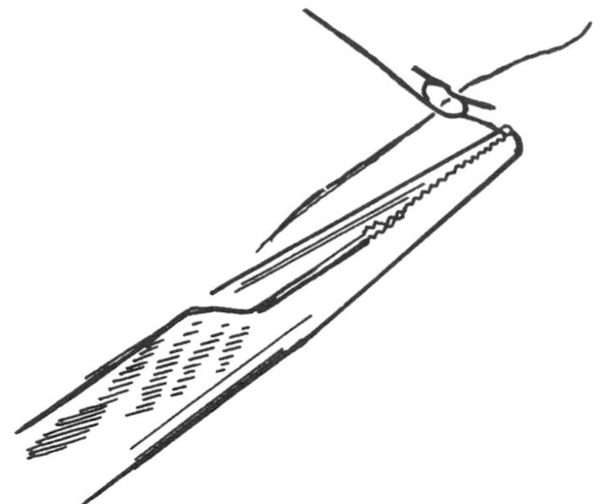

Figure 10.38. Open-loop simple interrupted suture. See text for discussion.

the knot. Introduced by Joseph Walike (99), the open loop simple interrupted suture is formed by using a knot as described earlier under Instrument Tie. On the first limb of the knot, tighten a *double throw* only until the suture lies flat against the skin surface. The second limb of the knot is a single knot *square* to the first that is tightened until the suture starts to deform the ends of the first double throw, thus creating an *open loop* (Fig. 10.38). A third single throw made square to the second throw completes the knot and, if properly tied, the loop will not close no matter how tightly the third throw is secured against the second. If the second and third throws are not square, a granny knot will result, and the loop will close. The 6-0 nylon used for this suture requires only three knots to secure the suture, rather than the usual four or five.

The open-loop technique has many advantages. If swelling occurs about the wound, the knot has some spring and will yield rather than cut into the tissue. The open loop technique also facilitates suture removal when sutures must be placed very close to the wound edge. Place the scissors simply into the loop; when the loop is cut open, the knot unravels. A major difficulty with this method is that, in closing some wounds, "perfect" approximation is achieved after the first double throw, only to be followed by deformation of the apposition of the edges when the second part of the knot is placed and secured. This problem is a common one, particularly in areas where the skin is thin and there is little subcutaneous supporting tissue, such as on the back of the hand.

INTERLOCKING SLIP KNOT

In a crying infant, it may be difficult to insert the point of a scissors under the knot to remove sutures. The interlocking slip knot introduced by Lucid (77) facilitates removal. The technique of placing this knot is shown in Fig. 10.39. Remove the suture with one hand without scissors. To remove, simply pull the longer end and then, if necessary, the shorter end.

CONTINUOUS OVER-AND-OVER

This suture is not commonly used in emergency medicine; however, if one becomes proficient in its use, one can achieve as adequate a closure as with the simple interrupted. It does have some disadvantages. There is more epithelialization of the suture track with this stitch, especially if the stitch is not removed early (40). Inclusion cysts may form in 3 to 4 weeks after the removal of these sutures (40). The stitch is most commonly used in the scalp, where lacerations and resulting scars are covered by hair and cosmetic repairs are not as necessary as elsewhere on the body. The primary advantage of this suture is the rapidity with which it can be placed, and it is especially useful in patients with multiple lacerations. The technique is shown in Fig. 10.40.

In a continuous over-and-over suture, place the first stitch similarly to a simple interrupted stitch (Fig. 10.40*A*). Instead of being cut, the suture is passed as a continuous running stitch (Fig. 10.40*A*). Each time it is passed through the skin to form a loop of the continuous stitch, pass the needle perpendicular to the skin edges, similar to the technique used in placing a simple interrupted stitch. This will aid in

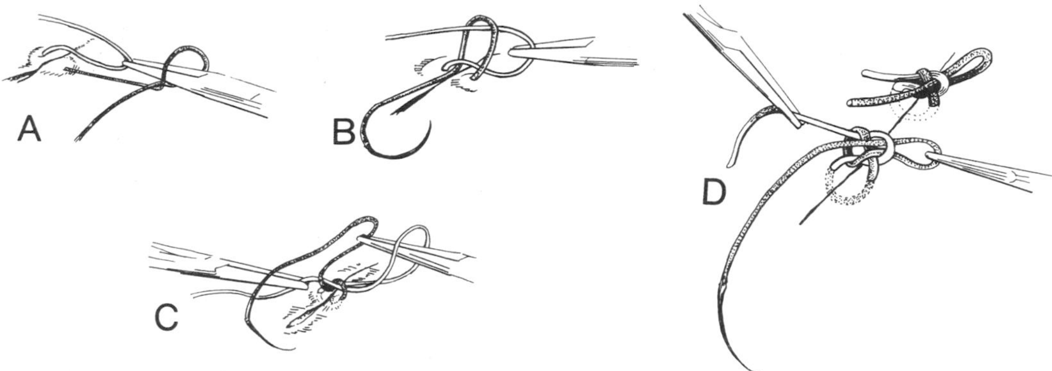

Figure 10.39. Interlocking slip knot. *A:* Make a loop around the needle holder with the free end of the suture material. *B:* Grasp the needle end of the suture material and pull through the loop and tie against the skin of the wound. *C, D:* Grasp the needle end of the suture material with the needle holder, and pass it through the loop while applying countertraction to the free end of the suture material. To remove the suture, pull the long end, and then, if necessary, the short end. One of the resulting tails of the suture may be trimmed at the skin edge before pulling it through the wound. (From Lucid ML: The interlocking slip knot. Plast Reconstr Surg 34:200, 1964, with permission.)

achieving eversion of the wound edges. The end of the wound is then approximated in similar fashion, and the suture is tied as a simple interrupted stitch (Fig. 10.40*B*). An alternate method of placing a continuous over-and-over suture is shown in Fig. 10.41.

CONTINUOUS SINGLE-LOCK

This suture may cause less epithelialization of the suture track while maintaining the advantage of a running suture. Place a simple interrupted suture first as with the continuous running stitch. Then hold this long end of the suture taut, and pass the needle through the skin, just as in the continuous over-and-over stitch, but, on coming out on the other side, pass the needle in front of the thread (Figs. 10.41*B* and 10.42). Once again, in placing the next stitch, hold the suture taut to maintain approximation of the sutured edges. As with the continuous over-and-over, in the final stitch, tie the terminal suture as a simple interrupted stitch.

This is a superior stitch to use when one desires to close the skin with a running stitch. It provides a more secure and regular apposition of the wound edges and less epithelialization of the tracks than does a continuous over-and-over stitch, because it combines basically the simple interrupted with the continuous over-and-over. It has the disadvantage of taking somewhat longer to place than does the continuous over-and-over stitch.

Mattress Closures

The mattress stitches all have in common their ability to secure good apposition and to produce the least amount of tension on the wound edges, because the basic principle in all mattress closures is that one provides a "two-in-one" closure. The "outside stitch" pulls in the wound to relieve tension from the edges and provides a "tensionless repair," while the "inside stitch" secures perfect apposition.

VERTICAL MATTRESS

This suture is unsurpassed in its ability to provide eversion of the wound edges. It provides the best apposition and the best control of the wound edge. Alternate this suture with a simple interrupted in large wounds to save time. The major disadvantage in this stitch is the time that it takes to

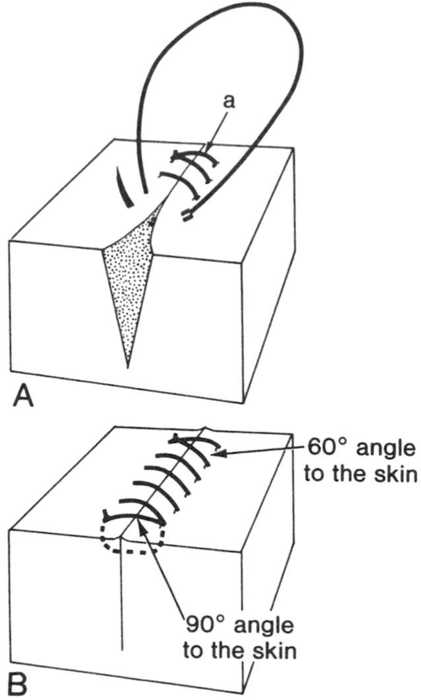

Figure 10.40. The continuous over-and-over suture. *A:* Begin this continuous suture with a single suture that is tied to anchor the rest of the suture. Pass the needle perpendicular to the skin edge; the suture threads lie perpendicular to the wound margin to maximize the effect of the suture on extrinsic wound tension, as with the simple interrupted suture. *B:* To finish and tie off this continuous suture, grab the loop formed at the free end after insertion of the needle through the skin at its midpoint with the needle holder, and pull on this loop. It will come together as if it were a single thread. Tie the needle end of the suture material and this "looped" free end as a simple interrupted suture would be tied. When one is proficient with this suture, eversion of the skin edges is quite adequate.

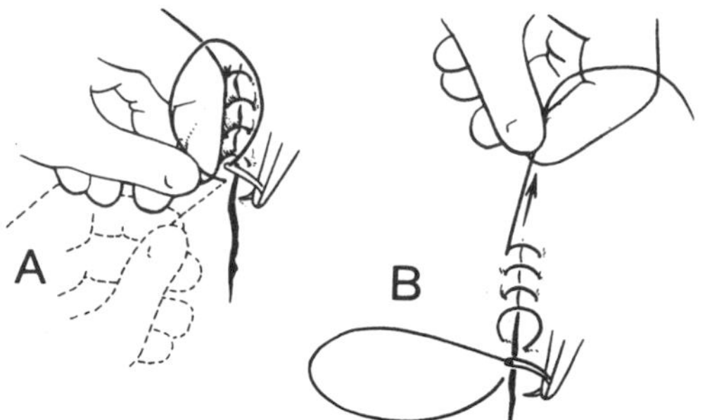

Figure 10.41. *A:* Conventional method of running a suture. *B:* By maintaining the initial cut end of the suture long, it can be used as a holding stitch. The advantage of this is that only one point must be held throughout the entire process of placing a continuous suture, thereby negating the continuous motion of regrasping with every stitch placement, the danger of forming a pursestring at the end of the wound, and the possibility of having placed sutures with altering tension along the wound. (From Noe JM, Goth DA: A technique for placement of a continuous suture. Surg Gynecol Obstet 150:404, 1980, with permission.)

place. The technique is shown in Fig. 10.43. The vertical mattress suture is basically a double suture, the first stitch of which is made by passing the needle more widely separated from the wound edges and deeper into the wound than usual (Fig. 10.43*A*). When the wound edges are approximated, this first suture loop will relieve the extrinsic tension from the wound edges and promote better healing. For a good cosmetic effect, make the second loop by passing the needle back through the epidermis and lower dermis close to the wound edge, taking a small bite of skin from both sides and approximating the edges (Fig. 10.43*B* and *C*). Then tie the suture to approximate the subcutaneous tissue (with the first suture loop) and the skin edges (second suture loop).

LOCKED VERTICAL MATTRESS

The locked vertical mattress stitch was introduced by Condon (23). In some patients (e.g., obese or elderly patients in whom there is diminished elasticity of the skin), approximation of the skin edges with a vertical mattress often is made by applying excessive tension to the deep portion of the suture. This excessive tension results in increased inflammation around the suture site and increased pain and scarring, producing the "railroad track" appearance of the healed wound. The locked vertical mattress obviates this tendency to apply excessive tension. Once

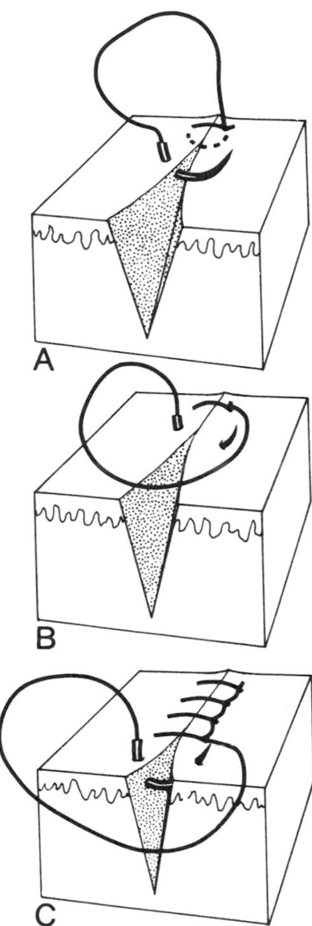

Figure 10.42. Continuous single-lock stitch. See text for discussion.

locked, the edges of the skin remain approximated without tension. The deep portion of the suture can then be tied loosely.

The technique is as follows (Fig. 10.44). The needle goes in 1 cm or more from the margin of the wound, the distance being approximately equal to the depth of the wound. After bringing it out with a similar bite on the far side of the wound, then return the needle, taking a very minute bite of skin at the wound edge (Fig. 10.44*A*). Then pass the needle end of the suture back through the loop formed on the far side of the wound, thus forming a locked portion of the stitch, as shown in Fig.

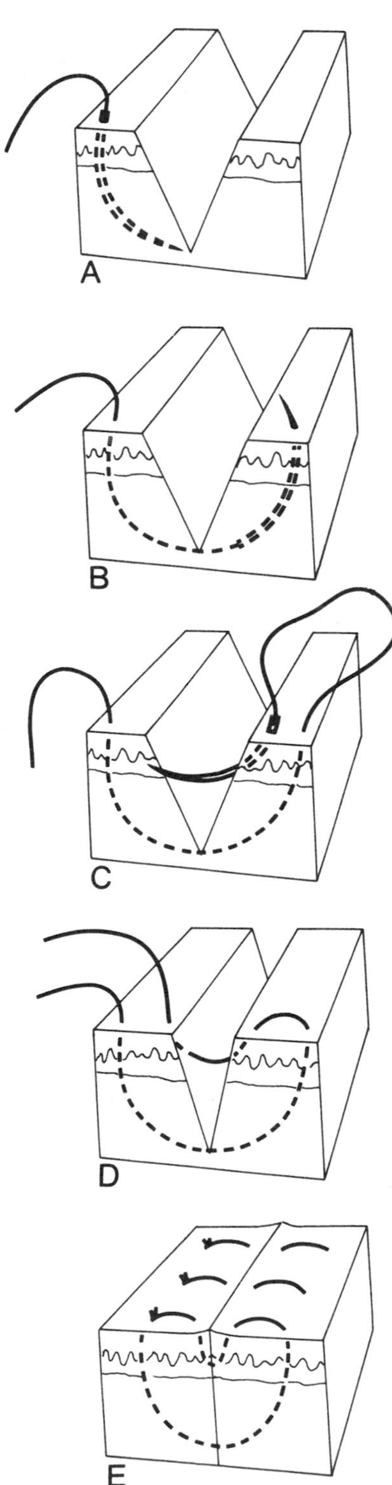

Figure 10.43. Vertical mattress stitch. See text for discussion.

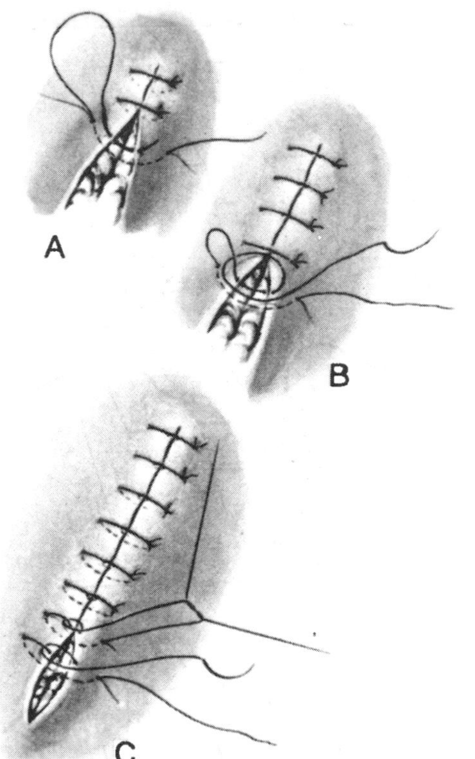

Figure 10.44. Locked vertical mattress stitch. *A:* Take a deep bite of the skin and subcutaneous tissue. The distance from the wound margin at which the needle enters should be approximately the same as the distance and depth at which the needle crosses the wound. The needle is brought out from the opposite side of the wound and is returned with only the most minute bite of skin being taken at the edge of the wound. *B:* Then pass the end of the suture back through the loop on the far side of the wound. This forms the locked portion of the stitch. This step is easily accomplished by passing the needle and suture back through the locking loop. *C:* Draw the suture taut to bring the margins of the skin together without any tension in the deeper portion of the wound. (From Condon RE: Locked vertical mattress stitch for skin closure. Surg Gynecol Obstet 127:839, 1968, with permission.)

10.44*B* and *C*. Draw the locking end of the suture taut to bring together the margins of the skin without any tension in the deeper portion of the wound. Then tie the two free ends of the suture loosely. To remove the suture, cut the end farthest from the knot and pull on the knot.

HORIZONTAL MATTRESS

The major advantage of this type of mattress stitch is that it reinforces the subcutaneous tissue by pulling it together across the length of the wound (Fig. 10.45*C*) and prevents stretching of the scar. Stretching is prevented because the horizontal mattress stitch removes more extrinsic tension from the wound margins than other stitches because of its placement along the axis of the wound. It is more rapidly placed than the vertical mattress, and fewer stitches are required to close a wound of a given length than would be required should a vertical mattress be used. The disadvantage is that although some eversion of the wound edges is provided, it is more difficult to achieve. The technique is shown in Fig. 10.45.

HALF-BURIED HORIZONTAL MATTRESS

This stitch is very commonly used in emergency medicine. It is especially useful in closing a flap when the corner has limited vascularity and perhaps questionable viability. A routine simple interrupted stitch, in approximating the corner to the opposite side, may damage the skin and cause vascular compromise because of the tension on the suture (Fig. 10.46). In placement of the half-buried horizontal mattress, the suture is buried in the flap so it may hold a thin flap in place without tension or vascular compromise. It is useful in closing a V-shaped wound and prevents necrosis of the tip of the V, which may occur with a simple interrupted suture. The technique of placing this stitch is shown in Fig. 10.47. Pass the needle through the lower dermis at the same level through the skin edges of both the V-shaped flap and the parent skin edge from which it came, as shown in Fig. 10.47*A*. There are numerous situations in which this stitch can be used, some of which are shown in Fig. 10.48.

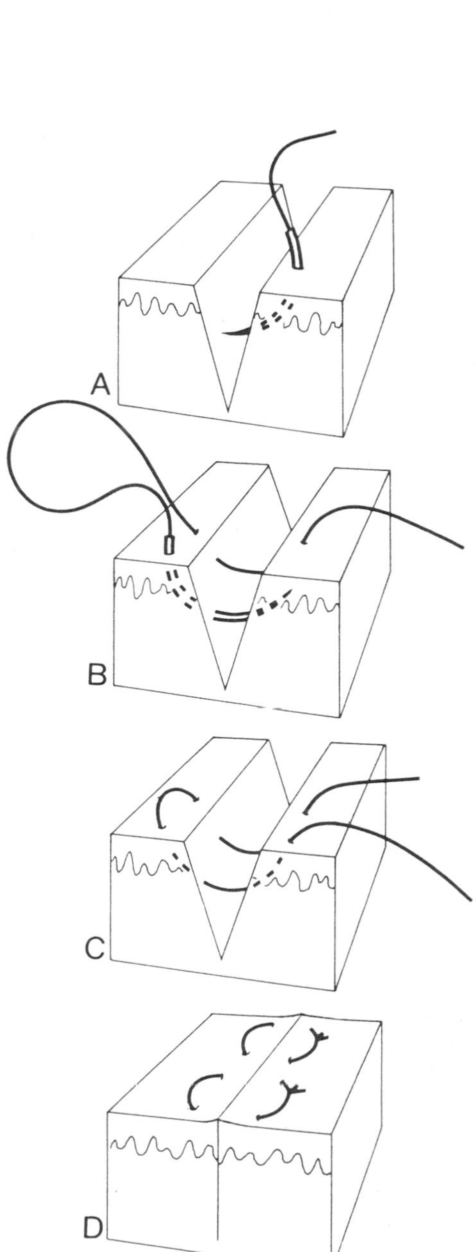

Figure 10.45. Horizontal mattress stitch. *A:* Pass the needle 0.5 to 1 cm away from wound edge deeply into the wound. *B:* Then pass the needle through the opposite side so it reenters the wound parallel to the initial suture. *C:* Enter the skin perpendicularly to provide some eversion of the wound edges, and enter and exit both the wound and skin at the same depth; otherwise, "buckling" and irregularities occur in the wound margin. *D:* Then tie the suture loop as shown.

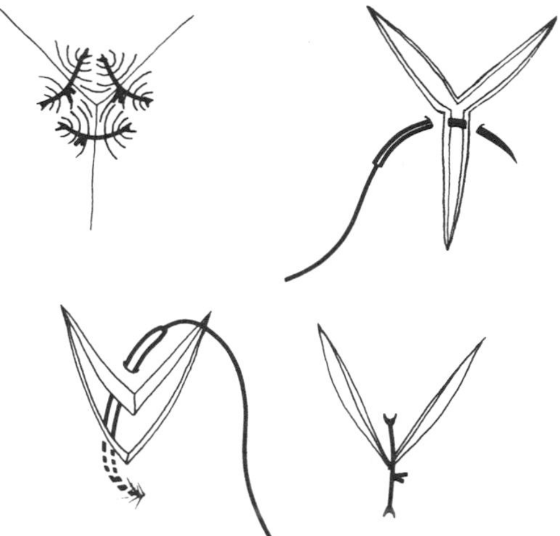

Figure 10.46. Simple suture producing vascular compromise at the V-shaped tip.

CONTINUOUS HORIZONTAL MATTRESS

The continuous mattress is not commonly used in emergency medicine. It has the advantage, like the horizontal mattress, of providing good apposition with less tension on the wound edges by pulling only the subcutaneous tension of the wound. The stitch has the added advantage that it is rapidly placed. Place the stitch equidistant on either side of the edges of a laceration, and then tie it (Fig. 10.49). Apposition is not so good with this stitch as with other sutures, and for this reason, it is not recommended for routine use.

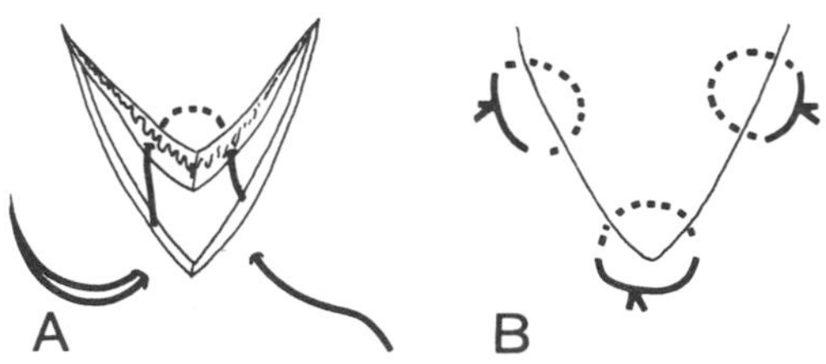

Figure 10.47. Half-buried horizontal mattress stitch. This minimizes the vascular compromise at a corner flap. See text for discussion.

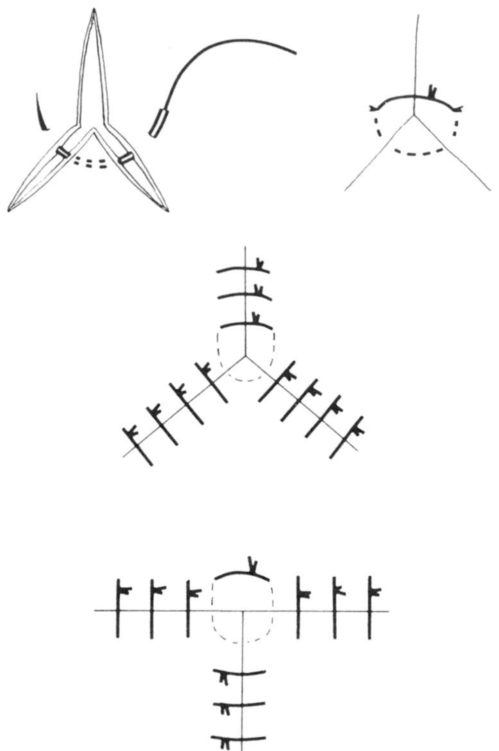

Figure 10.48. Half-buried horizontal mattress stitch used to approximate the center of a T-shaped laceration, a Y-shaped laceration, and a stellate laceration.

Subcutaneous and Buried Sutures

SUBCUTICULAR

The major advantage of this closure is that it provides superb cosmetic results when done properly. It requires more time and skill, however, to master. There is no possibility of suture marks because no sutures pass into the skin surface. Place the stitch by passing the suture horizontally, as shown in Fig. 10.50, through the dermis in small bites of about 0.5 cm. Adequately undermine the wound edges to achieve a good result (109). Alternate the stitch from one side to the other (Fig. 10.50). Several points should be mentioned about placing this suture. Maintain the same depth and level of placement of the suture in the opposing sides of the dermis (109). The exit and entrance sites of the needle on the opposing sides of the dermis should be at the same level. The entrance of the needle into the dermis may be backed up a little from the exit on the opposing side; however, this is not completely agreed on as yielding the best results. If the wound is very long

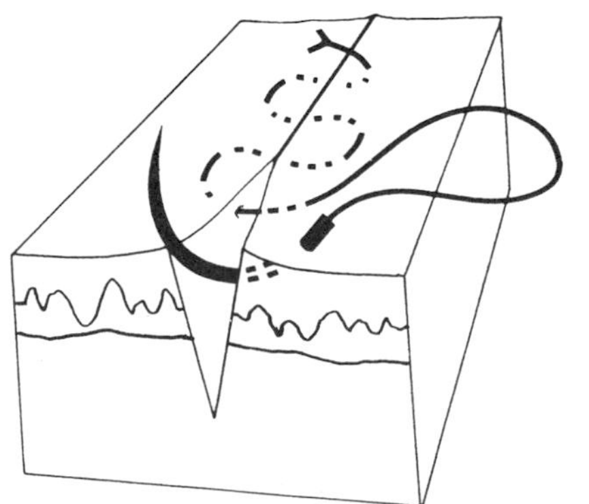

Figure 10.49. Continuous mattress stitch. See text for discussion.

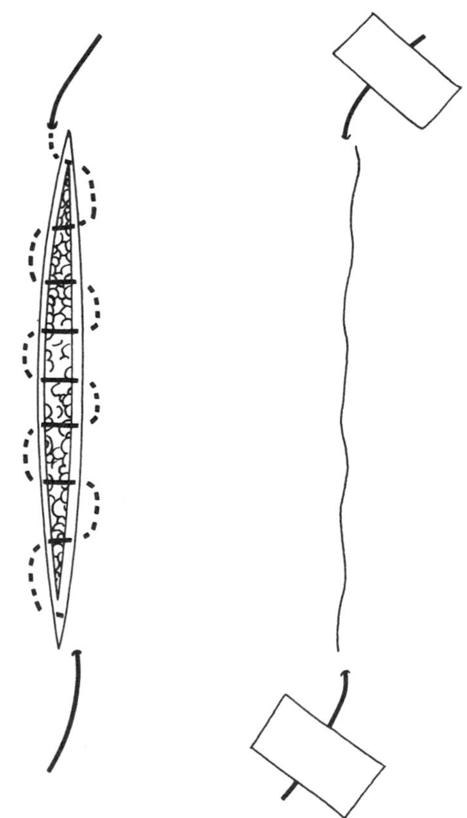

Figure 10.50. Subcuticular stitch. See text for discussion.

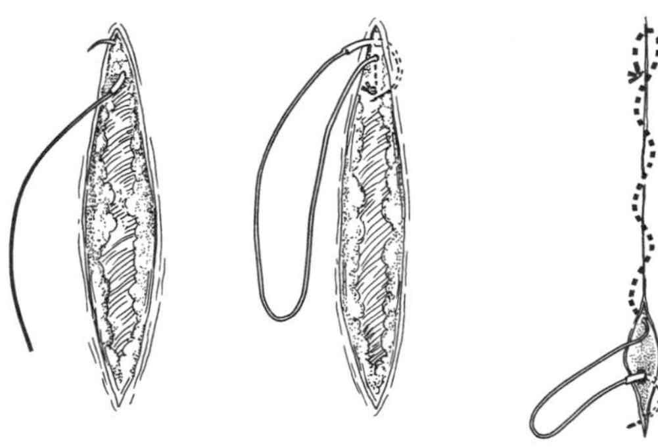

Figure 10.51. An alternative technique for placing a subcuticular stitch. To bury the initial stitch, place the first throw in the subdermal layer and then suture it. A layer-by-layer suture is shown.

and one elects to use this closure, then place the suture every 2 inches. A good suture material to use in this closure is 5-0 or 6-0 nylon. There are a number of techniques of beginning and ending the subcuticular suture. Another technique of doing this is shown in Fig. 10.51.

After completing the continuous subcuticular suture, add a simple interrupted suture or skin tape over the wound to secure more complete apposition or eversion of the wound edges.

An alternate method of using the continuous subcuticular was presented by Noe and Gloth (88). Leave the initial suture long, and use it to hold and stabilize the wound while the subcuticular suture is placed. Then tape the terminal ends securely in place (Fig. 10.50). Leave subcuticular stitches in place for a minimum of 7 days.

BURIED SUBCUTANEOUS

This suture is similar to the simple interrupted, but the suture is placed in such a manner as to bury the knot to avoid any irritation by the knot on the dermis of the skin edge. This suture is used to overcome tension at the wound edge from below and, thus, to decrease the chance for vascular compromise and scar spreading. Use this suture in the superficial layers under the skin surface and not necessarily in the deep fascial closure, where a simple interrupted suture or one of the running sutures described earlier can be used.

To place a buried stitch, pass the needle up from under the lower margin of the subcutaneous tissue on one side and then carry it over to the other side, passing the needle from above toward the lower portion of the wound, as shown in Fig. 10.52. This inverts the knot to avoid excessive tension at the wound edge.

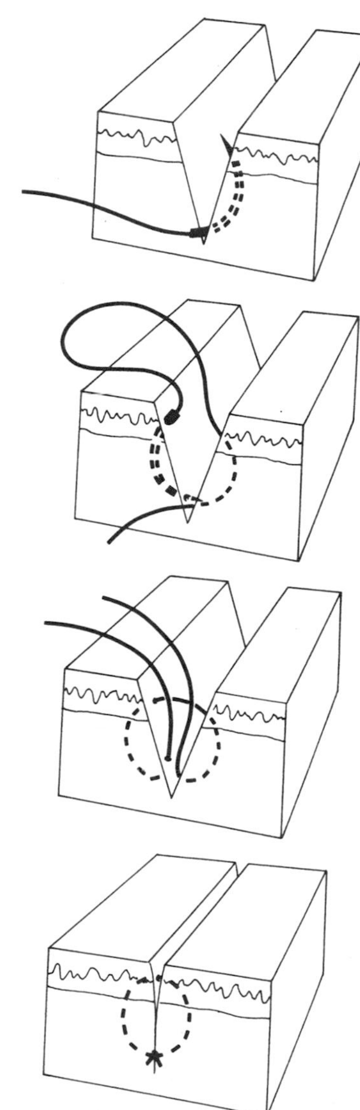

Figure 10.52. Buried subcutaneous stitch. This is particularly useful when approximating the subcutaneous tissue just beneath the skin edge, because it prevents irritation of the skin edge by the knot.

An alternate method first introduced by Straith et al. (109) permits more eversion of the wound edges. Excise the edges of the wound as shown in Fig. 10.53*A*. The subcutaneous stitch incorporates a piece of the lower dermis and takes a wider bite on the dermal side than on the deeper portion of the wound (Fig. 10.53*B* and *C*). This provides eversion of the skin edges when the suture is tied, because the lower dermis comes together before the subcutaneous tissue (Fig. 10.53*D*). This method, once mastered, is superior for closure of wounds and results in a wound whose skin edges can be apposed with skin tape, producing excellent results.

Reinforcing Sutures for Wounds under Tension

As discussed earlier, the mattress suture is good for closing wounds and for decreasing the tension on the wound edges. When there are very widely separated wound edges and closure cannot be accomplished without producing significant tension on the edges, the wound can be reinforced with either a button stitch or tape. The sterile buttons are present in most operating suites. A straight needle and 0 silk are usually used to place the stitch. Do not try to achieve apposition of the wound edges with this stitch, but rather approximation to a point where the

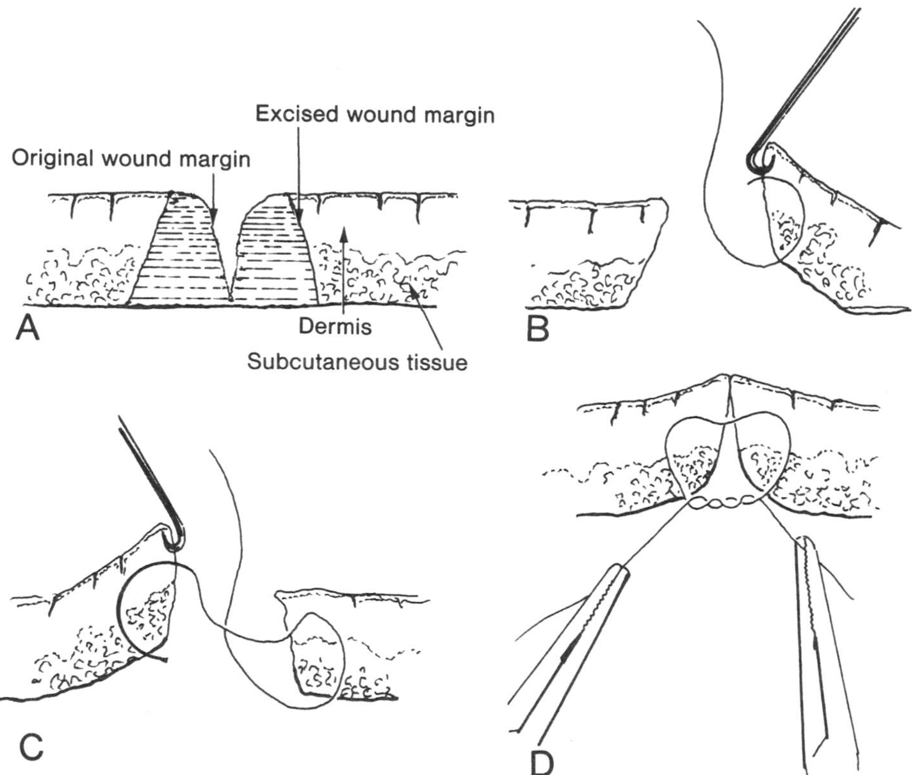

Figure 10.53. *A:* Sharply excise bruised skin edges. Then undermine the skin above the fascia. *B:* Buried suture passes up through the dermal layer of the skin. Notice that the suture emerges from the near skin, taking a larger "bite" from the dermal portion of the wound than the subcutaneous portion. *C:* Then pass the suture through the far skin edge. Path of the suture is a mirror image of the opposite side and emerges above the fascia in the undercut area. *D:* Then tie the knot as a double-hitch knot to prevent slipping. Illustration shows eversion of the skin edges over the previously buried sutures. (From Straith R, Lawson JM, Hipps CJ: The subcuticular suture. Postgrad Med 29:166, 1961, with permission.)

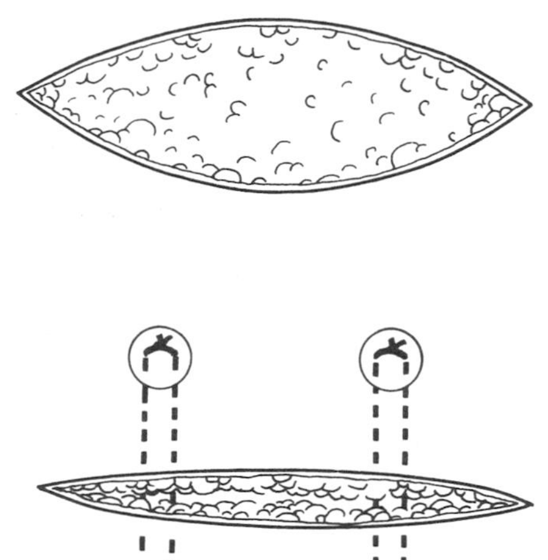

Figure 10.54. Reinforcing sutures for wounds under tension that cannot be closed. These are particularly useful in elderly patients who have pretibial lacerations that are widely gaping and in whom the skin is too atrophic to approximate without the suture cutting through the skin into the wound.

wound can be closed without significant tension by another technique. Leave the reinforcing sutures in place long after the skin sutures are removed, until adequate time has passed for the wound to gain strength. We have found this most useful in very elderly patients, whose skin is thin and friable with no elasticity, who have wide gaping lacerations of the lower extremity. Closure of these wounds results in tearing through the tissue and is fruitless until the edges are brought closer together (Fig. 10.54).

Summary

A compilation of the various basic closures and their advantages and disadvantages is found in Table 10.5.

Advanced Closures

The rotation of advancement flaps is quite useful when dealing with injuries in which there is significant tissue loss, making end-to-end approximation of the wound edges impossible. It is critical in performing these closures that there be adequate undermining. All of the area underneath the skin being rotated or advanced must be undermined, as well as the skin edges around the avulsed segment. Adequate undermining cannot be overly stressed. When to use one type of closure as opposed to another is often a matter of preference; however, it is guided by location of the wound, how adherent the skin is to the underlying surface, and the shape and type of wound.

THE "DOG EAR"

To correct the "dog ear" that occurs when one side of a sutured wound is longer than the other, do the following:

1. Make a superficial marking incision at a 45-degree angle to the line of the laceration.
2. Incise this marking with either a straight Iris scissors or a no. 15 blade (Fig. 10.55*A*).
3. Undermine the area.
4. Trim off the excess skin (Fig. 10.55*B*) of the dog ear so that the dog ear repair will fit in the area of skin that was excised.
5. Suture the wound (Fig. 10.55*C*).

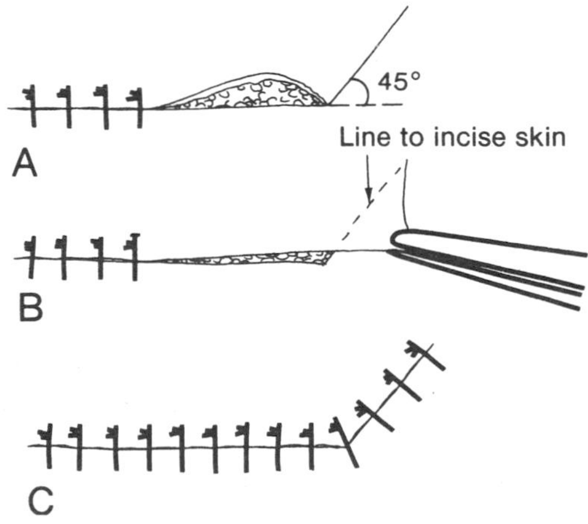

Figure 10.55. The dog ear. See text for discussion.

Table 10.5
Basic Closures and Their Advantages and Disadvantages

Suture	Advantages	Disadvantages
Simple interrupted	Permits good eversion of the wound edges. Is commonly used and can be applied rapidly.	Proper technique to provide eversion of edges requires practice to master. Eversion is not as good in difficult wounds as with other techniques. Does not relieve extrinsic tension from the wound edges.
Continuous over and over	Can be applied rapidly to close multiple lacerations and large wounds.	Apposition of the wound edges and eversion are more difficult to achieve. Inclusion cysts may form.
Continuous single-lock stitch	Can be applied rapidly. Apposition of the wound edges is more complete than with the continuous over and over stitch. Less epithelialization of the tracts.	Apposition of the wound edges is not as perfect as with the simple interrupted unless the procedure is mastered well.
Vertical mattress stitch	Unsurpassed in its ability to provide eversion of the wound edges and perfect apposition. Relieves tension from the skin edges.	Takes time to apply. Produces more cross-marks.
Horizontal mattress stitch	Reinforces the subcutaneous tissue. Relieves extrinsic tension from the wound edges more effectively than does the vertical mattress.	Does not provide as good apposition of the wound edges as does the vertical mattress.
Half-buried horizontal mattress	Relieves intrinsic tension and vascular compromise when approximating the tip of a flap.	Takes skill to master proper technique in order to provide perfect apposition of the wound edges.
Continuous mattress	Can be rapidly placed in order to approximate large lacerations in cosmetically unimportant areas.	Does not provide good apposition of the wound edges or eversion.

Z-PLASTY

Z-plasty is used to change the orientation of a wound to produce a better scar. This is most commonly used in the initial closure of a clean wound that extends vertically across the flexion crease of a joint or the mucosa of the lower lip.

The Z-plasty can be made at various angles to the original laceration, depending on the amount of lengthening one desires. The most common angle used is 60 degrees, which increases the wound length by 75%; the 45-degree angle Z-plasty increases the length of the wound by 50%; and the 30-degree Z-plasty increases the length of a laceration by 25%. Thus with a Z-plasty, one must increase the length of a laceration to overcome the effects of wound contracture as well as to change the orientation of the wound. The Z-plasty at an angle of 60 degrees is the most commonly used, because an increase in the length of a wound by 75% has been found in clinical practice to be optimal for preventing contractures at most sites. A Z-plasty can be performed in changing lacerations that run vertically across flexor creases such as the wrist, antecubital fossa, and popliteal fossa and vertical lacerations coursing across the anterior surface of the ankle. Z-plasties obviously increase the size of the wound by increasing the wound length. Z-plasty should not be done in contaminated wounds because it also decreases the blood supply, and therefore the possibility of infection is greater. Normally, Z-plasty should be reserved for secondary scar release and reconstruction. Many scars will not need release even though at the time of primary closure, it would appear this would be necessary.

The technique of performing a Z-plasty is shown in Fig. 10.56. Undermining is crucial in obtaining a good result. Measure the angle desired, and draw a line with a skin-marking pencil to plan the incision accurately. Measure a 60-degree angle at the ends of the original laceration, and extend the line at this angle from both ends, forming a "Z." Extend the line to the point where it meets a similar line drawn at the same angle from the opposite end, thus forming a diamond shape (stippled portion of Fig. 10.56*A*). Then undermine this area. With a no. 15 blade, make an incision carefully along the drawn lines, extending from the ends of the original laceration marked *a* and *b* in Fig. 10.55*A*. Then elevate and transpose the two Z-shaped flaps thus formed (Fig. 10.56*B*), as shown in Fig. 10.56*A* and *B*. Then close the Z-plasty (Fig. 10.56*C*).

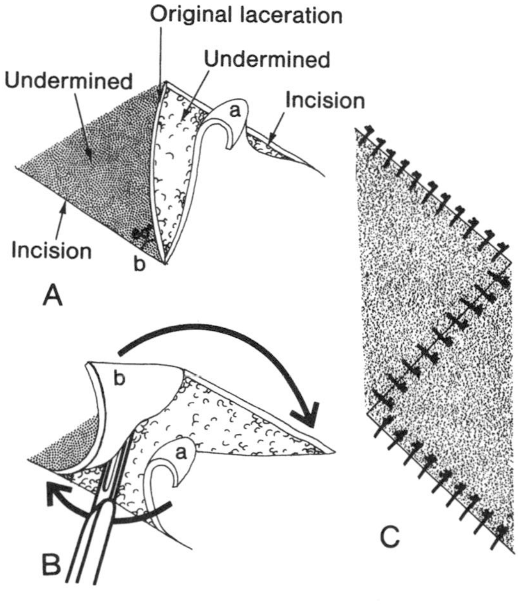

Original laceration
Undermined
Undermined
Incision
Incision
a
b
A
b
a
B
C

Figure 10.56. Z-plasty, 60-degree. The *stippled* area is undermined. *A:* Point (*a*) should be transposed to the position shown in *B*. Point (*b*) should likewise be transposed as shown above. The result is a laceration in which the orientation of the wound is changed from its original configuration to one that is parallel to the relaxed skin tension lines or skin creases. It also lengthens the laceration, thus decreasing the effective contracture.

Approximating the Edges of a Laceration with Grossly Unequal Lengths

Measure the width of the laceration across its widest point (A′B′ in Fig. 10.57), and excise an equilateral triangle from the center of the longer side such that the base of the triangle C′D′ is equal to the length of A′B′. Undermine and close the laceration, as shown in Fig. 10.57. The small vertical incision does not result in significant scarring.

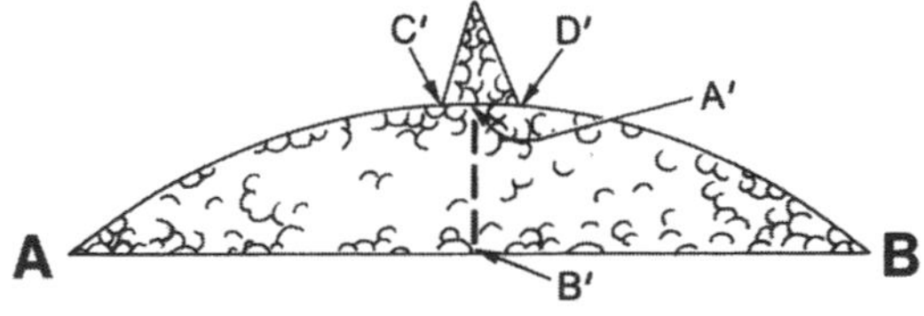

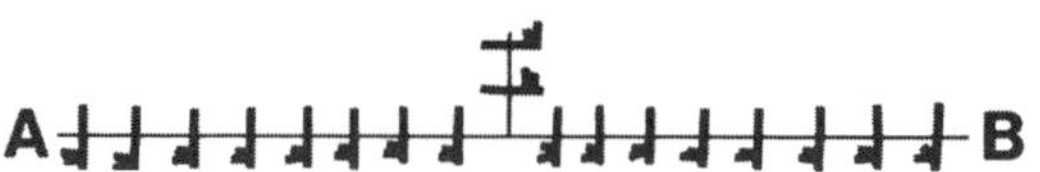

Figure 10.57. Approximating the edges of a laceration with grossly unequal lengths. See text for discussion.

Closing a Defect

SQUARE DEFECT

To close a square defect, an advancement flap may be needed. Make two parallel incisions approximately twice the length of the side of the square (Fig. 10.58). Undermine the stippled area widely, and excise small Burow's triangles at the ends of the incision that are half the length of one side of the original square. These triangles should be equilateral triangles. Then advance the flap, as shown in Fig. 10.58, to cover the defect. Approximate the edges by using simple interrupted sutures with the corners closed with half-buried mattress stitches. This method obviously works only with small defects.

DIAMOND-SHAPED DEFECT

A method of closing a diamond-shaped defect is to rotate a flap from alongside the wound. Measure and draw the following dimensions with a skin pencil (see Fig. 10.59):

Angle A = A′
Line BC = B′C′
Line CB′ = C′B″

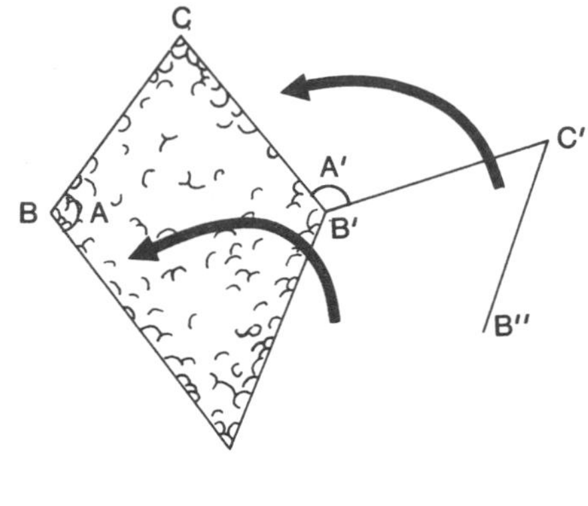

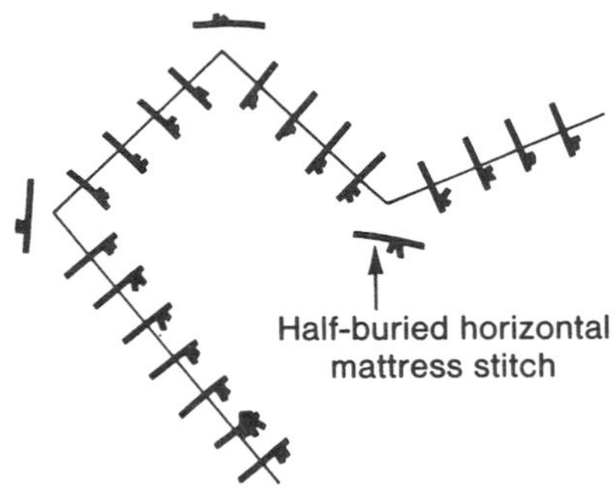

Figure 10.59. Closure of a diamond-shaped defect. This technique is especially useful in areas where the skin is tightly apposed to the underlying subcutaneous tissue, preventing advancement of a freed flap. See text for discussion.

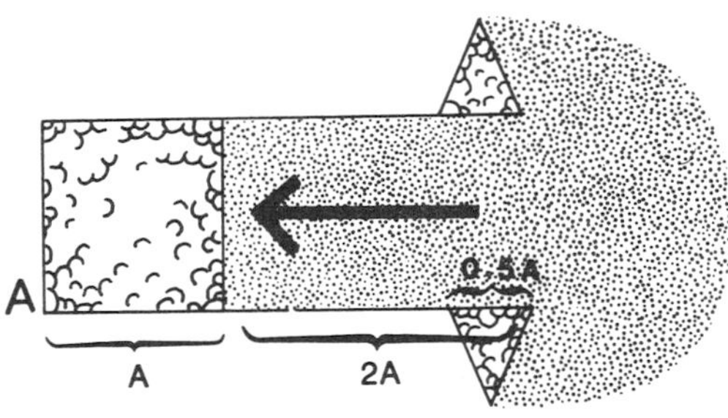

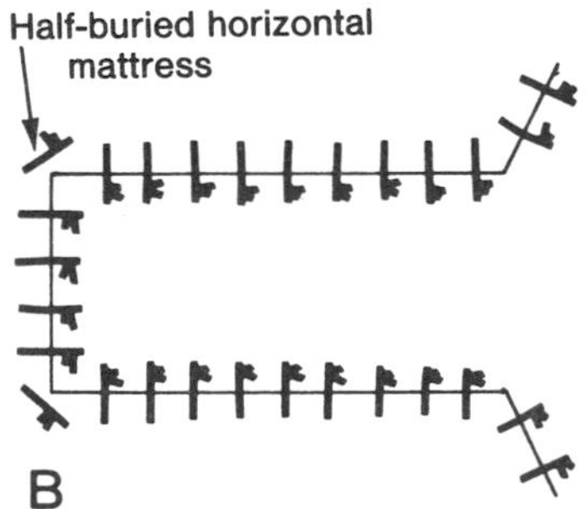

Figure 10.58. Closure of a square defect. See text for discussion.

Then incise, undermine, and rotate B′C′ and C′B″, as shown in Fig. 10.59.

ELLIPTICAL DEFECT

Elliptical defects placed over areas where the skin is adherent to the subcutaneous fascia may not permit approximation of the edges by simple means. A defect as shown in Fig. 10.60*A* can be closed by excising the margins of the wound to form an ellipse (Fig. 10.60*B*). Then extend the ends of the ellipse to form an "S" pattern (Fig. 10.60*B*). Widely undermine the area, as shown in Fig. 10.60*C*. This permits approximation of the ends of the ellipse. Then close the ellipse by bringing together the subcutaneous tissue with buried sutures. Place these buried sutures at the periphery of the undermined area to approximate the edges of the ellipse in a

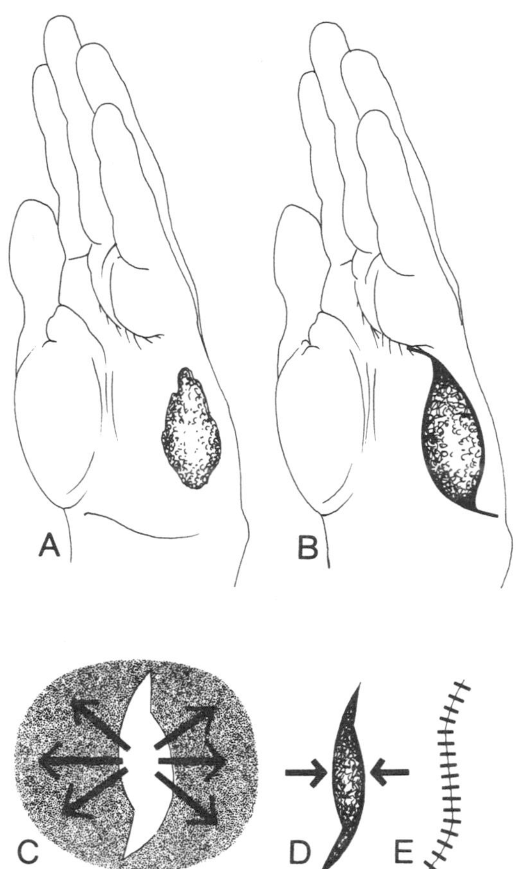

Figure 10.60. Closure of a wide ellipse. See text for discussion.

stepwise fashion, as the subcutaneous layers are brought closer and closer together. The result is an S-shaped laceration and that can be closed with little tension on the wound edges (Fig. 10.60*D*). Then close the wound with a simple interrupted stitch (Fig. 10.60*E*).

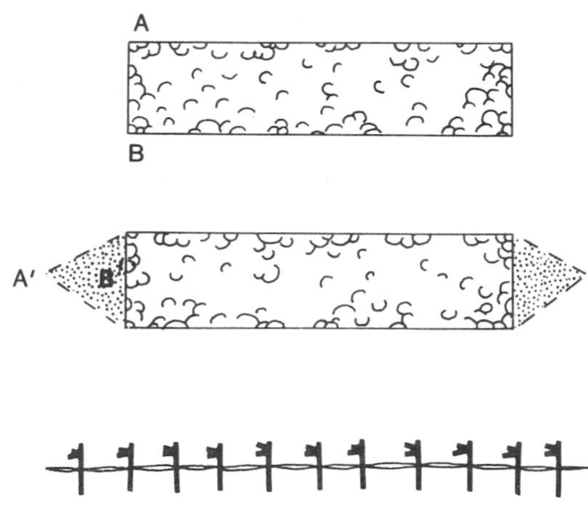

Figure 10.62. Closure of a rectangular defect. See text for discussion.

CLOSURE WITH A V–Y ADVANCEMENT FLAP

The V–Y advancement flap is used for repair of fingertip lacerations and is called the Kutler procedure. It is used to close an area where there is an elliptical defect (Fig. 10.61*A*). First excise the wound margins, as shown in the stippled area, to form an elliptical wound. Then incise a "V" at a distance slightly greater than the width of the elliptical defect at its widest point (Fig. 10.61*A*). Then close the ellipse with simple interrupted sutures after performing adequate undermining (Fig. 10.61*B*). Then the V-shaped incision is closed as a "Y" (Fig. 10.61*C*).

RECTANGULAR DEFECT

Close a rectangular defect by removing a skin triangle at both ends (Fig. 10.62). The

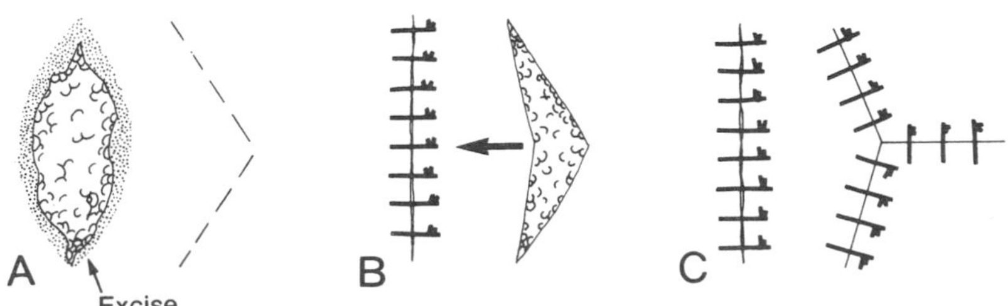

Figure 10.61. Closure of a defect with a V–Y advancement flap. See text for discussion.

length from the base to the apex of the triangle (A′B′) should be equal to the width of the rectangle (AB). Then undermine and close the wound, as shown in Fig. 10.62.

TRIANGULAR DEFECT (ROTATION FLAP)

A triangular defect can be closed with a rotation flap. Extend the base of the triangle in a wide circular fashion, as shown in Fig. 10.63. Draw an arched line extending from the base of the triangle that is approximately 4 times as long as the area it is to close. Rotation of the flap thus created is facilitated if this line is drawn beyond a line extending from the apex of the triangle perpendicularly (AD). Then extend the arc farther so that a triangle with the dimensions described later can be formed. In forming the triangle, try to place its base in such a position as to permit the secondary incisions to fall into favorable skin-tension lines. Make curved incisions to extend from one or more sides of the triangle. Excise the triangle so that the base is approximately half the length of the arms. After undermining, close the triangle by approximating point C to point B. This will create a dog ear that is then removed by creating a Burow's triangle. Undermine and close the defect, as shown in Fig. 10.63.

An alternate method is shown in Fig. 10.64. Use this alternate method when a

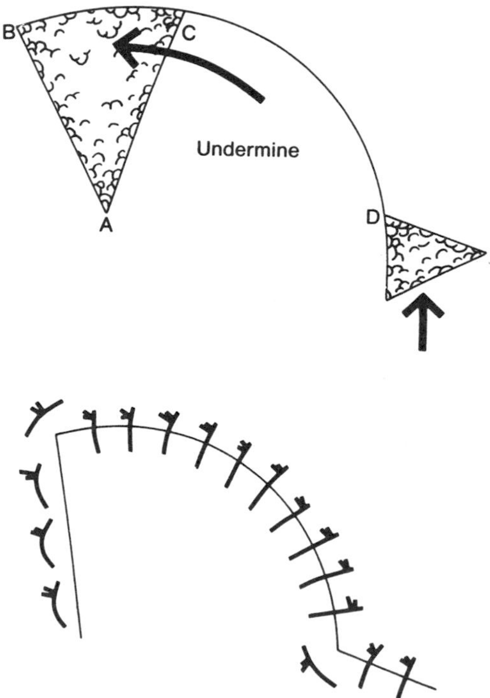

Figure 10.63. Closure of a triangular defect with a rotation flap. See text for discussion. Note that half-buried horizontal stitches are used in areas where vascular compromise may be present.

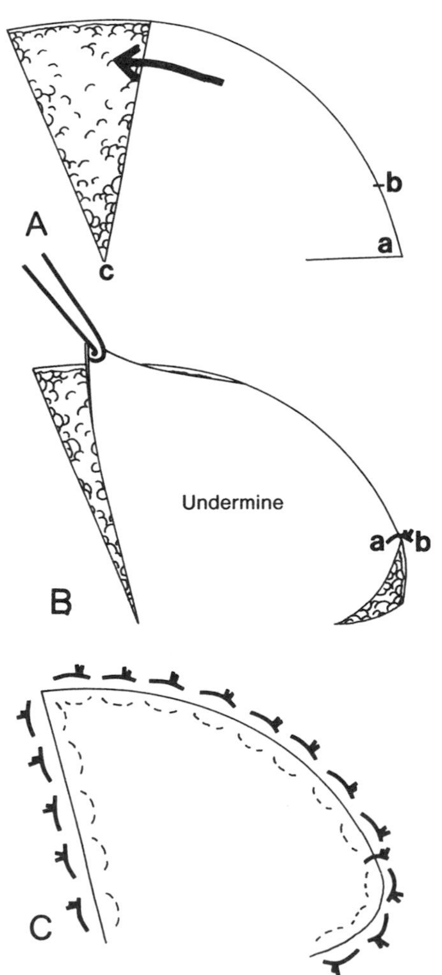

Figure 10.64. Alternate technique for closure of a triangular defect. Here, use half-buried horizontal mattress stitches throughout the closure.

triangle cannot be excised from the end of the arc, either for cosmetic considerations or because the region does not permit enough room for excision. Extend an arch from the base of a triangle similar to that previously described, ending at the same level as the point of the triangle (*c*), so that point *a* and point *c* are at the same level. Then mark point *b* on the arc so that the length of *ab* is equal to half the length of the base of the triangle. Undermine the area, and suture point *a* to point *b*, and close the original triangular defect (Fig. 10.64*B* and *C*). This alternative, however, cuts into the base of the flap and may compromise the flap's blood supply.

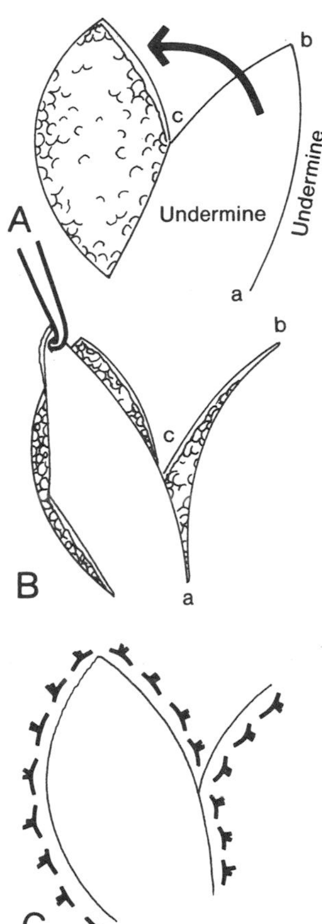

Figure 10.65. Interpolation flap. See text for discussion.

OVAL DEFECT (INTERPOLATION FLAP)

We believe that this flap should be commonly used in emergency medicine to close an oval defect. In this case, redraw the defect with a marking pencil over the site adjacent to it which is to be used (Fig. 10.65*A*). Incise and undermine the flap and tissue adjacent to it, as in Fig. 10.65*A*. The base of the flap must have a good vascular supply for the flap to survive. Then rotate the flap (Fig. 10.65*A* and *B*), which results in approximation of the upper half of line *ab* to line *cb*. Then close the defect by using half-buried horizontal mattress sutures, as shown in Fig. 10.65*C*.

REPAIR OF SPECIFIC TYPES OF WOUNDS

Closure of Wounds of Unequal Thickness

To approximate the edges of a wound in which the opposing sides are of unequal thickness, undermine both edges in the subcutaneous tissue plane at approximately the same depth. Then bring a "flap" of subcutaneous tissue from the thicker side to the thinner side beneath the area undermined. This "subcutaneous closure" elevates the depressed wound edge and permits good approximation of the wound.

Tangential lacerations can be closed in a number of ways, depending on the site and length of the laceration. An important factor is the angle at which the tangential wound is made. When the angle is not acute, resulting in a laceration such as the one shown in Fig. 10.66*A*, the optimal method of closure is to change the wound into a perpendicular laceration by excising the margins as shown in Fig. 10.66*B*. Do not use this on the face. Then undermine the subcutaneous tissue, and approximate the wound edges (Fig. 10.66*C*). When the angle of the tangential laceration is acute, then approximate the subcutaneous tissue, following which, bring together the deep dermal layers on the opposing edges of the wound by using ei-

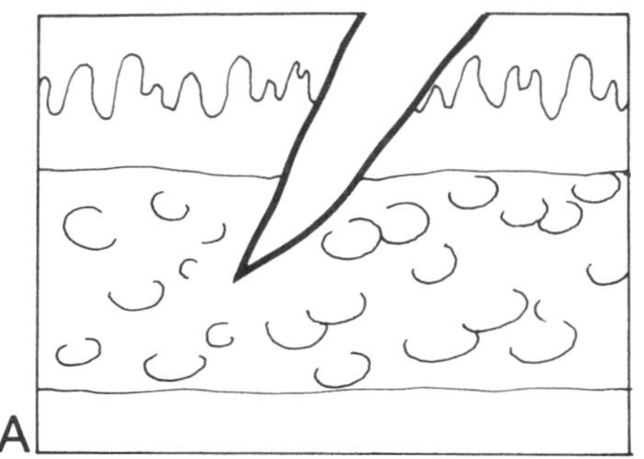

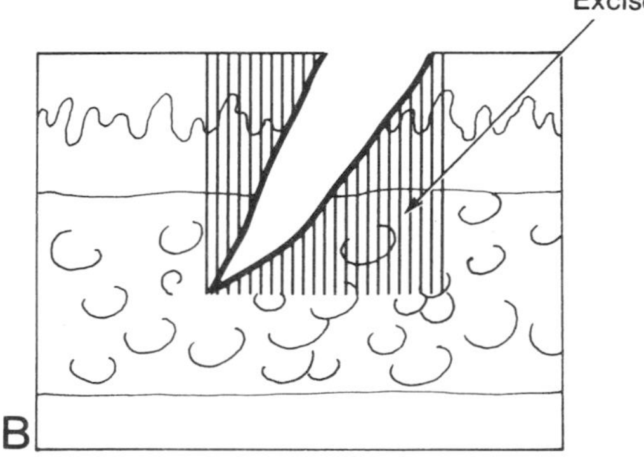

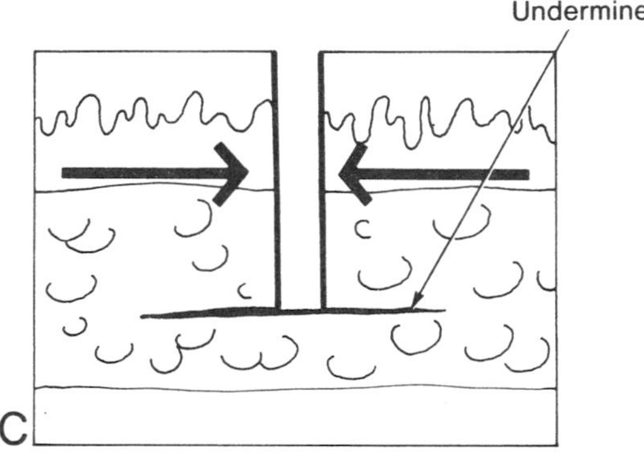

Figure 10.66. Repair of a tangential laceration. See text for discussion.

ther a buried suture or a half-buried horizontal mattress closure. Approximate the subcutaneous layer by using a buried technique for the knot, thus permitting the skin layer to be free (see Fig. 10.26, earlier). Then approximate the superficial dermis and epidermis with skin tape, because sutures placed at this site usually result in overriding of the wound edges. Apply a pressure dressing to all these lacerations, and leave it in place for a period of 1 or 2 days.

MULTIPLE LACERATIONS ON THE FOREHEAD

When lacerations on the forehead are adjacent to one another, suturing each may be impossible or may result in necrosis of the skin bridges and a poor outcome. Excise such multiple lacerations, and make them into one laceration parallel to the relaxed skin-tension lines (Fig. 10.67). Then close this wound, which will result in a better scar.

Suturing through Hair

Much has been stated about shaving hair and the deleterious effect of hair on a clean wound. As was discussed in the section, Contaminated Wounds Preparation, earlier, shaving is associated with an increased rate of infection when compared with the rate in similar wounds that are not shaved. We recommend suturing through areas such as the eyebrow; after completion of the repair, pull the entangled hair through the sutures and away from the wound. With this method, one study reported no problem with infection (107). We recommend shaving only to facilitate visualization of the wound edges for suturing. Eyebrows and eyelashes take months to grow back and should *never* be shaved or removed to close a laceration. When excising the edges of a laceration in the eyebrow or another hair-bearing area, such as the scalp, direct the excision obliquely to the hair follicles, not perpendicular to the skin edges, to reduce loss of hair follicles (Fig. 10.68). The scalp often must be shaved, but we do not advocate shaving wide areas around a scalp wound or other areas of the body where there is significant hair growth, unless such hair interferes with the closure.

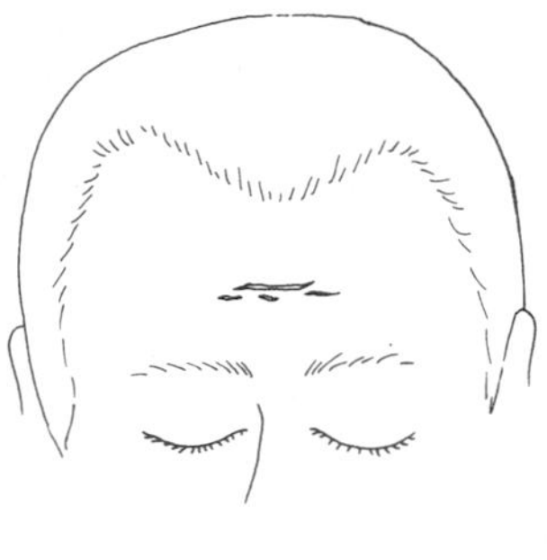
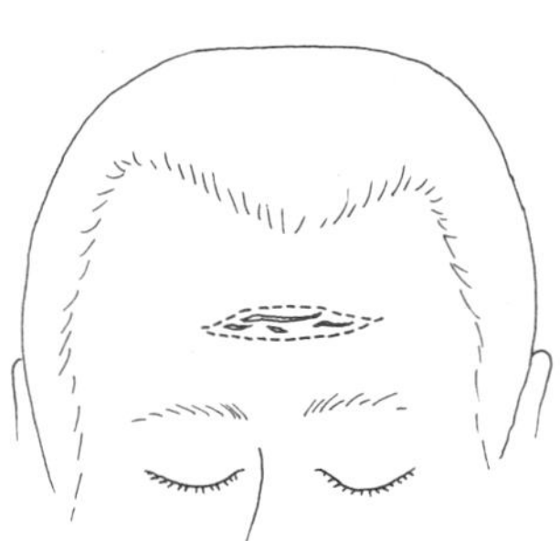

Figure 10.67. Excise multiple small lacerations of the forehead as a unit to create a single laceration. See text for discussion.

Abrasions

The debridement of abrasions was discussed in a previous section (Traumatic Wounds). Abrasions are commonly seen in areas such as the face, forehead, and extensor surfaces of major joints such as the knees and elbows. After thorough debridement has resulted in a clean surface, treat the abrasion like a burn and cover it with either Xeroform or Scarlet Red, which will seal over the abrasion with an antibacterial ointment gauze dressing. Permit this dressing to loosen spontaneously as the abrasion heals. Then apply sterile dry gauze dressings over the ointment gauze dressing and change them daily as they absorb exudate from the wound that comes through the porous surface dressings. Use a pressure bandage over certain areas where swelling is expected to occur, such as the forehead. Cleanse the area with a mild soap each day to remove exudate. In facial abrasions, leave these areas open, and apply an antibacterial ointment over them. Cleanse these abrasions 4 times a day to keep any exudate from accumulating.

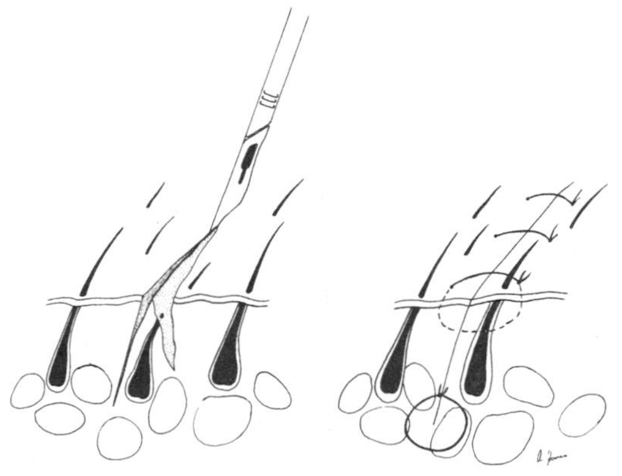

Figure 10.68. Debride lacerations along the eyebrow at an angle parallel to the hair bulb to reduce loss of hair follicles. See text for discussion.

Animal Bites

There continues to be much controversy surrounding the treatment of animal bites; some physicians advocate primary closure after irrigation, whereas others believe that a delayed closure should be performed in all cases (8, 59). We advocate the following regimen. Cleanse and debride the area. Ascertain if there may be joint penetration. If it is decided that joint penetration is not likely, irrigated the wound thoroughly with saline. Excise 1 mm of skin and subcutaneous tissue around the edges of the bite along the walls of the puncture wound. This resected tissue contains most of the bacterial contaminants. After this, close the elliptical wound site. This can be done in areas over joints and in all other areas of the body, including the face. In wounds that appear clean and superficial, irrigation without excision of the edges may be all that is needed; follow this by closure with either skin tape or sutures.

Avoid deep subcutaneous sutures in these wounds. These wounds must be carefully checked during follow-up for any signs of infection. If there is joint penetration, suggestion of deep structures being involved, or a severely contaminated wound, then perform irrigation, debridement, and a delayed primary closure. Give the patient oral antibiotics. Cephalosporins are an excellent choice for most animal bites. *Staphylococcus aureus* remains the most common cause of infection in most bites. Other common agents include *Streptococcus pyogenes* and *Pasteurella multocida* (particularly in cat bites).

Human Bites

Most human bites can be divided into those involving the face and those involving the hand. Controversy remains as to whether facial wounds should be closed primarily; however, because of the profuse vascularity of the face, infections have not been a problem in our experience. We recommend that bites over the head or the face should be cleansed, debrided, thoroughly irrigated, and closed loosely. Give these patients oral penicillin for treatment of infections from human mouth flora.

Bites of the hand are due to either a direct bite or a punch with metacarpophalangeal region striking an opponent's teeth. These latter "bites" are associated with a much higher incidence of infection. Debride and thoroughly irrigate these wounds, and give the patient oral penicillin without wound closure. If there is joint penetration or if there is any sign of infection in a patient seen more than 24 hours after the bite, admit the patient. Perform delayed closure of the wound 4 days later or longer if still not clean. Primary closure of human bites to the hand has been advocated by some; however, no harm is produced by a delayed closure, whereas significant harm may be produced with a primary closure. Therefore we advocate a delayed closure at 4 days or more for human bites of the hand.

In bites over other areas of the body, whether to close the wound primarily or do a delayed closure is contingent on the location of the wound and the depth. In areas such as the penis, we advocate loose approximation after thorough irrigation and administration of antibiotics. In regions where the skin is very close to bone and periosteum may have been penetrated (e.g., the pretibial region or ulnar border of the forearm or olecranon), delayed closure should be the procedure after thorough debridement and irrigation of the wound. The antibiotic of choice for the treatment of human bites is penicillin. Under no circumstances should subcutaneous sutures be placed in a human bite unless the bite is excised.

Avulsions of the Skin

There are a number of different types of avulsive injuries. When the skin is completely avulsed and is brought to the emergency center, remove the underlying fat of the avulsed skin, and trim the skin and replaced it as a free graft (66). Incomplete lacerations often involve the deep layer of the dermis.

Incomplete Lacerations

Treat windshield injury, in which the epidermis and papillary layer of the skin are sharply cut but the deep papillary layer is intact, producing a partial-thickness avulsion of the skin, by excision of the very loose epidermal pieces of skin. Place either a Xeroform or Scarlet Red dressing over the wounds, and apply a pressure bandage. These injuries are commonly seen on the forehead. An alternate way of treating these injuries is to apply an ointment dressing and a compression bandage for a few days; however, this method produces more scar because it involves leaving pieces of skin in place that are so small and "avascular" that they do not survive (107).

A curvilinear laceration, especially where there is a semicircular wound producing a trap-door type of flap, is a very difficult wound to manage, particularly when it occurs on the face. As the wound heals, contraction results, and a large amount of scar tissue develops (52). Excise the edges of a beveled wound to full-thickness skin so that a 90-degree angle is produced between the incision and the skin surface. In this fashion, a minimal amount of raw surface is present for healing by scar tissue, and the stage is set for optimal healing (Fig. 10.66) (52). Undermining in these beveled flap lacerations on the face presents a problem because of the compromise in lymphatic and venous drainage, which leads to elevation and congestion of the flap as it heals. For this reason, treat these lacerations with a compressive dressing (52). If the laceration is small or is in a "loose skin" area, complete excision and linear closure in the relaxed skin-tension lines will give the best results.

Complete Avulsions

There are five methods of treating avulsion injuries:

1. Debridement alone (abrasion).
2. Debridement and excision of soft tissue and repair primarily or secondarily.
3. Debridement and excision of avulsion flap and use of this flap as a free graft after defatting the undersurface.
4. Debridement and use of a split-thickness skin graft to cover the defect.
5. Debridement and covering the defect with a pedicle flap.

A question is always raised as to whether a flap with a small pedicle base can survive. A safe rule of thumb for extremities is that when the ratio of the width of the base of the pedicle to the length of the pedicle is 1:2 or more, the flap will usually survive. In the face, a base-to-pedicle length ratio of 1:5 or 1:6 is considered safe because of the heightened vascularity. If the pedicle appears tenuous (with the exception of the face), the safest approach is to remove it and replace it as a free graft after defatting the undersurface as suggested in no. 3 in the list. This maximizes the survivability of the pedicle.

GUNSHOT WOUNDS

Not all gunshot wounds appear to need debridement (50, 68, 111). With strict asepsis, placing the injured extremity in a splint with elevation may avoid infection in most gunshot wounds without debridement (50, 111). Debridement is unnecessary for wounds caused by bullets whose muzzle energy is less than 400 foot-pounds. Devitalized and contaminated tissue is more likely with higher-velocity wounds or shotgun wounds (111). When debridement is necessary, plan the incision so that it is done along the length of the track and so that all devitalized tissue can be debrided. After debridement, close the wound as a delayed closure. In some high-velocity wounds in which marked tissue destruction has occurred, a graft may be needed after adequate debridement.

ESCHAROTOMY FOR BURNS

Full-thickness burned skin has a leathery consistency and resists stretch. Edema develops beneath the burn, and a tourniquet-like effect occurs on an extremity or the chest (38), resulting in circulatory embarrassment and necrosis. If respiratory embarrassment due to limited respiratory excursion is caused by a constricting eschar on the anterior thorax, then escharotomy is imperative.

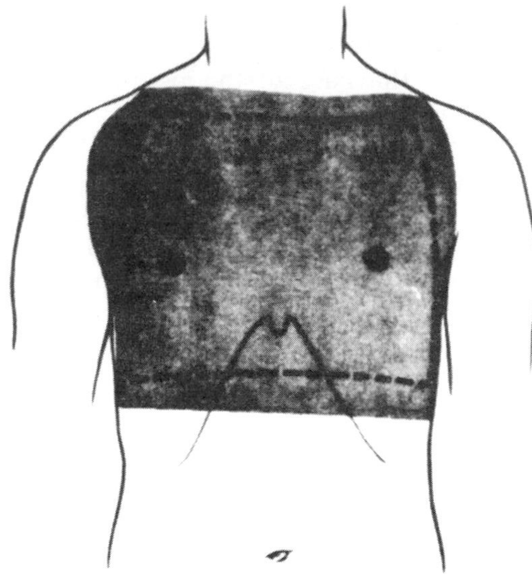

Figure 10.69. The site for escharotomy to relieve a constricting eschar of the anterior thorax. (From Edlich RF, Haynes BW, Larkham N, et al: Emergency department treatment, triage and transfer protocols for the burn patient. JACEP 7:153, 1978, with permission.)

TECHNIQUE

Make a lateral incision in the anterior axillary line extending from 2 cm below the clavicle to the ninth or tenth ribs on each side of the chest. Join the top and bottom of each incision transversely to form a square (Fig. 10.69) (10, 38, 64, 92). Hemorrhage from the incision is not usually a problem in these patients. Some may have an occasional bleeding vessel that needs ligation (10).

In circumferential burns of a limb, there may be a tourniquet-like effect on the extremity with subsequent circulatory embarrassment. During arterial tamponade, progressive loss of sensation and impaired joint proprioception are reliable early clinical signs of vascular insufficiency. Changes in digital blood flow can be monitored with a Doppler flowmeter. If it seems likely that the patient has circulatory embarrassment, then escharotomy through the burned skin restores circulation. Make the incision in the following manner. With the limb in the supine position, perform escharotomies midmedially and laterally (Fig. 10.70). Carry the incisions into the deep fascia to provide adequate decompression (10) only for burns extending through the dermis. Most burns extend only to the dermis and can be adequately decompressed by extending the incision only to the subcutaneous layer. In making these incisions, be careful to avoid the radial nerve at the wrist volarly and the superficial peroneal nerve at the fibular neck. The incision should extend from the proximal extent of the burn to its dis-

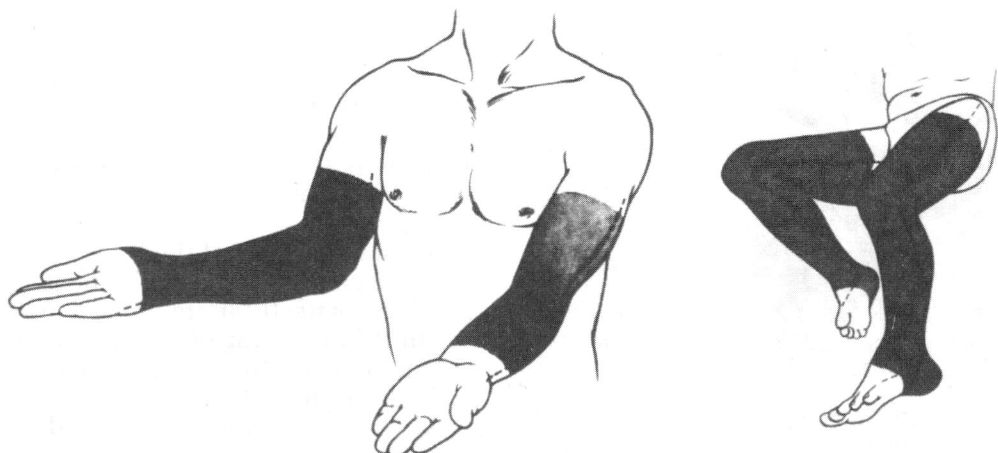

Figure 10.70. The midmedial and midlateral escharotomies for burns of arms and legs. The burned skin is the dark area. (From Edlich RF, Haynes BW, Larkham N, et al: Emergency department treatment, triage and transfer protocols for the burn patient. JACEP 7:155, 1978, with permission.)

tal margin and a short distance into normal skin. Carry midlateral and midmedial incisions over the involved joints (38). After decompression of the burn, rapid improvement in the color of the limb and return of distal pulses occur. The conscious patient often notes rapid disappearance in numbness and may experience brief, excruciating pain because of the sudden increase in blood flow. After decompression, apply adequate pressure dressings to the affected limb. Some authors believe that the extremity should be covered with a light plaster-of-paris shell and elevated (11, 44, 116). We do not think that a pressure dressing or a plaster splint should be applied after escharotomy. Instead, apply a burn dressing, and elevate the limb.

In the proximal and middle phalanges, the volar neurovascular bundles are straddled by two sheaths of fascia. The volar fascial sheath is called Grayson's ligament, the fibers of which join the flexor tendon. The dorsal ligament is called Cleland's ligament. The fibers of Cleland's ligament are oriented obliquely and secure the skin to the phalanx. Incise this ligament laterally to decompress the vascular compartment in a circumferentially burned finger. Extending the skin incision deep into the subcutaneous tissue of the finger and undermine dorsally and volarly (Fig. 10.71) (103).

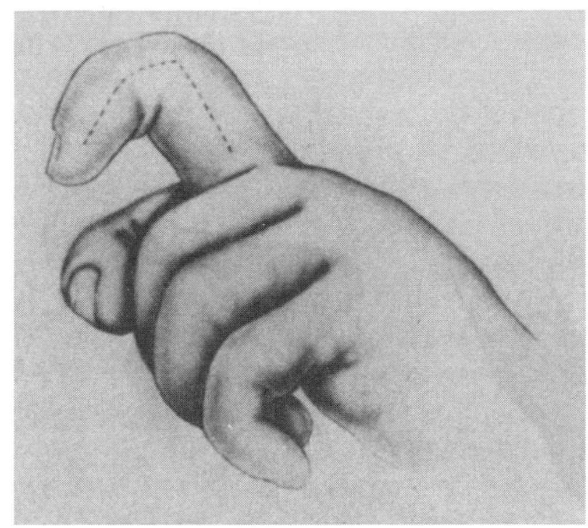

Figure 10.71. Medial skin incision from the metacarpophalangeal joint to the lateral edge of the nail to decompress a circumferentially burned finger. (From Edlich RF, Haynes BW, Larkham N, et al: Emergency department treatment, triage and transfer protocols for the burn patient. JACEP 7:156, 1978, with permission.)

SPECIAL REPAIRS

MULTIPLE SMALL SKIN FLAPS

Small skin flaps are commonly due to window glass shattered when a forehead strikes an automobile windshield. Such an accident produces U-shaped lacerations, which often contain fragments of glass. Bunched-up, small lacerations, such as these, can be excised together after removing the glass (Fig. 10.72).

Lacerations of the Eyelid

Eyelid lacerations can be classified as extramarginal (not involving the lid border) or intramarginal. Extramarginal lacerations can be superficial or deep. Intramarginal lacerations can be divided into those that are canalicular, usually avulsions, and those that are extracanalicular (85). Simple suturing of the edges is adequate for superficial extramarginal lacerations. When the laceration is horizontal, a simple layer-by-layer closure provides good results; however, when the laceration is vertical, contraction may occur, necessitating a Z-plasty at a later time. If less than one-third of the length of the lid is missing, minimal debridement and approximation will give good results (85). *For deep extramarginal lacerations of the upper lid, the levator palpebrae and the tarso-orbital fascia must be approximated to avoid ptosis.* Repair of the orbicularis oculi muscle also is a must. For these reasons, we recommend referral of all deep extramarginal lacerations that involve a large portion of the lid.

When the margin of the lid is involved and the canaliculi are not, perfectly approximate the margin to avoid notching or buckling of the lid margin, as shown in Fig. 10.73 (74). In most cases, 4% cocaine and epinephrine (1:2,000) can be in-

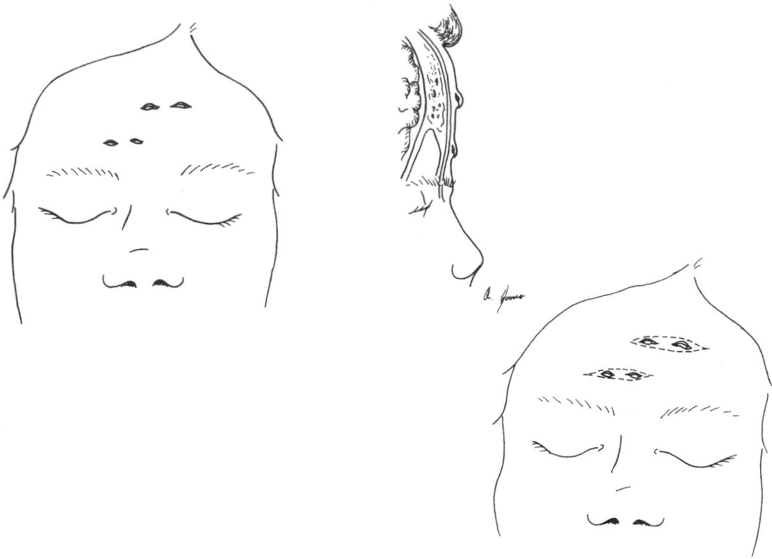

Figure 10.72. Multiple small avulsion flaps in the forehead, due to shattered auto window glass, often have glass particles embedded in the wound. After removing these particles, achieve a better result by excising the avulsion flap. See text for discussion.

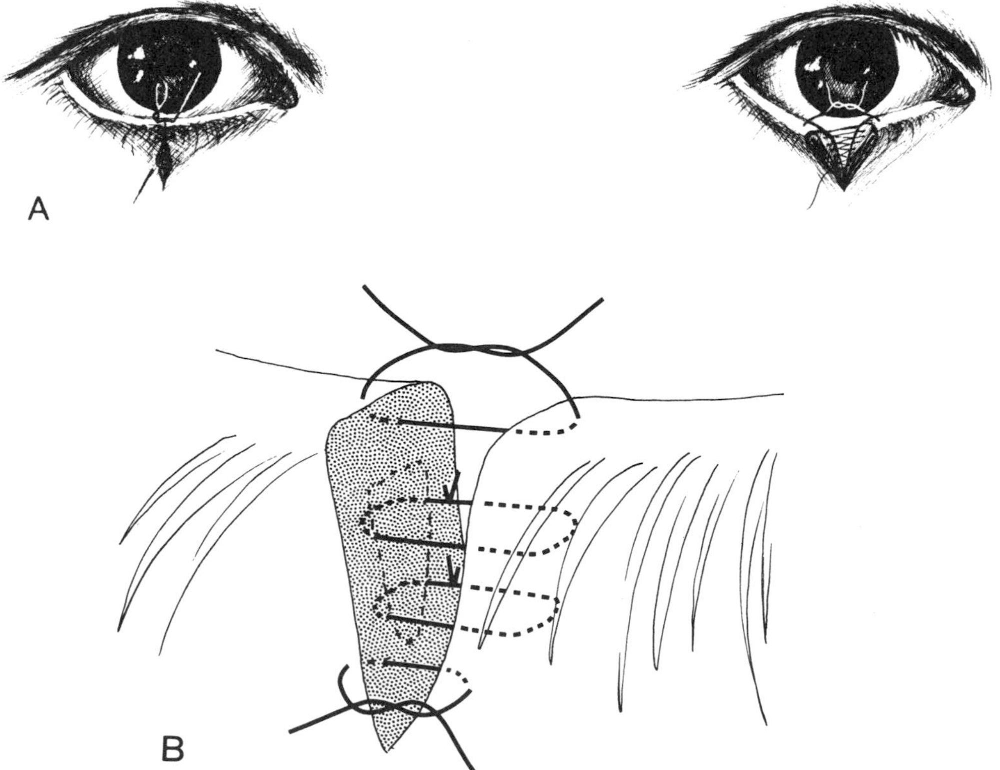

Figure 10.73. Repair of an eyelid laceration involving the margin of the lid. Approximate the tarsal plate with fine absorbable suture material. After this, approximate the skin and subcutaneous tissue with 6-0 or 7-0 nylon. See text for discussion.

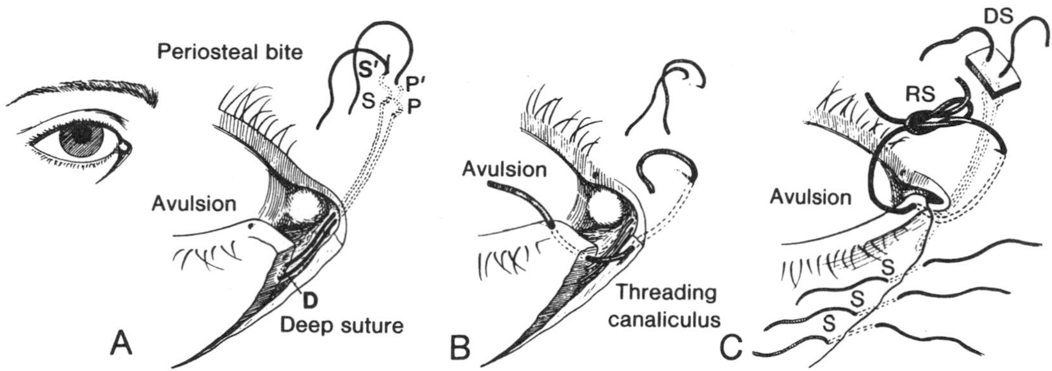

Figure 10.74. Avulsion of the medial aspect of the lower lid. Although this repair should be performed by a plastic surgeon or ophthalmologist, the technique should be familiar to the emergency physician. *A*: Insert a mattress suture beneath the canaliculus and secure the avulsion flap as shown. The points marked *S* and *P* indicate periosteum having been incorporated within the suture to provide a strong anchoring stitch. *B*: Then thread the canaliculus. Note that a suture needle is passed into the nasal aspect of the cut canaliculus and passes out of the skin on the lateral border of the nose. Use heavy chromic catgut suture for this procedure. *C*: Then repair the avulsion. Tie the thread through the canaliculus very loosely to form a loop as shown. (From Minsky H: Surgical repair of recent lid lacerations. Surg Gynecol Obstet 75:455, 1942, with permission.)

stilled in the conjunctiva for adequate anesthesia of the inner portion of the lid (85). Most of these lacerations are not painful (107). Therefore pain after an orbital or lid laceration usually indicates that a foreign body is present, or there is a hematoma within the orbit, and this must be evaluated. When an intramarginal laceration involves the canaliculus, perform a complex repair, as shown in Fig. 10.74. This repair requires meticulous care and, because it can be associated with injury to the lacrimal duct apparatus, should be performed by a specialist.

Treat defects of 1.5 cm or less with a releasing incision that extends into the lateral canthus. Such an incision should course inferior to the lateral canthus in a normal wrinkle line. It is essential that the canthus remain attached to the upper lid and bone. Excise a Burow's triangle, which will release the skin and allow the edges of the eyelid to be brought together to approximate the lower lid defect (Fig. 10.75).

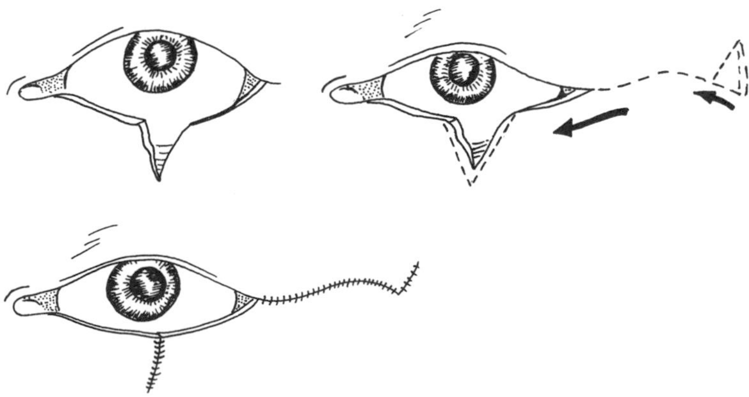

Figure 10.75. Accommodate loss of tissue in the lower lid relatively easily with the technique shown here and described in the text.

Approximate lacerations of the eyebrow regions in the usual manner, depending on the wound. Do not shave the eyebrows because shaving increases infection (see Contaminated Wounds Preparation, earlier), and the eyebrow is slow to regrow. If the laceration is deep and involves the orbicularis oculi, approximate this muscle before closure of the skin.

FLAP LACERATION
Malar Eminence

A U-shaped flap laceration along the malar eminence that has a deep oblique edge often has unequal wound edges. If one excises the wound in a traditional fashion, the shorter side will be of unequal length and will be difficult to bring together. Avoid this by excising only the dermis and a small amount of subcutaneous tissue (Fig. 10.67). The wound edges are "squared off" by this excision and then readily closed (Figs. 10.67 and 10.76).

Nasal Lacerations

The repair of nasal lacerations differs, depending on the area of the nose involved and the extent of the laceration. Provide anesthesia with an infraorbital nerve block or a nose block, as indicated in Chapter 3, Anesthesia and Regional Blocks. Achieve topical analgesia of the nasal mucosa with cocaine-soaked cotton pledgets. When dealing with small lacerations of the nose, use a local infiltration of lidocaine containing epinephrine.

Repair lacerations limited to the **outer aspect** of the nose (which are not through the nasal vestibule) as simple lacerations in the routine fashion. Scars placed across areas in which there is a hollowing of the skin, such as the side of the nose, along the nasolabial junction, inferior to the lower lid and below the eye, tend to shorten and obliterate the hollow and restrict normal motion of the skin as the skin adheres to underlying fascia. Never suture cartilage, and only minimally debride it when indicated, followed by closure of the mucosa, skin, and subcutaneous tissue, which will approximate the cartilage. When they are involved in a laceration, replace cartilaginous structures in their normal anatomic position and close the wound. Close wounds of the nose with

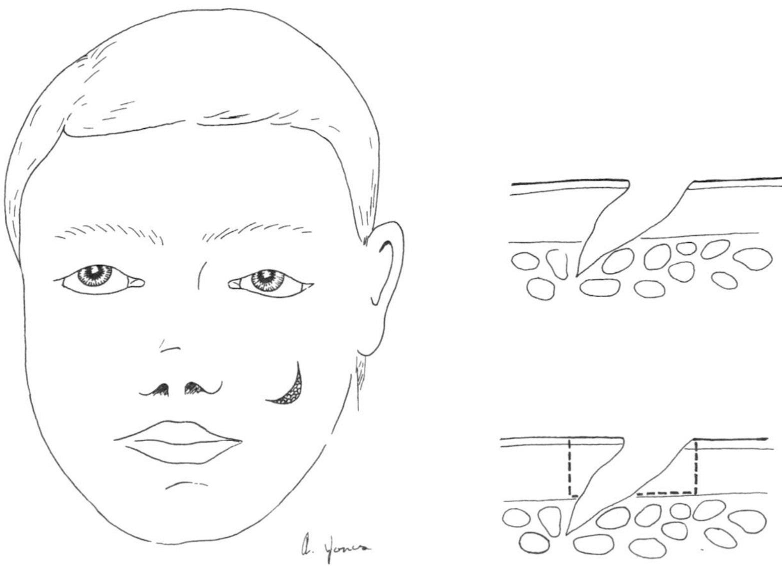

Figure 10.76. If lacerations of the malar eminence that are U-shaped flaps are closed without any revision, a hypertrophic area on the convex edge of the wound will result. Excise the edges as shown. See text for discussion.

very limited or no excision of vascularly embarrassed tissue (107). This is a key point in repairing nasal lacerations because very little "excess" tissue on the nose can be used. The subcutaneous tissue of the distal nose requires no approximation because the distance from the skin to the cartilaginous surface is very small, and there is very little subcutaneous tissue in the interspace. When dealing with extensive lacerations, place the nasal structures in an anatomic position with the wound edges approximated as closely as possible, and then suture them. Revisions can be made later, should they be required.

When the **nasal vestibule** is involved in a through-and-through laceration of the ala nasi or tip of the nose, only three or four fine Vicryl or catgut sutures are needed to approximate the nasal lining loosely. We prefer to use 5-0 or 6-0 suture material in this repair. After the approximation of the edges, place a pack of ½-inch gauze impregnated with an antibacterial in the vestibule to support the repair and promote hemostasis (107). Then repair the skin in the routine fashion, being careful not to incorporate the cartilaginous structures within the suture.

In **septal** injuries, use the minimal number of sutures necessary to approximate the wound edges. The important consideration in septal injuries is to provide adequate drainage to avoid the development of a septal hematoma or abscess. After repair of the septum, place an anterior nasal pack with ½-inch gauze impregnated with an antibacterial agent. Remove the pack in 2 days, and inspect the wound for any accumulation of hematoma or the development of infection. Place another anterior pack if indicated by continuing discharge from the wound.

In patients with **nasal bone or cartilage fractures**, realign and support the fragments with an intranasal packing as well as an external splint (see Chapter 8, Otolaryngologic and Ophthalmologic Procedures). Inspect the alar and lateral cartilages, minimally debride them if shredded, and reposition them anatomically. Repair first the lacerations of the nasal mucosa, followed by repair of the skin. Always inspect the septal mucosa in patients with either a nasal bone fracture or a contusion injury to the nose.

A **septal hematoma** is diagnosed when a soft and fluctuant bulge of the septal mucosa into the inferior meatus is seen. Septal hematomas are the same color as the septal mucosa and are not ecchymotic. Many of these will become infected with *Staphylococcus aureus*, and the ensuing abscess will necrose the cartilage and result in a nasal deformity or perforation (78). Perform incision and drainage to relieve the hematoma. Incise just posterior to the mucocutaneous junction after anesthetizing with 4% cocaine. The technique is as follows (78):

1. Begin the incision as high as possible on the septum and carry it down to the floor of the nose, as shown in Fig. 10.77.
2. Then make a horizontal incision along the floor of the nasal septum, forming an L-shaped flap. If the horizontal incision is not made, the initial vertical incision will close and result in little or no drainage. Some authors remove a piece of the septal membrane at the junction of the limbs of the "L" to assure adequate drainage.
3. Then insert a drain, begin antimicrobial therapy, and see the patient daily to evacuate any clots that may form (78).

If an avulsion of the skin is present at the tip of the nose, a full-thickness skin graft may be needed (Fig. 10.78). The donor graft usually selected is derived from behind the ear. Apply an external splint to these complex lacerations by using Xeroform ointment gauze, followed by a cotton-ball dressing and an anterior intranasal pack for support (52). Complex lacerations of the nose often involve some tissue loss. A small defect that measures less than 0.5 cm can be closed pri-

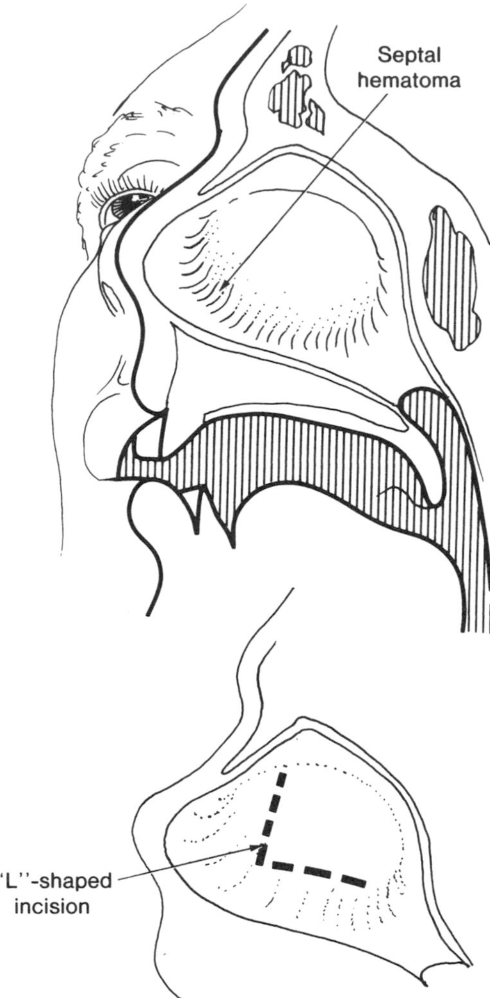

Figure 10.77. Use an L-shaped incision to drain a septal hematoma. Begin the incision as high as possible on the septum and carry it down to the floor of the nose. Then make a horizontal connecting incision along the floor of the nose, forming an "L." See text for discussion.

marily by elliptical incision and advancing the edges. This usually requires extending the laceration on both sides to prevent a dog-ear deformity (Fig. 10.79). When a defect is less than 2 cm in size, replace the tissue as a composite graft, which consists of skin, subcutaneous fat, and cartilage. A plastic surgeon should perform this procedure (Fig. 10.80). For tissue loss of the nasal margin producing a defect of less than 3 mm, use direct ap-

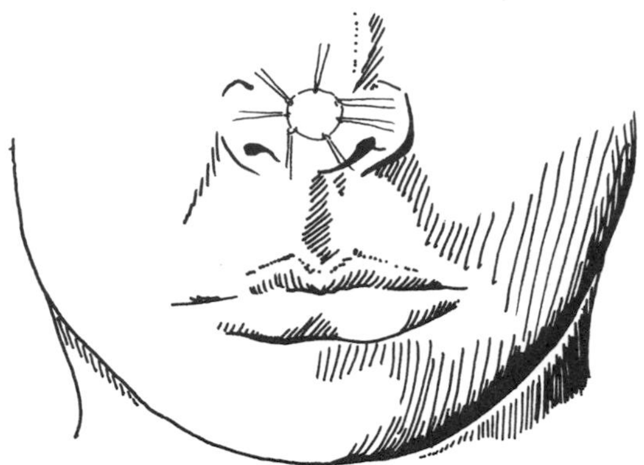

Figure 10.78. Treat avulsion of the tip of the nose with a full-thickness graft taken from behind the ear and applied to the tip of the nose. Secure the graft by using fine 6-0 nylon sutures and a cotton-ball dressing applied over the graft. Be certain to remove all fat from the skin graft before application.

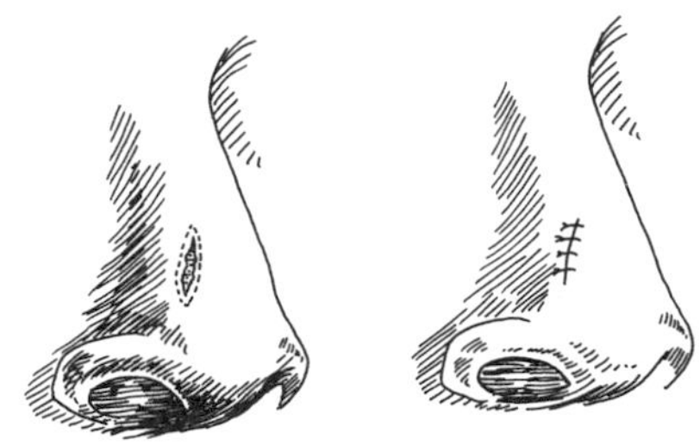

Figure 10.79. Debride a laceration with irregular edges on the nose. After minimal debridement, close the laceration primarily, provided the length-to-width ratio is 3:1 or greater.

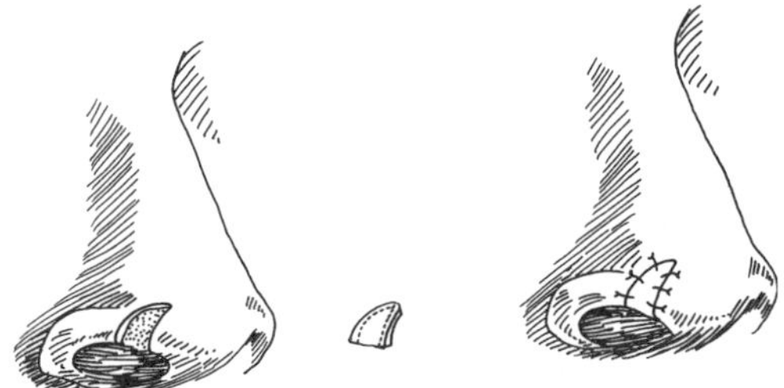

Figure 10.80. Place a composite graft by trimming the edges (see text). Then apply the graft, suturing the mucosal layer followed by the subcutaneous layer, and finally place the skin sutures.

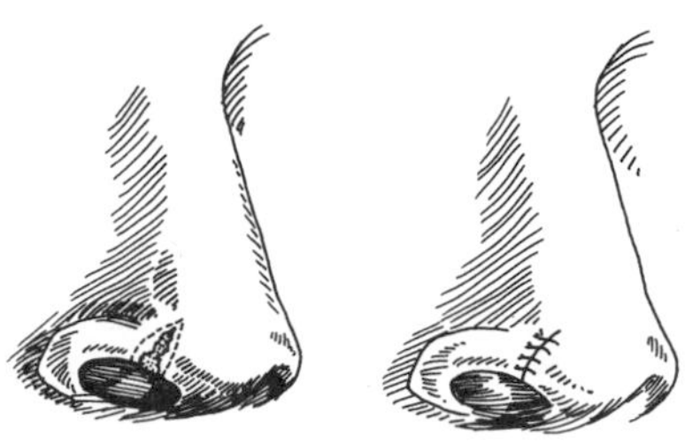

Figure 10.81. A V-shaped laceration of the nose may require minimal debridement; close the defect primarily when it is less than 0.5 cm in width at the base.

proximation (Fig. 10.81) with minimal debridement.

Lip and Oral Mucosa Lacerations

Repair deep lacerations of the lip in a two-layer closure. Approximate the deep musculature with either 5-0 plain catgut or Vicryl, followed by a surface closure of the skin and subcutaneous tissue (Fig. 10.82*A*) (74). Carefully approximate the

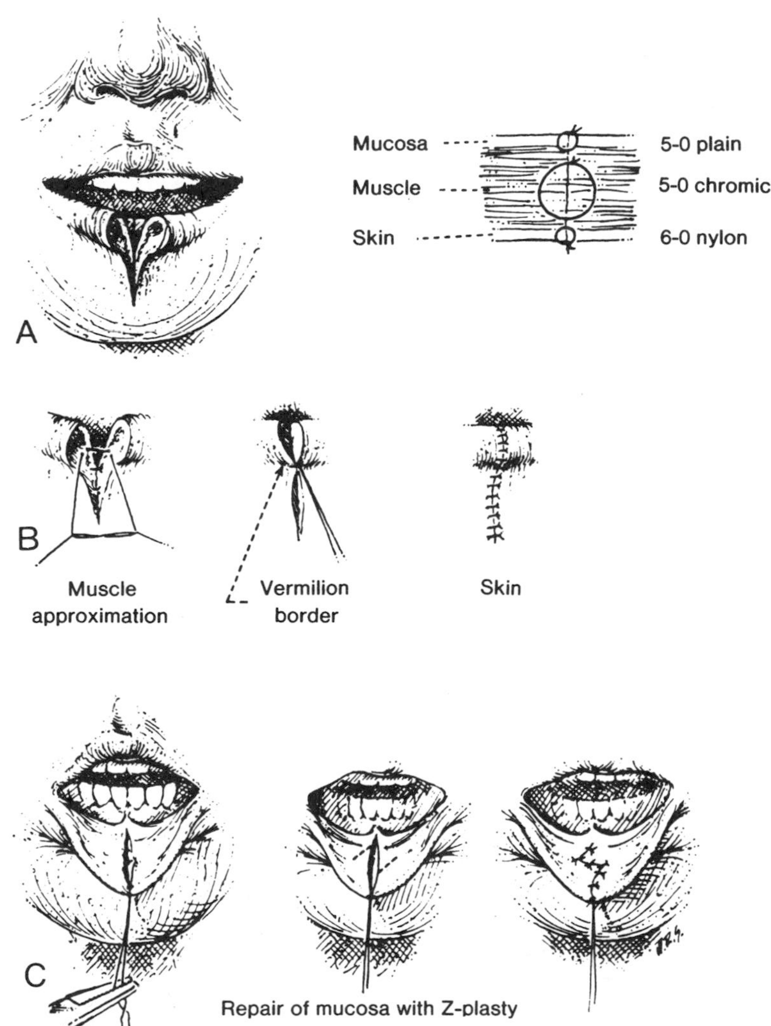

Figure 10.82. Repair the lower lip involved in a through-and-through laceration by three-layer closure, approximating the mucosa with 5-0 plain gut, muscle with 5-0 chromic, and skin with 6-0 nylon. Approximate the vermilion border carefully. Use a Z-plasty in the repair of a linear laceration involving the inner aspect of the lower lip to avoid contraction of the scar. (From Curtin J: Basic plastic surgical principles in repair of facial lacerations. Ill Med J 129:658, 1966, with permission.)

edges of the vermilion border to avoid a deformity. Approximate this border first, before placement of any other skin sutures (Fig. 10.82*B*). In linear lacerations that extend vertically along the mucosal border to the lower lip to the gingival margin, close the laceration with a Z-plasty primarily in the emergency center, as shown in Fig. 10.82*C*, to prevent contracture, which will result in a permanent deformity (49). If the wound is contaminated, do not perform a Z-plasty in the emergency center. Close a small defect with tissue loss of 1 to 1.5 cm primarily after debridement of the skin edges and careful approximation of the layers, as indicated earlier.

Gingival Lacerations

Gingival lacerations in which the gingiva is avulsed away from the teeth, exposing the root, are seen particularly in automobile accidents in which the passenger strikes the mouth against the dashboard or steering wheel. Suture the gingiva back into place in the manner shown in Fig. 10.83. Pass the needle 2 to 3 mm below the edge of the gingival margin so as to pass easily in the gap between the teeth. Loop the suture around the teeth, which are used to support the gingiva in its normal position, similar to a pole holding up a plant. Cut the knot short on the inner side of the teeth so as not to irritate the inner aspect of the lip.

LENGTHENING THE SHORTER SIDE OF A FOREHEAD LACERATION

With a forehead laceration that has a shorter side after debridement, lengthen the wound (as shown in Fig. 10.84). This lengthening will produce a longer scar. However, incisions made within relaxed skin-tension lines will achieve a good cosmetic result.

Ear Lacerations

The anatomy of the ear is shown in Fig. 10.85. Repair lacerations involving the pinna as with any other soft tissue injury. Lacerations of the helix, tragus, or external meatus are discussed later.

The blood supply to the ear is excellent, and incomplete avulsions heal well. Infec-

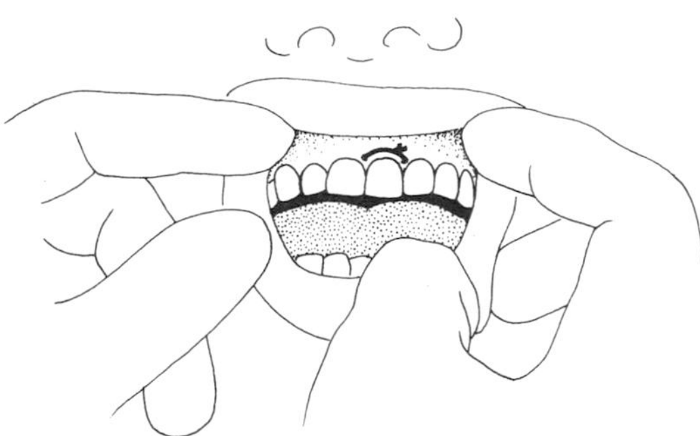

Figure 10.83. When the gingiva is avulsed away from a tooth, suture it by using the tooth as an anchoring point around which to hold the gingiva in place with the suture. Pass the suture 2 to 3 mm away from the edge of the gingival margin to pass in the gap between the teeth. Then wrap it around the posterior aspect and bring it out anteriorly. Achieve a more comfortable result by bringing the knot out posteriorly behind the teeth to avoid constant rubbing against the inner aspect of the lip.

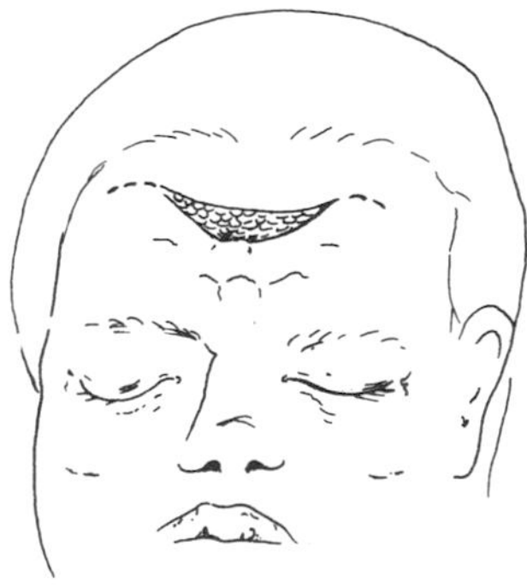

Figure 10.84. After debridement of a wound of the forehead with macerated edges, the wound edges may be of unequal length. Correct this by creating a gentle curve within the relaxed skin-tension lines of the forehead, as shown. When bringing the inferior edge toward the superior edge, excise the extra tissue along the incisions on either side while closing the wound. See text for discussion.

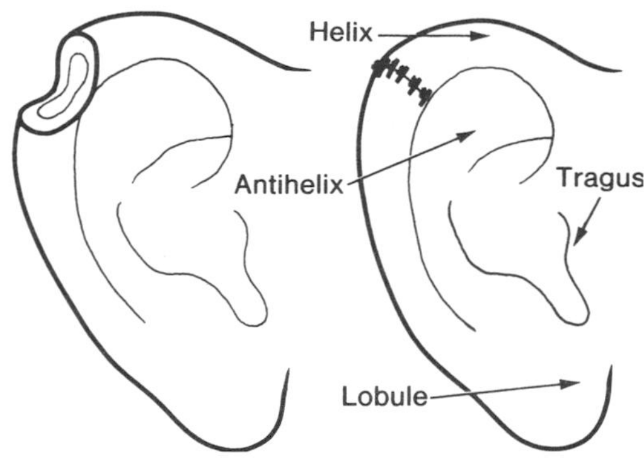

Figure 10.85. Repair of laceration involving a small segment of missing cartilage over the helix. See text for discussion.

tions are a hazard (75), because a chondritis may develop with even small lacerations; cleanse and repair minor lacerations meticulously. If cartilage is missing, approximation of the skin and maintenance of the anatomic configuration are important for good results (Fig. 10.85). A small defect of the ear that is less than 0.5 cm in length can be closed primarily. Perform the closure by excising small triangles in the antihelical fold, as shown in Fig. 10.86. The triangles permit primary closure of the defect. Remember not to place a suture within the cartilage but rather to include the perichondrium within the skin stitch.

In repairing extensive lacerations of the ear, trim the cartilage to the level of the skin and then close the wound by approximating the skin edges (Fig. 10.87). Incorporate the perichondrium in the skin suture, because closure with the perichondrium supports the skin closure and provides cartilaginous approximation. Do not suture the cartilage. The skin in the helix of the ear is adherent to the cartilage, and approximation of subcutaneous tissue (which is minimal in this area) is not indicated.

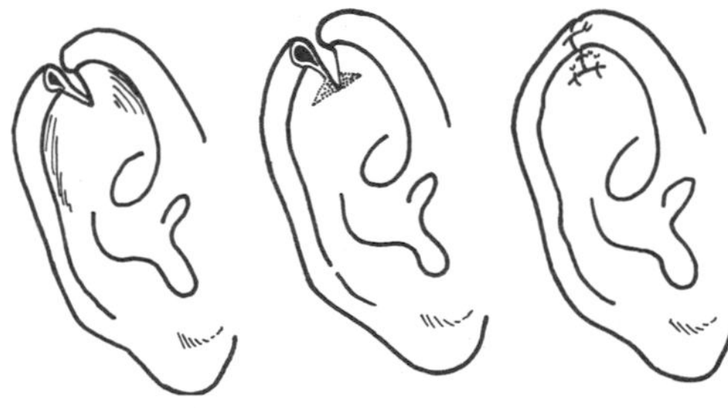

Figure 10.86. Close a defect of the ear primarily after excising two triangles from the apex of the wound. These triangles permit the wound edges to come together, which would otherwise be difficult to achieve because of the underlying cartilage.

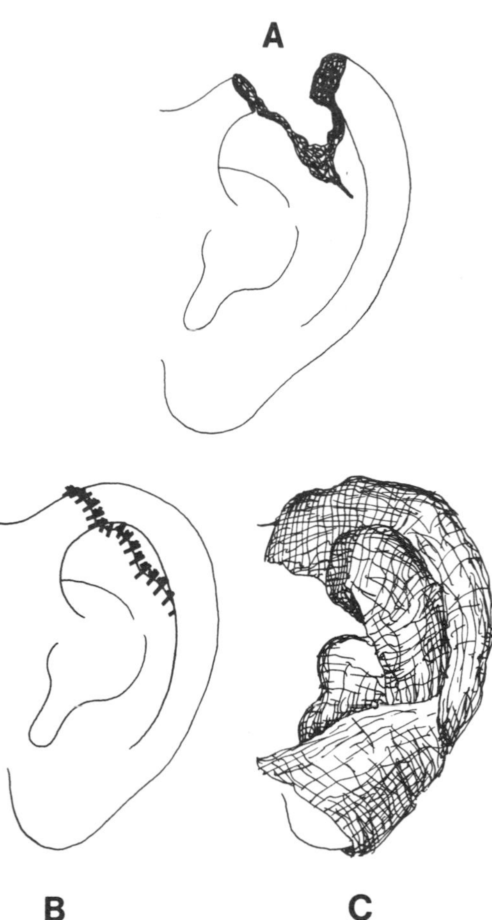

Figure 10.87. The repair of extensive lacerations of the ear. Trim the edges of the cartilage, and approximate the skin edges. Apply a Xeroform gauze dressing over the ear, followed by a bulky gauze dressing that maintains pressure over the ear to promote healing without hematoma formation. Place two folded 4 × 4-inch gauze pads behind the ear to provide a more secure dressing when wrapping the ear.

The dressing is the most important part of the repair of an ear laceration. Mold the dressing well to conform to the anatomic configuration of the ear to provide adequate support and prevent hematoma formation. Mineral oil–soaked cotton balls packed into the natural crevices of the auricle provide an excellent "cast," because the cotton balls retain their initial mold as a result of the oil. Use a single layer of Xeroform gauze to cover the sutures before application of the cotton balls. Hold this two-layered dressing in place with a bulky head dressing composed of gauze pads, providing support behind the ear as well as in front of it (108). Leave this dressing in place for 24 to 48 hours.

When a hematoma of the auricle is present, incise and drain it as shown in Fig. 10.88 (49). After the application of a Xeroform gauze dressing, saline-soaked cotton balls followed by a fluffy gauze pressure bandage encircling the head protect the ear from further hematoma formation. As the cotton balls dry, the cotton retains its shape and forms a well-molded firm cast over the ear. Leave this dressing in place for 24 to 48 hours. Serial drainage is usually necessary in these hematomas. Prescribe antibiotics for a perichondrial hematoma to prevent a perichondritis from developing.

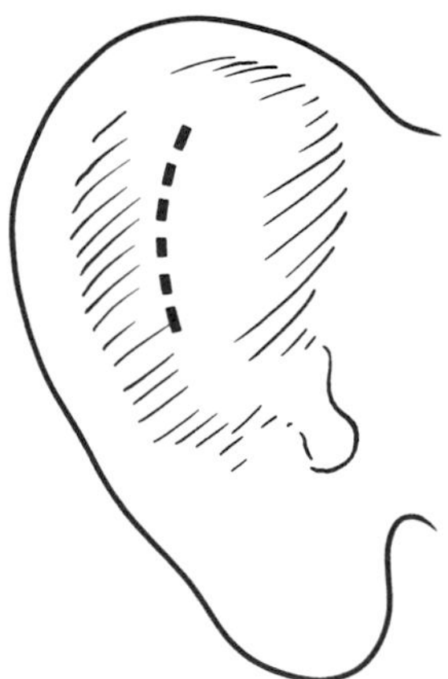

Figure 10.88. Drainage of a hematoma of the auricle. After the hematoma is drained, apply a Xeroform gauze dressing over the incision, and pack saline-soaked cotton balls over the Xeroform dressing to form a "cast" on the ear. Then cover this with a fluffy gauze pressure bandage encircling the head.

Lacerations may extend into the external meatus, usually as a result of a foreign object striking the ear. The skin in the external meatus is tightly adherent to the cartilage, and a cotton wick impregnated with an antibacterial otic solution will suffice to provide support as the laceration heals. Sutures are generally not indicated in this area. Be careful to check the tympanic membrane; if there are any signs of penetration, refer the patient for evaluation of injury to the ossicles.

MUSCLE INJURIES

With a laceration that penetrates into the muscle fascia, evaluate whether this injury is large or small and whether it is contaminated or clean (Fig. 10.89). Repair small rents in the fascia, if clean, because they can result in a hernia of the muscle, which can be symptomatic. If the wound is small and contaminated, open the fascia (Fig. 10.89*A*). Large fascial tears generally do not require repair. Repairing them may result in muscle compression and ischemia.

With a laceration into the muscle belly after debridement of devitalized muscle (devitalized muscle does not contract when incised), decide whether to do a delayed closure of the muscle and skin wound or to close primarily. If there is a possibility of severe contamination, it is best to pack the wound open with povidone–iodine (Betadine)-soaked gauze and to perform a delayed closure 3 to 5 days after the injury. Antibiotics are usually recommended. If suturing of the muscle is necessary, use horizontal mattress sutures, and pull the fascia together with absorbable sutures. If one approximates the edges with simple sutures, they will pull through the muscle fibers and not hold (Fig. 10.90).

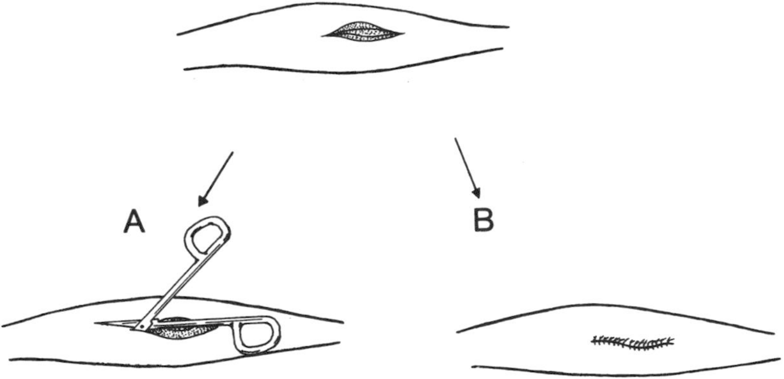

Figure 10.89. Small lacerations in muscle fascia can result in muscle herniation. Treat them as shown above and described in the text.

Fingertip Injuries

A number of reports exist in the literature on the various ways to manage fingertip injuries. Five ways currently exist:

1. Primary closure.
2. Healing by secondary intention.
3. Local advancement flap.
4. Skin graft.
5. Pedicle flap.

Primary closure, when possible, is the treatment of choice (55). When primary closure of a fingertip amputation will result in shortening and tenderness of the digit, use alternative methods. Skin grafts tend to contract and pose problems with regard to loss of normal sensation over the grafted skin. In 67% of cases, induration and fissuring occur at the site of the graft, and there is a decrease in sensation at the site (55).

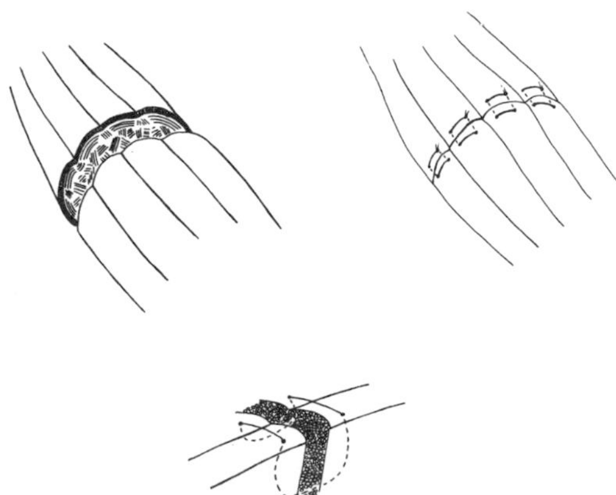

Figure 10.90. Repair large transverse lacerations through the belly of a muscle with horizontal mattress sutures. See text for discussion.

Healing by secondary intention is a conservative approach advocated by many authors and by us (6, 33, 45, 55, 63). When the avulsion exceeds 10 mm in the adult, some prefer the use of other procedures indicated later. Remarkably good results are achieved in children, including regrowth of amputated nails and phalanges, with healing by secondary intention (33). Dress the fingertip with Xeroform gauze and Telfa, followed by a fine-mesh gauze dressing. Then elevate the hand for 24 hours, and keep the dressing dry. Give the patient oral penicillinase-resistant antibiotics in the emergency center. See the patient in 48 hours, and remove the dressing. The patient subsequently soaks his hand in warm water for 15 minutes, 4 times a day, for 1 week, and permits the wound to epithelialize completely (33, 45). In a child, even with bone exposure, the wound heals without the development of osteomyelitis (33). Occasionally the stump may be painful, and, at times, troublesome remnants of the fingernail persist. It may take 1 month for healing to occur (33). Most adults treated conservatively are able to return to work within a few days (41). Indurated scars occur in 48% of patients treated conservatively, with reduced sensation in only 13% of patients (55). With conservative open treatment of fingertip amputations, the average healing time was 29 days (71). This treatment was used even when bone was exposed. Amputations of the fingertips were successfully treated with preservation of finger length and contour with retention of sensation and healing without loss of sensation or functional stability of the pad (71). Block the finger and cleanse the wound. Achieve hemostasis by a pressure dressing or with small sutures. Then cover the open wound with Bacitracin ointment and a dressing of tubular gauze. Place a four-pronged plastic splint over the gauze dressing for immobilization and protection (45). Although other techniques are described later, we strongly recommend conservative therapy whenever possible.

When a transverse amputation results in the bone of the distal phalanx being exposed, a number of alternative methods of closure exist. In the Kutler method of repair, a **local advancement flap** is transferred as a triangular flap from the proximal volar side of a finger amputation to the center of the wound, with good results (46). It is important to round off the bone by removing a small amount of phalanx with a rongeur to prevent tension on the flap (46). This method is illustrated in Figs. 10.61 and 10.91.

Skin grafts are commonly used to cover amputations of the distal phalanx, and some authors believe they are the treatment of choice (17). Skin grafts may be either split thickness, incorporating only a portion of the dermis, or full thickness. Split-thickness grafts have a tendency to shrink as much as 70%, which draws normally tactile skin over most of the defect (17). Contraction of the graft is minimal when a thicker graft is used (9). In the emergency center, a full-thickness graft is

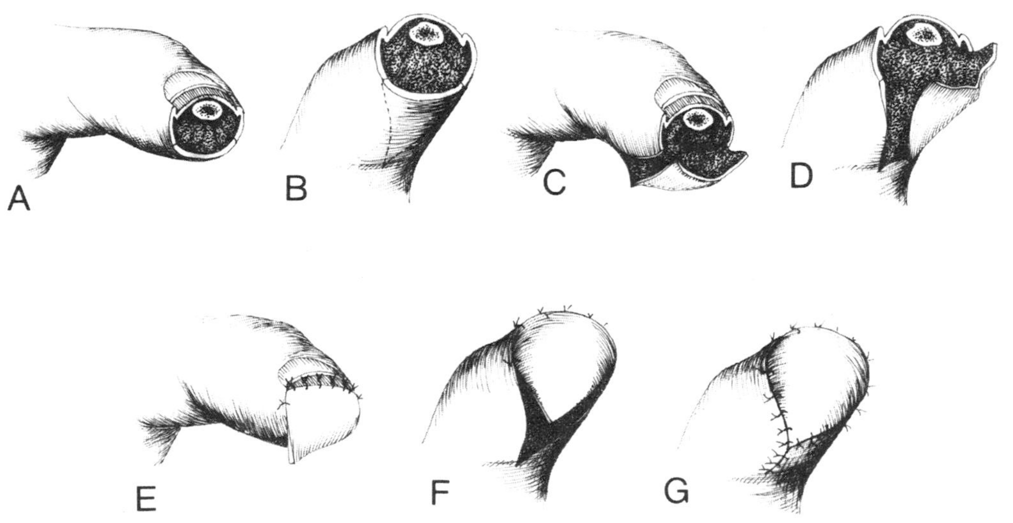

Figure 10.91. An advancement flap or Kutler procedure. *A:* Amputation of the distal tip of the finger with bone exposed. *B:* Excise a small piece of the tip. Then make a V-shaped incision on the volar surface of the finger with the point of the "V" just distal to the interphalangeal joint. *C:* Pull the V-shaped flap distally. *D:* Do not undermine the base of the flap; it should remain in contact with the septi that nourish the flap. *E:* Then trim the flap slightly and carry it distally to the nail margin. *F:* Use fine sutures to secure the distal pole of the flap to the nailbed and skin folds. *G:* Then suture the lateral edges, resulting in a Y-shaped repaired wound.

more commonly used. When applying a skin graft, be certain there is no protruding bone. The bone must be at least flush with the amputated tissue and preferably recessed for the graft to be accepted. As the graft shrinks, it pulls surrounding skin over the bone. The volar surface of the forearm and the wrist are excellent sites for grafting donor skin (Fig. 10.92). Hemostasis is mandatory to ensure an adequate take of the graft. After the graft is applied over the defect, suture it in place with 5-0 or 6-0 nylon, and tie the ends of each suture over a bolus of moist cotton, thus providing a stent dressing. Place a small piece of Xeroform gauze dressing over the grafted skin, between it and the cotton balls. Close the donor site primarily by undermining the skin edges. Continuous elevation of the finger for the first 5 days is extremely important.

A cross-finger **pedicle flap** is used in some amputations and provides a good result with regard to tactile sensation and return to normal function (63). This procedure is not one that is performed in the emergency center, and it is not discussed here.

A review of 151 partial and total amputations of fingertips showed that the best results were achieved with early primary closure and the use of the local advancement flap with the avoidance of skin grafts (63).

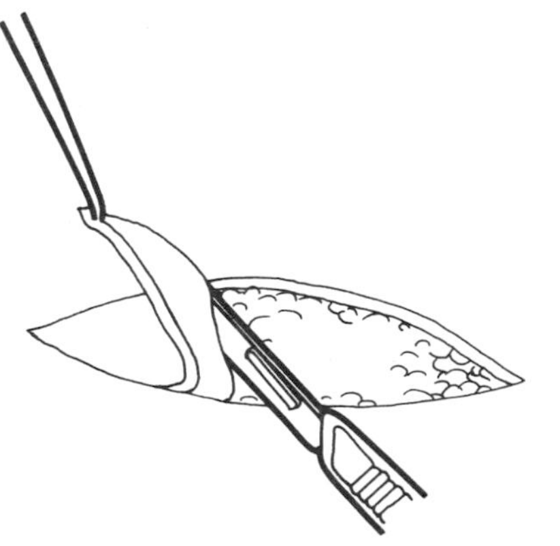

Figure 10.92. Excise a full-thickness graft as an ellipse, leaving behind as much of the fat as possible. Grafts are commonly obtained from the volar surface of the forearm or wrist.

In summary, individualize treatment for each patient, depending on occupation, age, and health. In the child, treat most fingertip injuries conservatively with healing by secondary intention, with excellent results. In the adult, conservative therapy remains our treatment of choice whenever possible. An advancement flap, as illustrated in Figs. 10.61 and 10.91, yields excellent results in patients with distal or middle phalangeal amputations. Be careful to leave an adequate attachment of the flap to its base and to resect an adequate amount of bone so that the flap may be advanced without tension.

Ingrown Nails

Several procedures have been recommended for treating ingrown toenails. These include

1. Surgical procedures, such as total nail avulsion.
2. Nail-edge excision.
3. Phenol ablation of the nailbed, with or without surgical ablation (110).

In one study, wedge resection of granulation tissue in the ingrown nail was performed and sutures applied (87). The standard therapy recommended is excision of the nail and nailbed using a wedged recession technique and excision of all granulation tissue. After this, either sterile strips or sutures are used to bring the edges together (118).

Several studies have recommended phenol cauterization as a treatment of choice (5, 48, 110, 113). In a study that compared phenol with surgical therapies of recurrent ingrown toenails, phenol ablation of the nailbed was the more successful therapy (5). In a random trial of surgical versus phenol ablation of the nailbed to treat ingrown nails, the results again confirmed the superiority of phenol over surgical ablation. In this study, when phenol was used, the affected nail edge was avulsed, and an 80% phenol in aqueous solution was applied to the nailbed for 3 minutes. The phenol was then neutralized with 70% alcohol, and the toe was dressed (110).

When 249 patients were treated randomly with phenol or surgical therapy, the recurrence of ingrown toenails after surgical therapy with wedge resection was 16% versus 9.6% recurrence with phenol ablation (113). In another study, the recurrence rate after surgical removal with wedge resection was 73% without phenol versus 9% with phenol (48). Phenol is an excellent antiseptic, and thus can be used on infected toes (48). In yet another study, pledgets were inserted under the ingrown toenails of children. The success rate using this technique was reported at 72% (24, 104).

We recommend phenol ablation, as demonstrated in Figs. 10.93 and 10.94. When there is granulation tissue and the nail is deeply embedded, we recommend wedge resection followed by phenol ablation for 3 minutes to destroy all of the nailbed. Follow this with alcohol neutralization of the wound using 70% alcohol. Leave the wound open, and dress it.

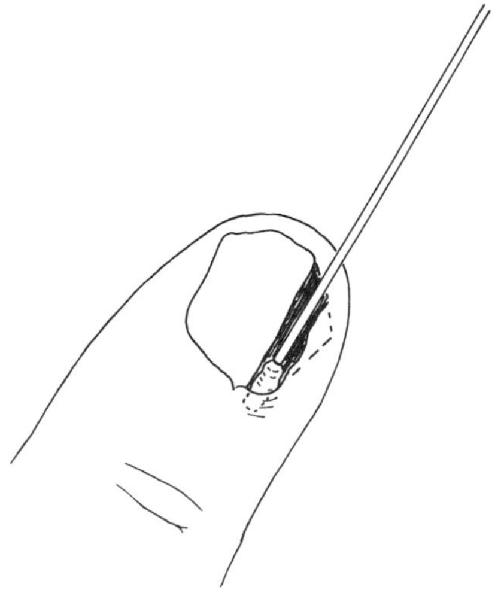

Figure 10.93. Phenol ablation for an ingrown toenail. See text for discussion.

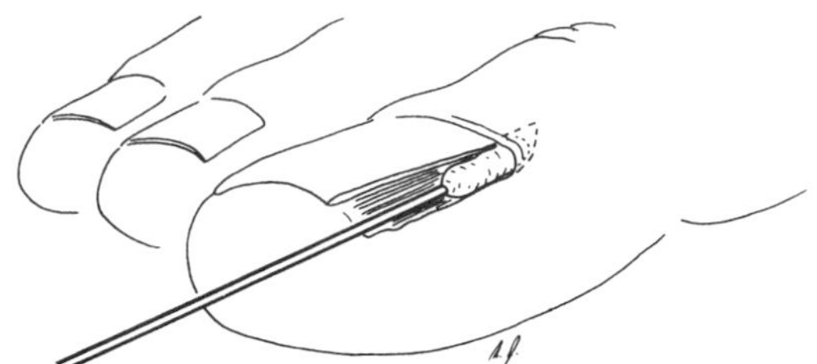

Figure 10.94. Use a cotton-tipped applicator for phenol ablation. Insert the applicator between the roof and root matrix. See text for discussion.

Nailbed Injuries

Based on the evaluation of the repairs of more than 3,000 nailbed injuries, certain principles can be summarized regarding this common injury (6):

1. Use very minimal debridement.
2. Remove the nail and accurately appose and repair the lacerated nailbed and root with 6-0 absorbable gut or other absorbable suture. If the root is not replaced, the pouch deep to the proximal skin fold is obliterated within a few days. (If the root cannot be replaced easily, follow the procedure in the legend to Fig. 10.99.)
3. Preserve skin folds surrounding the nail margins. Prevent adhesions between skin folds, nailbed, and root by preserving these spaces with a nonadherent gauze packing, such as Xeroform, molded to the contour of the skin folds.

Immediate primary reconstruction of the nailbed and root is the treatment of choice. Before a discussion of the methods of repairing the various injuries of the nailbed, understand the anatomy and generation of the nail. The nail matrix is formed from three sites, the nailbed, the roof matrix at the eponychial region (Fig. 10.95), and the root matrix. The most important areas to be preserved for the generation of a normal nail are the roof and root matrices. In a child, if the nailbed is destroyed, an entirely normal nail will

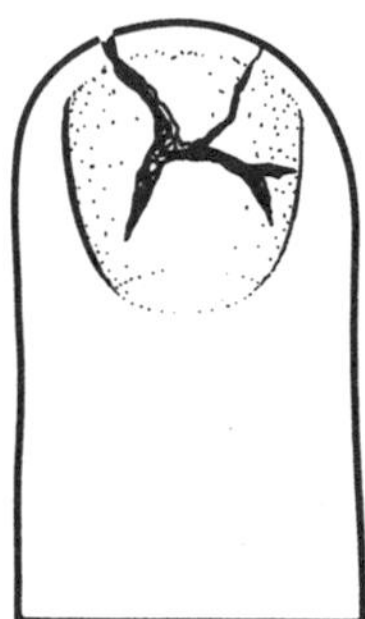

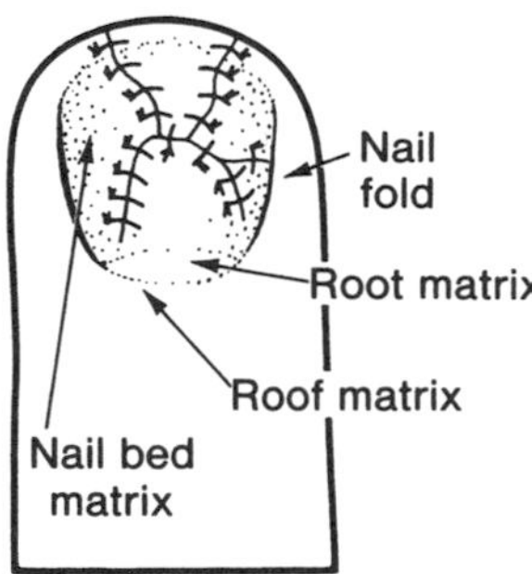

Figure 10.95. Repair of a complex nailbed injury. Often these patients have a large subungual hematoma that necessitates removal of the nail to repair the nailbed. After removal of the nail, approximate the bed with fine plain gut suture. Little debridement is necessary.

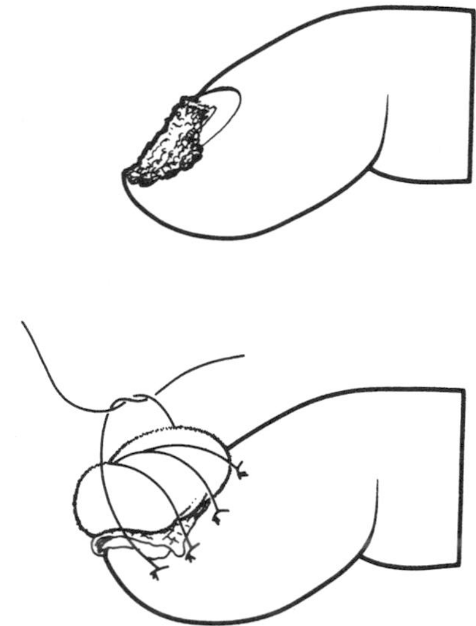

Figure 10.97. An avulsion of the nail involving the dorsal aspect of the distal tip. Treat this with a simple Xeroform dressing held in place with nylon sutures. Leave this gauze in place for 10 days.

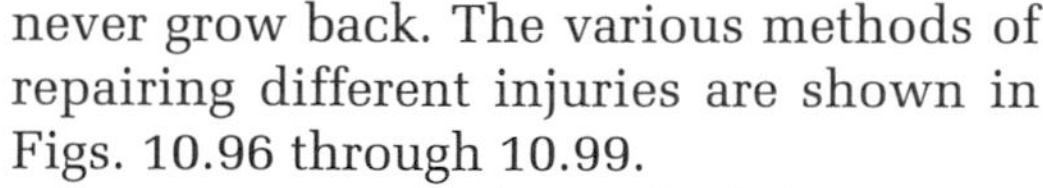

never grow back. The various methods of repairing different injuries are shown in Figs. 10.96 through 10.99.

Leave sutures in the nailbed for approximately 7 days. Leave in place the nonadherent Xeroform gauze dressing that is instilled in the nail folds, as shown in Figs. 10.91 and 10.96, for 4 days. After the wound is sutured, cover it with a piece of Telfa, which will not adhere to the secretions produced by the nailbed, followed by a thick gauze dressing. Splint the finger, and elevate the hand whenever possible. Remove the outer dressing, excluding the Telfa, and check the wound in 2 days. Advise the patient that, although the chances of forming a new nail are good when the injury is not severe, there is no guarantee as to what the final outcome will be.

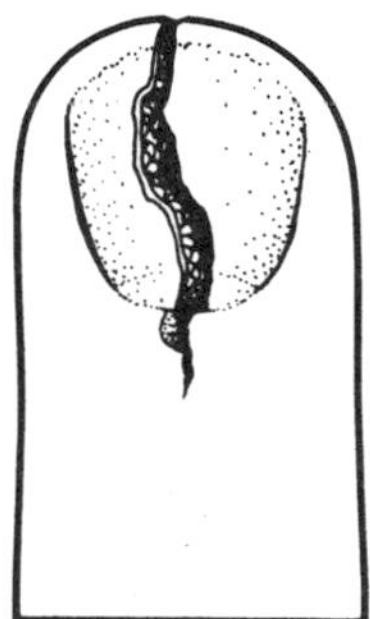

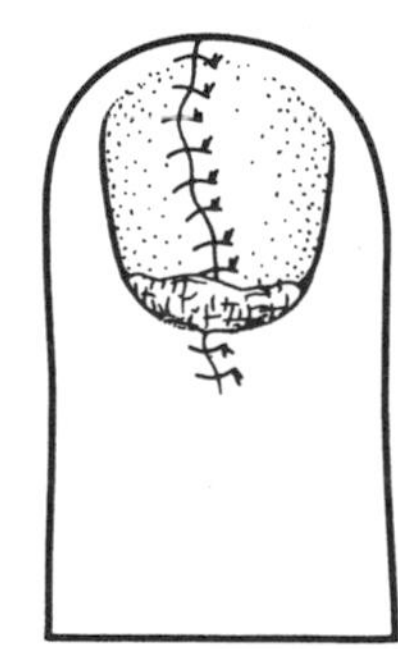

Figure 10.96. When lacerations are vertical and traverse the root of the nail as well as the distal tip, remove the nail and repair the nailbed separately from the skin over the eponychial portion of the nail. To maintain the integrity of the space between the roof and root matrix, pack Xeroform gauze in that space.

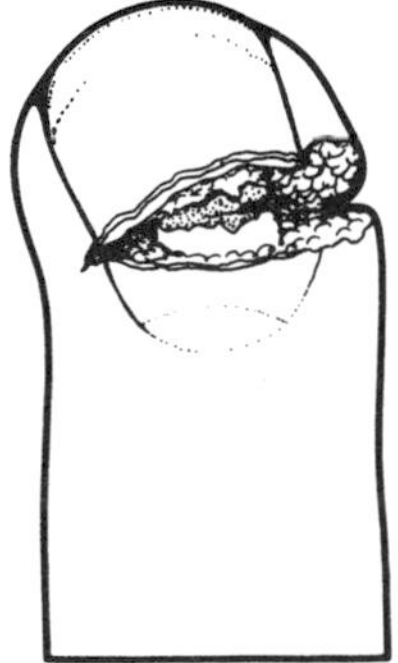

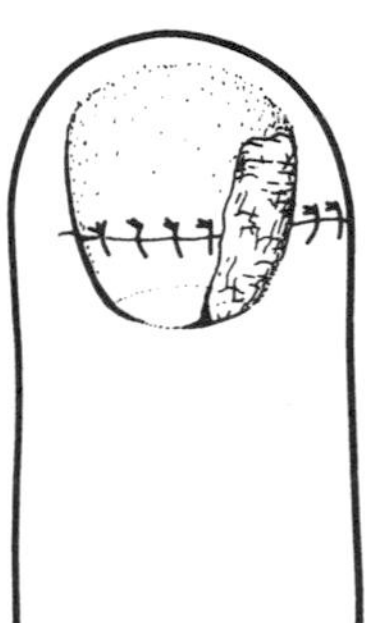

Figure 10.98. When a transverse laceration extends across the nail, remove the distal nail, and repair the nailbed as shown. Similar to the vertical laceration that extends across the eponychia of the nail, pack the lateral nail folds with Xeroform gauze to maintain the integrity of this space. Leave this gauze in place for a period of 10 days.

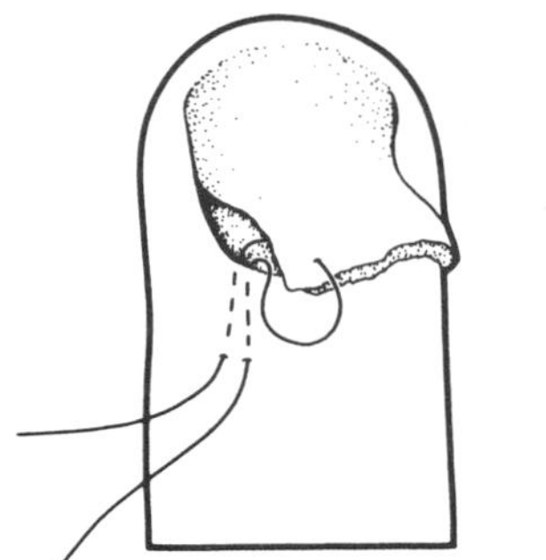
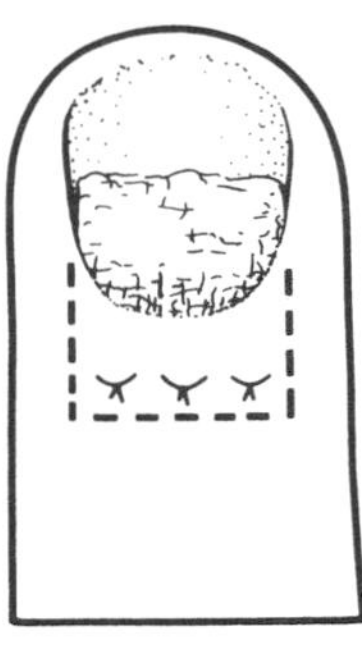

Figure 10.99. Proximal avulsion of the nailbed. When this occurs, reattach the nailbed in its anatomic location. Pass a suture through the skin, pick up the avulsed bed by the suture loop, and secure it back under the eponychia. Do not return the nailbed to its normal location until two to three sutures are first applied, and then pulled to reapproximate the nailbed to its normal position, and tied. Apply a Xeroform dressing to separate the roof and root matrix.

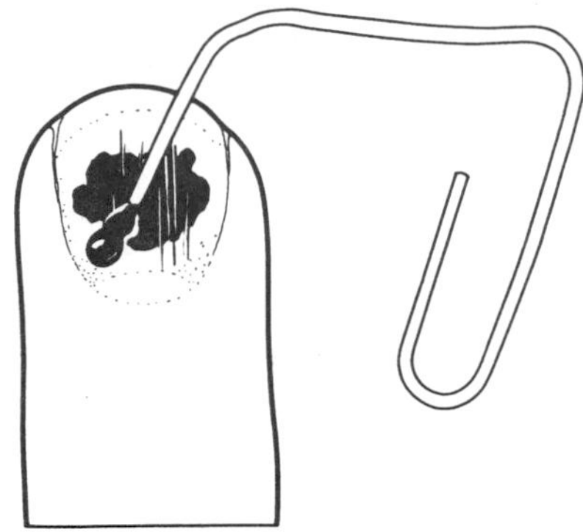

Figure 10.100. Drainage of a subungual hematoma.

Complications that arise from improper treatment include the following:

1. **Split nail.** A split nail occurs when the root is improperly approximated, resulting in a wide scar that produces splitting.
2. **Adhesions.** Adhesions of the skin fold to the nail root occur when a laceration involves both the skin fold and the nail matrix, and they are not repaired separately, resulting in obliteration of the space. Pack the space with nonadherent gauze packing.

Removal of a Nail

When and whether removal of a nail should take place has been a controversial issue. No good data in the literature support opinions regarding when to remove a nail. It would appear logical that because the base of the nail contains epithelial cells from the roof and root matrices, the base should be preserved when possible. We advocate preservation of the base of the nail to repair a laceration when the laceration extends across the nail transversely. When the nail has been removed traumatically and is intact and clean, reapply it in its normal anatomic position because it provides an excellent stent over the nailbed. When open fractures occur in patients with a nail or nailbed injury, repair the injury as would be routine, and treat the fractures separately. Give these patients oral antibiotics, although osteomyelitis in the distal phalanx after an open fracture is quite uncommon.

When a subungual hematoma is present, drain this by a simple puncture of the nail with either a hot paper clip or a small drill (Fig. 10.100). A subungual hematoma that is large is almost always associated with a nailbed laceration. We believe the nail should be removed and the bed repaired. Then replace the nail as an anatomic stent. If one does not repair the nailbed, a step-off may occur with ridging of the nail when it grows back.

AFTERCARE OF SELECTED WOUND INJURIES

Suture Removal

Remove sutures as soon as possible, because they serve as a foreign body in the wound and a nidus for infection, as well as permitting suture marks to form when left in place an excessively long time. Nylon sutures can get wet for brief periods and should be dried after exposure to

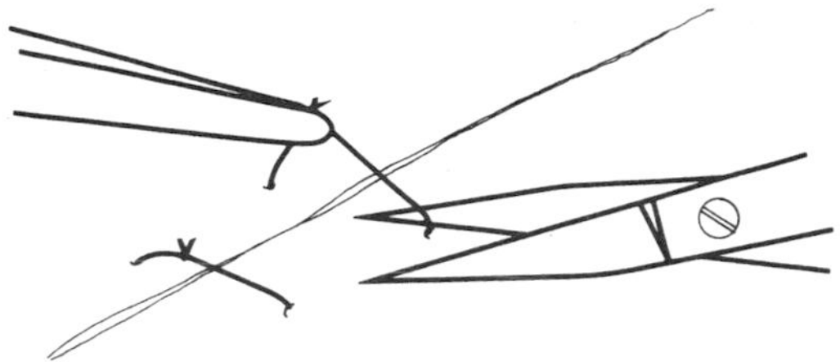

Figure 10.101. Correct method of removing a suture. Remove the suture by cutting the end away from the knot near the skin to prevent passage of the contaminated outer portion of the stitch back through the skin. When fine sutures are used and are close to the skin, use a no. 11 blade rather than a scissors for suture removal. Insert the tip of the blade under the suture loop, and cut the suture.

Table 10.6
Suture Removal

Location	Time of removal (days)
Face	3–4 (Adult) 2–3 (Children)
Lower extremity	8–10
Upper extremity	7–10
Extensor surface of joints	10–14
Delayed closure	8–12

moisture. The technique of suture removal is shown in Fig. 10.101. This method avoids pulling the outside portion of the suture back through the wound and causing contamination. Sutures left in place for 3 or 4 days are unlikely to leave a permanent suture mark (74). If one removes a suture by the eighth day, the epithelial track will regress and leave no significant mark; however, the earlier the suture is removed, the better (29). During the first 8 days, there is very little tensile strength in the wound. The closure is held by vessels crossing the wound, epithelialization, and a fibrin coagulant. In some areas of the body (such as around the joints), when sutures are removed at 8 days, support the wound by the use of Steri-Strips (7). In the face, remove sutures in 3 or 4 days. In extensive facial lacerations, provide support for longer than 3 days. Remove alternating sutures on day 3 and the remainder by day 5, and apply Steri-Strips for added support for 5 to 7 days.

In the lower extremity, where healing is slower, leave sutures for 14 days to assure adequate strength, especially around joints. In the upper extremity, remove sutures in 7 to 10 days (Table 10.6). Although sutures are removed earlier, the tensile strength of the wound does not return to normal until 21 days after closure.

Primary closure of a wound carries with it the obligation to maintain optimal conditions for wound healing (79). If sutures are removed too early, the wound may be disrupted even with minimal activity unless supported by Steri-Strips. Separation may occur when an overwhelming force breaks the laceration open, when absorbable sutures dissolve too quickly, or when tight sutures cut through the tissue. **Dehiscence** represents the failure of the wound to gain sufficient strength to withstand stresses. When dehiscence does occur, it does so on the third to the fifth day after incision, and about half of the cases are associated with infection. Perform *delayed closure* on wounds that are heavily contaminated with saliva, dirt, or grease and that cannot be adequately cleansed and debrided. Delay closure of these wounds to permit the wound to gain sufficient resistance against infection, at which time closure can be performed safely. In these cases, pack the wound with fine-mesh gauze and dress it with a pressure dressing, and elevate the limb. Close the wound at 4 days. This time can be altered, depending on the area of the body. When these wounds subsequently are closed, splint them and apply a pressure dressing. The sutures should remain in place for 12 days, particularly on extremity wounds (79). Delayed closure usually is not necessary on facial wounds, and we do not advocate it. Because of the profuse vascularity of the face, wounds tend to heal well after being adequately cleansed and debrided.

Delayed wound closure can be accomplished by one of three techniques: secondary suturing after a local anesthetic is infiltrated, tying previously placed untied sutures, or pulling the wound edges together after adhesive tape is applied parallel to the wound margins. This latter method is used in closing large, gaping, linear lacerations and can be used for both delayed wound closure and primary wound closure, especially in somewhat contaminated wounds. In using this method of closure, place 2- to 3-inch wide strips of adhesive tape parallel to the wound margins, approximately 5 mm from the margin on both sides of the wound. Apply a thin layer of benzoin tincture to the skin on both sides of the incision before applying the tape. Lay the two strips of adhesive tape adjacent to the wound edges, and fold the longitudinal edge of the tape bordering the wound ¼-inch under each strip, thus providing a "hem" in which sutures can be placed. Then pass a running stitch through the "hems" on both sides of the wound to close the wound. This technique combines the advantages that no anesthesia is required, no skin sutures are placed that may become infected, and no strips of tape are applied over the wound, thus permitting adequate drainage of secretions.

Elevation and Pressure Dressings

A snug pressure dressing and elevation are desirable in most instances to minimize edema formation and to prevent collection of blood and serum, hematoma formation, lymphedema, and venous congestion (7, 74). A pressure dressing also supports and protects the tissue by avoiding pull on the approximated edges (74). In certain areas (such as the lips and eyelids), use cold compresses for 48 to 72 hours after the injury to minimize pain and swelling. In the scalp and forehead, use a firm pressure dressing for 48 hours to prevent hematoma formation (107). A pressure dressing is extremely important, particularly in regions that are highly vascular, to prevent hematoma formation, which may disrupt the wound closure as well as be a source for infection. The scalp, forehead, periorbital and pretibial regions, and dorsal surface of the hand are common sites for hematoma formation. Apply pressure dressings to lacerations in these areas. In addition, apply pressure dressings to wounds over the extensor surfaces of the major joints to prevent hematoma formation. In children, the best way to immobilize joints is to provide a big bulky dressing over the area of laceration. Accompany a pressure dressing, whenever practical, by elevation of the injured part to accomplish the aforementioned objectives. In facial lacerations, advise the patient to sleep upright on many pillows or in a reclining chair.

Dressings

A single layer of ointment gauze, Xeroform, or Vaseline can be used under the pressure dressing (7). To have an optimally aesthetic wound, prevention of desiccation of the wound margins with these ointments is critical and one of the most important parts of aftercare. Where a pressure dressing is impractical (e.g., on the face), clean the wound daily with a mild soap, and Xeroform cut to the appropriate size should be placed over the wound. After 12 to 24 hours, use a mild soap 4 times a day to cleanse the area around the wound and to remove any exudate over the Xeroform dressing. After this, use a hair blow-dryer to dry the surface of the wound. Leave the Xeroform dressing in place for 7 to 14 days when dealing with a facial abrasion. Remove all dried blood from the surface of the wound and from around the sutures, because this debris may serve as a nidus for infection (107, 115). This can be accomplished with the use of a cotton-tipped applicator. Apply a thin layer of Bacitracin or similar ointment to keep the surface free of crusting. Do not use a neomycin-containing oint-

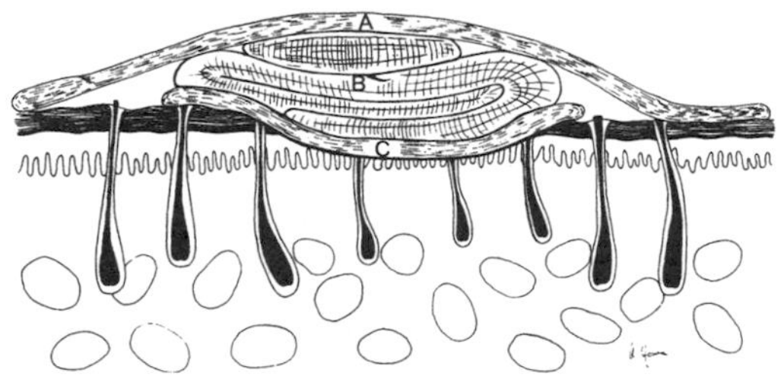

Figure 10.102. Treat deep abrasions with a three-layer dressing, as shown. Apply a fine-mesh gauze with an antibacterial ointment first *(C)*. Follow this with a loose gauze *(B)*. The outer dressing is elastic tape or a gauze roll *(A)*. See text for discussion.

ment because this may result in a contact dermatitis.

In patients with abrasions, after cleansing the wounds and debriding any foreign material, apply a three-layer dressing (Fig. 10.102). The inner layer (Fig. 10.102*C*) should be an antibiotic, such as Xeroform or nitrofurazone (Furacin), impregnated gauze dressing. The second layer (Fig. 10.102*B*) should be a gauze dressing that will absorb moisture and protect the wound from further trauma. The outer layer (Fig. 10.102*A*) should be an elastic wrap or tape that will hold the dressing over the wound surface.

Treat patients with contaminated lacerations that cannot be debrided and closed primarily with a three-layer dressing, and perform a delayed closure. The inner layer should be of fine-mesh gauze impregnated with povidone–iodine. The second layer should be a gauze pad, which will absorb secretions from the wound. The outer layer should be a gauze wrap, which will provide pressure and hemostasis. Remove and replace this three-layered gauze dressing within 12 hours. The inner fine-mesh gauze will debride the necrotic tissue on removal. Repack the wound on a daily basis and then close it in 3 to 7 days.

When covering special areas, such as the ear, first apply a nonadherent gauze dressing. Next place 4 × 4-cm gauze pads behind and in front of the ear (Fig. 10.103). After this, place a wrap around the ear and head to hold the dressing in place (Fig. 10.104).

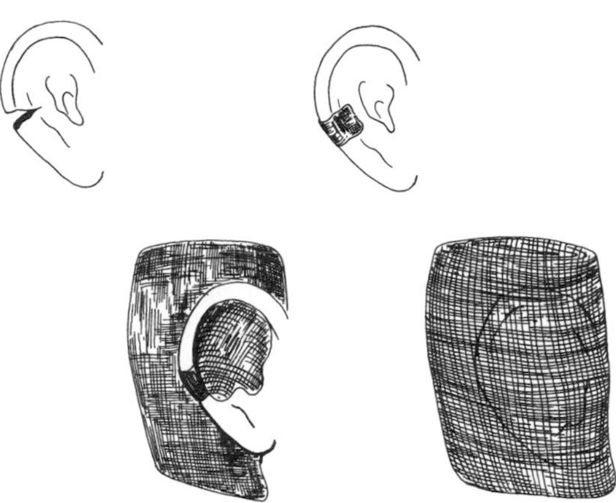

Figure 10.103. To dress a wound of the auricle after packing the wound with a loose gauze dressing, place gauze both behind and in front of the ear. See text for discussion.

Infection

When a sutured wound becomes infected, relieve the constriction, provide adequate drainage, and remove the sutures, which provide a nidus for infection. Always consider an undiscovered foreign body as the source of infection. Remove the sutures in part or totally, which im-

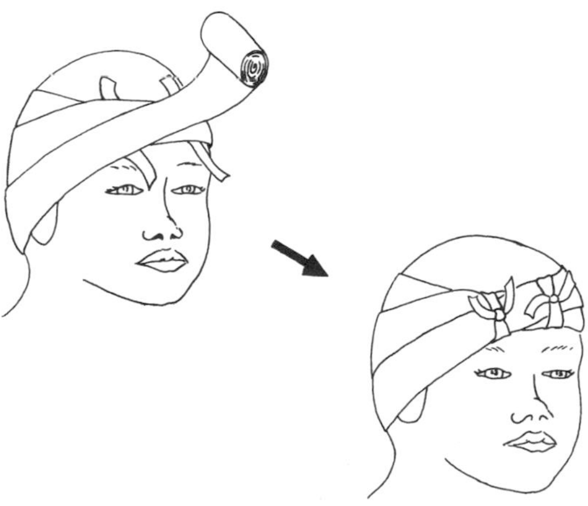

Figure 10.104. Use a gauze wrap-around, as shown, to hold an ear dressing in place. See text for discussion.

proves drainage and circulation and removes a foreign body. Apply warm packs, and give the patient penicillinase-resistant penicillins. Always follow up wounds closed by an emergency physician, preferably by the same physician, in 48 hours. Instruct all patients to watch for signs of infection and to return immediately if any of the signs are noted. If the incidence of infection is greater than 5%, reevaluate the technique of wound preparation and suturing and investigate possible sources of contamination during wound closures.

Suture sinuses form when a suture site becomes infected. A suture sinus is a tract leading from suture material within the wound to the skin surface that continually drains serous or purulent material. A small abscess called a *stitch abscess* often forms beneath the sinus. A suture sinus or suture abscess usually indicates that a foreign body, which may be the suture material itself, is present and has become infected in the wound. As long as the suture remains in place, the sinus will persist. These infections occur most commonly with silk and other multifilament sutures and are least often seen with monofilament synthetics. Explore the sinus tract gently with a probe, and remove the suture with a skin hook when possible; if this is not possible, wait a few weeks for spontaneous ejection to occur.

Scar Revision

Occasionally the result of a repair will be poor because of the nature of the wound itself. The patient may complain of a bad cosmetic result. Scar revision is not usually performed before 6 months, to allow scar maturation to occur, and the patient should be so advised (74, 107). In young children and in the elderly, maturation of a scar to its final appearance may take a year or more (65, 107).

Modalities such as compression dressings and steroids injected in the interim may be helpful in these patients; therefore, refer these patients. Posttraumatic scars can usually be improved with surgical excision and revision because these revisions are carried out in wounds that are not traumatically induced.

ABSCESSES

Abscesses are commonly seen in the emergency center. Too often, physicians treating an abscess incise in the most "convenient" location and give the patient oral antibiotics. Anesthesia is difficult to provide, especially when dividing the septi within the cavity of the abscess. In the treatment of abscesses, the important anatomic structures underlying the abscess must be appreciated. The location of the abscess is critical to the direction of the incision.

In seven locations in the body, abscesses are in close proximity to major vessels:

1. Peritonsillar and retropharyngeal regions.
2. The anterior triangle of the neck (an area enclosed by the sternocleidomastoid muscle, mandible, and anterior midline of the neck).
3. The supraclavicular fossa.
4. Deep in the axilla.
5. The antecubital space.
6. The groin.
7. The popliteal space.

Aspirate abscesses that occur in any of these seven locations with an 18-gauge needle attached to a 10-mL syringe before drainage. The aspiration is only for diagnostic confirmation. Too often, what was thought to be an abscess has been incised, only to find a mycotic aneurysm and imminent exsanguination. The aspiration should not drain the abscess cavity entirely, because the purulent material serves as a marker for the hollow of the abscess cavity. The aspiration merely confirms that the material contained within the cavity is purulent and not serosanguinous or pure blood. If the latter material (mycotic aneurysm) is found, drain the abscess more judiciously in the operating room.

Antiseptic Preparation and Technique of Anesthesia

Surgically prepare the area with a topical anesthetic such as povidone–iodine. Use a regional field block anesthetic technique to anesthetize the abscess (3). Inject a ring of anesthetic material approximately 1 cm away from the perimeter of the erythematous border of the abscess. The entire lesion is thus anesthetized circumferentially. In providing a ring of anesthesia around the abscess, be certain to inject the anesthetic solution subcutaneously. Then inject a small amount of anesthetic solution into the roof of the abscess in a linear fashion along the line of the projected incision. The onset of action of the anesthetic in this location is approximately 5 minutes and is quite successful in relieving pain.

Incision

Perform the incision along the relaxed skin-tension lines to reduce scarring. When purulent material drains, obtain a specimen for culture if desired, especially in immunosuppressed patients. Insert a hemostat into the abscess cavity and spread to break up the septi and loculations and to release any further pockets of purulent material. Irrigate the cavity with normal saline before inserting any gauze to pack the cavity. Then insert iodoform gauze into the abscess cavity with 1 cm of gauze exiting from the cavity. Apply a sterile dressing. Remove the Iodoform gauze in 24 to 48 hours. The Iodoform gauze serves two purposes: it prevents the incision from sealing over and provides for adequate drainage of the abscess cavity. After removal of the Iodoform pack, apply warm wet soaks to the area several times a day for a few days. The incision will heal in approximately 7 to 10 days in most cases.

In a large study, abscesses were treated with and without antibiotics (84). All the abscesses were treated with incision and drainage, and all were found to heal without complications, including approximately three fourths of those cases that were treated without adjunctive antibiotics. It was concluded that the primary management of abscesses should be incision and drainage and that routine culture and antibiotic therapy were not indicated for the typical abscess in patients with normal host defenses. Abscesses that we believe should be treated with oral antibiotic therapy are those that are surrounded by lymphangitis or a large area of cellulitis. The cellulitis is determined by tenderness peripheral to the area of the abscess as well as increased warmth and redness, as opposed to the nontender induration palpated around an abscess that is well localized and that would not be benefited by the addition of oral antibiotics. Culture purulent material from immunosuppressed patients; give the patient oral antibiotics pending the culture results (84).

Special Considerations

FELONS

A felon is an infection or abscess occurring in the pulp of the volar surface of the distal phalanx. The proper technique of draining a felon has been controversial (43). The incision that is associated with the lowest rate of complications is a simple vertical incision carried out over the center of the abscess (Fig. 10.105). The fishmouth incision and the lateral con-

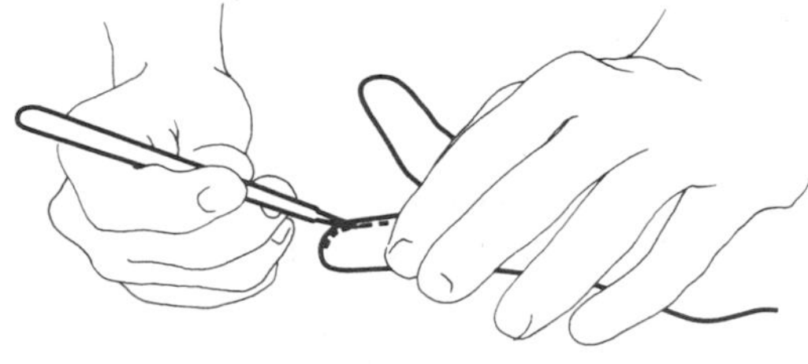

Figure 10.105. Correct incision for a felon. See text for discussion.

necting incisions that have been used in the past have been found to produce a higher incidence of fingertip anesthesia and instability (67).

PARONYCHIAL AND EPONYCHIAL ABSCESSES

A paronychia, as referred to here, is an abscess under the lateral nail fold. An eponychia is an abscess under the roof matrix.

For the common paronychia, an incision is unnecessary. Instead, insert the tip of a no. 11 blade approximately 5 mm under the surface of the nail, uplifting the cuticle (Fig. 10.106), thus providing an escape for the collected suppurative material. This procedure alone provides adequate drainage in most paronychia and eponychia.

HIDRADENITIS SUPPURATIVA

This is an infection leading to multiple abscess formation in the apocrine glands of the axilla. The matted and indurated dermis contains the apocrine glands, and multiple drainage sites from these abscesses are noted. Incise and drain these as described earlier; pack a large abscess cavity in the manner described earlier. Refer these patients to a general surgeon for follow-up care, because surgical excision may be needed to prevent recurrence.

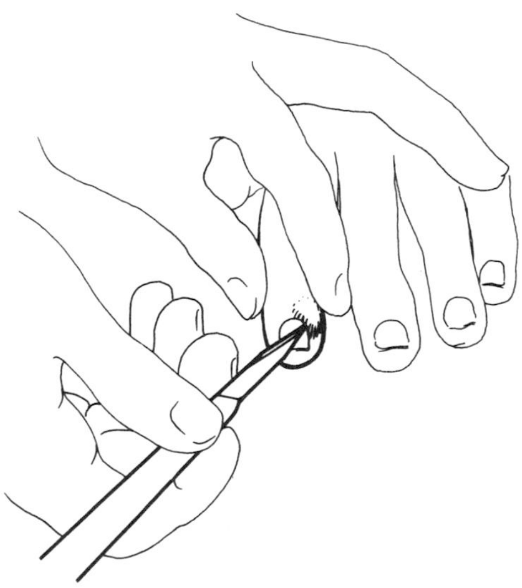

Figure 10.106. Drain a paronychial or eponychial abscess by inserting a no. 11 blade along the surface of the nail and uplifting the nail fold under which lies the paronychia. An incision is not necessary to drain this abscess unless it extends or is very large. We have found no increased incidence of recurrences with this technique. After this, use warm saline soaks.

PERITONSILLAR ABSCESSES

A peritonsillar abscess usually dissects into the soft palate above the tonsillar pillars; the abscess that forms forces the uvula to deviate to the opposite side. Drain this abscess with a transverse incision at the site of maximal fluctuation, which is usually superior and lateral to the tonsil. To prevent pulmonary aspiration of the purulent material, make a small stab initially into the abscess cavity, and hold a suction tip at the site of the stab to aspirate the majority of the purulent material as it exudes from the stab. Once the majority of the suppurative material has been evacuated, extend the incision. These abscesses are not packed routinely. Advise the patient to sleep face down rather than on the back to provide adequate drainage of the purulent material and to avoid aspiration. This procedure is more completely discussed in Chapter 8, Otolaryngologic and Ophthalmologic Procedures.

PERIODONTAL ABSCESSES

A periodontal abscess is usually seen along the border of the premolars and molars and is drained by an incision that parallels the gingival border at the site of maximal fluctuance within the oral cavity (Fig. 10.107). It is usually packed with plain gauze; remove the packing within 24 to 48 hours. Give these patients oral penicillin to protect the surrounding sinuses from secondary infection and to treat the usual cellulitis that is seen accompanying these abscesses.

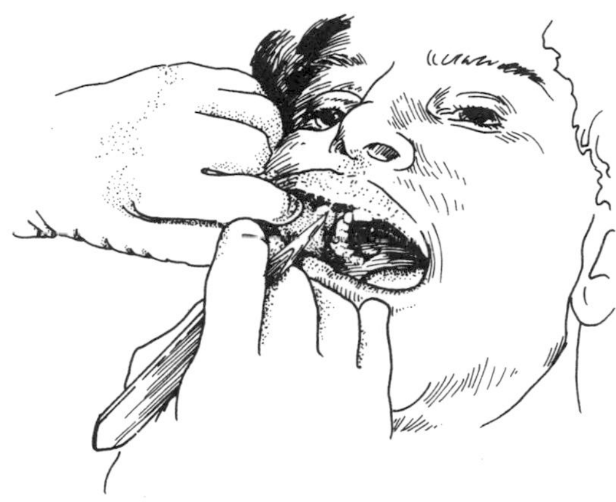

Figure 10.107. Drain a periodontal abscess with an incision made in the sulcus of the mouth where the gingiva meets the buccal mucosa. Make the incision over the point of maximal fluctuance.

PERIRECTAL ABSCESSES

Drain perirectal abscesses with a radial incision that is carried into the abscess cavity and can be extended through the subcutaneous portion of the external sphincter. Be careful not to extend the incision through the deep portion of the sphincter because this may produce complications, such as fecal incontinence, when the incision heals. Then pack these abscesses with Iodoform gauze, and advise the patient to sit in a sitz bath for 20 minutes, 3 times a day for the first day, and to remove the packing while in the bath. The healing is usually complete within approximately 10 days, during the course of which, advise the patient to take sitz baths twice daily. This procedure is more completely discussed in Chapter 1, Abdominal Procedures.

PILONIDAL ABSCESSES

A pilonidal abscess occurs in the midline posteriorly in the region of the coccyx. Most pilonidal abscesses contain hair (96); after excision and drainage, refer the patient to a surgeon for definitive treatment, which includes excision of the sinus. Some authors believe that definitive treatment with incision of the sinus and drainage of the abscess can be performed in the office or the hospital as a single procedure (51). Definitive treatment of repeated pilonidal abscesses during the initial visit can be done by a plastic surgeon, with total excision of the abscess and primary closure of the defect.

FOREIGN-BODY REMOVAL

Embedded Needle

A broken needle embedded in the foot is a common problem seen by the emergency physician. This foreign body can engage the physician for hours in an attempt to remove the elusive "needle in a haystack." When it is available, fluoroscopy offers an excellent aid in removal of these foreign bodies. Transport the patient to the fluoroscopy suite, and under sterile conditions, make an incision over the needle, as judged from the anteroposterior and lateral films; localize the particle under fluoroscopic visualization, and remove it with a curved hemostat.

An alternate method has been described (73). Place a radiopaque marker at the point of entry of the particle. A bent paper clip serves as an excellent marker. Take posteroanterior films to show the exact size of the particle, its relation and orientation to the marker, and its configuration; a lateral projection shows its exact length. After the posteroanterior and lateral films are taken, leave the marker in place. Prepare, drape, and anesthetize the area, preferably with a regional nerve block (as described in Chapter 3, Anesthesia and Regional Blocks). Because the posteroanterior and lateral films are obtained perpendicular to each other, with the marker in place, one can discern the exact length and orientation of the needle. With a no. 11 blade, make a stab incision at a 90-degree angle to the middle of the foreign body. Because of the width of the blade, one can insert a small hemostat in the wound and, with minimal probing, remove the needle. Cover the resulting stab wound with a single dressing after the needle is removed.

Another method is to use two 19-gauge needles placed perpendicular to each other to localize the needle particle. Use these to guide a no. 11 blade into position near the particle by intermittent exposure with a fluoroscope to pinpoint the particle. Ask the patient to move the extremity when needed, and turn off the radiograph beam for each manipulation of the localized needle. Once the particle is localized between the two needles, make a small incision between the needles, and remove the particle found at the tips.

NAILBED SPLINTERS

When a splinter is embedded deep into the nail, incise the nail longitudinally with a no. 11 blade. With an 18-gauge needle, tease out the splinter (Fig. 10.108).

Fishhook

Remove a fishhook embedded in the subcutaneous tissue by passing the barb out through the skin as if completing its passage through the tissue. After doing this, simply cut the eye of the hook and grasp the point and barb with a needle holder or pliers, and withdraw the hook. Be careful not to cut the eye from the hook until the point and barb have passed through the skin, or the embedded portion of the hook and barb may disappear beneath the skin, preventing removal. In situations in which the hook is small and embedded in the face, it may be preferable to back the hook out rather than add an extra wound. When doing so, pass a large-bore needle over the entrance track of the barb, and then insert it over the barb as the hook is being withdrawn (42). Advance the hook slightly to dislodge the barb from the tissue. Pull and twist the hook so that the barb is "housed" by the lumen of the large-bore needle. Place the hook and barb, along with the large-bore needle, over the barb, and then withdraw them through the entrance wound as a single unit. In situations in which the hook is quite large, it may be better to pass the barb through the skin even when the face is involved, because a barb may produce a sizable irregular tear. If a fishhook is embedded in cartilage but has not passed through the skin on the opposite side, as in the ear, then back the

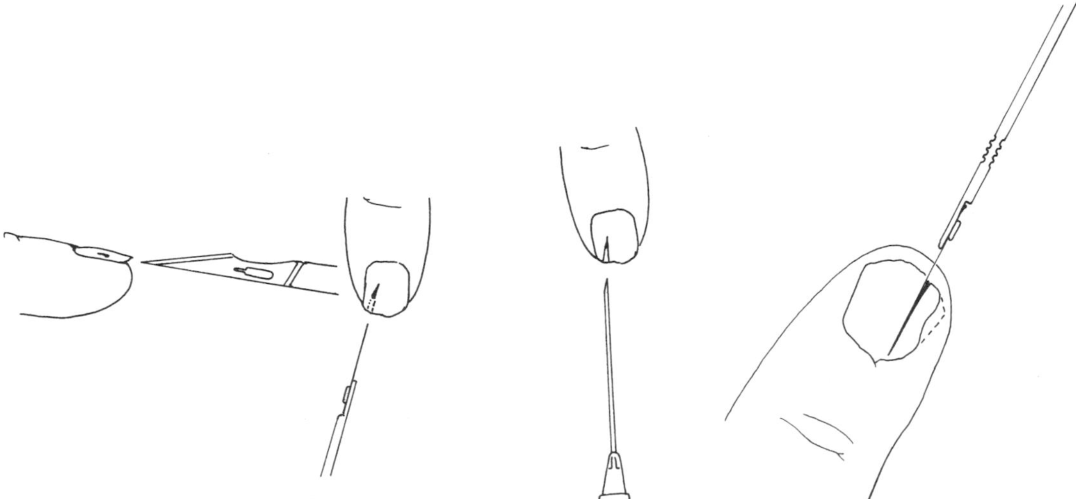

Figure 10.108. Removal of a difficult-to-remove thorn or foreign body under the nail. Incise the wound with a no. 11 blade and tease the foreign body out with an 18-gauge needle, as shown. See text for discussion.

hook out in manner similar to that described earlier, by using the large-bore needle. If the hook has passed through the cartilage, but has not passed through the other side of the skin, then pass the barb through the skin on the opposite side, the eye of the hook clipped, and the rest of the fishhook pulled out of the skin.

The best method for removal of a fishhook is a technique popularized by Cooke (23). This method requires no anesthesia, and the only material necessary is a 3-foot-long piece of sewing thread or silk. Place the silk or thread around the curve of the fishhook (Fig. 10.109*A*) with the other end wrapped around the physician's hand

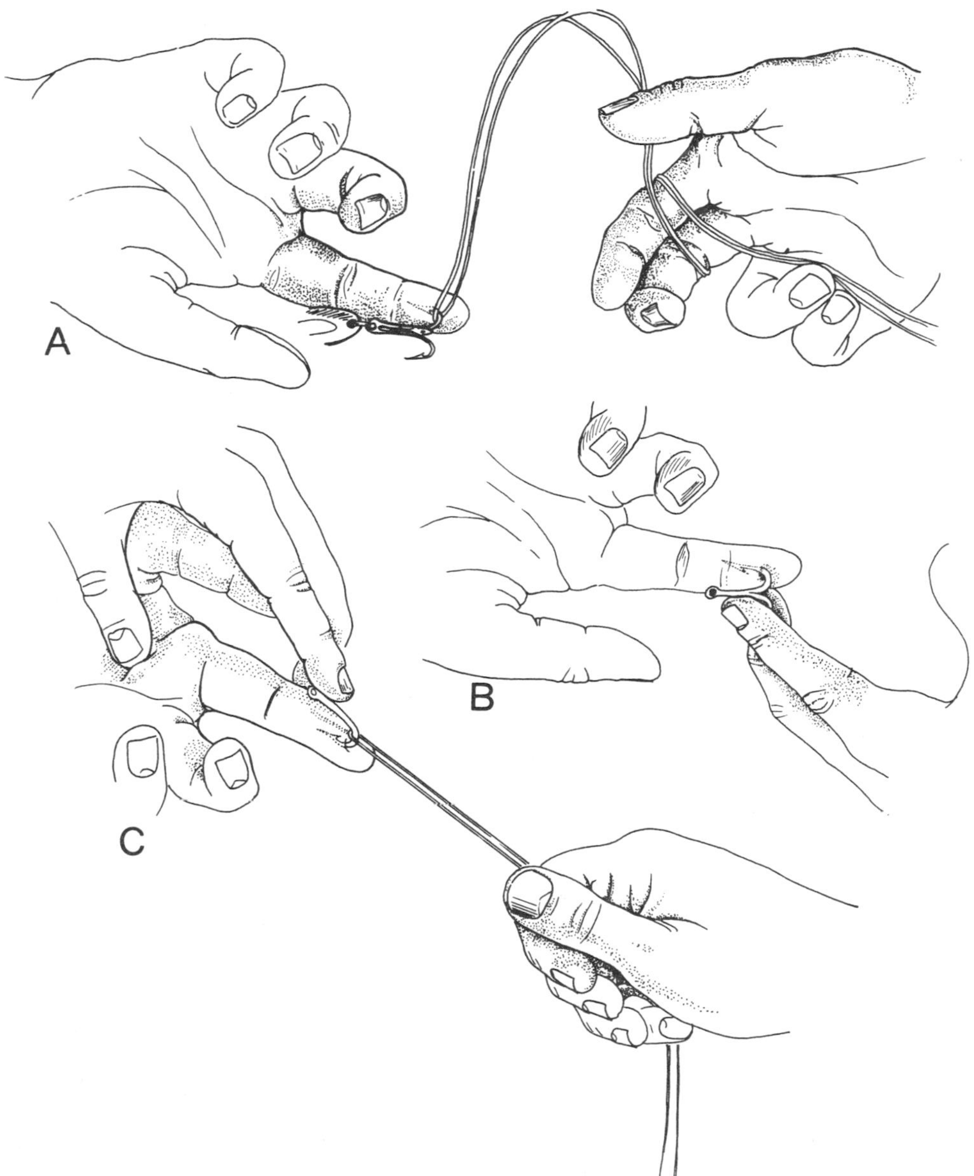

Figure 10.109. *A:* Place silk suture material or a string around the curve of the fishhook. *B:* Hold the involved digit firmly against a flat surface, and depress the shank until resistance is met. *C:* While the shank is depressed and the string is held taut, apply a quick jerk to dislodge the needle.

several times to prevent slippage. Then depress the shank of the hook, as shown in (Fig. 10.109*B*) until it meets a resistance. To provide stability, hold the involved digit or adjacent tissue flatly against a firm surface during the procedure. Then depress the shank, and jerk the thread in one forceful move parallel to the shank, which dislodges the hook (Fig. 10.109*C*). This technique is effective and produces no additional puncture wound for the patient.

References

1. Agris J: Traumatic tattooing. J Trauma 16:798, 1976.
2. Albert J, Lofstrom B: Effects of epinephrine in solutions of local anesthetic agents. Acta Anaesth Scand Suppl 16:71, 1965.
3. Albom M: Surgical gems. J Dermatol Surg 2:2, 1976.
4. Alexander JW, Kaplan JZ, Altemeier WA: Role of suture materials in the development of wound infection. Ann Surg 165:192, 1967.
5. Anderson JH, Greig JD, Ireland AJ, et al: Randomized prospective study of nailbed ablation for recurrent ingrowing toenails. J R Coll Surg Edinb 35:240–242, 1990.
6. Ashbell TS, Kleinhert HE: The deformed fingernail: A frequent result of failure to repair nailbed injuries. J Trauma 7:177, 1967.
7. Backpus LH, DeFelice CA: Treatment of accidental wounds. Postgrad Med 27:209, 1960.
8. Baxter CR: Surgical management of soft tissue infections. Surg Clin North Am 52:1483, 1972.
9. Bennett JE: Fingertip avulsions. J Trauma 6:249, 1966.
10. Bennett JE, Lewis E: Operative decompression of constricting burns. Surgery 43:949, 1958.
11. Blocker TG Jr, Moyer CA: In: Womack NA, ed. On Burns. Springfield, IL: Charles C Thomas, 172, 1953.
12. Borges AF, Alexander JE: Relaxed skin tension lines: Z-plasties on scars, and fusiform excision of lesions. Br J Plast Surg 15:242, 1962.
13. Borges AF, Alexander JE, Black LI: Z-plasty treatment of unesthetic scars. Eye Ear Nose Throat 44:39, 1965.
14. Branemark PI: Proceedings of the American Society for Surgery of the Hand: 21st Annual Meeting, Jan. 21 and 22. Chicago: 1966.
15. Branemark PI, Albrekisson B, Lindstrom J, et al: Local tissue effects of wound disinfectants. Acta Chir Scand Suppl 357:166, 1966.
16. Brickman KR, Lambert RW. Evaluation of skin stapling for wound closure in the emergency department. Ann Emerg Med 18:1122–1125, 1989.
17. Broday GS, Cloutier McL, Woolhouse FM: The fingertip injury: an assessment of management. Plast Reconstr Surg 26:80, 1960.
18. Bruns TB, Robinson BS, Smith RJ, et al. A new tissue adhesive for laceration repair in children. J Pediatr 132:1067–1070, 1998.
19. Bruns TB, Worthington JM: Using tissue adhesive for wound repair: A practical guide to dermabond. Am Fam Physician 61:1383–1388, 2000.
20. Byrne DS, Caldwell D: Phenol cauterization for ingrowing toenails: A review of five years' experience. Br J Surg 76:598–599, 1989.
21. Carpendale MTF, Sereda W: The role of the percutaneous suture in surgical wound infection. Surgery 58:672, 1965.
22. Condie JD, Ferguson DJ: Experimental wound infections: Contamination versus surgical technique. Surgery 50:367, 1961.
23. Condon RE: Locked vertical mattress stitch for skin closure. Surg Gynecol Obstet 127:839, 1968.
24. Connolly B, Fitzgerald RJ, et al.: Pledgets in ingrowing toenails. Arch Dis Child 63:71–72, 1988.
25. Conolly WB, Hunt TK, Zederfedt B, et al: Clinical comparison of surgical wounds closed by suture and adhesive tapes. Ann Surg 117:318, 1969.
26. Cooke T: How to remove fish-hooks with a bit of string. Med J Aust 48:815, 1961.
27. Coover HN, Joyner FB, Sheere NH, et al: Chemistry and performance of cyanoacrylate adhesive. J Soc Plast Surg Engl 15:5–6, 1959.
28. Covino BG: Comparative clinical pharmacology of local anesthetic agents. Anesthesiology 35:158, 1971.
29. Crikelair GF: Skin suture marks. Am J Surg 96: 631, 1958.
30. Cruse PJE, Foord R: A five-year prospective study of 23,649 surgical wounds. Arch Surg 107:206, 1973.
31. Davis JS: Plastic Surgery. Philadelphia: P Blakiston, 26, 1919.
32. Demling RH, Buerstatte WR, Perea A: Management of hot tar burns. J Trauma 20:242, 1980.
33. Douglas BS: Conservative management of guillotine amputation of the finger in children. Aust Paediatr J 8:86, 1972.
34. Douglas DM: Tensile strength of sutures, II: Loss when implanted in living tissue. Lancet 2: 499, 1949.
35. Downs TM: The healing of wound. Surg Clin North Am 20:1859, 1940.
36. Duke WR, Robson MC, Krizek TJ: Civilian wounds: Their bacterial flora and rate of infection. Surg Forum 23:518, 1972.
37. DuMortier JJ: The resistance of healing wounds to infection. Surg Gynecol Obstet 56:762, 1933.
38. Edlich RF, Haynes BW, Larkham N, et al: Emergency department, triage and transfer protocols for the burn patient. JACEP 7:152, 1978.
39. Edlich RF, Panek PH, Rodeheaver GT, et al: Physical and chemical configuration of sutures in the development of surgical infection. Ann Surg 177:679, 1973.
40. Edlich RF, Rodeheaver GT, Thacker JG, et al: Fundamentals of Wound Management in Surgery: Technical Factors in Wound Management. South Plainfield, NJ: Chirurgecom, Inc., 1977.
41. Elek SD, Conen PE: The virulence of *Staphylococcus pyogenes* for man: Study of the prob-

lems of wound infection. Br J Exp Pathol 38: 573, 1957.
42. Emerson EB: Fishhooks. NY State J Med 66:2414, 1966.
43. Entin MA: Infections of the hand. Surg Clin North Am 44:981, 1964.
44. Evans AJ: Experience of the burns unit: A review of 520 cases. Br Med J 8:547, 1956.
45. Farrell RG, Disher WA, Nesland RS, et al: Conservative management of fingertip amputations. JACEP 6:243, 1977.
46. Fisher RH: The Kutler method of repair of fingertip amputations. J Bone Joint Surg 48:606, 1966.
47. Gant T: A suturing refresher for family doctors. Patient Care 13:34, 1979.
48. Greig JD, Anderson JH, Ireland AJ, et al: The surgical treatment of ingrowing toenails. J Bone Joint Surg Br 73:1, 131–133, 1991.
49. Gross CW: Soft tissue injuries of the lip, nose, ears, and preauricular area. Otolaryngol Clin North Am 2:292, 1969.
50. Hampton OP: The indications for debridement of gunshot (bullet) wounds of the extremities in civilian practice. J Trauma 1:368, 1961.
51. Hanley PH: Acute pilonidal abscess. Surg Gynecol Obstet 50:9, 1980.
52. Hoehn RJ: Agents, mechanisms, and incidence of facial injury. Surg Clin North Am 53:1479, 1973.
53. Hollander JE, Singer AJ: Application of tissue adhesives: Rapid attainment of proficiency. Acad Emerg Med 5:1012–1017, 1998.
54. Hollander JE, Singer AJ, Valentine S, Henry MC: Wound registry: Development and validation. Ann Emerg Med 25:675–685, 1995.
55. Holm A, Zachariae L: Fingertip lesions: An evaluation of conservative treatment versus free skin grafting. Acta Orthop Scand 45:382, 1974.
56. Hoover NW, Ivins JC: Wound debridement. Arch Surg 79:701, 1959.
57. Howell JM: Current and future trends in wound healing. Emerg Med Clin North Am 10:655–663, 1992.
58. Howes EL: A renaissance of suture technique needed. Ann Surg 48:548, 1940.
59. Huang TT, Lynch JB, Larson DL, et al: The use of excisional therapy in the management of snakebite. Ann Surg 179:598, 1974.
60. Hunt TK: Fundamentals of Wound Management in Surgery: Wound Healing: Disorders of Repair. South Plainfield, NJ: Chirurgecom, 1976.
61. Hunt TK: Fundamentals of Wound Management in Surgery: Wound Healing: Normal Repair. South Plainfield, NJ: Chirurgecom, 1976.
62. James RC, MacLeod CJ: Induction of staphylococcal infections in mice with small inocula introduced on sutures. Br J Exp Pathol 42:266, 1961.
63. Jamra FNA, Khuri S: The treatment of fingertip injuries. J Trauma 11:749, 1970.
64. Jelenko C, McKinley JC: Post-burn respiratory injury. JACEP 5:455, 1976.
65. Jones LT: An anatomical approach to problems of the eyelids and lacrimal apparatus. Arch Ophthalmol 66:137, 1961.
66. Ketchum LD, Cohen IK, Masters FW: Hypertrophic scars and keloids: A collective review. Plast Reconstr Surg 53:140, 1974.
67. Kilgore ES, Graham WP: The Hand. Philadelphia: Lea & Febiger, 1977.
68. Kim Y-S: A new surgical suture technique. Surg Gynecol Obstet 137:669, 1973.
69. Kraissl CJ: The selection of appropriate lines for elective surgical incisions. Plast Reconstr Surg 8:1, 1951.
70. LaBagnara J: A review of absorbable suture materials in head and neck surgery and introduction of Monocryl: A new absorbable suture. ENT J 74:409–415, 1995.
71. Lamon RP, Cicero JJ, Frascone RJ, et al: Open treatment of fingertip amputations. Ann Emerg Med 12:358, 1983.
72. Larsen JS, Ulin AW: Tensile strength advantage of the far-and-near suture technique. Surg Gynecol Obstet 131:123, 1970.
73. Leidelmeyer R: The embedded broken-off needle. JACEP 5:362, 1976.
74. Lewis JR: Management of soft tissue injuries of the face. J Int Coll Surg 44:441, 1965.
75. Liston SL, Cortez EA, McNabney WK: External ear injuries. JACEP 7:233, 1978.
76. Localio SA, Casale W, Hinton JW: Wound healing: Experimental and statistical study. Surg Gynecol Obstet 77:481, 1943.
77. Lucid ML: The interlocking slip knot. Plast Reconstr Surg 34:200, 1964.
78. Lynch G: Minor surgery of the ear, nose and throat. Surg Clin North Am 31:1315, 1951.
79. Lyons C, Upchurch SE: The management of common superficial wounds. Surg Clin North Am 31:1271, 1951.
80. Macomber DW: Lacerations and incisions: Technical considerations. Am J Surg 26:145, 1960.
81. Madden JC, Edlich RD, Schauerhamer R, et al: Application of principles of fluid dynamics to surgical wound irrigation. Curr Top Surg Res 3: 85, 1971.
82. Maw JL, Quinn JV, Wells GA, et al: A prospective comparison of octylcyanoacrylate tissue adhesive and suture for the closure of head and neck incisions. J Otolaryngol 26:26–30, 1997.
83. McCaig LF, Stussman BJ: National Hospital Ambulatory Medical Care Survey: 1996 Emergency Department Summary: Advance Data from Vital and Health Statistics no. 293. Hyattsville, MD: National Center for Health Statistics, 1997.
84. Meislin HW, Lerner SA, Graves MH, et al: Anaerobic and aerobic bacteriology and outpatient management. Ann Intern Med 87:145, 1977.
85. Minsky H: Surgical repair of recent lid lacerations. Surg Gynecol Obstet 75:449, 1942.
86. Myers MB: Functional and angiographic vasculature in healing wounds. Am J Surg 36:750, 1970.
87. Nakajima T, Yoshimura Y, Yoneda K: Open treatment with drainage for ingrowing toenail. Surg Gynecol Obstet 170:223–224, 1990.
88. Noe JM, Gloth DA: A technique for the placement of a continuous suture. Surg Gynecol Obstet 150:404, 1980.

89. Orlinsky M, Goldberg RM, Chan L, et al. Cost analysis of stapling versus suturing for skin closure. Am J Emerg Med. 13:77–81, 1995.
90. Price PB: Stress, strain and sutures. Ann Surg 128:408, 1948.
91. Pryor GT: Local anesthesia in minor lacerations: Topical TAC vs lidocaine infiltration. Ann Emerg Med 9:568, 1980.
92. Quinby WC: Restrictive effects of thoracic burns in children. J Trauma 12:646, 1972.
93. Quinn, J, Wells G, Sutcliffe T, et al: Tissue adhesive versus suture repair at 1 year: Randomized clinical trial correlating early, 3-month, and 1-year cosmetic outcome. Ann Emerg Med 32:645–649, 1998.
94. Quinn J, Wells G, Sutcliff T, et al: A randomized trial comparing octylcyanoacrylate tissue adhesive and sutures in the management of lacerations, JAMA 277:1527–1530, 1997.
95. Quinn JV, Drzewiecki A, Li MM, et al: A randomized, controlled trial comparing a tissue adhesive with suturing in the repair of pediatric lacerations. Ann Emerg Med 22:1130–1135, 1993.
96. Raffman RA: A re-evaluation of the pathogenesis of pilonidal sinus. Am J Surg 150:895, 1959.
97. Robson MC, Lea CE, Dalton JB, et al: Quantitative bacteriology and delayed wound closure. Forum 19:501, 1968.
98. Rocha Moreira RC, Abrao E: Modified mattress suture for closure of difficult wounds. Surg Gynecol Obstet 168:545, 1989.
99. Rodeheaver GT: Pluronic F-68: A promising new skin cleanser. Ann Emerg Med 9:572, 1980.
100. Rodeheaver GT, Pettry D, Thacker JG, et al: Wound cleansing by high-pressure irrigation. Surg Gynecol Obstet 141:357, 1975.
101. Roettinger W, Edgerton MT, Kurtz LD, et al: Role of inoculation site as a determinant of infection in soft tissue wounds. Am J Surg 126: 354, 1973.
102. Rubin LR: Langer's lines and facial scars. Plast Reconstr Surg 3:147, 1948.
103. Salisbury RE, Taylor JW, Levine NS: Evaluation of digital escharotomy in burned hands. Plast Reconstr Surg 58:440, 1976.
104. Senapati A: Conservative outpatient management of ingrowing toenails. J R Soc Med 70: 339–340, 1986.
105. Seropian R, Reynolds BM: Wound infections after preoperative depilatory versus razor preparation. Am J Surg 121:251, 1971.
106. Singer AJ, Clark RAF: Mechanisms of disease: Cutaneous wound healing II. N Engl J Med 341: 738–746, 1999.
107. Spira M, Gerow FJ, Hardy SB: Windshield injuries of the face. J Trauma 8:513, 1968.
108. Spira M, Hardy SB: Management of the injured ear. Am J Surg 106:678, 1963.
109. Straith RE, Lawson JM, Hipps CJ: The subcuticular suture. Postgrad Med 29:164, 1961.
110. Tait GR, Tuck JS: Surgical or phenol ablation of the nailbed for ingrowing toenails: A randomized controlled trial. J R Coll Surg Edinb 32:6:358–360, 1987.
111. Tejani F, Aufses AH: A new technique for skin closure. Surg Gynecol Obstet 142:407, 1976.
112. Trott AT: Cyanoacrylate tissue adhesives: An advance in wound care [Editorial]. JAMA 277:1559–1560, 1997.
113. VanDerHam AC, Hackeng CAH, Tiklen Yo, et al: The treatment of ingrowing toenails. J Bone Joint Surg Br 72:3, 507–509, 1990.
114. Van Winkle W Jr, Hastings JC: Consideration in the choice of suture materials for various tissues. Surg Gynecol Obstet 135:113, 1972.
115. Walike JW: Suturing technique in facial soft tissue injuries. Otolaryngol Clin North Am 12: 415, 1979.
116. Wallace AB: Assessment and emergency treatment of burns. Br Med J 2:1136, 1955.
117. Williams DF: The reactions of tissues to materials. Biomed Eng 6:152, 1971.
118. Williams RS: A better technique for wedge resection of ingrown toenail. Aust N Z J Surg 56: 437–438, 1986.
119. Yamamoto LG: Preventing adverse events and outcomes encountered using Dermabond [Letter]. Am J Emerg Med 18:511–515, 2000.

Suggested Reading

Ariyan S: A simple sterotactic method to isolate and remove foreign bodies. Arch Surg 112:857, 1977.
Beasley RW: Reconstruction of amputated fingertips. Plast Reconstr Surg 44:349, 1969.
Bennett JE, Thompson LW: The role of aggressive surgical treatment in the severely burned patient. J Trauma 9:776, 1969.
Berger RS: A critical look at therapy for the brown recluse spider bite. Arch Dermatol 107:298, 1973.
Burke JF, Bondoc CC: A method of secondary closure of heavily contaminated wounds providing "physiologic primary closure." J Trauma 8:228, 1968.
Dupertuis SM, Musgrave RH: Burns of the hand. Plast Reconstr Surg 40:490, 1967.
Dziemian AJ, Mendelson JA, Lindsey D: Comparison of the wounding characteristics of some commonly encountered bullets. J Trauma 1:341, 1961.
Edlich RF, Rodeheaver G, Kuphal J, et al: Technique of closure: Contaminated wounds. JACEP 2:375, 1974.
Fardon DW, Wingo CW, Robinson DW, et al: The treatment of brown spider bites. Plast Reconstr Surg 40:482, 1967.
Forrest JF: An improved technique for delayed primary closure of potentially infected lesions. Surg Gynecol Obstet 149:401, 1979.
Fryer MP, Brown JB, Bin JW: Repair of trauma about the orbit. J Trauma 12:290, 1972.
Glass TG: Early debridement in pit viper bites. JAMA 235:2513, 1976.
Kleinert HE: Fingertip injuries and their management. Plast Reconstr Surg 25:41, 1959.
Lehr HB, Fitts WT: The management of avulsion injuries of soft tissue. J Trauma 9:261, 1969.
Mawr B: The healing of wounds. Surg Clin North Am 20:1859, 1940.
Morgan MM, Spencer AD, Hershey FB: Debridement of civilian gunshot wounds of soft tissue. J Trauma 1:354, 1961.
Paradies LH, Gregory CF: The early treatment of close-range shotgun wounds to the extremities. J Bone Joint Surg Am 48:425, 1966.

Peloso OA, Wilkinson LH: The chain stitch knot. Surg Gynecol Obstet 139:599, 1974.

Ramsay G, Caldwell D: Phenol cauterization for ingrowing toenails. Arch Emerg Med 3:243–246, 1986.

Richards KE, Feller I: Grid escharotomy for debriding burns. Surg Gynecol Obstet 137:843, 1973.

Russell FE, Carlson RW, Wainschel J, et al: Snake venom poisoning in the United States. JAMA 233:341, 1975.

Scatliff JH, Camnitz PS, Partain CL: Claw hammer technique for extraction of knives. J Trauma 18:742, 1978.

Scott JE: Amputation of the finger. Br J Surg 61:574, 1974.

Sherman RT, Parrish RA: Management of shotgun injuries: A review of 152 cases. J Trauma 3:76, 1963.

Snyder CC, Straight R, Glenn J: The snakebitten hand. Plast Reconstr Surg 49:275, 1972.

Stevenson TR, Thacker JG, Rodeheaver GT, et al: Cleansing the traumatic wound by high-pressure syringe irrigation. JACEP 5:17, 1976.

Tabor GL: Trauma to eye and orbit. J Trauma 8:1089, 1968.

Tanner JC, Vandeput J, Olley JF: The mesh skin graft. Plast Reconstr Surg 34:287, 1964.

Trevaskis AE, Rempel J, Okunski W, et al: Sliding subcutaneous-pedicle flaps to close a circular defect. Plast Reconstr Surg 46:155, 1970.

Wee GC, Shieber W: Painless evacuation of subungual hematoma. Surg Gynecol Obstet 131:535, 1970.

Ziperman HH: The management of soft tissue missile wounds in war and peace. J Trauma 1:361, 1961.

11

Urologic Procedures

ANATOMY

The Male Anatomy

The structure of the male urethra is rather complex. It consists of three parts: the prostatic, membranous, and spongy parts. It is about 8 inches in total length. The prostatic urethra commences at the internal urinary meatus. It is embedded within the prostate gland. The urethra exits the prostate gland just anterior to the apex of the gland, and at this point, it becomes the membranous urethra. The urethra is at its widest through the prostatic part. The ejaculatory ducts and the prostatic ducts open into the prostatic part of the urethra.

The shortest and least dilatable part of the urethra is the membranous part. The membranous part is about ¾-inch long, and passes through the deep peroneal pouch. The urogenital diaphragm is the muscle that fills the deep peroneal pouch. This muscle comprises the sphincter urethrae (also called the external urethral sphincter) and the deep transverse perineal muscles. The sphincter urethrae is a pear-shaped muscle that encircles the urethra. The upper part of the "pear" envelops the lower part of the prostatic urethra, whereas the globular part is just above the perineal membrane.

The spongy urethra, also called the penile or anterior urethra, is about 6 inches long. It is within the corpus spongiosum of the penis (q.v.). The spongy urethra can be divided into the bulbous and the pendulous parts. The bulbous part, continuous with the membranous urethra, passes through the perineal membrane and enters the bulb of the corpus spongiosum. It takes a right-angled curve forward into the root of the penis. It then passes down the penis as the pendulous part. Just before the external urethral meatus is a small, dilated part: the navicular fossa.

The urethra is narrowest at the external urethral meatus, at the proximal part of the navicular fossa, in the membranous part, and at the bladder neck. It also is important to be aware of the 90-degree turn at the base of the penis.

The shaft of the penis consists of the two corpora cavernosa, with the corpus spongiosum between and behind (with the penis flaccid). The corpus spongiosum contains the urethra, and the distal end of the corpus spongiosum enlarges to form the glans of the penis. The whole is surrounded by strong fascia, and, with the exception of the glans, by skin.

Female Anatomy

The female urethra passes from the lower angle of the trigone of the bladder to the external urethral meatus. The external urethral meatus is in the vestibule of the vagina, anterior to the vaginal opening, and about 1 inch behind the clitoris. The urethra is about 1.5 inches long. It is important to note that the urethra is not just in front of the vagina, but is actually embedded within the vaginal wall for all except the part immediately after leaving the bladder. Unlike that in the male, there is no internal urethral sphincter in the female.

Special Anatomic Considerations

In addition to the obvious differences in size, there are some differences between the pediatric and the adult male anatomy. In the penis, the foreskin of uncircumcised males is adherent to the glans until the age of between 3 and 5 years. At this time it separates, and the foreskin should be retractable.

It also is important to be aware of changes in urethral anatomy related to pregnancy. There may be significant stretching of the urethra during the later stages of pregnancy to as much as 10 cm in length.

Specimen Collection

- Clean catch: A clean-catch urine specimen is obtained from patients who are continent, are well enough to go to a rest room, and are toilet trained. The patient cleanses the urethral area with an antiseptic solution, and then voids into a sterile receptacle. A special example of the clean catch is the "midstream" clean catch. This requires that after careful cleaning, the patient start to void into the toilet. After the stream has started, the patient then passes a specimen into the sterile collection receptacle, and then completes urination into the toilet. Thoroughly instruct the patient for this procedure.
- Urine collection in children: Bag collection of urine in young children has been shown to be inaccurate, with higher white cell and bacterial counts from bag specimens than from catheter specimens from the same patient. It may be possible to obtain a specimen directly from the urine stream. Alternatively, suprapubic collection or catheterization may be needed.

BLADDER CATHETERIZATION

Many types of catheters are used to catheterize the bladder, including Foley catheters, Coudé-tip Foley catheters, Robinson, Malecot, and Pezzer catheters.

INDICATIONS

As many as 25% of patients who are admitted to hospital in the United States require a urinary catheter at some stage during the hospitalization. Urinary catheters are placed to relieve urinary retention, to enable accurate measurement of urinary output, to protect against skin breakdown, and for numerous other nursing and medical reasons.

1. To relieve acute urinary retention.
2. To monitor urinary output in a critically ill or injured patient.
3. To obtain urine for diagnostic purposes.
4. To enable patients with either a neurogenic or a mechanical inability to void.

CONTRAINDICATIONS

The major contraindication to the passage of a urethral catheter is the possibility of trauma to the urethra. Patients who have experienced significant trauma should have an examination of the perineum for bruising, the urethral meatus for evidence of bleeding, and a digital examination of the prostate to ensure it is not displaced, before attempting the passage of a urinary catheter. If there is evidence of perineal bruising, bleeding at the meatus, or a displaced or high-riding prostate, defer urethral catheterization until the continuity of the urethra can be confirmed.

Suspicion of urethral trauma. A number of signs indicate the possibility of urethral injury:

1. Prostatic displacement on rectal examination.
2. Perineal hematoma.
3. Blood present at the urethral meatus.

NOTE

A number of relative contraindications exist for bladder catheterization in patients who have sustained trauma. In these patients, catheterization may be attempted; if obstruction is encountered, attempt an alternative approach (suprapubic catheterization) or make a radiographic study of the distal urinary tract to ascertain patency of the urethra. These contraindications include the patient who has sustained a severe fracture of the pelvis, particularly a straddle fracture, and traumatized patients who have the desire to void but are unable.

Risks and Benefits

In hospitalized patients, urinary catheters are a leading cause of nosocomial infections and of gram-negative bacteremia. Infections originating in the urinary tract represent as many as 40% of nosocomial infections. An estimated 800,000 patients annually are affected. The development of urinary infections in catheterized patients is directly related to the length of time that the catheter is in place. Bacteria can readily invade the urinary tract along the external surface of the catheter, or in the urine within the lumen of the catheter. Because of the high risk of infection, insert all catheters with a scrupulous sterile technique. Careful care of patients already catheterized is important. Infections are often found in clusters and are probably related to a lack of adequate sterile measures, including hand washing, when managing patients. The prophylactic use of antibiotics is not indicated, as it appears simply to encourage infection with resistant organisms. Recently the use of a povidone–iodine cream on the meatus has been associated with a lower risk of infection, but further study must confirm definite benefit (18).

EQUIPMENT

Equipment to perform a urinary catheterization adequately can be found in commercially available kits. Essential equipment includes drapes, sterile lubricant, an appropriate sized catheter, a cleansing solution [povidone–iodine (Betadine)], sterile gloves, and a syringe with 10 mL of saline for inflating the balloon.

Most of the equipment necessary for a catheterization is contained in commercially available sets.

Drapes
Sterile lubricant
Catheter for the average adult, a 16-French Foley catheter; for a child, an 8- to 10-French Foley (1 French is equal to 1 mm circumference.)
Cotton balls
Iodinated (Betadine) solution
Sterile disposable gloves
Syringe (10 mL) and saline for inflating the balloon

Male Catheterization

PREPARATORY STEPS

1. Lay all of the needed materials on a sterile field.
2. Check the Foley catheter balloon for leaks.
3. Spread a sterile towel below the urethra.

PROCEDURAL STEPS

1. Place the patient supine with the legs separated and the head of the bed as close to the horizontal position as is comfortable for the patient.

2. Place drapes above and below the penis and put on sterile gloves.
3. Immobilize the penis with the nondominant hand, and retract the foreskin.
4. With the dominant hand, cleanse the glans penis with cotton balls dipped in povidone–iodine solution.
5. Lubricate the catheter tip with a topical anesthetic.
6. Insert the catheter into the urethra, and apply constant gentle pressure. This pressure will guide the catheter up to the point of the external urethral sphincter, unless there are urethral strictures, diverticuli, or false passages.
7. When resistance is felt, bring the penis parallel to the bed. Ask the patient to try to relax his pelvic floor and rectum, and continue with gentle pressure to overcome the urethral sphincter (Fig. 11.1).
8. Insert the catheter up to the hub, if possible. If this is not possible or if there is no return of urine after 1 minute, irrigate the catheter with 50 to 100 mL of sterile saline, because the lubricant (topical anesthetic) may have occluded the drainage ports.
9. Once the urine returns or the catheter irrigates freely without obstruction, slowly inflated the balloon and withdraw the catheter gently until the balloon is positioned at the bladder neck. If the patient experiences pain when the balloon is inflated, the balloon is located in the urethra and must be deflated and withdrawn.

NOTE

A 20-French catheter is used in the average adult because a larger catheter may prevent urethral exudates from draining properly and lead to urethritis. Using a smaller catheter is a mistake; they are pliable and may curl in the urethra. In some patients in whom catheterization may be difficult, a larger catheter may be used and not uncommonly can be passed because it is stiffer, even though a smaller one cannot. A mandarin guide, although rarely indicated, can be inserted inside the catheter and bent into the desired shape. Then insert the catheter as though it were a urethral sound, with digital pressure over the perineal region (Fig. 11.2) to aid in advancing the catheter through the posterior urethra.

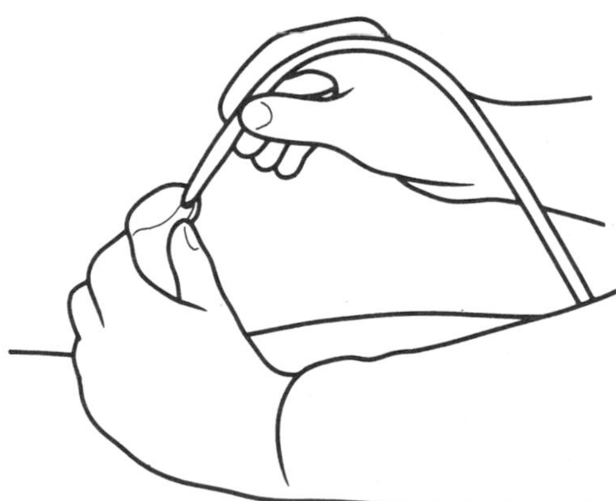

Figure 11.1. Insert a Foley catheter into the urethra with the right hand as the penis is held firmly in position with the left hand. See text for details.

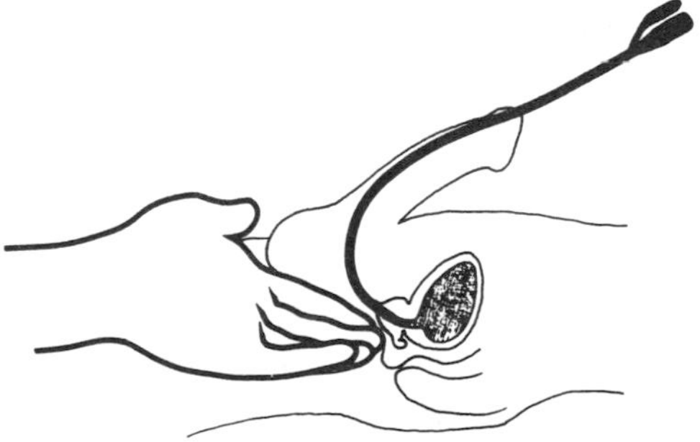

Figure 11.2. Insert a mandarin guide inside the Foley catheter and bend it into the desired shape. This stiffens the catheter; then insert the catheter as a urethral sound with perineal digital pressure applied, which aids in advancing the catheter through the posterior urethra. (The mandarin guide is not shown in the diagram.)

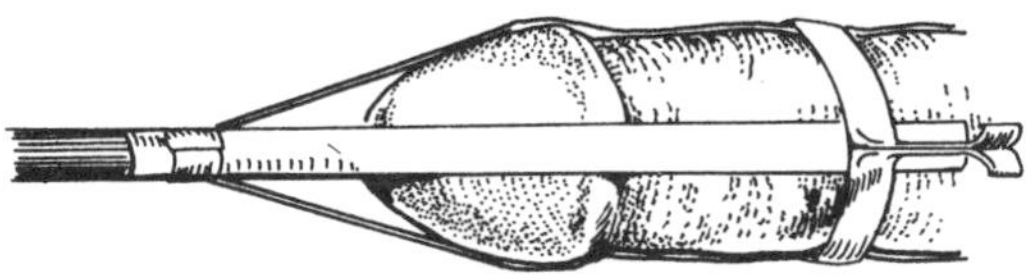

Figure 11.3. A method for securing a catheter to the penis.

NOTE

When a catheter type is used that is not self-retaining, secure the catheter to the penis with two strips of tape opposite one another, extending from the sides of the catheter to the penis (16). Then place an encircling strip of tape around the catheter at the point where the catheter enters the penis. This prevents forward and backward displacement of the catheter into and out of the urethra; this displacement introduces bacterial contaminants into the urinary tract. Figure 11.3 shows a method for securing a catheter to the penis.

NOTE

When difficulties are encountered in catheterization, install 2% lidocaine (Xylocaine) jelly into the meatus, under constant gentle pressure, to allow the passage of a catheter. If the lubricant does not easily pass, then there may be an anatomic (urethral stricture) or a physiologic (sphincter spasm) obstruction.

Female Catheterization

PREPARATORY STEPS

1. Place the patient in the dorsolithotomy position.
2. Use the left hand to spread the labia apart to reveal the urethral orifice, above the introitus and just inferior to the clitoris.
3. Identify the urethral meatus and cleanse it with cotton balls dipped in povidone–iodine solution, using a single wipe directed from anterior to posterior. Discard each cotton ball after the single wipe.

PROCEDURAL STEPS

1. Lubricate the tip of the catheter, and with the thumb and index finger, hold the catheter 1 to 2 inches from the tip, and insert it into the meatal orifice.
2. After the bladder has been entered, as indicated by urine flow through the catheter, inflate the balloon with 5 mL of saline.

CAUTION

If the catheter inadvertently enters the vagina, use a new catheter to prevent vaginal contaminants from entering the bladder and causing cystitis.

---

3. Then securely tape the catheter to the patient's thigh.
4. After inserting the Foley catheter, wash the hands because these catheters are a major source of nosocomial infections. Also wash the hands after any urine sample is removed from the drainage bag or catheter (20).

COMPLICATIONS

1. **Urethritis.** Urethritis is a common complication after catheterization, particularly in a patient with strictures or prostatic enlargement.
2. **Epididymitis.** This is an uncommon problem after catheterization; however, it may be encountered in a patient who has cystitis or urethritis before catheterization.
3. **Bacteremia.**
4. **Trauma to the urethra,** leading to urethral strictures.
5. **Conversion of a partial urethral tear to a complete one** in a traumatized patient.

6. **Hemorrhage from urethral trauma** during catheter insertion.
7. **Creation of a false passage** by inserting the catheter alongside the urethra.
8. **Cystitis and pyelonephritis.** Infectious complications may be unavoidable with prolonged catheterizations. Avoid many complications by the use of sterile technique during insertion. The urinary drainage should remain as a closed system with removal of urine from the bag or sterilely from connecting tubing with a needle and syringe (7, 13). The urine in the collecting bag should *never* be elevated and permitted to drain retrogradely into the bladder.

Coudé Catheters

Experience is required to learn the atraumatic use of a Coudé catheter. In unusual circumstances in which a suprapubic cystostomy is contraindicated and the bladder must be catheterized, pass a 20-French Coudé catheter with the elbow pointing anteriorly to negotiate the enlarged prostatic urethra. In some cases, use a finger in the rectum to push the tip of the catheter anteriorly, while an assistant exerts gentle forward pressure, permitting entry into an elevated bladder neck.

Newer suprapubic catheters use the "Seldinger" wire technique. Advance a long spinal needle with a syringe attached into the bladder. Once urine is aspirated, remove the syringe, and pass a guidewire passed down into the bladder. Then place one of the commercially available "over the wire" suprapubic catheters over the wire and advance it into the bladder.

The elderly are at increased risk of a difficult catheterization due to prostatic hypertrophy or to anatomic changes related to surgery. Give careful consideration to the necessity for catheterization in this group. In male patients, a slightly larger, but firmer, catheter may make catheterization easier. Consider suprapubic catheterization if there are problems with urethral catheterization.

Removal of the Nondeflating Catheter

Occasionally a patient has a catheter in the bladder that cannot be removed. In these cases, a number of techniques can be used to try to remove the catheter. The inability to remove the catheter may be due to a problem at one of the following points. First, the valve where water is injected into the catheter may be blocked. Second, external clamping or kinking may have damaged the tube. Finally, crystallization of the fluid used to inflate the balloon may cause a problem, preventing the balloon from deflating (19).

The first step is to cut the balloon port proximal to the inflation valve. If this does not result in a release of water, and ability to remove the catheter, then pass a wire through the inflation channel. The wire from a central venous cannula set is appropriate for this task. Pass the wire into the balloon to perforate it. However, sometimes a firmer structure is needed, and in this case, use the venous catheter itself. Pass it over the guidewire into the balloon.

If the venous catheter does not rupture the balloon, leave the catheter in place and use it to introduce chemicals into the balloon. The chemicals chosen work by degrading the balloon sufficiently that it ruptures, but not to the extent that it totally disintegrates. Use chemicals such as ether, chloroform, acetone, or mineral oil. Of these, we recommend mineral oil, 10 mL, drawn up into a syringe, and introduced into the catheter balloon. After waiting for about 15 minutes, make an attempt to remove the urinary catheter. If this is unsuccessful, instill a further 10 mL.

If the balloon ruptures, inspect it carefully, and ensure that no bits have been left behind. They can act as a nidus for infection, or calculus formation, and can produce significant irritation when voiding.

SUPRAPUBIC CATHETERIZATION AND ASPIRATION

Suprapubic catheterization is an easy and reliable method of both obtaining urine for diagnostic procedures and draining the urinary bladder in patients in whom urethral catheterization cannot be performed. Obtain urine from the bladder for diagnostic purposes by simple needle aspiration, particularly in children.

INDICATIONS

1. For diagnostic purposes in children, when a clean-catch urine specimen is unobtainable or contamination exists.
2. To relieve urinary obstruction when one is unable to pass a urethral catheter in a patient with acute urinary retention.
3. In trauma patients who have sustained major urethral injury (rupture), in which case it is not possible to pass a urethral catheter.

CONTRAINDICATIONS

1. A small or nonpalpable bladder.
2. Scars from previous lower abdominal surgery.

Suprapubic Aspiration

EQUIPMENT

22-gauge 1-inch needle for children or 20-gauge needle for adults
10-mL syringe
Prep solution
Anesthetic with 1% lidocaine with epinephrine
25-gauge needle
3-mL syringe

TECHNIQUE

Percuss the abdomen to determine the level of the bladder. Do not perform suprapubic aspiration of the bladder unless the bladder is at least partially filled with urine. Determine this by palpation, percussion, or by the physician pressing with fingers above the pubic symphysis and checking whether this gives the patient the desire to void. Prepare and shave the suprapubic region. Attach a needle (as indicated earlier) to the syringe, and insert it in the midline approximately 2 cm above the symphysis of the pubis. Direct the needle at an angle of approximately 45 to 60 degrees to the skin and aim it caudally. A "pop" can be felt when the bladder is entered. Then aspirate the urine and send it for analysis.

Suprapubic Catheterization

EQUIPMENT

In addition to the equipment listed earlier:

Percutaneous suprapubic cystostomy kit
Gauze dressings and wide cloth tape
Sterile drapes
20-gauge spinal needle
No. 11 and 15 scalpels and blades
3-0 nylon on a cutting needle, needle holder, and scissors
Closed system urinary drainage bag

TECHNIQUE (4, 8, 13, 15)

1. Percuss the abdomen to determine the level of the bladder as indicated under suprapubic aspiration.

NOTE

Do not attempt to catheterize the bladder if it is not at least partially filled with urine.

---

2. Shave the hair in the midline of the suprapubic region, and then prepare and drape the skin.
3. With 1% lidocaine in the midline, two finger breadths (3 to 4 cm) cephalad to the superior border of the symphysis pubis, raise a skin wheal. Anesthetize the subcutaneous tissue.
4. Use a 20-gauge spinal needle to anes-

thetize the abdominal wall with 1% lidocaine. With continuous pressure, insert the needle directly posteriorly, until urine is aspirated. If there has been prior lower abdominal surgery, angle the needle 30 degrees caudad to enter the bladder at a lower level and to avoid bowel loops that may be adherent to the surface of the bladder. If no urine is retrieved and air is aspirated, terminate the procedure (1, 7).

5. After waiting a few minutes and checking that the anesthetic has worked, make a 1-cm horizontal incision in the midline of the suprapubic region.
6. Stretch a mushroom-tipped suprapubic catheter over a trocar. Be sure that the trocar and catheter are directed as was the spinal needle previously (Fig. 11.4).
7. Puncture the linea alba with the trocar with a controlled stabbing motion. Place the operator's nondominant hand on the patient's abdomen, gently grasping the tube between the thumb and forefinger. Thus, one is able to stabilize the trocar, support the suprapubic catheter, and control the depth of the trocar penetration.
8. The trocar traverses the prevesical space without resistance; guide it to the surface of the dome of the bladder. A short rapid stabbing motion is most effective for puncturing the pliable bladder wall.
9. Aspirate urine from the trocar to confirm placement in the bladder, unless urine in the bladder is under high pressure.
10. Then advance the mushroom-tipped catheter 3 cm over the trocar, and remove the trocar (12).
11. Connect a drainage adapter and urinary collection bag to the catheter.
12. With a 3-0 nylon suture, secure the cystostomy tube to the skin. Place folded gauze dressings lateral to the catheter to prevent kinking. Secure the dressings with tape, and tape the catheter to the patient's lateral abdominal wall (Fig. 11.5).

Inadvertent penetration of a normal bowel with a spinal needle does not appear to cause any morbidity. Frequently one has to go approximately 3 cm deeper with the mushroom catheter and trocar than the distance with the spinal needle. The Stamey trocar has a black line to mark the depth of penetration that should not be exceeded beyond the surface, except in patients who are markedly obese. The Stamey trocar (Cook Urological, Spencer, Indiana) kit seems the easiest to use. We recommend

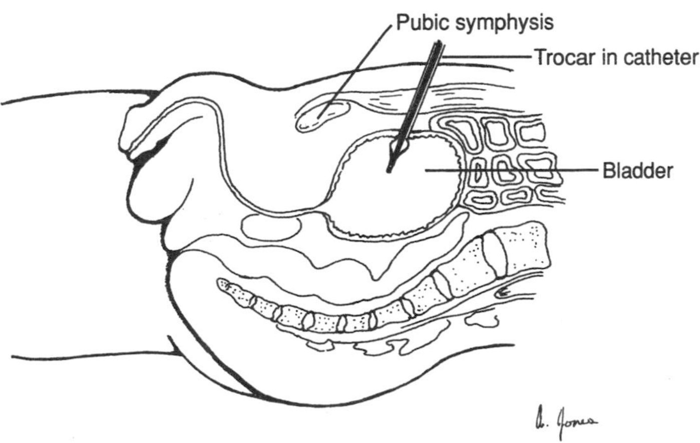

Figure 11.4. Technique of suprapubic catheterization by using a trocar with a catheter. See text for discussion.

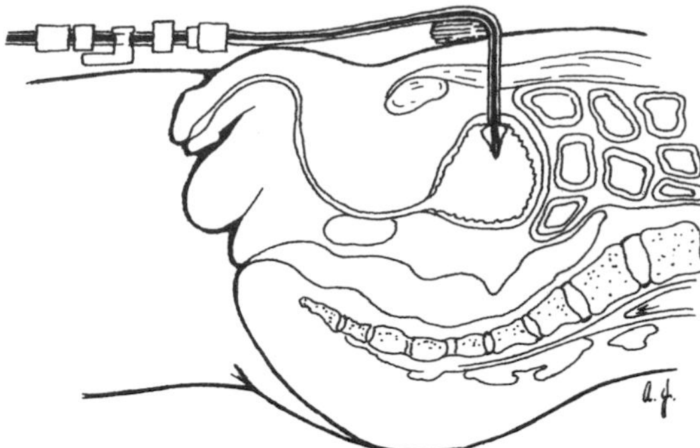

Figure 11.5. Trocar taped over 4 × 4-cm gauze pads after insertion. See text for discussion.

using a 14-French catheter in adults and a 10-French catheter in children.

Occasionally a suprapubic cystostomy is indicated when a patient either has a coagulopathy or had prior abdominal surgery. An emergency physician may feel uncomfortable doing this procedure with a trocar and a mushroom-tipped catheter. In these instances, use a small-gauge Intracath to enter the bladder and drain urine temporarily until a urologist can be consulted (Fig. 11.6).

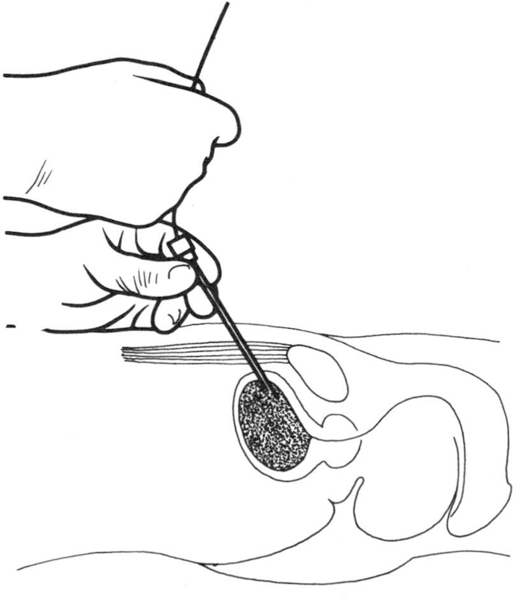

Figure 11.6. Technique of suprapubic catheterization with a small-gauge Intracath. See text for discussion.

COMPLICATIONS

1. **Leakage around the catheter** (8, 15).
2. **Kinking of the catheter** or suprapubic tube (8).
3. **Hematuria** induced by the catheter or tube irritating the bladder.
4. **Bowel puncture** (15).
5. **Puncture of a large vessel** (15).
6. **Anterior abdominal wall abscess** after suprapubic aspiration (15). In the cases reported, the needle was inserted into dehydrated patients in the midline about 1 cm above the suprapubic skin crease and perpendicular to the anterior abdominal wall. The needle was advanced 2.5 cm, the syringe plunger withdrawn, and intestinal contents were aspirated.
7. **The tip of the plastic catheter may be voided through the urethra** (8).

NOTE

Some authors stated that suprapubic tube cystostomy can be performed in patients with a ruptured bladder (4). Most believe, however, that it should not be done in patients with small or shrunken bladders or in patients with infected urine (11). With a suspected bladder rupture, instill about 250 mL of opaque contrast medium through a patent urethra and into the bladder to perform a cystogram. Be certain rupture has not occurred before aspiration (3).

CATHETERIZATION OF THE INFANT

The urethra of the female infant is C-shaped (21). The incidence of bacteremia after catheterization is remarkably high (22), approaching 30% of cases. A disposable, polyethylene urine-collecting bag is commercially available; this bag has a conical shape and fits well between the legs of male and female infants (9). The collecting bag has adhesive on the sides, which sticks well to the baby. This bag can be applied and removed from the child with little discomfort (9).

URETHRAL SOUNDING

Urethral sounding may be necessary in a patient who has stricture and urinary retention and in whom one is unable to bypass the obstruction with a urethral catheter. A sound is a firm J-shaped instrument that is used to facilitate passage into the bladder.

INDICATIONS

Patients with stricture causing obstruction in whom one is unable to insert a urethral catheter.

EQUIPMENT

Urethral sounds in assortment of sizes, 18 French and larger.

TECHNIQUE

1. Hold the penis in a manner similar to that used for urethral catheterization.
2. Cleanse the glans with cotton balls impregnated with povidone–iodine solution.
3. Select the size of the sound desired. In an adult male, first attempt a 24 French. Never use a smaller sound than an 18 French in the man. When an 18-French sound or larger cannot be passed through the urethra, then use a filiform and follower catheter because this is a safer technique in bypassing an obstruction.
4. Lubricate the sound.
5. Instill a topical anesthetic through the penis and use a penile clamp to aid in retaining the anesthetic gel for several minutes before the procedure.
6. With the penis stretched taut and stabilized with the left hand, advance the tip of the sound into the meatus with the sound held parallel to the patient's abdomen. Introduce the sound through the meatus of the penis with the handle of the sound positioned over the left iliac crest to facilitate passage (Fig. 11.7*A*).
7. Advance the sound into the urethra as the penis is drawn over the instrument (Fig. 11.7*B*). Resistance is often encountered by the sound at the bulbomembranous junction. Gently maneuver the sound to the vertical position to facilitate advancement through the external sphincter and bladder vesicle neck. Digital pressure may assist in passage at this point (Fig. 11.7*C*). As the sound is passed toward the prostate, depress the handle so the instrument can be advanced smoothly (Fig. 11.7*D*). In this manner, the tip of the sound easily follows the curve of the posterior urethra. Never use force in passing the sound or the urethra may be injured. Aid in the passage of the sound by applying downward pressure over the anterior aspect of the root of the penis as it passes the posterior urethra to relax the penile suspensory ligaments.

CATHETERIZATION WITH A FILIFORM AND FOLLOWER

In a patient with severe urethral strictures, insert a filiform and follower catheter through the urethral meatus. The filiforms come in various sizes, as do the follower catheters. The follower catheter has a special tip that should be screwed into the filiform after the latter is passed into the bladder.

EQUIPMENT

Several filiforms, sizes 4, 5, and 6 French, some with Coudé or corkscrew-tipped curves and some without. The follower screws onto the filiform catheter as shown in Fig. 11.8.

TECHNIQUE

1. Prepare and drape the penis as for catheterization. Follow the steps indicated under strict aseptic technique.

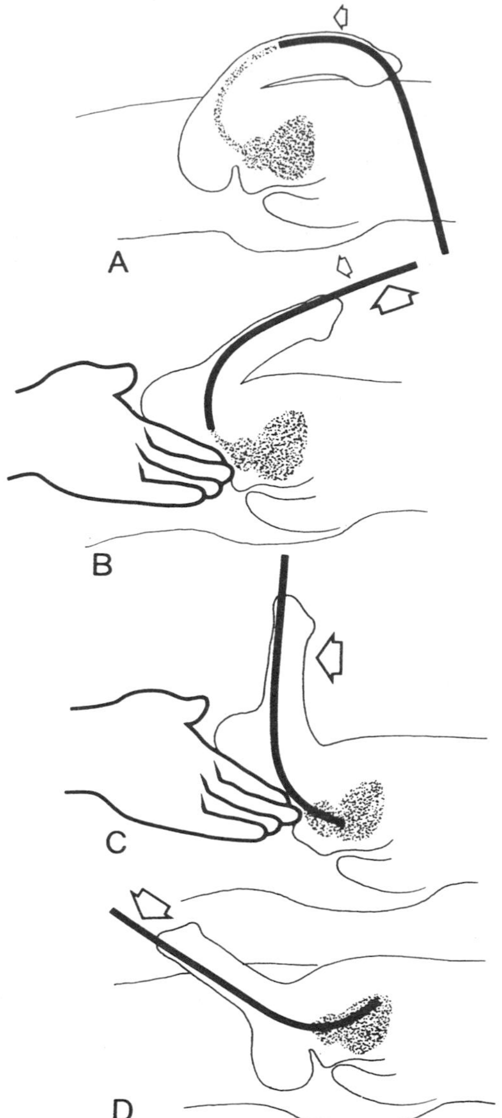

Figure 11.7. Urethral sounding technique: *A:* Hold the penis with the left hand, and insert the tip of the urethral sound into the meatus. Hold the handle of the sound over the left iliac crest to facilitate passage. *B:* Advance the sound into the urethra by drawing the penis up over the instrument. Maneuver the sound to the midline vertical position, and advance it to the level of the urethral bulb. *C:* Resistance is encountered by the sound at the bulbomembranous junction. Maneuver the sound gently to facilitate passage of the point. Digital pressure often assists in passing the sound. *D:* Depress the handle of the sound slowly. The tip of the sound is advanced more easily over the curve of the posterior urethra. Then advance the sound through the bladder neck.

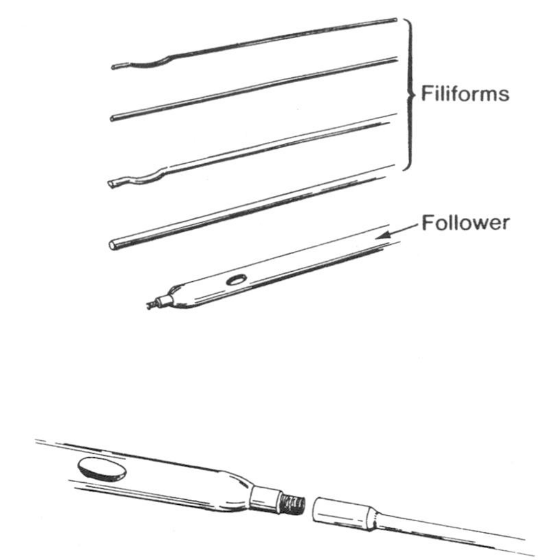

Figure 11.8. Filiforms come in many sizes. A follower catheter may be screwed into the base of a filiform catheter that has been previously inserted into the bladder.

2. After the urethra has been anesthetized with lidocaine jelly, pass one filiform until an obstruction is encountered. The filiform should be well lubricated. Do not attempt to force the filiform past the obstruction (Fig. 11.9*A*). Gently rotate the catheter in a twisting motion (Fig. 11.10) to see if the obstruction can easily be bypassed.
3. Lubricate several filiforms generously and place in the urethra up to the point of obstruction (Fig. 11.9). Stretch the penis to its full length at right angles to the patient's body.
4. Gently manipulate each filiform sequentially with a twisting motion, until one of the catheters enters the bladder without force (Fig. 11.9*B*, *C*).
5. Remove all filiform catheters, leaving the filiform that entered the bladder in place (Fig. 11.9*D*).
6. Then lubricate a follower catheter of approximate size and thread it onto the end of the filiform. Gently advance the catheter into the bladder until urine returns through the channel (Fig. 11.10).

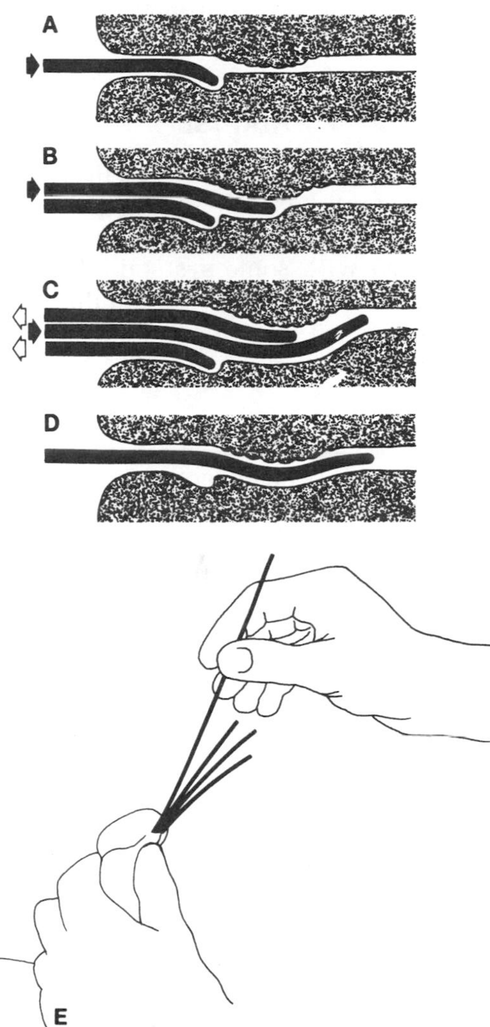

Figure 11.9. The insertion of urethral filiforms. Multiple filiforms are often required to bypass a stricture. Insert several filiforms, which obliterate the closed passages, only to the point where obstruction is met (*A, B*). Gently manipulate each filiform in a twisting motion until one enters (*C*). Then stabilize the filiform that enters the bladder, and remove the remaining filiforms (*D, E*).

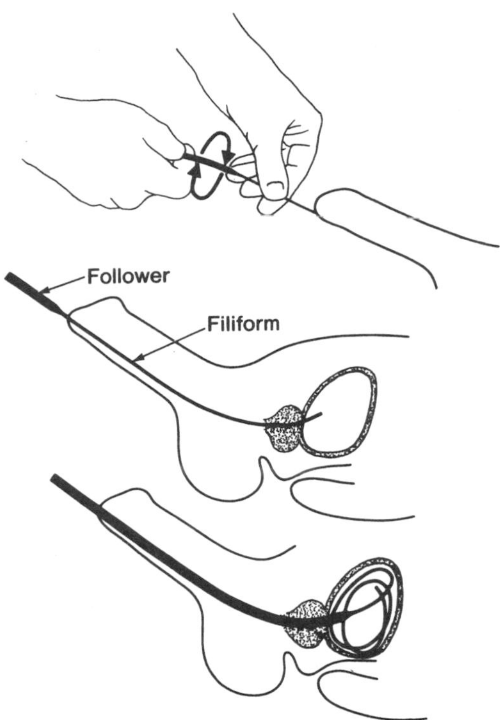

Figure 11.10. Screw the follower catheter onto the filiform, and advance the catheter into the bladder. The filiform functions as a guide for the advancement of the follower catheter. The filiform remains coiled within the bladder during the time of drainage.

EMERGENCY URETHROGRAM

Emergency urethrography can be performed in the emergency center in selected cases. In patients with severe pelvic fractures in whom there is blood at the meatus, emergency urethrography should probably be performed before insertion of a urethral catheter. The simple technique we prefer is illustrated in Fig. 11.11. Insert a 50-mL Toomey syringe into the tip of the meatus. Pull the penis forward into the catheter tip, and slowly inject 10 mL of a 10% solution of contrast material. Take a radiograph, and search for the leakage of dye around the meatus or blockage of the meatus.

An alternative technique involves placing an 8-inch urethral catheter into the meatus and passing it only enough so that the balloon is through the tip of the meatus. Instill approximately 2 mL of sterile saline into the balloon, and then slowly inject approximately 10 mL of contrast material through the lumen as shown in Fig. 11.12.

If a tear is detected and the urethra is totally obstructed, then perform a suprapu-

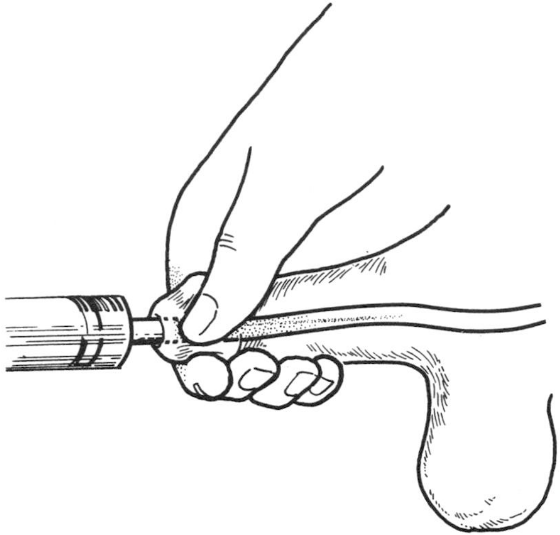

Figure 11.11. Insert a Toomey syringe into the tip of the meatus, and inject 10 mL of contrast material into the urethra. Place fingers around the meatus to prevent seepage of the contrast material from around the tip, as shown.

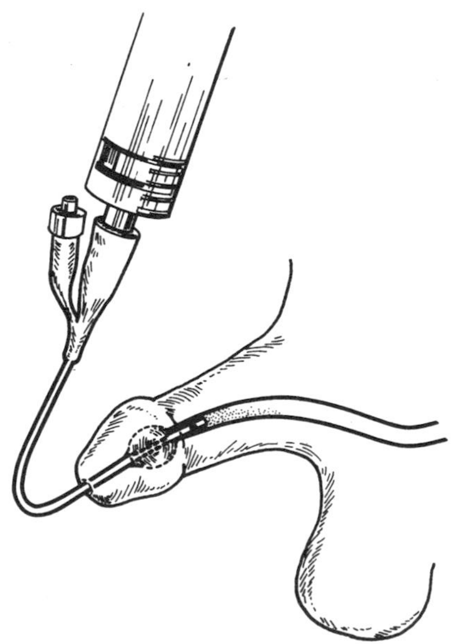

Figure 11.12. Insert a urethral catheter so that the balloon is just into the tip of the meatus, and inject 10 mL of contrast material after the balloon has been inflated with 2 mL of sterile saline.

bic cystostomy for a continual drainage, as discussed earlier.

PRIAPISM

Priapism is the presence of a persistent, usually painful, erection of the penis. Although frequently idiopathic, priapism is associated with some systemic diseases. Priapism also is associated with the use of intracavernosal injections of medications to treat impotence.

PATHOPHYSIOLOGY

Priapism is a persistent erection of the corpora cavernosa of the penis, originating from disturbances to the mechanisms that control penile detumescence. This process affects only the corpora cavernosa. The corpora spongiosum of the glans penis and surrounding the urethra remain flaccid.

Two types of priapism are described.

1. Arterial high flow priapism usually is secondary to a rupture of a cavernous artery and unregulated flow into the lacunar spaces. This type of priapism is usually not painful. In general, surgical management is required for this type of priapism, as other treatment options have a high rate of recurrence of priapism. Temporizing measures in the emergency department may include the use of ice packs.
2. Veno-occlusive priapism usually is due to full and unremitting corporeal veno-occlusion. Prolonged veno-occlusive priapism results in fibrosis of the penis and a loss of the ability to achieve an erection. Significant changes at the cellular level are noted within 24 hours in veno-occlusive priapism, whereas arterial priapism is not associated with fibrotic change. Some patients may use chemical agents to induce an erection. In these patients, excessive use may produce priapism. Examples of agents used to

induce an erection include papaverine, phentolamine, and prostaglandin E_1. The most common cause of veno-occlusive priapism is idiopathic. Other causes include leukemia and multiple myeloma, sickle cell disease and thalassemia, tumor infiltration, spinal cord injury and spinal anesthesia, Fabry disease, recent infection with *Mycoplasma pneumoniae*, amyloidosis, carbon monoxide poisoning, malaria, black widow spider bites, and numerous drugs including many psychotropic medications, especially chlorpromazine, trazodone, and thioridazine. Other drugs implicated include hydralazine, metoclopramide, omeprazole, and hydroxyzine, calcium channel blockers, anticoagulants, cocaine, marijuana, and ethanol abuse.

NONINVASIVE MANAGEMENT

A couple of techniques have been described to relieve priapism. The first involves the use of ice packs to the penis, scrotum, and perineum. The second is having the patient run or walk briskly up stairs. The mechanism of action for the latter technique is related to a "steal" phenomenon. However, if these conservative methods are not effective, the patient should have more aggressive medical management.

Some studies suggested that the use of terbutaline orally, at a dose of 5.0 mg, followed by another 5.0 mg 15 minutes later, if required, will produce resolution in about one third of patients. This may be a reasonable treatment option while preparing to perform more invasive measures. If no resolution occurs within 30 minutes, injection therapy will be required.

INVASIVE MANAGEMENT

Equipment and Medications

Intracavernous injection of an α-adrenergic agonist can rapidly reverse the vascular effects of phentolamine or papaverine. Phenylephrine is the most selective and potent α_1-adrenergic vasoconstrictor. It has a rapid onset of action at less than 1 minute, and its duration of action is 7 to 20 minutes. As phenylephrine has no clinically significant β-adrenergic receptor activity, it is unlikely to produce systemic cardiovascular toxicity after intracavernous injection.

TECHNIQUE

Preparation

The dose of phenylephrine is 100 to 500 μg per dose, up to a total of 10 doses. The drug is best administered in a dilute solution. Add 10 mg (usually 1.0 mL) of phenylephrine to 499 mL of saline, 0.9%. This will yield a solution with 20 μg/mL. Use 10 to 20 mL of this solution via intracavernous injection every 5 to 10 minutes.

Procedure

If medical management is not successful, then aspiration of the corpus cavernosum may be required. Clean the shaft of the penis, and drape the area. Perform a penile nerve block, injecting around the base of the penile shaft with 1% plain lidocaine. After anesthesia is assured, attach a 19-gauge needle to a large syringe to puncture the corpus cavernosum through the shaft of the penis, not through the corpus spongiosum. The aspiration site should be at the 2 or the 10 o'clock position. Initially, aspirate 20 to 30 mL of blood. Milking the shaft of the penis to empty the corpora may be necessary. As there are multiple communications from one corpus to the other, aspiration usually is required only at one side or the other. After detumescence is obtained, dress the penis with an elasticized bandage to ensure continued emptying of the corpora and to compress the puncture site. If this procedure is not successful, repeat the aspiration, with the instillation of an equal volume of a solution of phenylephrine (10 mg phenylephrine in 500 mL of 0.9%

saline). Phenylephrine is contraindicated in cases of known hypersensitivity, severe hypertension, and in patients with ventricular tachycardia. If aspiration of the corpus cavernosum reveals bright red blood initially rather than the dark blood expected, this represents high-flow priapism. In this situation, consult a urologist.

MANAGEMENT OF PHIMOSIS AND PARAPHIMOSIS

Phimosis

Phimosis is the inability to retract a previously retractable foreskin, or the inability to retract the foreskin of a male patient after puberty. In young male patients, the foreskin usually becomes retractable between the ages of 3 and 5 years. In older children or adolescents, the presence of a thickened margin between the glans penis and the foreskin when it is retracted as far as possible indicates the presence of infection, and a true phimosis. In these cases, circumcision is usually required; refer the patient to a surgeon.

Paraphimosis

A paraphimosis occurs when the foreskin has been retracted and then remains proximal to the glans penis. Significant swelling can ensue, and the viability of the foreskin and of the glans can be compromised because of restriction of blood flow. Causes of paraphimosis include failure to retract the foreskin over the glans after catheterization, and failure to retract the foreskin after it has been retracted in patients with adhesions between the foreskin and the glans. Reduction of paraphimosis can be difficult. The most effective technique is to place the index and middle fingers of each hand behind the paraphimotic ring, with the shaft of the penis between the digits. The thumbs then exert firm, constant pressure on the glans penis, pushing it gently back through the paraphimotic ring, which is supported by the four fingers. The technique can be painful, and a penile anesthetic block may be required. If reduction is not successful, then make an urgent referral for a dorsal slit through the foreskin. A newer technique involves the use of a 20-gauge needle to make 15 to 20 holes in the edematous prepuce. Then gently compress the prepuce, and express the edema fluid. Reduction is then described as being significantly easier (17).

Urethral Meatotomy

Meatal stenosis is rarely an emergency. More often the child will have a poor stream noted after toilet training. However, it may be noted in the emergency room when a child has a history of discomfort during micturition, or the finding of blood on the underwear due to meatal inflammation. Examination will reveal a very small meatus when the foreskin is gently retracted. Observation of the child voiding will reveal a very thin, forceful stream, which may be deflected dorsally.

This procedure can be performed under general or local anesthesia. Local anesthesia can be accomplished by the injection of a small quantity of lidocaine directly into the foreskin in the midline a few millimeters down the ventrum of the penis away from the meatus. This procedure is very uncomfortable. The use of a topical anesthetic cream to the foreskin may alleviate much of this discomfort. Apply the cream liberally to the glans penis, with an occlusive dressing over the penis. Leave this dressing in place for about an hour.

Once anesthesia has been achieved, grasp the skin in the midline of the ventrum of the penis in a clamp for a distance of a few millimeters. Hold the clamp in place for a minute or so. This crushes the skin, and results in less bleeding. Release the clamp, and incise the skin with a pair of fine-point scissors. This will reopen the meatus. Instruct the parents to keep the meatus open by using gentle pressure, especially at bath time.

Complications from the procedure include bleeding. Manage this with the aid of a suture to the bleeding edge. Restenosis can occur, but is prevented by the methods noted earlier. Recurrent stenosis is more common in patients who remain wet, due to the increased risk of inflammation.

MANAGEMENT OF TESTICULAR TORSION

The incidence of torsion of the testis is about 1 in 4,000 males younger than 25 years. The majority of cases occur in late childhood and early adolescence. As many as 50% of patients with an acute torsion will have a history of recurrent, self-limited episodes of lower abdominal or scrotal pain. Torsion can occur, though, at any age.

In older children, torsion is due to an anatomic abnormality of the attachment of the testis within the scrotum. The tunica vaginalis inserts high on the spermatic cord instead of on the lower pole of the testis. This results in the testis lying abnormally, and allows the testis to rotate freely within the tunica vaginalis. This is the so-called "bell-clapper" deformity. It is important to remember that this abnormality is usually bilateral, and this is why surgeons detort one testis and then surgically anchor the other testis (orchiopexy). With torsion, the testis will rise within the hemiscrotum from spermatic cord shortening. Usually the cremasteric reflex (a movement of the scrotum with firm stroking of the inside of the thigh on the same side) is absent in cases of acute torsion. However, the presence of this reflex does not exclude the diagnosis (5, 10, 14).

Manual detorsion can be attempted, but may be very difficult because of pain and scrotal edema. It is important to note that manual detorsion of the testis does not mean that the testis does not need to be explored. Contact a surgeon urgently.

TECHNIQUE

Attempt the reduction of a testicular torsion only if immediate access to a urologist is not possible. Anesthetize the spermatic cord in the following manner. Grasp the cord, just distal to the external inguinal canal, between thumb and index finger. Insert a small needle, attached to a 5-mL syringe filled with 1% lidocaine, into the cord. Aspirate the syringe to ensure that it has not been inserted into a vessel. If not, 3 to 5 mL of lidocaine is injected into the cord. Anesthesia of the testis should occur within a few minutes.

Once the cord is anesthetized, make an attempt to reduce the torsion. Hold the testis gently, and rotate it laterally and superiorly. If reduction is successful, the testis will drop into its normal position. Do not attempt this maneuver repeatedly. As noted, the patient will still require immediate referral to an urologist.

RADIOLOGIC TECHNIQUES

Retrograde Urethrography

This is covered in the current section on the Emergency Urethrogram.

Retrograde Cystography

A retrograde cystogram is performed only when it is certain that the urethra is intact, but there are doubts about the integrity of the bladder. Pass a Foley catheter into the bladder. Place a large (60 mL) syringe on the catheter, with the plunger removed. Instill an initial total of 100 mL of diluted contrast into the bladder. Allow the contrast to drain into the bladder under gravity drainage. Take an initial film. If this film is negative, instill a total of 400 mL of diluted contrast (in the adult), again by gravity drainage, and take a repeated view. Failure to complete the study with 400 mL has been associated with a significant false-negative rate. In children, the formula (age in years + 2) × 30 is used to estimate the volume of contrast solution to be instilled. If the volume initiates a bladder contraction, then instill a further 50 mL of contrast very gently under hand pressure.

References

1. Bonnanno PJ, Landers DE, Rock DE: Bladder drainage with the suprapubic catheter needle. Obstet Gynecol 35:807, 1970.
2. Brown MR, Cartwright PC, Snow BW: Common office problems in pediatric urology and gynecology. Pediatr Clin North Am 44:1091–1113, 1997.
3. Charron JW, Brault J-P: Recognition and early management of injuries to the urinary tract. J Trauma 4:702, 1964.
4. Clark SS, Prudencio FR: Lower urinary tract injuries associated with pelvic fractures. Surg Clin North Am 52:183, 1972.
5. Cuckow PM, Frank JD: Torsion of the testis. BJU Int 86:349–353, 2000.
6. Finkelberg Z, Kunin CM: Clinical evaluation of closed urinary drainage systems. JAMA 207: 1657, 1969.
7. Freeman S, Chapman J: Urologic procedures. Emerg Med Clin North Am 4:543, 1986.
8. Hale RW, McCorriston CC: Suprapubic cystotomy with a polyethylene tube. Am J Obstet Gynecol 105:1181, 1969.
9. Hill EJ: New method for collecting urine samples in infants. Plast Reconstr Surg 22:567, 1958.
10. Kass EJ, Lundak B: The acute scrotum. Pediatr Clin North Am 44:1251–1266, 1997.
11. Kunin CM, McCormack RC: Prevention of catheter-induced urinary tract infections by sterile closed drainage. N Engl J Med 274:1155, 1966.
12. Neuwirth H, Frasier B, Cochran T, et al: Genitourinary imaging and procedures by the emergency physician. Emerg Med Clin North Am 7:1, 1989.
13. Nystrom K, Bjerle P, Lindqvist B: Suprapubic catheterization of the urinary bladder as a diagnostic procedure. Scand J Urol Nephrol 7:160, 1973.
14. Pillai SB, Besner GE: Pediatric testicular problems. Pediatr Clin North Am 45:813–828, 1998.
15. Polnay L, Fraser AM, Lewis JM: Complication of suprapubic bladder aspiration. Arch Dis Child 50:80, 1975.
16. Reinarz JA: Nosocomial infections. CIBA Clin Symp 30:6, 1978.
17. Reynard JM, Barua JM: Reduction of paraphimosis the simple way: The Dundee technique. BJU Int 83:859–860, 1999.
18. Sedor J, Mulholland SG: Hospital-acquired urinary tract infections associated with the indwelling catheter. Urol Clin North Am 26: 821–827, 1999.
19. Shapiro AJ, Soderdahl DW, Stack RS, et al: Managing the non-deflating urethral catheter. J Am Board Fam Pract 13:116–119, 2000.
20. Steere A, Mallison GF: Handwashing practice for the prevention of nosocomial infections. Ann Intern Med 83:683, 1975.
21. Storts BP: Equipment for catheterization of female infants. Pediatrics 23:149, 1959.
22. Sullivan NM, Sutter VL, Mims MM, et al: Clinical aspects of bacteremia after manipulation of the genitourinary tract. J Infect Dis 127:49, 1973.

12

Vascular Procedures

BASIC PRINCIPLES IN INTRAVENOUS CANNULATION

The establishment of a "lifeline" is one of the essential procedures at which an emergency physician must be as skilled as any expert practitioner. In the ensuing discussion, we present a didactic presentation of the various types of intravenous catheters, site of insertion, and complications.

Intravenous cannulation is a means of access to the venous circulation and is useful for the administration of fluids or drugs, as well as for obtaining samples of blood for laboratory evaluation. Insert a cannula into either the peripheral system or the central system, and centrally either through a long peripheral line or through a separate site in one of the larger central veins.

Intravenous Cannulas

GENERAL FEATURES AND COMPLICATIONS

Three types of cannulas are available for use: hollow needles ("butterfly-type"), over-the-needle catheters (plastic catheters inserted over a hollow needle, e.g., Angiocath), and through-the-needle catheters (indwelling plastic catheters inserted through a hollow needle, e.g., Intracath). Plastic catheters are more commonly used for intravenous therapy than are hollow needles because these catheters can be better secured and are less easily displaced than are butterfly catheters. Butterfly catheters are more commonly used in infants and children.

Over-the-needle catheters are available in Teflon and polyethylene and in sizes ranging from 14 to 20 gauge. The needle and catheter are inserted together; then the needle is removed, leaving the catheter in the vein. This technique prevents catheter embolism and puncture of the back wall of the vein. Through-the-needle catheters are made of the same materials. The needle must be larger than the catheter, necessitating a large needle that may make insertion difficult. Catheter embolism is a risk with through-the-needle catheters.

STIFFNESS AND THROMBOGENICITY

When comparing catheters, two properties must be mentioned: stiffness and thrombogenicity. The *stiffer* the catheter, the higher the incidence of intimal trauma and subsequent phlebitis (26). In addition, perforation of the vein during either insertion or subsequent displacement is another hazard of a stiff catheter. The Medi-Cath polymeric silicone (Silastic) catheter (over-the-needle catheter) is flexible, virtually eliminates the risk of vessel perforation, and decreases the risk of intimal damage (26).

Plastic catheters initiate thrombus formation. A fibrin layer is seen over the site of contact of the plastic with the vessel. This fibrin, in general, is not thrombogenic; the clot begins at areas of intimal contact and injury and propagates circumferentially along the catheter (26). Hoshal et al. (104) demonstrated that fibrin sleeves are present around both polyethylene and Teflon subclavian catheters. In a study by Formanek et al. (75), Teflon catheters were about twice as thrombogenic as were polyethylene or siliconized polyethylene arterial catheters.

INFUSION RATES

The amount of fluid or blood one may infuse per unit time is directly related to the diameter of the catheter and its length. Obviously, the greater the diameter, the faster one can infuse a solution. The reverse is true with the length: the shorter the catheter, the faster one can infuse a solution. Reports indicate that the time required for 500 mL of whole blood to be infused through an 18-gauge 1.5-inch catheter is 15 minutes (184). When the catheter size is increased to a 12 gauge, it requires only 4 minutes. Select as short and as large a bore catheter as possible for most urgent uses. Blood should be passed only through a catheter that is 18-gauge or larger, preferably a 14 to 16 gauge. For cannulation of a peripheral vein, use a needle and catheter length of 5 cm. In central vein cannulations, we prefer a length of 8 cm.

A number of studies have been published on infusion rates. Table 12.1 shows the cannula size and infusion rates in liters per hour of several popular cannulas. The UMI 8-French catheter introducer has a flow rate of 11.05 L/h. This is by far the fastest flow rate (60). The Cordis 8 French, which is of comparable length, has one third of this flow rate, or approximately 3.05 L/h (60).

CATHETER SHEARING

Another problem with catheters is catheter shearing, which occurs with the use of through-the-needle catheters when the catheter is pulled back after being advanced through the needle. The sharp point of the needle may shear off a piece of catheter, which may remain in the skin or may act as an embolus. This is eliminated by the use of over-the-needle catheters (Argyle Medicut cannula and Deseret EZ Cath). Shearing also has been reduced by adding a device that retards catheter withdrawal in a through-the-needle unit (26).

AIR EMBOLISM

The possibility of air embolism is reduced by using a closed vacuum system (Medi-Cath, Intrafusor, Intracath using a closed technique). If a catheter is left open, air embolism is possible with any catheter design (2,149).

PHLEBITIS AND CELLULITIS

Reduce contamination of the catheter by preventing contact with the skin as the

Table 12.1.
Infusion Rates

Cannula	Diameter	Length	Liters per hour ± SD
Medicut	14 gauge	5.1 cm (2 in)	9.67 ± 0.28
	16 gauge	5.1 cm (2 in)	7.45 ± 0.08
	18 gauge	5.1 cm (2 in)	4.81 ± 0.13
Bard-I-Cath	16 gauge	20.3 cm (8 in)	3.51 ± 0.07
	16 gauge	30.5 cm (12 in)	2.87 ± 0.16
	16 gauge	61.0 cm (24 in)	2.02 ± 0.07
UMI	8 Fr	12.7 cm (5 in)	11.05 ± 0.05
Cordis	8 Fr	10.2 cm (4 in) (+22 cm sideport)	3.05 ± 0.02

catheter is threaded into the vein (through-the-needle catheters) or by preventing exposure of the catheter in a closed system. Intimal trauma is a source of phlebitis and is decreased by use of a soft, pliable catheter (Medi-Cath) (26).

Phlebitis may be difficult to prevent. Remove a catheter at 48 hours to prevent phlebitis (40, 105). Catheter infection may be as high as 50% at 3 days and increases with time (23). The more prolonged the cannulation, the greater is the risk of sepsis; thus it is important that emergency personnel place the data regarding catheter insertion (gauge of needle, date of insertion) on the tubing for subsequent reference (46,192). Sometimes no clinical signs of inflammation are present at the catheter site despite the presence of infection (20). Venous microabscesses have been shown to develop in septic phlebitis (18). In catheter-associated sepsis in which the catheter was in place for 5 days, the chief organism culture was *Staphylococcus aureus* (20). Survival after catheter-induced sepsis is influenced by the time of removal of the catheter (20). It has been shown that colonization of the plastic cannula occurs within 48 hours, phlebitis in 48 to 96 hours, and septicemia in longer than 96 hours (20).

Prevention and Treatment

Date the catheter on insertion. Place a dressing with an antibacterial ointment over the cannula, and treat the puncture site as any wound (192). In one study, it was shown that phlebitis could be prevented by the use of 1 mg/dL hydrocortisone cream over the insertion site (150). The use of topical antibiotics prolongs the time one may use an intravenous cutdown site to 4 days and may decrease infection and the number of pathogens cultured in all intravenous catheter sites (161). Phlebitis, however, is unaffected by the use of topical antibiotics (226). Seventy percent of intravenous cannulas associated with sepsis were placed in the emergency center and remained in place for longer than 4 days; thus we advise removal of plastic intravenous cannulas at 48 hours (18).

SEPSIS

The majority of catheter-associated infections are due to skin flora entering the wound as a result of insertion of a cannula with nonsterile technique (106, 140). The primary disadvantage of the percutaneous technique of catheterization is the possibility of contaminating the catheter. Catheter contamination is primarily a function of breakdown in sterile technique, which, in turn, is a function of the experience of the operator. In patients in whom sepsis developed from intravenous catheters, one study in which house physicians placed only 10% of the intravenous catheters found that these cannulas resulted in 90% of the infections (20). Infection at the catheter site and subsequent septic phlebitis are characterized by tenderness at the puncture site, proximal erythema that takes a linear course along the tract of the vein, and lymphadenitis with proximal adenopathy. In more advanced cases, the tenderness may be noted along the length of the vein for large distances from the puncture site.

The clot that forms around the cannula tip may trap organisms and lead to sepsis (140). Septic emboli occur twice as often with intravenous catheters as compared with intravenous drug abuse. Aspiration of the vein, culture, and a Gram stain of any purulent material is helpful in identifying the organism (20).

Prevention and Treatment

Use of sterile technique is mandatory. Begin heat, elevation, and antibiotics when septic phlebitis develops in an extremity. We advise oxacillin and gentamicin for staphylococcus and gram-negative organisms for the first 24 hours; if no response is noted, excise the vein and drain any abscess (14).

Heparin-impregnated catheters are now in wide use. Controversy continues surrounding the use of femoral catheters as they relate to the development of a deep venous thrombosis (DVT). A recent study of 140 patients showed a sixfold increase in the rate of DVTs associated with femoral vein cannulation (113). Interestingly, there was no significant difference in rates between heparin-impregnated and nonheparinized catheters. Furthermore, the notion that a safe duration of catheterization exists is false, in the earlier study, a DVT was reported from day 1 up to 1 week after catheter removal.

Given the increased rate of DVT formation regardless of the use of heparin-impregnated catheters, no effective preventive measures can be recommended. Maintain a high index of suspicion under these circumstances, and evaluate the involved leg frequently for signs and symptoms consistent with a DVT.

VENOPULMONARY FISTULA

This quite uncommon complication is described for central venous insertions (179, 217). Venopulmonary fistula occurs when the tip of a catheter erodes through the central venous system or atria, or a fistula is formed with the pulmonary vasculature.

CATHETER FRAGMENT EMBOLISM

Intravascular embolization of polyethylene catheter fragments is a significant problem. It is caused in the majority of cases by intravenous indwelling catheters (72).

Prevention and Treatment

Be careful in the use of through-the-needle catheters. If one must remove the catheter after an unsuccessful attempt, remove the catheter and needle together as a single unit. Sixty-nine nonsurgical retrievals of embolized fragments have been reported, and a number of techniques have been used (72). The most common technique uses a loop snare, in which a guidewire-like device, folded in half at its midsection, is inserted through a catheter to snare the fragment. Hooked catheters, helical baskets, and Fogarty catheters also have been used for retrieval of an embolized fragment (72).

ARRHYTHMIA

In some patients, central venous pressure (CVP) catheter insertion can result in arrhythmias, particularly in atrial arrhythmias. Forty-one percent of patients examined with a CVP catheter experienced arrhythmias during the course of the line placement (172, 217). Twenty-five percent had ventricular ectopy. Ventricular ectopy was more common in shorter patients, in whom the catheter was inserted from the right subclavian (43% vs. 10% from the left side) (172, 217). The wire used to insert and guide the catheter is thought to cause many of the problems encountered in CVP insertion. Thus after insertion of the catheter, remove the wire once the venous system is accessed.

HEMATOMA FORMATION

Hematoma formation is due either to unsuccessful cannulation in which pressure was not applied over the site for an adequate period or to puncture of both the anterior and posterior walls of the vein with the needle. Use an oblique angle when advancing the needle into a vein to minimize puncturing the posterior wall of the vein. When hematoma occurs, remove the needle and apply pressure over the site. Alternately, leave the needle in the vein, and select a more proximal site, after which, remove the original needle and apply pressure. This method permits one to use the same arm after an unsuccessful attempt.

INFILTRATION

Infiltration occurs when the cannula is not in the vein. When this occurs, remove the cannula and apply pressure over the site. Alternatively, leave the needle in place, and use a proximal site, and then remove the first needle.

NEUROLOGIC COMPLICATIONS

Several neurologic complications have been described after insertion of central venous catheters (49). These include brachial plexus injury, phrenic or recurrent nerve palsies, and compression injuries to nerves located in nearby veins (49).

INJURY TO NEARBY NERVES

The median nerve at the elbow may be injured with cannulation of a medial antecubital vein. Avoid injury to the median nerve by avoiding deep penetration when attempting to enter the vein. The superficial radial nerve, a sensory nerve, may be injured by cannulation of the superficial radial vein. Other nerve injuries are reported but are quite uncommon.

PERIPHERAL INTRAVENOUS TECHNIQUES

Various techniques are common to all the procedures whether in the upper or lower extremity veins; the differences are only with the type of catheter used. Do not use veins in the legs except under urgent circumstances, because the risk of provoking thromboembolic complications is significant.

Peripheral Veins of the Upper and Lower Extremity

In the upper extremity, the dorsum of the hand is a good site to find a vein for cannulation because a number of veins arise from the digital veins, which are interconnected, forming a dorsal plexus. Several sites along the forearm can be used, probably the best of which is the branch of the cephalic vein called the superficial radial vein. This vein courses laterally and joins the median cephalic vein to form the cephalic vein proper in the antecubital space (Fig. 12.1). Four sites can be searched for in the patient in whom it is difficult to locate a vein. These include the ulnar veins, superficial radial vein, median basilic vein, and median cephalic vein (Fig. 12.1). These veins are large and relatively constant. In the obese patient in whom veins may not be visible, these veins are not always palpable; however, one may enter them "blindly." Their constant position makes them useful to the emergency physician seeking a peripheral intravenous route. When passing a long Intracath into the central system, it is best to use the median basilic vein (Fig. 12.2) because the cephalic vein courses deep in the interval between the pectoralis major and deltoid muscles and undergoes a

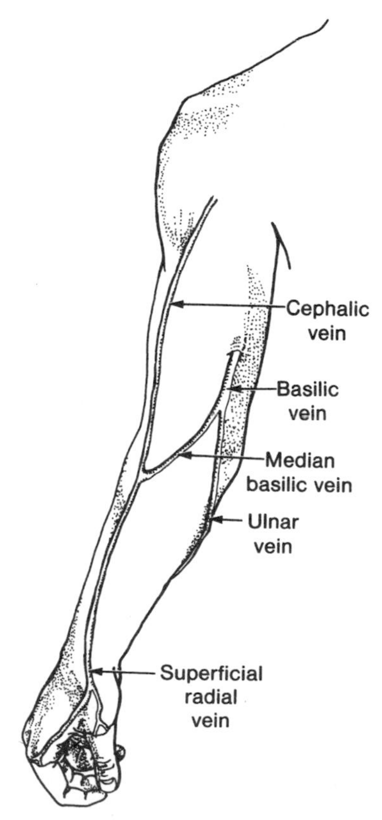

Figure 12.1. Peripheral veins of the upper extremity.

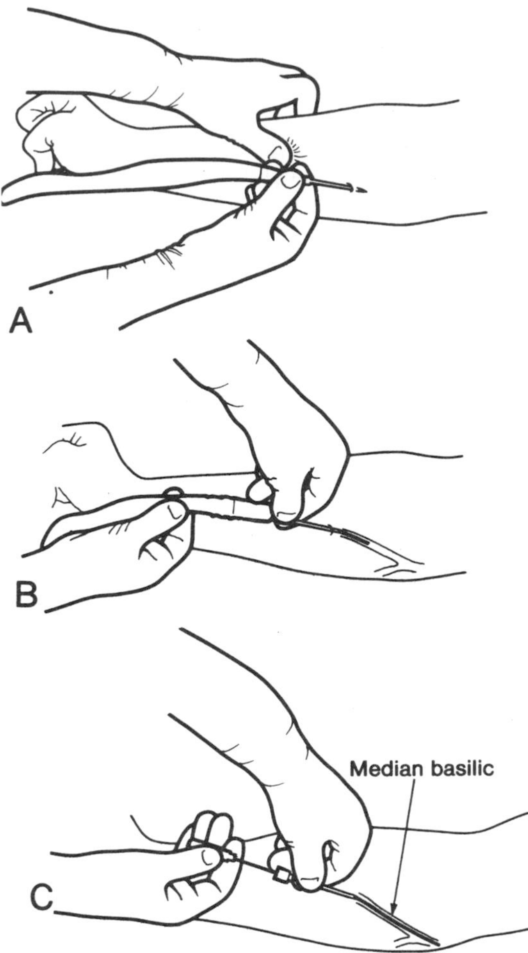

Figure 12.2. When passing a long Intracath into the central system from a peripheral site, it is best to use the medial basilic vein in the upper extremity. *A:* Insert the Intracath through a skin puncture site after applying traction with the thumb of the left hand to retract the skin. *B:* Thread the Intracath into the vein after the vein is entered and blood is noted to return into the lumen of the catheter. The plastic housing on the outside of the catheter keeps the catheter sterile during the process of threading the catheter into the vein. *C:* Then remove the plastic sheath, and secure the catheter into the needle hub.

sharp angulation, after which it joins the axillary vein. It is often difficult to pass the catheter around this angulation.

A cannula may be inserted blindly into the basilic vein. When other peripheral routes fail, this procedure has an 80% success rate (199). At the antecubital fossa, 1 to 2 cm proximal to the crease, palpate the brachial artery. On entering the skin at a 45-degree angle, just medial and slightly deep to the artery, is the basilic vein, which can be cannulated at this site. Use a 16-gauge Angiocath or smaller.

In the lower extremity, the long saphenous vein and the femoral vein are the two vessels most commonly cannulated. The long saphenous vein receives branches from the dorsal venous plexus of the foot and courses anteriorly to the medial malleolus, where it lies very superficially; it continues in the groove between the upper medial aspect of the tibia and the gastrocnemius. From here, it passes posteriorly behind the medial femoral condyle, courses proximally to pierce the femoral fascia at the saphenous opening, and enters the femoral vein approximately 1.5 inches below the inguinal ligament.

EQUIPMENT

Skin preparation
Alcohol swabs
Povidone–iodine (Betadine) solution
4 × 4-inch gauze pads
Intravenous cannula: Select a plastic cannula, which can be either an over-the-needle cannula (Angiocath) or a through-the-needle cannula (Intracath) of appropriate size. Butterfly needles are useful, particularly in children.
Intravenous solution and tubing
Tourniquet
Blood pressure cuff (optional)
Dressing
Antibacterial ointment
Paper tape
Sterile gauze of appropriate size
Armboard
Lidocaine (Xylocaine) 1%
25-gauge needle, 18-gauge needle, and 3-mL syringe

TECHNIQUE

The discussion of the technique refers to the upper extremity, but it is applicable to the lower extremity also.

1. Select the site. In the average patient, the best site is the cephalic vein approximately 10 cm proximal to the wrist in the adult. In the infant, scalp veins are commonly used. In selecting an optimal site, observe four points:
   a. Use a distal site in the extremity rather than a more proximal site. If unable to enter the vein at this distal site, ascend to a more proximal site. If a proximal vein is used first and perforation through the venous wall occurs, distal locations along that vein can no longer be used.
   b. Use the nondominant hand ideally; however, in an emergency situation, the extremity with the largest veins is used.
   c. Avoid veins over joint surfaces.
   d. The optimal site in which to enter a vein is where two feeding veins join forming a Y. The junction of the three arms of the Y is a stable part of the vein, permitting entrance without lateral motion of the vein as the needle penetrates its wall, which is commonly a problem.

NOTE

If unable to find a vein, apply a tourniquet to the extremity to distend the veins. Apply warm, soaked towels to the extremity held in a dependent position. An alternative method of bringing a vein out is to apply a blood pressure cuff on the extremity and inflate to above systolic pressure for about 5 minutes. Then deflate the cuff to below systolic pressure but above diastolic, with the patient advised to open and close the fist while the arm is held in a dependent position. This may bring out a hidden vein.

---

2. Apply a tourniquet around the patient's arm and apply restraints with infants.
3. Prepare the skin. First prepare the skin with alcohol swabs. Venipuncture is less painful and more bacteriostatic once the alcohol has dried (170). Then prepare the same area with povidone–iodine solution.
4. Infiltrate with 1% lidocaine. The site of infiltration should be distal to the site at which one intends to enter the vein so that there is a few millimeters' distance between the skin-entry site and the venipuncture site to decrease the risk of bacterial contamination at the venipuncture. The pain resulting from the injection of lidocaine intradermally through a 25-gauge needle is trivial, particularly when compared with the pain from the cutaneous insertion of a large-bore cannula (57, 170).
5. Puncture the vein.

   Butterfly needle: Enter the vein with a smooth motion by placing the needle flat alongside the skin. A return of blood into the tubing will be noted. Advance the needle carefully, following the course of the vein.

   Over-the-needle cannula (Angiocath): Select a cannula of appropriate size. An 18-gauge or larger cannula is needed for blood infusions. While maintaining traction on the skin (Fig. 12.3), enter the vein with a sudden motion at a 15-degree angle with the bevel up at site a few millimeters distal to the site of entry into the vein. Advance the needle and cannula as a unit until the vein is punctured. Once there is a free backflow of blood, advance the cannula and needle a few millimeters into the vein. Slide the catheter over the needle into the vein. If difficulty is encountered, a rotating motion of the catheter back and forth will sometimes aid in entering the smaller puncture site produced by the needle. Withdraw the needle and connect the intravenous tubing. Direct pressure over the venipuncture site will control bleeding from the cannula while connecting the tubing.

   Through-the-needle cannula (Intracath): The needle will be larger than

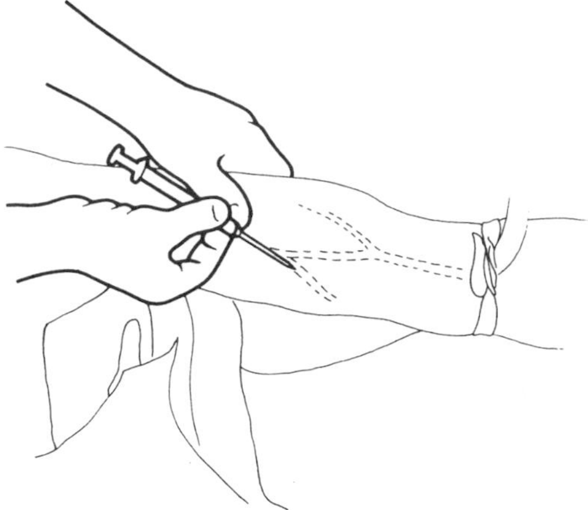

Figure 12.3. To insert a needle or catheter into a vein, hold the needle at a 15-degree angle to the skin with the bevel pointing upward at a site a few millimeters distal to the site of preferred entry into the vein. Apply traction to the skin with the thumb of the left hand to stabilize the vein, and then puncture the vein along its side.

the cannula, and, if blood is to be infused, use a 16-gauge or larger catheter. While maintaining traction on the skin, enter the vein at a 15-degree angle. Advance the needle into the vein a few millimeters. The flow of blood into the cannula confirms entry into the vein. Advance the catheter through the needle. Withdraw the wire stylet from the catheter hub. Engage hub of the cannula into the plastic casing, and then connect to intravenous tubing.

CAUTION

Do not withdraw the catheter back through the needle at any time because this may result in shearing of a piece of the catheter and a catheter embolism. If the catheter must be withdrawn during the procedure, withdraw the catheter and needle simultaneously as a single unit.

CAUTION

If swelling or a hematoma develops, stop the procedure and remove the cannula with any of the previously described techniques. Apply local pressure to the site and locate an alternate site. To avoid pulling out the cannula to control bleeding, apply pressure to the site, leaving the needle in place; place the tourniquet and another cannula at a more proximal site along the vein. Once a vein is cannulated, remove the first needle and apply pressure over the site.

---

6. Apply antibiotic ointment and dressing at the puncture site.
7. Secure the line with adhesive tape or paper tape; with an upper extremity vein, use an armboard to immobilize the wrist or elbow. Secure a butterfly catheter as shown in Fig. 12.4.

BASILIC VEIN VENIPUNCTURE

The basilic vein can be entered percutaneously in approximately 80% of the patients, even though it is not palpated (217). The brachial artery provides access to the basilic vein. To enter the vein, palpate the brachial artery at the antecubital crease. Insert a needle just medial to the fingertips of the palpating hand at an angle of 45 degrees (Fig. 12.5). Perform aspiration as the needle is inserted.

Heparin Lock

This cannulation is simply a butterfly needle inserted into a vein without a continuous fluid infusion maintaining the pa-

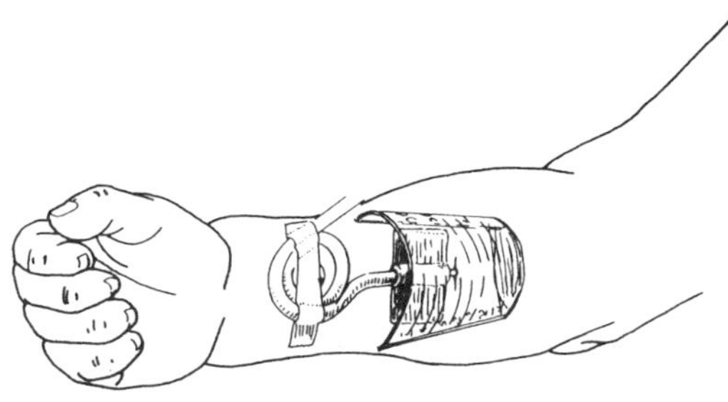

Figure 12.4. Method for securing a butterfly needle in place in a small child. Cut a routine plastic medicine cup in half and use it to cover the catheter and puncture site. This protects the site from a dislodging force.

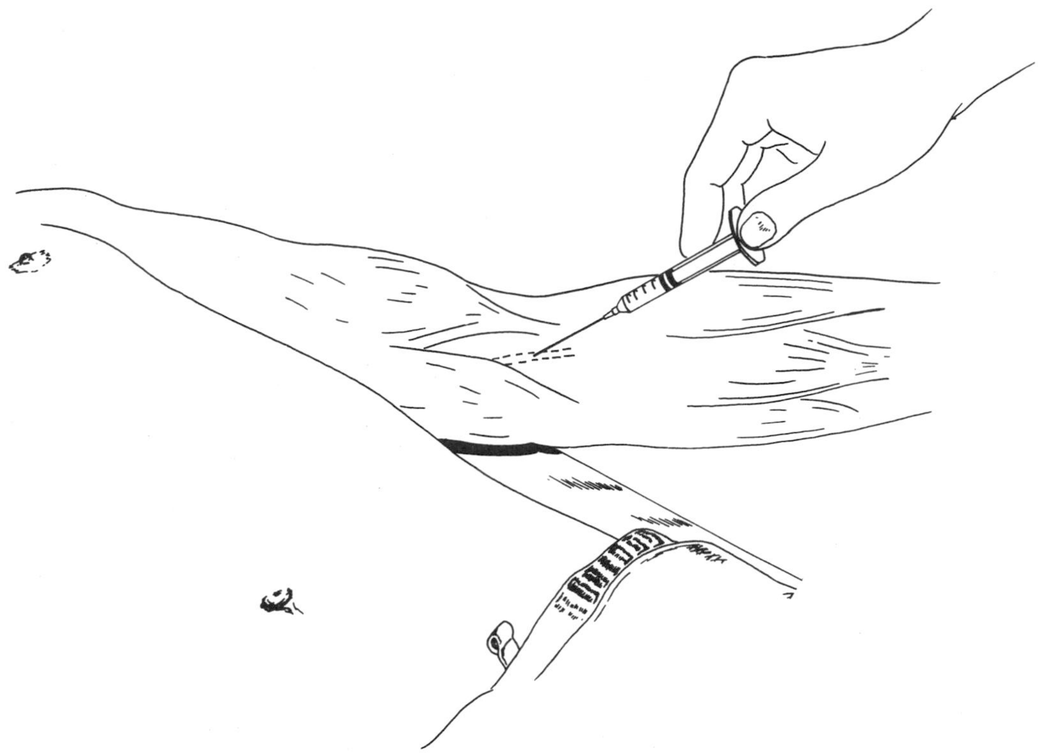

Figure 12.5. Percutaneous basilic vein catheterization can be achieved by inserting a 2-inch needle, attached to a syringe, just medial to the insertion of the biceps tendon, which is easily palpable. Aspirate as the needle is passed in the direction shown. See text for discussion.

tency of the needle lumen. The cannulation proceeds in the same fashion as for a "butterfly" needle. Maintain this cannula by using 1 to 2 mL of a solution of 10 units of heparin per milliliter of saline flushed through the "butterfly" to keep the needle lumen patent. Higher concentrations increase the partial thromboplastin time (170). Three times per day and after each use, flush the line with 1 mL of the heparin flush solution. The heparin lock can be used for 4 days with minimal risk of infection (69). The heparin lock is especially useful for patients receiving intermittent intravenous drugs (e.g., antibiotics).

Peripheral Veins of the Head and Neck

The external jugular vein, formed behind the angle of the mandible by the joining of the posterior facial vein and the posterior auricular vein, is the site most commonly used in the neck. The vein passes downward across the surface of the sternocleidomastoid muscle. At a level just above the middle of the clavicle, the vein pierces the deep fascia of the neck to end in the subclavian vein. Several valves may be encountered in passing a catheter through this vein. One valve lies at the entrance into the subclavian vein, and another, approximately 4 cm above the clavicle.

TECHNIQUE

1. Place the patient in a Trendelenburg position to fill the external jugular vein; turn the patient's head toward the opposite side.
2. Prepare the skin in the manner described earlier for upper and lower extremity cannulation.
3. Select the cannula type and size.

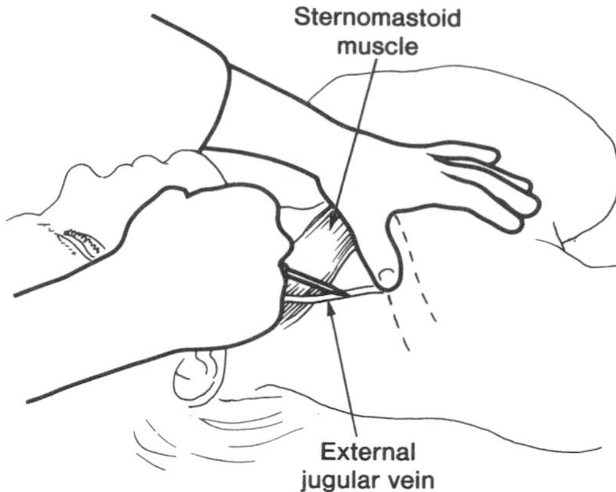

Figure 12.6. Optimal site of entry into the external jugular vein. Distend the vein by applying pressure over it with the thumb placed just above the clavicle. A Valsalva maneuver or the Trendelenburg position may aid in distending the vein.

4. Puncture the skin at a site distal to the site of entry into the vein.
5. Align the cannula parallel to the direction of the vein with the bevel pointing upward. The optimal site of entry into the vein is at a point midway between the angle of the jaw and the midclavicular line (Fig. 12.6).
6. Obstruct the outflow of the vein proximally to distend it by lightly placing a finger about the clavicle and pressing over the midclavicular region, as shown in Fig. 12.6.
7. Perform cannulation of the vein rapidly during inspiration when the valves are open.
8. Cover the cannula orifice at all times to prevent air embolism.
9. Insert a Cordis catheter into this vessel by the modified Seldinger technique (see technique under Swan–Ganz Catheterization of the Pulmonary Artery).

CENTRAL INTRAVENOUS TECHNIQUES

Percutaneous Central Venous Access

Percutaneous central venous access to the cephalic or basilic veins with a through-the-needle 91-cm cannula is not described here. We believe that in the emergency setting, when central venous access is needed, it must be rapid and reliable. Central venous access by a peripheral arm vein resulted in 25% to 40% unsuccessful cannulation of the central circulation (112, 119, 218). Many of the unsuccessful cannulations went into the internal jugular vein; this risk may be reduced by turning the head of the patient so that the chin rests on the ipsilateral shoulder during cannulation (31).

Infraclavicular Subclavian Vein Cannulation

The subclavian is a large vein located in the root of the neck, sometimes reaching a diameter of 2 cm or more (47). The axillary vein becomes the subclavian vein as it crosses the first rib. The subclavian vein joins the internal jugular vein behind the sternoclavicular joint to form the innominate vein (47, 154). Just lateral to this point, the subclavian vein lies immediately posterior to the medial third of the clavicle (12). It is separated from the subclavian artery by the anterior scalene muscle (the artery lies posterior to this muscle). The brachial plexus courses posterior and superior to the subclavian artery. The pleura of the lung lies behind the vein as it approaches the midline. The vein courses in close proximity to the undersurface of the medial one third of the clavicle; this relation makes possible cannulation of the vein at this point (148). Other important structures related to the course of the vein are the vagus and phrenic nerves, which course medially in front of the subclavian artery. The trachea and esophagus lie medial to the vein. No vital structures are crossed in entering the vein at the medial one third of the clavicle between the subclavian vein and the skin. The structures coursing at this point include the pectoralis major and subclavius muscles and the costoclavicular ligament.

INDICATIONS

1. Emergency intravenous route in seriously ill or injured patient.
2. Hyperalimentation.
3. Vasopressor administration.
4. CVP measurement and monitoring.
5. Rapid administration of large volumes of fluid (48).
6. Insertion of a transvenous pacemaker (48).
7. Passage of a Swan–Ganz catheter (67, 144).
8. Intravenous access in patients without peripheral veins (67).
9. Infusion of hypertonic or irritant solutions (57, 150).

CONTRAINDICATIONS

1. A patient who is agitated and uncooperative; in such patients there is an increased incidence of serious complications (210).
2. Distorted landmarks due to obesity (37), trauma to shoulder girdle, fibrotic changes, deformity of the chest wall, previous surgery, or fracture of the clavicle.
3. Radiation therapy in the region (150, 154).
4. Vasculitis and coagulopathies (150).

EQUIPMENT

Skin preparation
Anesthetic preparation
Sterile field
Towels
14-gauge Bard Intracath (8 or 12 inch) (80)
Intravenous solution and tubing
Three-way stopcock (for CVP monitoring)
Extension intravenous tubing
Adhesive tape
Antibiotic ointment
Dressing
Tuberculin syringe

TECHNIQUE

Preparatory Steps

1. Place the patient in 10 to 20 degrees of Trendelenburg (80, 171, 189, 209). When this is not feasible, elevate the patient's feet to transfer blood from the lower extremity into the central circulation (165). If the patient is able, a forced expiration against a closed glottis (Valsalva maneuver) held for a brief time will distend the veins in the neck.

   Place a folded sheet under the patient's upper back, between the shoulder blades (Fig. 12.7). This will allow the shoulders to fall back and widen the space between the first rib and the clavicle, thus allowing easier entrance into the subclavian vein. In addition, it prevents the humerus from interfering with cannulation (154, 179).

   Locate the site of entrance and turn the patient's head to the opposite side (154, 171, 209). We prefer the right side, to avoid the thoracic duct (47, 154). Turning the head does not alter the clavicle–vein relation (150).
2. Prepare and drape the patient (165, 189). Place the drapes in the shape of a "V" so that the suprasternal notch is easily visible and palpable (80, 154).

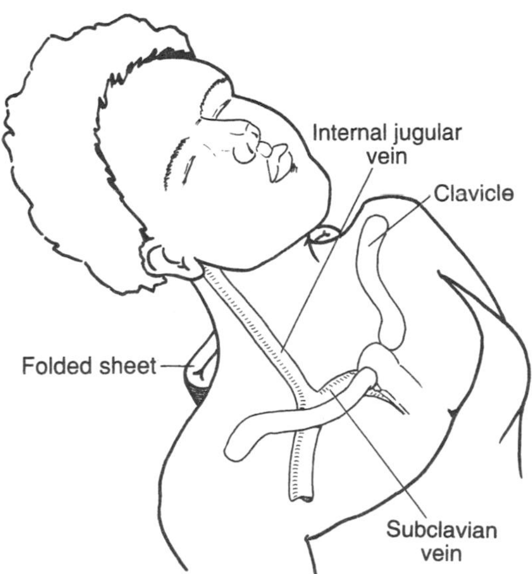

Figure 12.7. Place a folded sheet placed between the scapular blades to allow the shoulders to retract posteriorly and allow easier entrance into the neck veins. See text for discussion.

3. Attach the needle to the tuberculin syringe. Detach the Intracath from the needle of the Bard Intracath and attach the needle to a tuberculin syringe. Use a syringe to aspirate blood to ascertain that the vein has been entered (41). We prefer a tuberculin syringe because of the low pressure generated when aspirating to determine entrance into the vein. In many patients, the higher pressures generated by larger syringes will cause collapse of the subclavian vein, particularly in the presence of hypovolemia, resulting in the inability to ascertain whether the vein has been entered.

Procedural Steps

1. Locate the point of insertion. A number of articles have been published indicating the "optimal" site of entrance (41, 118, 171, 189, 209). The left subclavian vein passes posterior to the clavicle near the junction of the inner and second quarters of that bone in most patients (150). The subclavian vein is more medial on the left side than on the right side, where it runs along the medial one third (209). The site of entrance can be located by any of the following methods:
   a. The point just lateral to the midclavicular line along the inferior surface of the clavicle (209).
   b. One centimeter below the junction of the middle and medial third of the clavicle (41, 118).
   c. At the inferior surface of the clavicle at the point where the lateral head of the sternocleidomastoid muscle inserts.
   d. (Our preferred method) Palpating along the inferior surface of the clavicle at about one third to one half the length of the clavicle from the sternoclavicular joint, find a tubercle on the clavicle that corresponds to the site of entrance (189). The advantage of using the tubercle in identifying the point of insertion of the needle is that it is a definite landmark and does not involve approximating distances, as does the use of the midclavicular line, junction of the middle and medial thirds of the clavicle, or other methods indicated earlier. One of the authors (R.S.) noted a remarkably high success rate when inexperienced personnel performed the procedure for the first time (184).

NOTE

Measure the length of the catheter that is needed by estimating the distance between the manubrial–sternal junction and the point of insertion. Do this by placing the catheter over the path that it will traverse. If the catheter is too long, complications such as ventricular dysrhythmias may occur.

---

2. Using 1% lidocaine, anesthetize the skin at the site of entrance and infiltrate around the clavicular periosteum (154).
3. Insert the needle and syringe. Place the fingertip of the index finger into the suprasternal notch as a point of reference (8, 154, 189). With the bevel pointing inferiorly, puncture the skin at the site located earlier. "Walk" the needle inferiorly and under the clavicle until the subclavius muscle is entered.

   Aspirate the syringe and advance the needle toward the midpoint of the suprasternal notch, holding the needle and syringe parallel to the frontal plane (the back of the patient) (Fig. 12.8) (154). Hug the undersurface of the clavicle.

NOTE

In elderly patients, the direction of the subclavian often is more inferior, so aim to-

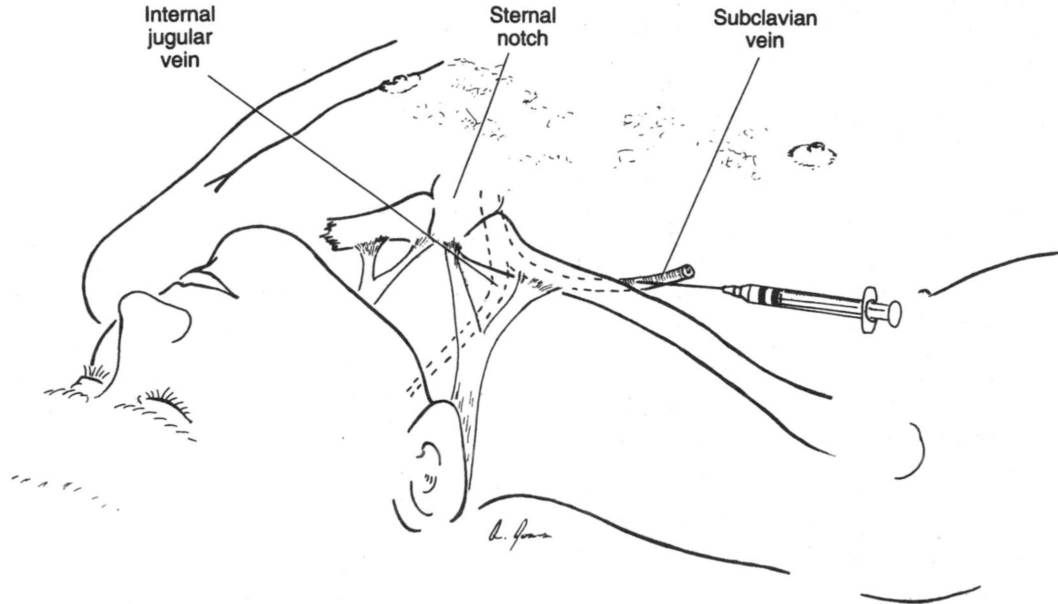

Figure 12.8. To locate the subclavian vein using the infraclavicular approach, place the index finger in the sternal notch and the thumb at the point of insertion of the needle, as discussed in the text. After inserting the needle under the clavicle, aim the syringe and needle at the suprasternal notch, which should be at the tip of the index finger, while holding the syringe and needle parallel to the table. See text for discussion.

ward the inferior margin of the suprasternal notch if the initial attempt is unsuccessful (165).

NOTE

If the first rib is struck, remove the needle and reinsert farther laterally (41).

NOTE

During cutaneous insertion, a skin plug may pass into the needle because of its large bore, resulting in a dermoid cyst or plugging of the needle and inability to aspirate blood on entry into the vein. Remove the skin plug by removing the needle after penetrating only the skin and "squirting" the plug out by forcefully expelling air through the needle. Then pass the needle through the same puncture site, and continue the procedure.

CAUTION

A pulsatile resistance, if noted, indicates the subclavian artery. If this should be felt, withdraw the needle and reinsert.

NOTE

An alternate method published by Asimacopoulos et al. (9) is useful in locating the vein in the obese, uncooperative, or poorly positioned patient in whom the needle cannot be sufficiently depressed to pass under the clavicle into the vein, resulting in the needle coursing inferior to the vein. To avoid this problem, smoothly bend the standard no. 14 Intracath needle over its entire length to form an arc of about 30 degrees (30 degrees from the point of the needle to a horizontal line extended at a tangent to the midpoint of the arc). Then place the needle at a 45-degree angle to the skin at the point of insertion under the clavicle, and as the needle follows its 30 degree arc, enter the vein.

NOTE

In difficult cases, ultrasonic guidance has been used to cannulate the subclavian vein (65, 117, 198). With the growing availability of bedside ultrasonography, the emergency physician skilled in this modality may find it helpful in patients with excessive body habitus or those that have clotting abnormalities. A study of 43 patients who had relative contraindications to central venous access or abnormal landmarks due to extreme body habitus were all successfully cannulated with ultrasonographic guidance (78).

In those skilled with ultrasonography, the key elements of the approach are highlighted.

---

a. We recommend either a 5- or 7-MHz linear probe after preparation with povidone–iodine.
b. First apply sterile ultrasound gel, and place the probe in the infraclavicular region.
c. Once the vein is located and confirmed to be patent, perform real-time guidance of the access needle with the free hand.
d. Once the needle has entered the vein, as confirmed by aspiration of blood and with ultrasonographic imaging, insert the catheter via the Seldinger technique.

4. Grasp the needle firmly and remove the syringe. Grasp the needle between the thumb and long finger of the left hand or with a hemostat and remove the syringe.

NOTE

When the syringe is difficult to remove, hold the needle with a hemostat and then remove the syringe. This prevents moving the needle from its position in the vein. Place the index finger of the left hand over the orifice of the needle hub immediately on removing the syringe to prevent an air embolism.

---

5. Advance the catheter (Fig. 12.9). Insert the catheter through the needle into the vein and remove the stylet. Do this while the patient is holding their breath to avoid entrance of air into the vein and air embolism.

   If the catheter does not advance, rotate the needle and continue to attempt advancing it. If it still does not advance, hold the needle closer to the skin. If one is able to withdraw blood from the needle but the catheter will not advance, the following may be tried:

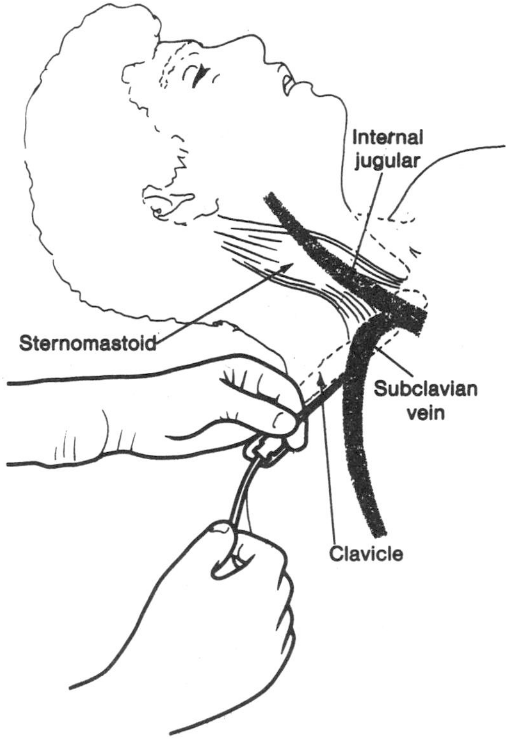

Figure 12.9. Subclavian vein catheterization by the infraclavicular approach. See text for discussion.

a. Rotate the needle and angle it so that it enters the vein more acutely (hold closer to the skin with the needle more vertical and closer to the ear of the patient).
b. Bend the tip of the catheter and then introduce it with the bent tip pointing inferiorly.
c. Pass a guidewire through the needle with a flexible tip, and then slide the catheter over the wire (Seldinger technique). If the catheter does not advance, remove the catheter and needle *as a single unit.*

CAUTION

Withdrawing the catheter through the needle alone may result in a catheter embolism (8, 165, 171, 189). Always withdraw the needle and catheter together and never the catheter alone. Advance the catheter until it sits in the hub of the needle.

---

6. Aspirate for blood.

NOTE

If blood is not returned, the catheter is either outside the lumen of the vein, kinked, blocked by a thrombus, or lodged against the posterior wall of the vein (154). If this should occur, partially withdraw the catheter and needle while maintaining negative pressure on the syringe. If blood still is not returned, then remove the catheter (154). Remember that if the negative pressure is too strong on the syringe, the vein will collapse, and no blood will return even when the catheter is in the proper place (171). This is the main reason we recommend a tuberculin syringe.

---

7. Attach the intravenous tubing and withdraw the needle, securing it within the needle guard. After attaching the guard to the needle, lower the intravenous bottle below the level of the chest; blood should return in the tubing if the catheter is within the vein (189).

CAUTION

Be certain to place the catheter carefully in the guard. If the catheter is malpositioned in the guard, the catheter may be severed or torn.

AFTERCARE

1. Suture the catheter in place with 4-0 suture (Fig. 12.10). Apply tincture of benzoin around the site and antibacterial ointment to the puncture site; cover the area with a 4 × 4-inch dressing, and tape with 3-inch adhesive taping.

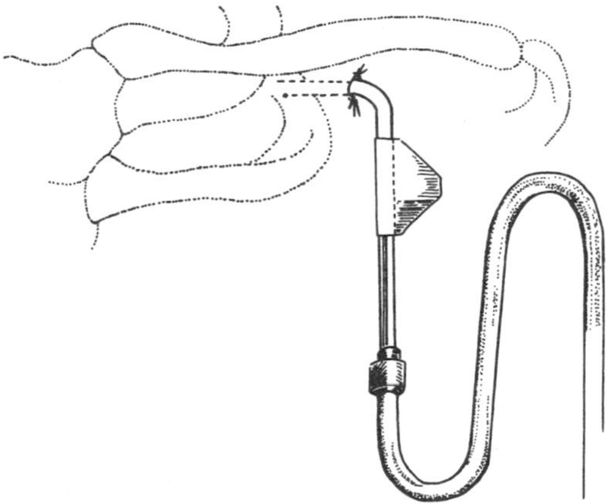

Figure 12.10. Secure the subclavian catheter in place with a suture placed around the catheter close to the puncture site. This will minimize back-and-forth motion between the catheter and skin, which may carry skin contaminants from the puncture site into the vein. Then shape the intravenous tubing into an "S" curve, and secure it into position with adhesive tape. The purpose of the double loop or S-shaped curve is that, if a pulling force is applied to the intravenous tubing, it will be transmitted to the first loop, thus protecting the second loop from transmitting the force to the catheter and causing dislodgment.

NOTE

In studies in which the catheter was left in place for weeks, no infection was noted over a 2-week period when the dressing was changed every 2 days, the skin was cleansed with iodine, and Neosporin ointment was applied to the site before a sterile dressing was placed (209). Change the intravenous tubing every 2 or 3 days (209). The most important precautions are (a) to close the intravenous system completely from the bottle to the patient by taping all connections, and (b) to provide meticulous catheter care (148).

---

2. Check the catheter position. Attach a CVP manometer to a three-way stopcock, and fill the manometer with intravenous fluid from a bottle by turning the three-way stopcock "off" to the patient. Fill the tubing to approximately the 10-cm level. After this, turn the three-way stopcock so that it is open between the patient and the manometer. With inspiration, the fluid level should fall below 2.5 cm (in the normal patient), and with each expiration, it should rise again, if the catheter is patent and located in the superior vena cava (154). In up to 20% of non–central catheter placement, normal respiratory variation occurred (119). A Valsalva maneuver also will raise the fluid level in the manometer.
3. In all cases, take chest radiographs to ascertain that the catheter tip is in the superior vena cava and to check for a pneumothorax; intravenous fluids have flowed freely even when catheters were in poor positions. Obtain a chest radiograph even if all attempts to cannulate the subclavian were unsuccessful.

COMPLICATIONS

Forty-four percent of complications occur when the procedure is performed as an emergency (101). Those physicians who have placed more than 50 subclavian vein cannulations have an insignificant complication rate when compared with those who have placed fewer than 50, who had a complication rate of 5% to 10% (22). Thus, although the list of complications is long, the complications become uncommon as one performs the procedure more often.

1. Pneumothorax (8, 67, 110, 144, 215). This is one of the most common complications from subclavian vein catheterization. Pleural laceration with air leak occurs with a lung laceration. In one study, it occurred in five of 98 catheterizations (37). Positive-pressure ventilation in a patient with a pneumothorax secondary to subclavian vein catheterization increases the chance of a tension pneumothorax within 48 hours (37, 110). Three cases have been reported; two of the three patients with tension pneumothorax due to subclavian vein cannulation died of the pneumothorax (182). Delayed pneumothorax is a described complication of subclavian vein catheterization (172). Small pneumothoraces may be missed if radiographs are not obtained later. If the patient has symptoms of dyspnea, obtain radiographs 1 to 2 hours after venipuncture (172), because this is the time required before one can visualize a delayed pneumothorax.

Prevent pneumothorax by avoiding multiple attempts at cannulation. If one is unsuccessful after three attempts, select another site. If the patient is receiving mechanical ventilation, place the patient on bag ventilation, if possible, before performance of the procedure. The risk of pneumothorax is greater in children, in whom the pleural reflection is higher than that in the adult. In addition, in the thin emphysematous patient, the risk is markedly increased because of the increased size of the lung in the anteroposterior diameter (171). One probably should attempt another approach in such a patient; we recommend the internal jugular route.

2. Air embolism (67, 144). Air can enter the vein through an opening during disconnection of the intravenous infusion tubing or during the initial puncture (65). During the initial puncture of the subclavian vein, place the index finger over the hub of the needle when the syringe is withdrawn to prevent air entry into the vein. A markedly increased incidence of air embolism occurs with hypovolemia (110). In subclavian punctures performed in dogs, only those with hypovolemia developed air embolism (27). Prevent this complication by positioning the patient in the Trendelenburg position and maintaining a closed system at all times. Approximately 100 mL of air per second can pass through a 14-gauge needle (27). Patients with hyperalimentation lines, cachexia, and/or hypovolemia are at a high risk for air embolism, even after the subclavian catheter has been removed (169)! Prevent this by covering the wound and track with Vaseline-impregnated gauze (169) after removal of the catheter.

Air can pass from the right side of the heart to the left through a patent foramen ovale, resulting in coronary, cerebral, or renal infarcts. In arterial air embolism, air in the retinal vessels on ophthalmoscopic examination is termed *Liebermeister's sign*. A sharply defined area of pallor on the patient's tongue, marbling of the skin (especially over the superior parts of the body), and air bubbles on incision of skin (termed *air-bleeding*) (54) are associated clinical signs of arterial air embolism.

Symptoms and signs of cyanosis, tachypnea, hypotension, and a mill-wheel murmur (sounding like a washing machine) over the precordium, caused by the air and water mixing, are indicative of venous air embolism (55, 67). Death due to air in the pulmonary outflow tract may ensue shortly (55). If symptoms of air embolism develop, immediately turn the patient to the *left lateral Trendelenburg position*, and aspirate through the catheter (97). This will allow air to enter the right ventricle from the pulmonary outflow track. The air can be "churned" into small bubbles in the right ventricle, which can then possibly pass through the pulmonary circulation without complication. Give the patient oxygen (67). Finally, aspirate blood quickly from the central venous catheter, which permits aspiration of the air from the ventricle (99, 188).

3. Catheter embolism (67, 144). This complication may be due to traction on the bevel tip of the catheter while inserting the needle (67) or, occasionally, may be due to excessive motion of the patient (67). To prevent this complication, during unsuccessful cannulation, remove the needle and catheter together as a single unit to avoid shearing the catheter (67). If this complication does occur, remove the catheter fragments to prevent the common complications of catheter embolism (68, 201, 204), which include myocardial thrombi, recurrent septicemia, endocarditis, coronary artery thrombosis, and cardiac perforation with pericardial tamponade (51).

Treat this complication by many methods. An infraclavicular incision along the path of the catheter fragment may occasionally be successful in retrieving it if it is lodged in the subcutaneous tissue (67). Subclavian venography may demonstrate the catheter, and one then may remove the catheter with wire loops, baskets, hooked catheters, or endoscopic forceps (56, 141, 142, 193). If these techniques are unsuccessful, use a supraclavicular approach to remove the cannula (67).

NOTE

Make a medial supraclavicular incision; divide the clavicular head of the sternocleidomastoid, freeing the medial clavicle. Then divide the clavicle at the junction of the medial and middle thirds. Elevation of the ends of the bone and retrieval of the catheter fragment by using vascular clamps is then possible. If angiographic studies localize the catheter fragment in the superior vena cava or the pulmonary outflow tract, then a right thoracotomy to remove the catheter is necessary to prevent pulmonary hypertension, pulmonary infarction, or endocarditis.

---

4. Infection (67, 144, 191). Infections have been described after subclavian vein insertion. The incidence of infections is 1.6% within the first few days and typically 4.9% after long-term insertion of the catheter (179). There is an increased incidence of infection with catheter-induced sepsis in catheters remaining in place for more than 48 hours (17, 214). Osteomyelitis caused by *Pseudomonas* (131) and by *Staphylococcus aureus* has been reported involving the clavicle. Septic arthritis of the sternoclavicular joint secondary to *Pseudomonas* also has been reported (131).

5. Hemothorax (67, 191). Hemothorax may occur as a result of penetration of the vein wall by the catheter tip (144). A pleural rent with secondary bleeding also may cause this complication. Excessive motion during insertion can cause laceration of the internal mammary artery near its origin, resulting in a hemothorax (210). Lethal exsanguination has been reported after subclavian vein penetration (67). If the catheter tip has penetrated the vein wall, bleeding may not necessarily occur. Administration of blood through such a cannula may simulate a hemothorax. Indigo carmine dye may be injected into the subclavian catheter; the presence of the indigo dye in a thoracostomy bottle is indicative of this complication (144). This test is useful in the patient who is injured and has a hemothorax, but its association with the subclavian catheter is not certain.

6. Hydrothorax (6, 11, 24, 144, 182, 215). Perforation of the catheter tip through the subclavian vein and into the thorax may cause a hydrothorax. Prevent this complication by demonstrating free backflow of blood immediately after placing the catheter (6, 37). One cannot tell on the radiograph if the cannula is extraluminal, because the catheter may advance along the vein from an intraluminal position to then become extraluminal (6). In addition, with intrapleural insertion, respiratory variation of the CVP may be misleading. In part, to prevent this complication, do not insert a subclavian cannula in a patient with suspected injury to the subclavian vein (67).

7. Hydromediastinum (144, 191). Perforation of the catheter tip through the innominate vein may lead to a hydromediastinum. Injection of radiopaque dye through the cannula will confirm this complication (52). The onset of symptoms may be delayed for 30 hours after cannulation. Treatment is to aspirate the mediastinum (by suctioning what one can), if cardiopulmonary embarrassment occurs, and to withdraw the catheter.

8. Hydropericardium (1, 67, 101, 184). Perforation of the catheter tip through the right atrium into the pericardial space causes hydropericardium (52, 205) and pericardial tamponade. During cardiac tamponade, one may see only a moderately increased CVP but massively increased neck veins 24 to 48 hours after insertion. Injection of radiopaque dye through the cannula will confirm this entity (52). Catheters initially in normal position may move (101) to an abnormal position such as the pericardial space, so be certain that normal respiratory movement occurs with each CVP reading. The treatment is to withdraw all fluid from the pericardial space through the cannula, and then to remove the catheter and to treat tamponade, if still present. To prevent this complication, place the catheter not in the right atrium but in the superior vena cava (52, 205).

9. Venous thrombosis (65, 139, 170, 207). A late complication of central vein cannulation is venous thrombosis. In a prospective study, three types were found in 90% of cases: sleeve thrombus, which accounted for 80% of cases, mural thrombus in 13%, and major venous thrombosis in 7%; pulmonary emboli occurred in three cases (4). Thrombosis in this instance was not prevented by anticoagulation (17, 214). There is a high association between thrombosis and suppuration at the catheter site (216). Superior vena cava thrombosis secondary to central vein cannulation has been reported (216).

10. Pulmonary emboli (4, 64). See earlier.

11. Subclavian artery puncture (40, 88). No serious complications are associated with this puncture, according to some authors (37); however, hemothorax (88, 132), arteriovenous fistula, false aneurysms, and compressive hematomas have been reported as a result of inadvertent subclavian artery puncture (66, 132). Repair any subclavian arterial puncture that causes a hemothorax; for most subclavian artery punctures, observation is all that is needed (132).

12. Internal mammary artery laceration (130, 210). The internal mammary artery may be lacerated, resulting in an upper mediastinal mass due to the hematoma formation. Obtain a chest radiograph to diagnose this condition, even in those situations in which all attempts to cannulate the subclavian vein are unsuccessful (132).

13. Diaphragmatic paralysis. Diaphragmatic paralysis from phrenic nerve injury may result from attempts at subclavian vein cannulation. A raised hemidiaphragm is seen with paralysis and lack of diaphragmatic motion confirmed by fluoroscopy. This complication can be prevented by directing the needle as anteriorly as possible (63) when entering the vein.

14. Puncture of the cuff of the endotracheal (ET) tube. This is seen as a sudden persistent air leak (29) in patients with an ET tube. Sudden extubation of the patient with motion also may occur.

15. Faulty positioning of the catheter tip. The subclavian catheter may proceed retrograde into the internal jugular vein, which may result in swelling of the neck (37). If this occurs, the line can still be used for infusion of fluids but cannot be used to register a CVP. This complication can be prevented by turning the patient's head to the ipsilateral side when advancing the cannula, thereby increasing the acuteness of the subclavian–internal jugular vein angle.

16. Brachial plexus injury (151).

17. Knotting and kinking. This complication may be seen as difficulty in withdrawing the catheter (24). Prevent this by not using too long a catheter, which coils around itself in the atria.

18. Arrhythmias (120, 144). Atrial or ventricular arrhythmias may result with intracardiac positioning of the catheter. These arrhythmias are usually resistant to standard antiarrhythmics and can be stopped promptly by withdrawal of the catheter.

19. Ascites. Abnormal communication between the chest wall and the abdominal cavity with concomitant intrapleural administration of fluid results in this complication. Lack of recognition of this abnormal communication led to the administration of 12 L of fluid "intraabdominally" in one case (6).

20. Hematoma at puncture site. Raise the head of the bed to reduce pressure in the hematoma after the procedure is completed. A pressure dressing aids in the management of this complication.

21. Chylothorax. This complication occurs secondary to puncture of the thoracic duct during subclavian vein cannulation. Avoid the left side, when feasible, in central vein cannulation where the thoracic duct may be accessible. Extrinsic compression can be used (207) to treat this complication. Use a pleural drain, and measure losses of medium-chain triglycerides, and replace if needed.

22. Dermoid cysts. Dermoid cysts can occur from skin plugs "squirted" subcutaneously (83); therefore, the practice of removing the skin plug by squirting it into the subcutaneous tissue is not encouraged. When a skin plug is a problem, expel it by withdrawing the needle and "squirting" out the plug, and then reinsert the needle into the same puncture site.

23. Cortical blindness. Air embolism and neurologic complications during insertion of CVP catheters is well documented. A few cases of cortical blindness due to the procedure have been described (1).

Supraclavicular Subclavian Vein Cannulation

An alternate approach to central venous cannulation is the supraclavicular subclavian approach. Advocates of this method state that the primary advantage is that it avoids the major complication associated with the infraclavicular approach: pneumothorax (81, 125, 223, 228). Furthermore, this approach is best suited during cardiac arrest resuscitation situations where space is limited [i.e., physician at the head performing intubation, nurse on one side obtaining peripheral i.v. access, and a tech performing cardiopulmonary resuscitation (CPR) on the other side]. This approach is indicated when the infraclavicular subclavian approach cannot be performed.

There are numerous advantages to this approach:

1. The junction of the subclavian vein and internal jugular vein make a larger "target" (125).
2. The needle is directed away from the pleura and toward the mediastinum (81, 125).
3. It is less painful, for the needle avoids the clavicle periosteum (81, 223).
4. The distance between the skin and the vein is shorter than in the infraclavicular vein technique (81).
5. The variability of the space between the first rib and the clavicle is avoided (81, 223).
6. A much greater success rate in inserting the catheter into the proper position is achieved because of a more direct course taken by the catheter into the superior vena cava. In contrast, the infraclavicular approach may result in the catheter tip positioned within the internal jugular vein or the left subclavian vein.
7. This procedure can be performed on patients in the sitting position. This is advantageous in patients with orthopnea or severe respiratory distress.

TECHNIQUE

Preparatory Steps

1. Place the patient in the Trendelenburg position, which minimizes the risk of air embolism and allows venous distention. Note that this position is not mandatory, for cannulation can be obtained in the supine as well as upright position. Have the patient's head turned approximately 30 degrees to the opposite side.
2. Prepare and drape the supraclavicular region.
3. Identify the site of entry (Fig. 12.11). The site of entry is 1 cm cephalad and 1 cm lateral to the junction of the clavicular head of the sternocleidomastoid muscle with the superior border of the clavicle, which is called the clavisternomastoid angle (81, 125, 223). Identification of this angle is essential for procedural success. This angle can be identified by asking the patient to raise the head off the stretcher.

NOTE

The right side is preferred for two reasons: (a) the thoracic duct may be injured on the left (81), and (b) the right subclavian vein has a straighter course in relation to the innominate vein and the superior vena cava, which may result in more successful catheterization when compared with that on the left side (223).

---

4. Anesthetize the site of entrance.

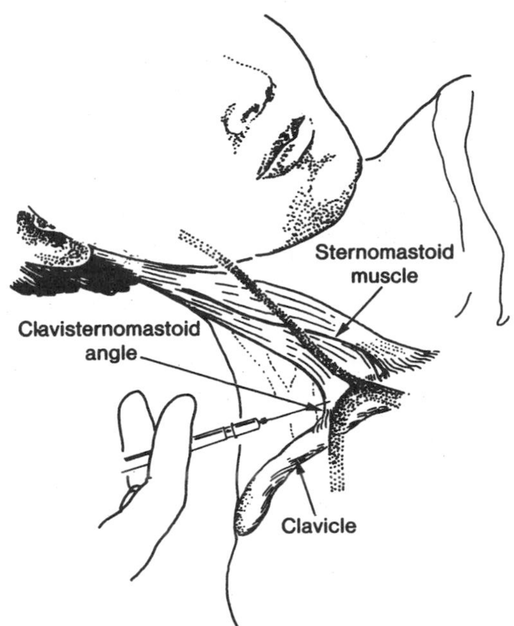

Figure 12.11. Supraclavicular subclavian approach. The site of entry is at the junction of the lateral aspect of the clavicular head of the sternocleidomastoid muscle with the superior border of the clavicle, called the clavisternomastoid angle. Direct the needle at a 5-degree angle from the coronal plane, at 50 degrees from the sagittal plane, and at 40 degrees from the transverse plane. See alternative method in text.

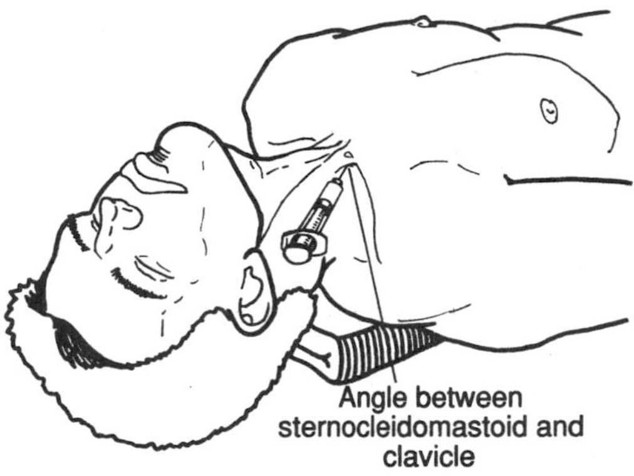

Figure 12.12. In supraclavicular subclavian vein insertion, note the angle at which the syringe is directed to the contralateral nipple. See text for discussion.

Procedural Steps

1. Puncture the site indicated earlier with a standard 14-gauge introducer needle attached to a 5-mL syringe. Align the bevel of the needle with the graduated markings on the syringe; this will serve as a reminder to the orientation of the bevel. Ensure that the bevel is facing anteriorly on penetration of the skin.
2. While applying negative pressure to the syringe, advance the needle, directing it toward the contralateral nipple (Fig. 12.12). In addition, angle the needle anteriorly 10 to 15 degrees from the horizontal plane. In the average adult, the junction of the internal jugular and subclavian veins should be reached within 2 to 3 cm. If flashback is not obtained within 3 cm, withdraw the needle to a point just beneath the skin, and redirect in a slightly more cephalad direction.
3. Once flashback is obtained, rotate the syringe 90 degrees clockwise so that the graduated markings are now directed caudad. This will orient the bevel of the needle caudally and facilitate proper positioning of the guidewire into the superior vena cava.
4. Secure the needle and detach the syringe. Cover the hub with your thumb to prevent air entry. Pass the guidewire through the introducer needle, and insert the catheter as outlined by the Seldinger technique.

NOTE

Difficulty passing the guidewire may occur on occasion. In this event, have an assistant apply traction to the upper extremity on the ipsilateral side.

---

5. Secure the catheter in place.

COMPLICATIONS

Complications are uncommon with this procedure (37). Those complications noted include

1. **Phrenic nerve paralysis.**
2. **Hemothorax** (104).
3. **Pneumothorax.**
4. **Hydrothorax.**
5. **Arteriovenous fistula.**
6. **Brachial plexus injury.**
7. **Air embolism** (104).
8. **Arrhythmias.**
9. **Pulmonary artery laceration.** This occurs from penetration into the superior pulmonary vessels during passage of the needle.

Internal Jugular Vein Cannulation

Because of the incidence of complications with the subclavian approach, the internal jugular vein is the site preferred by many authors for access to the central circulation (48, 62, 109, 174).

The internal jugular vein emerges from the base of the skull posterior to the internal carotid artery. During its course through the neck, it lies lateral and then anterolateral to the carotid artery and is covered superficially throughout its length by the sternomastoid muscle (62). With the head turned to the opposite side, the internal jugular vein, in the lower part of the neck, lies just lateral to a line joining the medial portion of the clavicular head of the sternomastoid to the mastoid process. The vein is subject to almost no anomalies or positional variations.

The vein has two valves immediately above the inferior bulb (a bulge formed by the junction of the subclavian and internal jugular veins). The vein can be cannulated quickly despite profound shock or even obesity. Catheterization of the right side is preferred because the internal jugular, the innominate, and the superior vena cava form a nearly straight line into the right atrium. In addition, in the adult, the right internal jugular vein is larger, and when distended, it may reach a diameter of 2.5 cm. Finally, the apex of the pleura is higher on the left than on the right (48, 86, 174).

DeFalque (48) listed the advantages and disadvantages of internal jugular venous cannulation over the subclavian route as follows:

ADVANTAGES

1. Lower risk of pleural puncture.
2. If a hematoma forms in the neck, it is visible and easily compressible.
3. It has a superficial and constant position. It is particularly useful in the elderly or the obese patient. In the patient with a short, thick neck, the infraclavicular subclavian route is preferred.
4. Malpositioning of the catheter is rare with internal jugular vein cannulation, but can be as high as 25% by the subclavian route.

DISADVANTAGES

1. Failure rate is higher with internal jugular than with subclavian route.
2. Internal jugular vein may collapse in the hypovolemic patient. Alleviate this by placing the patient in the Trendelenburg position.
3. It is more uncomfortable for the patient than is the subclavian route and may dislodge or kink as a result of neck motion.

INDICATIONS

Same as for infraclavicular subclavian cannulation.

EQUIPMENT

Same as for infraclavicular subclavian cannulation.

TECHNIQUE

Two approaches are used in entering the internal jugular vein: the anterior approach and the posterior approach. Both are described.

Preparatory Steps

1. Position the patient in 15 to 20 degrees of Trendelenburg (28, 174). Maintain the head in as neutral a po-

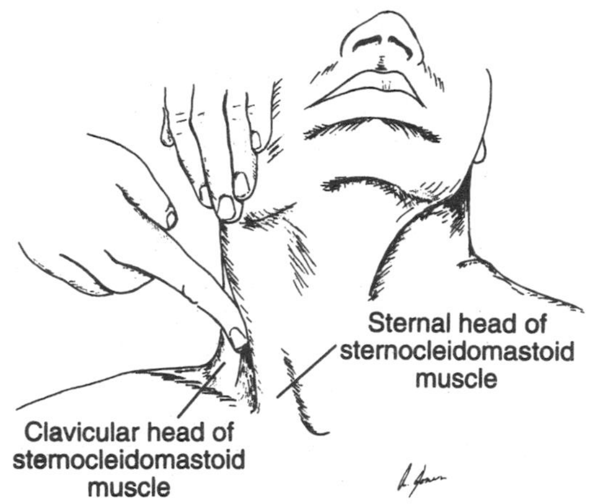

Figure 12.13. An important triangle (in which the internal jugular vein passes) is formed by the medial and lateral heads of the sternocleidomastoid on two sides and the clavicle on the third side. In attempting an internal jugular vein insertion by the central approach, place the finger in the apex of the triangle as shown. See text for discussion

sition as possible, not to exceed 40 degrees of rotation (200).

NOTE

In infants and small children in whom the head is relatively large and the neck short, it is best to have the neck well extended by placing the body on a pillow or placing a folded towel beneath the shoulders. Place a rolled towel or pad under the shoulders to enhance the neck structures (28).

---

2. Prepare and drape the neck.
3. Locate the site of entrance.

   Anterior approach: Locate the triangle formed by the sternal and clavicular heads of the sternocleidomastoid muscle superiorly and the clavicle inferiorly (Fig. 12.13). The point of insertion is at the apex of this triangle (Fig. 12.14).

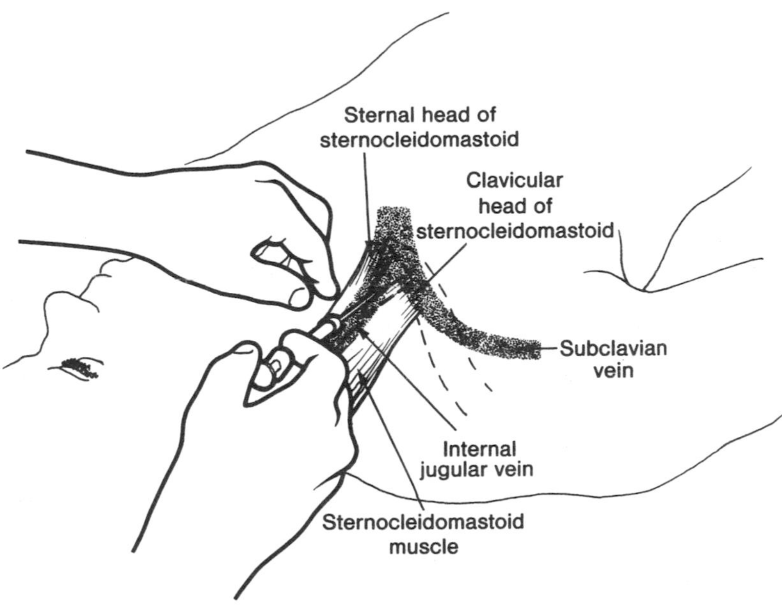

Figure 12.14. Anterior approach for internal jugular vein cannulation. The point of insertion is at the apex of the triangle formed by the junction of the sternal and clavicular heads of the sternocleidomastoid muscle superiorly and the clavicle inferiorly. Insert the needle at an angle of 30 to 40 degrees to the skin, and direct the needle slightly laterally and caudad toward the ipsilateral nipple. See text for discussion.

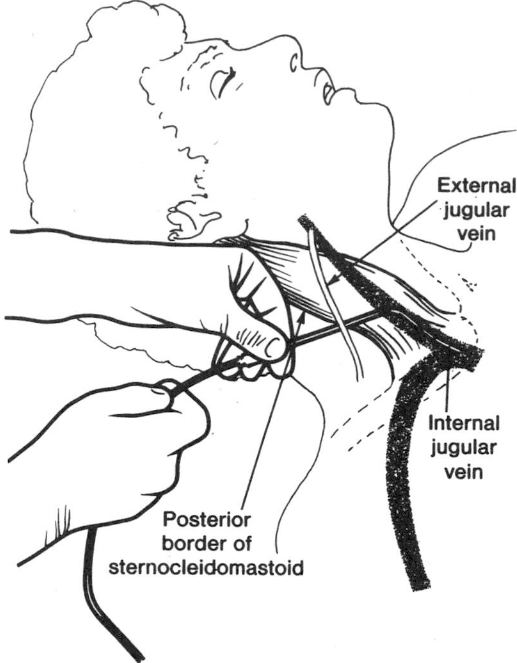

Figure 12.15. Posterior approach to cannulation of the internal jugular vein. Insert the needle along the posterior border of the sternocleidomastoid muscle just above the site where the external jugular vein crosses that border. Alternatively, when one cannot see the external jugular vein, introduce the catheter at the junction of the medial and lower one third of the posterior margin of the sternocleidomastoid muscle. The vein should be entered in 5 to 7 cm. See text for discussion.

Posterior approach (Fig. 12.15): The site of insertion with this approach is along the posterior border of the sternocleidomastoid muscle just cephalad to where the external jugular vein crosses that border (28). Alternatively, when the external jugular vein cannot be visualized, introduce the needle under the sternocleidomastoid muscle at the junction of the medial and lower thirds of the posterior margin (48, 159).

4. Anesthetize the site.

Procedural Steps

1. *Anterior approach* (Fig. 12.14): With a needle connected to a tuberculin syringe, puncture the skin at the apex of the triangle as indicated earlier. Insert the needle at an angle of 30 to 40 degrees to the skin. Direct the needle laterally and caudad toward the ipsilateral nipple or midclavicular line (Fig. 12.16) (44, 174). Enter the vein after 1 to 2 cm because it is quite superficial in this location. If one misses the vein, direct the needle 5 to 10 degrees more laterally (48). If by 4 to 5 cm, the vein is not entered, remove the needle.

   Aspirate as the needle is advanced. If the vein is not entered, aspirate as one withdraws.

   Posterior approach: Insert the needle at the site indicated earlier. Advance the needle and syringe under the sternocleidomastoid, aiming at the midpoint of the suprasternal notch (48). Enter the vein in 5 to 7 cm (28).

NOTE

Some authors advocated the use of a small-gauge needle and syringe to locate the vein before cannulating with the large Intracath needle (174). We believe this is

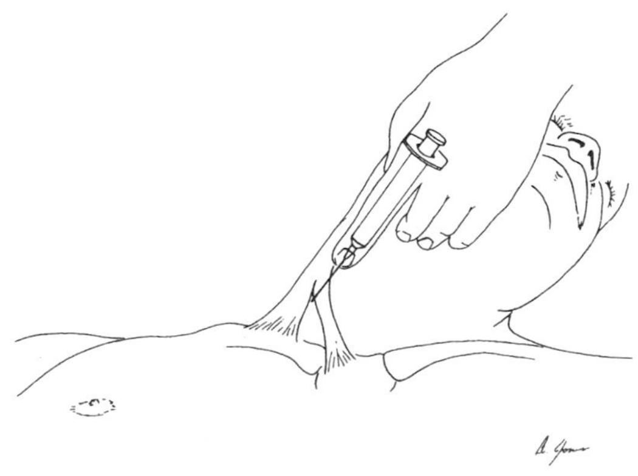

Figure 12.16. With the tip of the index finger at the apex of the triangle formed by the two heads of the sternocleidomastoid muscle, pass the needle just in front of the index finger (as shown), directing it toward the ipsilateral nipple at approximately a 30-degree angle to the skin. See text for discussion.

helpful in the difficult patient whose anatomy is not discerned readily.

---

2. Insert the cannula (Fig. 12.15). Advance the cannula through the needle. If resistance is met, remove the catheter and needle together so that the catheter is not sheared, resulting in a catheter embolism (174). Advance the catheter while the patient holds their breath to prevent air entrance into the vein (48). Advance the catheter until it is lodged in the hub of the needle.
3. Withdraw the needle and aspirate for blood. If blood does not return into the tuberculin syringe, this may be because of hypovolemia and vascular collapse. Withdraw the catheter a centimeter or so, and aspirate again. If one still cannot aspirate blood, then assume improper positioning, and remove the catheter.
4. Attach the intravenous tubing, and secure the needle guard.

Aftercare

1. Lower the intravenous bottle to check that the catheter is in the vein. Blood should return into the tubing.
2. Anchor the cannula to the skin with sutures, and apply antibiotic dressing.
3. Loop the plastic intravenous tubing behind and over the patient's ear, and tape into position (28).

Internal Jugular Vein Cannulation: Direct Anterior Approach (The Schaider Approach)

A technique for cannulating the internal jugular vein was described by Schaider (personal communication, J. Schaider, Emergency Medicine, Chicago Medical School, 1993). It combines several of the advantages of the commonly called "anterior approach," which involves palpation of the carotid artery, and the middle approach, which is referred to as the anterior approach in this chapter.

TECHNIQUE

Preparatory Steps

1. Positioning of the patient: Position the patient in 15 to 20 degrees of Trendelenburg. Keep the patient's head in a neutral position or turned minimally (5 degrees) toward the contralateral side.
2. Prepare and drape the neck as described earlier.
3. Identify the site of entrance. Locate the triangle formed by the sternal and clavicular heads of the sternocleidomastoid muscle superiorly and the clavicle inferiorly. The point of insertion is at the apex of this triangle.

Procedural Steps

1. With a 3-mL syringe filled with lidocaine and fitted with a 25-gauge needle, inject a small amount of lidocaine intradermally at the insertion site. Remove the syringe and fit it with a 21-gauge needle. Palpate the carotid artery with the index finger of the left hand. As with other procedures involving the neck, it is preferable to use the patient's right side. Insert the needle at the apex of the triangle at a 60-degree angle to the skin, directing the needle toward the ipsilateral nipple. Advance the needle while aspirating. To anesthetize the tissue, inject a small amount of lidocaine each 3 mm of needle advancement. Enter the internal jugular vein within 1.5 cm of needle advancement. If one misses the vein, withdraw and redirect the needle more medially. Palpate the carotid artery to demonstrate the most medial structure that must be avoided at all times.
2. After the internal jugular vein is located and anesthetized by using a 21-gauge needle, withdraw the needle. As the needle leaves the skin, drag the needle along the skin and deposit a small line of blood on the same line along which one entered the skin. This will serve as a guide when one

reenters the neck with the catheter set needle by using the Seldinger technique.

3. Using the guideline, reenter the skin with a catheter set needle, attached to a tuberculin syringe, again at the apex of the triangle. Direct the needle in the same direction as the locator needle while aspirating for blood. After blood is aspirated, fix the position of the needle to insert the cannula.
4. Insert a cannula as described elsewhere in the text.

COMPLICATIONS

1. **Hematoma.** Hematoma can occur from either venous or arterial bleeding. This complication may result from inadvertent puncture of the carotid artery (48, 174). If one side of the neck develops a large hematoma, do not cannulate the other side because a bilateral hematoma can result and compromise the patient's airway. Treat the hematoma with a compression dressing (48).
2. **Thoracic duct injury.** This complication is rare. A case of chylothorax necessitating surgery has been described (121). If this occurs, treat the resulting chylothorax with repeated thoracocentesis and replacement of lost proteins with medium-chain triglycerides.
3. **Hemothorax.** Hemothorax is secondary to puncture of either the lung or a major vessel such as a subclavian artery, aorta, or carotid artery. Deaths as a result of hemothorax have been reported (174). Treat hemothorax with chest tube drainage, and, if it is secondary to arterial injury, repair the artery.
4. **Pneumothorax.** Pneumothorax is secondary to puncture of the lung. This is much less common with internal jugular vein cannulation than with subclavian puncture.
5. **Pneumomediastinum and hydromediastinum.** This is more common in infants, in whom laceration of the trachea may occur (48). To prevent hydromediastinum, carefully insert the catheter and check for blood reflux into the intravenous tubing on lowering the bottle. Avoid directing the needle medially in the infant.
6. **Air embolism.** This is especially common in hypovolemic patients (188). Always make certain that the connections in the intravenous tubing are tight. Place the index finger over the hub of the needle when the syringe is withdrawn. For therapy see "Air Embolism" in the section on "Infraclavicular Subclavian Vein Cannulation."
7. **Phlebitis.**
8. **Infection.** Catheter tips cultured for organisms were found to have an 11% incidence of pathogenic organisms; however, only one patient in 70 did clinical infection develop (137, 177).
9. **Catheter embolism.** See "Complications" discussion, under "Infraclavicular Subclavian Vein Cannulation," earlier (98).
10. **Myocardial puncture.** See subclavian discussion.
11. **Cerebral infarction**. This results as a consequence of inadvertent carotid artery puncture (225).
12. **Nerve damage**. In 1988 Defalque (50) identified 19 cases within a 20-year period. These cases involve damage to the phrenic nerve, recurrent laryngeal nerve, cervical roots, brachial plexus, cervical sympathetic chain, and cranial nerves. Furthermore, Burns (32) reported a case of spinal accessory nerve injury after right internal jugular vein catheterization. The mechanism for injury is postulated to result from either direct needle trauma or compression from a hematoma.

Femoral Vein Cannulation

Femoral vein catheterization has many advantages over subclavian vein catheterization, particularly in situations of cardiac arrest. The reported success rate for femoral vein catheterization is 77%, compared with 94% for subclavian vein catheterization (61).

INDICATIONS

1. Rapid placement of a large-bore intravenous route, especially during external cardiac compression when motion of the neck and subclavian region necessitates cessation of cardiac compression for central venous cannulation.
2. Drawing blood when unable to locate a vein elsewhere.
3. Radiographic procedure.
4. Emergency intravenous route when unable to find access elsewhere or when there is clinical contraindication to use of an upper extremity vessel.
5. Rapid placement of a transvenous pacemaker.

TECHNIQUE

Preparatory Steps

1. Meticulously prepare the overlying skin because contamination is a significant problem.
2. Locate vein. Palpate the pulse of the femoral artery. The vein is located 1 cm medial to the artery (82). In the patient with vascular collapse or cardiac arrest in whom the femoral artery pulse cannot be palpated, find the vein by extending an imaginary line between the pubic tubercle and the anterior superior iliac spine. The vein will be located midway between these two structures (168).
3. Anesthetize with 1% lidocaine.

Procedural Steps

1. When the catheter and needle are chosen, position the needle two finger breadths (2 to 3 cm) below the inguinal ligament (25) and medial to the artery; direct the needle cephalad at a 45-degree angle with the skin, and aim the bevel of the needle toward the umbilicus. In difficult cases, enter the vein perpendicular to the skin and then change the direction of the needle to 45 degrees to cannulate the vein.
2. Attach intravenous tubing.
3. Apply dressing with antibacterial ointment and sterile gauze.

COMPLICATIONS

1. **Thrombosis and phlebitis.** A very common problem with prolonged femoral cannulation is thrombosis, which may extend proximally into the deep veins and into the inferior vena cava (25, 87). Twenty-four patients with femoral catheterizations that remained in place 3 to 14 days were studied (214). In five patients, caval thrombosis developed, and two patients had pulmonary emboli. In four of the patients, suppurative thrombophlebitis and sepsis developed. Patients with serious complications had the catheter in place for 13 days, whereas those without complications had the catheter in place for 6 or fewer days.

   In the *prevention and treatment* of these complications, remember to remove the femoral cannula as early as possible. Use strict aseptic technique, and change the fluid infusion sets every 48 hours (16, 33). Use heparin in a bottle as indicated in the section "Intravenous Cannulas General Features and Complications," earlier, for patients undergoing prolonged cannulation of central veins, especially the femoral.
2. **Hematoma.** This is a common problem (10). In *preventing and treating* this complication, apply a good pressure dressing over an unsuccessful cannulation site. When the vein is entered and the cannula removed, apply pressure for a full 5 minutes. Avoid the use of the femoral vein in patients with coagulopathies (138).

3. **Septic arthritis of the hip** (10, 25, 138). This results from piercing the hip capsule, which lies under the vein. The development of anterior thigh edema and decreased extension and internal rotation of the hip joint should suggest this complication. The most common organism is *Staphylococcus aureus* (10).

   The *prevention and treatment* of this complication involves avoidance of piercing the posterior wall of the femoral vein and avoidance of contact with bone. Strict aseptic technique is encouraged so that, if the capsule is penetrated, septic arthritis does not result (10).
4. **Femoral nerve damage** (10, 25). The femoral nerve courses lateral to the femoral artery. In the obese patient in whom landmarks are difficult to define and arterial pulsation is difficult to identify, one may cause damage to the femoral nerve by inadvertently aiming the needle too far laterally.
5. **Penetration of a viscus** in an unrecognized femoral hernia (10, 25).
6. **Psoas abscess** (10, 25). A psoas abscess may result from introduction of skin bacteria into the psoas fascia, which lies beneath the femoral artery and vein.
7. **Cervical dural puncture** (152). Although uncommon in the adult, this rare complication has been reported in neonates.

VEIN CUTDOWN TECHNIQUES

Saphenous Vein Cutdown at the Ankle

The saphenous vein in the ankle is probably the ideal vein for cannulation. It is the only vessel of importance in this location, and its constant location just anterior to the medial malleolus permits ready access. Its elasticity permits the vein to be dissected easily through a short incision without rupture (178). The disadvantages of this site are the greater risk of phlebitis, the difficulty in rapidly infusing fluids via this route because of the valves in the leg veins, and the low flow rates through these relatively small-caliber veins (171).

In addition to the ankle, other sites can be used for cannulation (Fig. 12.17). The

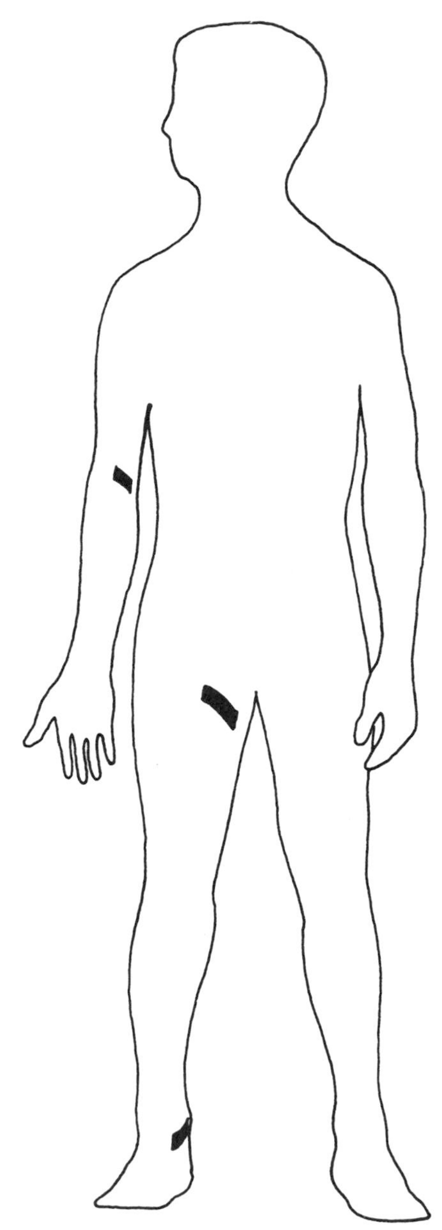

Figure 12.17. Antecubital, groin, and ankle cutdowns are perhaps the most commonly performed.

saphenous vein in the groin is especially useful to place a large-bore line, such as intravenous tubing, for voluminous fluid and blood administration in a patient with a traumatic cardiopulmonary arrest. In addition, the saphenous vein in the groin is easily accessible and can be cannulated rapidly in infants and children. The basilic vein, located in the medial antecubital fossa, is another site that can be cannulated. Catheters can be inserted through this route for central monitoring. This site is the most commonly used cutdown site in the upper extremity. The cephalic vein, located on the lateral aspect of the antecubital fossa, is another available site; however, it is infrequently used because of the difficulty in passing a catheter (if a CVP line is needed) past the sharp angulation as this vein enters the axillary vein. There also is the possibility of injury to the lateral cutaneous nerve at the cutdown site. According to some authors (45), in the upper extremity, the cutdown site of first choice is the median basilic because of its superficial location and large caliber; the brachial vein is the second choice, and the median cephalic is the third choice (Fig. 12.1).

INDICATIONS

1. Poor peripheral sites for intravenous cannulation, for example, in obese patients and drug addicts, in whom a central line cannot be placed.
2. Hypovolemic shock in which rapid volume replacement through a large-bore cannula is needed (162).
3. Placement of a CVP monitor or Swan–Ganz catheter, in patients in whom a central line is not preferred.
4. Pacemaker insertion.
5. Cardiac arrest in infants and small children, in whom access to a central line is unsuccessful.

CONTRAINDICATIONS

1. Injury to vessels proximal to the site of cutdown.
2. Unstable fractures proximal to the site of the cutdown that may increase the risk of phlebitis because of swelling proximally.

EQUIPMENT

One scalpel with no. 10 and 11 blades
One curved Kelley hemostat
One small mosquito hemostat
Fine-toothed forceps
Scissors, Iris and sharp cutting
Anesthetic prep
Skin prep
Drapes and towel clips
At least two sizes of polyethylene tubing
One sterile intravenous extension tubing
Sterile sponges, 4 × 4
Syringes, 5 mL
Self-retaining retractors
Small rake
Needle holder
Silk 3-0 and 4-0 sutures
Injectable saline
Intravenous tubing and solution
Dressings with antibiotic ointment

TECHNIQUE

The technique discussed here is for the saphenous vein at the ankle. The same principles are applicable to other sites, and the differences between this site and the others are discussed separately.

Preparatory Steps

1. Select a site approximately two finger breadths above the medial malleolus (Fig. 12.18).
2. Prepare and drape.
3. Infiltrate with local anesthetic if necessary.

Procedural Steps

1. Incise the skin and subcutaneous tissue. Make a transverse incision over the vein, extending from the anterior border of the tibia above the medial malleolus posteriorly to the posterior border of the medial malleolus (Fig. 12.19). Be certain to hold the skin

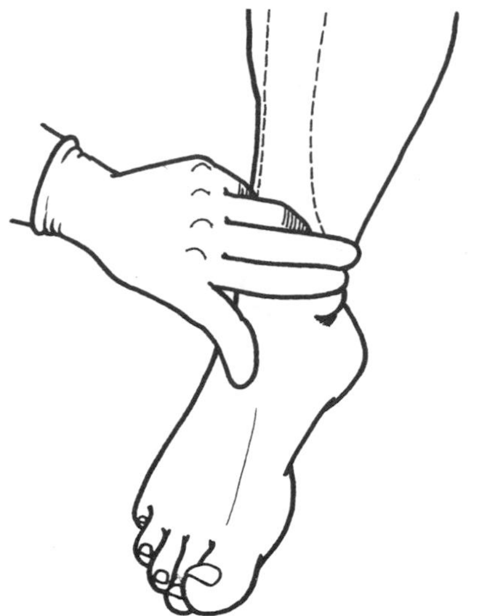

Figure 12.18. Enter the saphenous vein two finger breaths above the medial malleolus. See text for discussion.

apart as shown in Fig. 12.19. The incision should barely penetrate into the subcutaneous tissue to avoid incising the vein.

2. Using a curved hemostat, "scoop" all of the tissue from one end of the wound to the other. To do so, direct the closed curved hemostat downward into the wound, to be certain to pick up all of the tissue along the tibia. Do this in one single maneuver. The hemostat is then turned upward, so that the point faces the physician (Fig. 12.20).
3. Open the hemostat (Fig. 12.21). The tissue will part, and the saphenous vein should be easily identified. If it is difficult to identify the vein, squeeze the foot, and blood will fill the saphenous vein. Using a straight Kelly, separate the vein from the other structures (Fig. 12.21).
4. Insert a closed straight hemostat under the vein (Fig. 12.22).
5. Isolate the vein between two ligatures, as in Fig. 12.23.

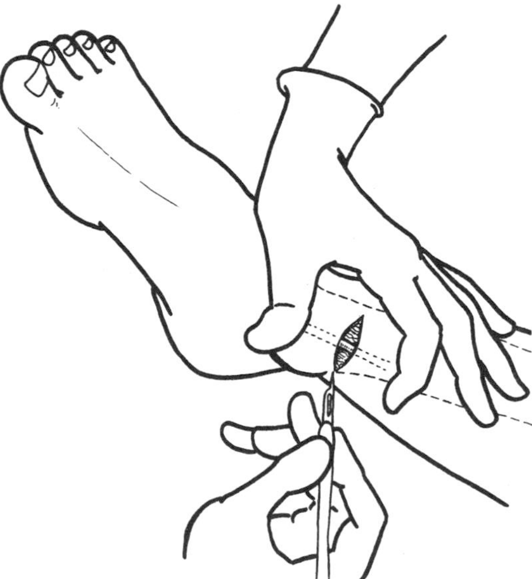

Figure 12.19. Saphenous vein cutdown in the ankle. Make an incision from the anterior to the posterior border of the tibia. See text for discussion.

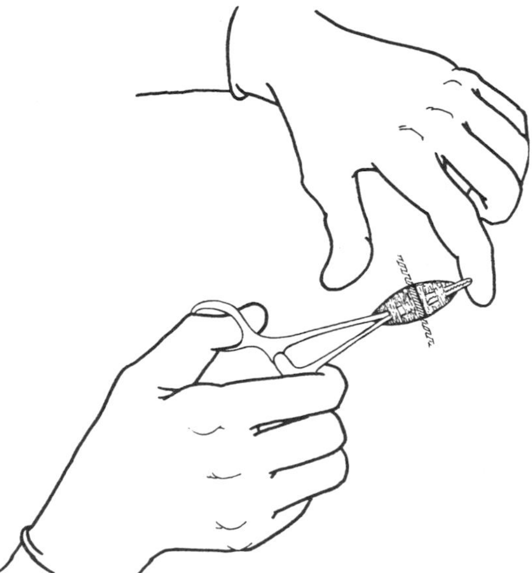

Figure 12.20. To find the saphenous vein, pass a hemostat under all of the tissue within the incision. See text for discussion.

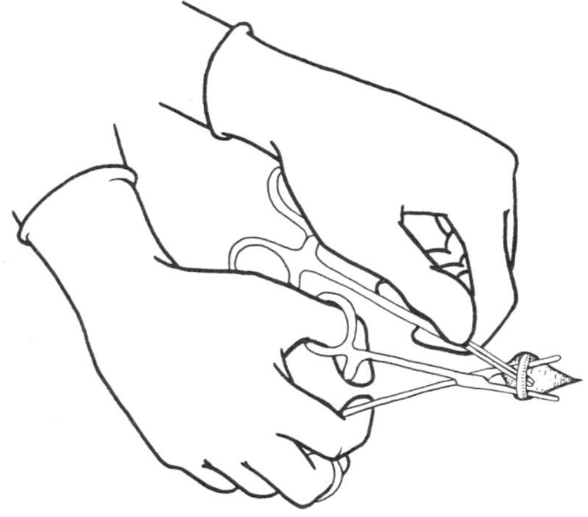

Figure 12.21. Separate the saphenous vein as shown. See text for discussion.

6. Select a cannula approximately one size larger than the vein appears. Use extension tubing from an intravenous line set if the end that inserts into an Angiocath is cut off at an angle, thus creating a bevel. This will result in a large port, equivalent to an 8-gauge intravenous line, through which a prodigious volume of fluid can be administered.

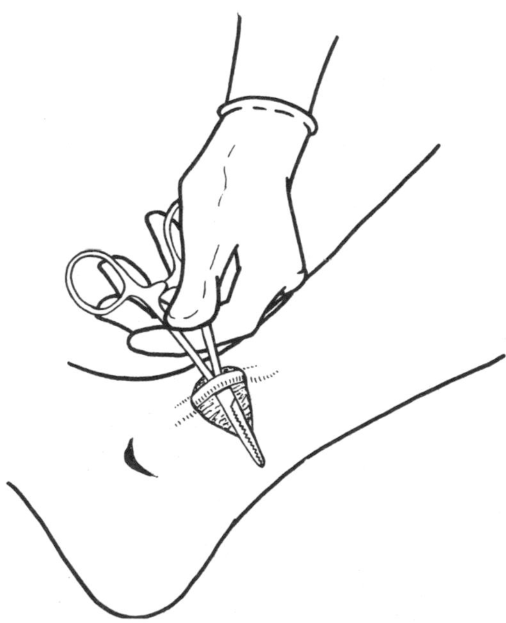

Figure 12.22. Isolate the saphenous vein, and place a closed hemostat under it. This hemostat will act as a "cutting board" for insertion of the catheter. See text for discussion.

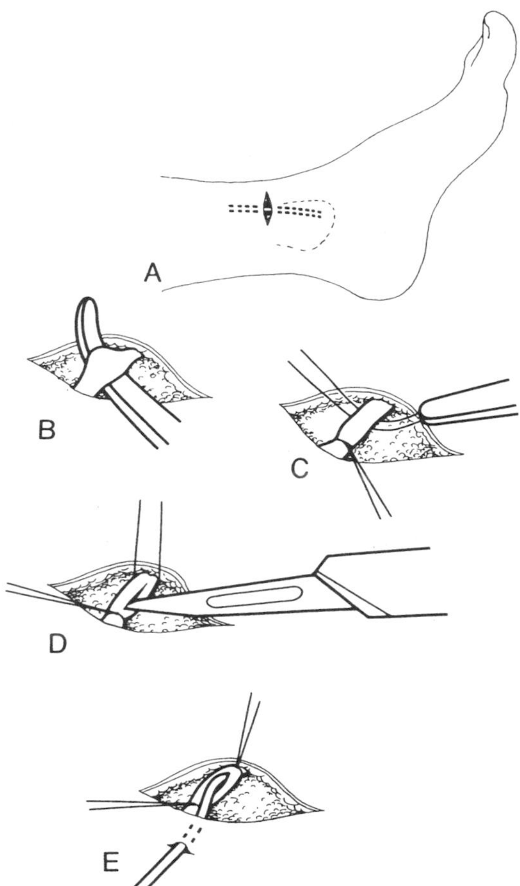

Figure 12.23. Procedure for a cutdown over the saphenous vein at the ankle. See text for discussion.

7. Multiple techniques have been described to cannulate the saphenous vein. Lift the vein, as shown in Fig. 12.23, and make a longitudinal incision between the two suture ligatures. Insert iris scissors into the vein, and spread apart to facilitate inserting a catheter into the lumen.

   Another technique is to incise, with the tip of a no. 11 blade, the vein from its midpoint laterally. This transverse incision, through half the diameter of the vein, can then be cannulated by inserting either an Iris scissors or vein introducer followed by a catheter. We prefer a vein introducer, because it causes less trauma to the tissues and more easily facilitates passage of the catheter.

8. Insert the cannula into the vein. A vein introducer (small plastic insert) can be inserted into the venotomy site to aid in cannulation. With the bevel facing the posterior wall of the vein, relax the proximal ligature and gently advance the cannula. Stabilize the vein with gentle traction of the distal suture.

   Alternative method: An alternative technique is to pass the cannula through a separate stab wound distal to the site of the incision for the cutdown. A 14-gauge needle or larger is passed through the skin from inside the incision to the skin distal to the cutdown site so as not to introduce bacteria from the skin. Then pass a cannula through the needle, after which, remove the needle. Then insert the cannula into the vein as discussed earlier. This decreases the incidence of infection at the incision site and at the vein, because the cannula does not pass through the incision, acting effectively as a "drain within an abscess cavity." This is our preferred approach; however, one may not be able to use this technique in an emergency situation when time is of the essence.
9. Aspirate to confirm that one is in the vein and not in a false passage in the wall of the vein. After this, inject a few millimeters of sterile saline so as to prevent clot formation at the tip and to assure free flow.
10. Attach the cannula to the intravenous solution.
11. Secure the proximal ligature around the cannula now within the vein, and ligate distally.
12. Close the wound.

Aftercare

1. Suture the cannula to the skin, using nylon or silk suture.
2. Apply antibiotic ointment over the incision site and site of cannula exit, and dress with 4 × 4-inch gauze. Tape securely and immobilize the ankle in a splint.

Saphenous Vein Cutdown at the Groin

Through a saphenous vein cutdown at the groin, infuse 500 mL of whole blood within 5 minutes (163) with a large-bore cannula. We believe this is the best route for patients with massive trauma in whom large volumes of fluid are needed over a short period. In such a situation, use a sterile intravenous extension tubing with the tip cut off at a 45-degree angle as the cannula. In a dire emergency, perform a cutdown at this site within 60 seconds (163). Catheters at this site should, however, be removed within 24 hours to avoid phlebitis, because this is not a sterile area.

TECHNIQUES

It is important to recognize that, at the groin, the saphenous vein is superficial and lies in the subcutaneous fat, well above the femoral artery and vein (Fig. 12.24).

1. Make an incision that begins at the point where the scrotal or labial fold meets the medial aspect of the thigh (Fig. 12.25). Carry the incision laterally in a transverse direction approximately 6 cm. The saphenous vein lies at the point where this transverse incision meets an imaginary line that extends perpendicularly from the lateral edge of the hairline (Fig. 12.26). If one imagines the hair on the mons pubis as forming a triangle, then the imaginary line is formed from the lateral point of this triangle directly inferiorly (Fig. 12.26).

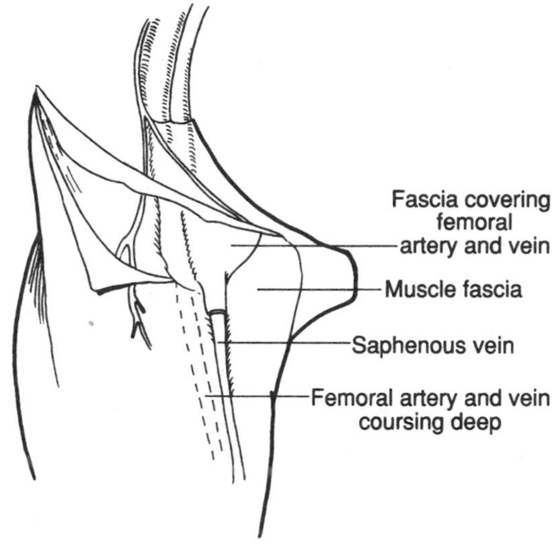

Figure 12.24. The saphenous vein in the groin is superficial to the fascia, the femoral artery, and the femoral vein.

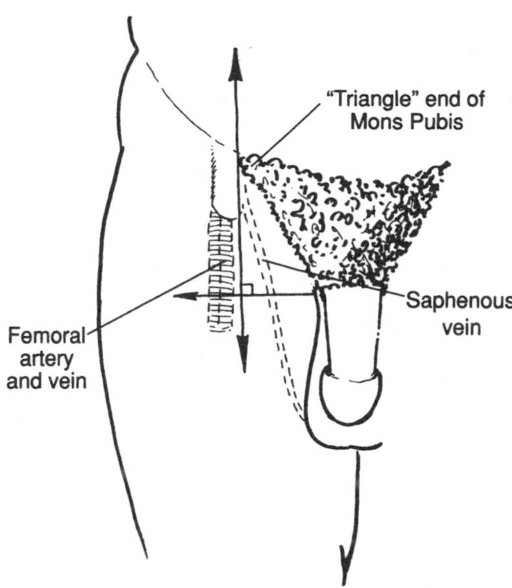

Figure 12.26. The saphenous vein is superficial and medial to the femoral artery and vein. See text for discussion.

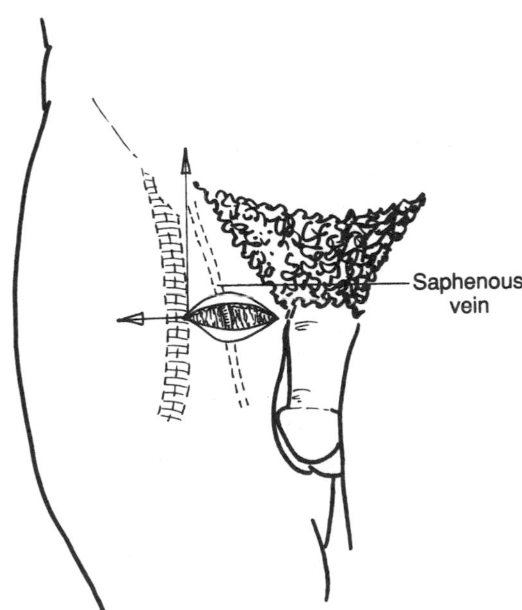

Figure 12.25. The incision extends from the junction of the scrotal or labial fold, where the fold meets the thigh laterally, to an imaginary line coursing down from the mons pubis. See text for discussion.

2. Dissect out the saphenous vein at the point where the transverse incision and the imaginary line, described earlier, cross. The vein is located in the fat superficial to the muscle, fascia, artery, and femoral vein. Thus if one reaches these structures, one has progressed too deep.
3. After the vein is isolated, make a venotomy and pass intravenous extension tubing.

Basilic Vein Cutdown

Perform this cutdown with the patient's elbow extended and the forearm supinated. It is traditionally taught that, in this cutdown, a 2.5-cm incision is made two finger breadths superior to the medial epicondyle with the center of the incision being over the brachial pulse (Fig. 12.27). When this pulse is not palpable, extend the transverse incision between the biceps and triceps muscles at the junction of the distal one fourth and proximal three fourths of the arm. The

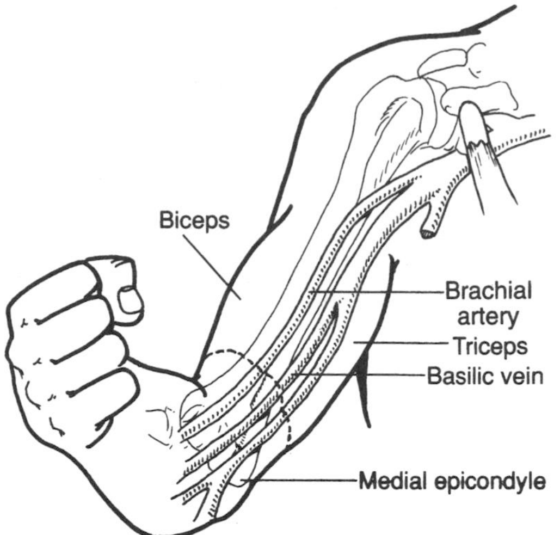

Figure 12.27. The basilic vein is located two finger breaths above the medial epicondyle, midway between the biceps and triceps muscles.

vein courses just over the triceps muscle. The vein will be found superficial to the neuromuscular bundle between the biceps and the triceps on the medial side of the arm (Fig. 12.28). The vein will lie just medial and superficial to the brachial artery and median nerve. It is important to note that the vein is superficial to the median nerve and brachial artery. Thus if one enters the plane where these structures are found or where muscle fascia is identified, one is too deep. Once the vein is identified, its cannulation is similar to that described for a saphenous vein cutdown in the ankle.

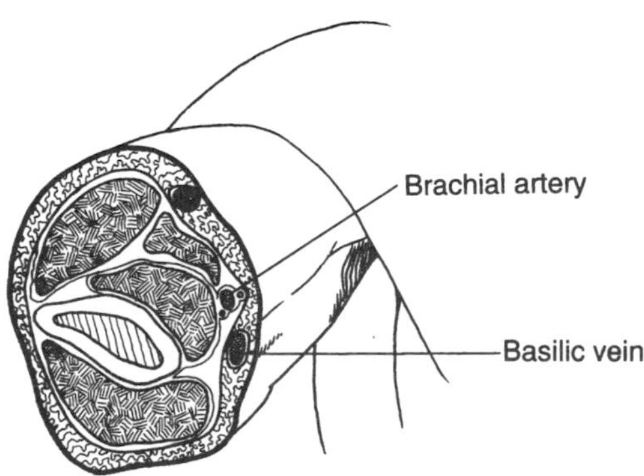

Figure 12.28. Note that the basilic vein is superficial to the brachial artery, which is located with the median nerve in the deeper fascia.

COMPLICATIONS

1. **Thromboembolism and phlebitis.** This complication can occur from prolonged catheterization, infection from the cutdown site extending into the vein, or irritation from the cannula against the vein wall. It is more common with lower-extremity cutdowns than with those in an upper extremity (163).
2. **Infection.** In a double-blind study using Neosporin (not recommended here), bacteria were cultured from the cutdown wound in 18% of Neosporin-treated patients as compared with 78% in a placebo group. Some patients in whom phlebitis developed subsequently had sterile wounds, and some benign-appearing wounds grew pathogenic bacteria (106, 156). Use aseptic technique, and if possible, bring the cannula out through a separate stab wound. We prefer bacitracin ointment to cover the cutdown site.
3. **Injury to associated arteries and nerves.** The median nerve lies in close proximity to the basilic vein and can be injured. The saphenous nerve courses adjacent to the saphenous vein at the ankle. The lateral antecubital nerve courses close to the cephalic vein at the elbow. There are cases in which the artery is mistaken for a vein. To avoid this, feel for arterial pulsation in the vessel. This may be a problem, especially in a child or in a patient in shock in whom pulsations may not be evident.
4. **Catheter embolism.** See "Complications" discussed under "Infraclavicular Subclavian Vein Cannulation," earlier.
5. **Air embolism.** See "Complications" discussed under "Infraclavicular Subclavian Vein Cannulation," earlier.

6. **Perforation of vein proximal to puncture site,** resulting in fluid infusion into the subcutaneous tissue proximally. This occurs from puncture of the vein wall with a sharp cannula or previous attempts at intravenous insertion proximally, or as a result of traumatic injury.

Cephalic Vein Cutdown at the Wrist

Recently Talan (217) described a cutdown technique for the cephalic vein at the wrist. The cephalic vein runs alongside the radius and courses subcutaneously. Make a horizontal incision 1 to 2 cm proximal to the radial styloid in the midlateral line, and isolate the vein (Fig. 12.29*A*, *B*). Be certain not to make the incision too deeply, in that the cephalic vein is very superficial. The vein is large enough to introduce a large-bore catheter without difficulty.

This approach has not gained popularity because, in patients who have had multiple intravenous lines or injections, the vein is often scarred proximally. However, there are multiple connecting veins throughout its route and thus, we recommend using this approach as an alternative to the basilic vein cutdown more proximally.

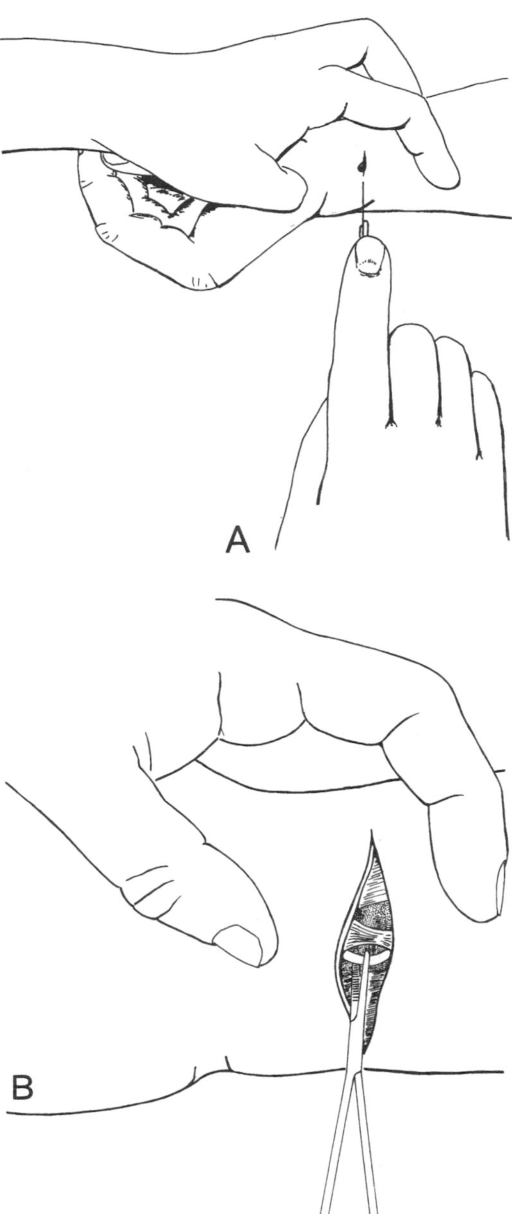

Figure 12.29. Cephalic vein cutdown at the wrist. The cephalic vein courses along the radius. Make an incision as shown, and find the cephalic vein superficially. See text for discussion.

INTRAVENOUS CANNULATION OF THE INFANT

Several sites of cannulation are available on the infant, both peripherally and centrally. However, because of the relatively infrequent need of a large intravenous cannula in an infant, experience with these approaches is limited; therefore, the physician often is somewhat fearful when central cannulation becomes necessary. To avoid redundancy, we concentrate on those procedures that are useful in establishing an intravenous route, and discuss both peripheral and central approaches. The reader should be familiar with the techniques for intravenous cannulation in adults, such as subclavian and internal jugular veins, because only the pertinent dissimilarities or striking similarities are discussed in this section on intravenous cannulation in the infant. Because cutdowns are used in emergency medicine in difficult infant intravenous cannulations, these also are discussed here.

Several primary sites exist where veins have a constant position in the infant (221) and can be used for peripheral, central, or cutdown venous cannulations. These include the long saphenous vein at the ankle (anterior to the medial malleolus) and the cephalic vein at the wrist over the lateral surface of the distal end of the radius. Secondary sites are on the back of the hand and in the antecubital fossa (basilic and median antecubital veins). The external jugular vein in the neck and the long saphenous vein at the medial knee and in the groin also are places where access to the circulation can be attained in the infant.

Perhaps the most commonly used veins in small infants are the scalp veins, because they are readily accessible (42). When one dresses these venous sites with antibiotic ointment, there is a decreased incidence of colonization, and the infection rate decreases from 36% to 3.7% (21). Infection associated with scalp vein cannulation is infrequent, even when the cannula remains in place for 3 or 4 days (43). Scalp veins have a lower incidence of phlebitis than do other veins and can be used repeatedly (43).

Use as large a catheter as possible. Generally a vein will take a catheter one size larger than it appears (221). This is especially true in dealing with a cutdown. A 2-French catheter will not permit even saline to flow well without an infusion pump (221). A 3 French allows saline to pass, but not blood, whereas a 4 French is a good all-purpose catheter (221). This is the smallest size recommended for most cutdowns performed on infants. The long saphenous in the full-term neonate generally takes a 4-French catheter easily.

Peripheral Intravenous Lines in the Infant

Select a site, usually a scalp vein or a vein on the dorsum of the hand initially. The technique using a butterfly is discussed later. For intravenous cannulation, use a small-gauge Angiocath; the technique is similar to that in the adult.

1. In starting an intravenous line in a child with small veins, it is important to connect the butterfly needle to the intravenous tubing first. Fill the tubing with the intravenous solution.
2. Apply a tourniquet to the forearm or a rubber band to the scalp.
3. Secure the arm and hand to an armboard when one of these veins is used. With scalp veins, the covering used over the site (Fig. 12.4) should protect the needle or cannula from dislodging.
4. Flush a small amount of solution into the site by pressing on the end of the tubing after the needle has penetrated the skin. This creates a negative pressure in the system and assures prompt blood return once the vein is entered.
5. Cannulate the vein at a 15-degree angle, and once the vein is entered, do not advance the needle farther. The exception to this is when a large vein is cannulated and advancement can be performed under direct vision without the hazard of going through the vein.
6. Begin the intravenous infusion.
7. Secure the line in place, wrapping several loops of the tubing (attached to the butterfly needle) adjacent to the site.
8. Cut a small plastic disposable medication cup (15 mL) in half vertically. Cover the site with half-cup forming a "hood" over the puncture site to protect the needle from displacement (see Fig. 12.4).

Internal Jugular Vein Cannulation in the Infant

English et al. (62) reported a success rate of 91% in cannulation of the internal jugular vein in a group of 85 infants and children. In another study, 100 children underwent cannulation between the ages of 2 weeks and 9 years without any complications (93). The reader is referred to the adult section for a full discussion of the procedure.

TECHNIQUE

Preparatory Steps

1. Place the child in 15 to 20 degrees of Trendelenburg, with the head held firmly over the edge of the table (121, 168). Turn the infant's head to the opposite side, and have an assistant hold it, hyperextending the neck to tense the sternocleidomastoid muscle (95, 126, 174).
2. Prepare and drape as routine (95, 175), and place three towels under the shoulders (212).
3. Select a catheter. Various authors have recommended different sizes; however, generally use either a 16-gauge Abbott or Deseret Venocath (95) or a 17-gauge Intracath (126).

Estimate the length of the cannula before insertion by "eyeballing" the length needed to pass from the puncture site to the sternal notch.

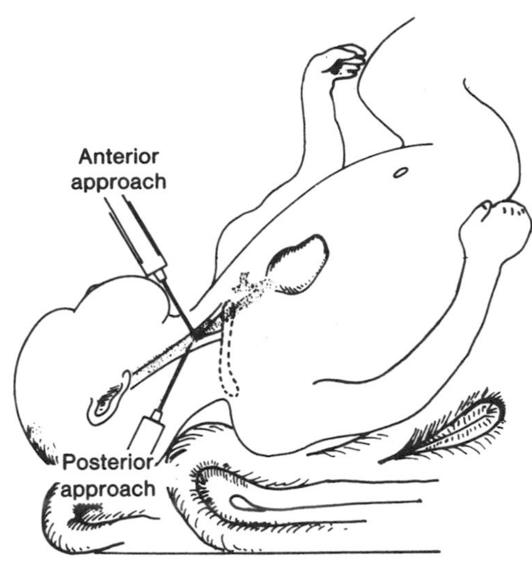

Figure 12.30. Catheterization of the internal jugular vein by the anterior and the posterior approach in the infant. With the anterior approach, the apex of the triangle formed by the two heads of the sternocleidomastoid is the site of insertion. Direct the needle at a 45-degree angle to the skin caudally. In the posterior approach, the site of entrance is at the junction of the middle and lower thirds of the sternocleidomastoid muscle. Hold the needle at a 30-degree angle to the skin. (From Craux MM: Percutaneous cannulation of the internal jugular vein in infants and children. Surg Gynecol Obstet 148:593, 1979, with permission.)

Procedural Steps (same as in adults)

1. Insert needle attached to a tuberculin syringe at the site.

   Anterior approach (Fig. 12.30): The apex of the triangle formed by the two heads (sternal and clavicular) of the sternocleidomastoid is the site of insertion. Direct the needle at a 45-degree angle to the skin caudally, and aim it toward the ipsilateral nipple (Fig. 12.14) (157, 174).

   Posterior approach (Fig. 12.30): The site of entrance is at the junction of the middle and lower thirds of the posterior border of the sternocleidomastoid muscle (126). Advance the catheter to the midpoint of the suprasternal notch (95, 126). Hold the needle at a 30-degree angle to the skin (95).

   SmartNeedle method. The SmartNeedle has a built-in Doppler at the tip of the catheter that allows differentiation between the artery and vein. Arterial flow is pulsatile and high-pitched, whereas venous flow is of low frequency, "blowing," and varies with respiration. After skin puncture, pan the catheter until the loudest venous sound is identified. Slowly insert the catheter as the sound intensity increases until the vein is cannulated. At this point, note a "pop." If the sound intensity on the other hand decreases, redirect the catheter until the sound intensity is regained, and readvance (212).

   Ultrasonographic-guided approach. The use of bedside ultrasonography to localize the internal jugular vein has been shown to be more precise and efficient than either the landmark or SmartNeedle techniques. We recommend a 7.5-MHz probe; the carotid artery and right internal jugular vein can be visually distinguished by their relative position, compressibility of the vein, and pulsatile nature of the artery. Position the ultrasound probe on the neck perpendicular to the vessels, lateral to the trachea, and superior to the clavicle. Advance the needle into the vein under direct ultrasound visualization (212).

NOTE

Some authors prefer to use a 22- or 23-gauge needle attached to a 5-mL syringe to locate the vein before introducing the cannula, as previously mentioned (95).

---

2. Aspirate and advance. With the anterior approach, one usually enters the vein in 1 to 2 cm (114, 157); if not, aspirate during withdrawal.
3. Remove the syringe and insert the catheter. Place the thumb or index finger over the hub of the needle as the syringe is removed to prevent air entry. Thread the catheter into the superior vena cava. Aspirate after the catheter is in place to check position, and withdraw the needle and catheter out of the puncture site once the catheter is securely locked into the hub of the needle.

CAUTION

The same precautions apply in infant cannulations as in the adult. Should it be necessary to remove the catheter, remove the needle and catheter as a single unit, and never withdraw the catheter through the needle, because this may result in shearing and catheter embolism.

---

4. Connect the intravenous solution and lower the infusion bottle to check for return of blood into the tubing, indicating the proper location in the vein (126, 174).

Aftercare

Tape and secure the line. Obtain radiographs to check proper location in the superior vena cava. If one has difficulty seeing the catheter tip, inject 5 mL of contrast material to visualize the position (126). Change the antibiotic ointment and the dressing 3 times a week, and the intravenous tubing once a day.

Subclavian Vein Cannulation in the Infant

There seems to be an inordinate amount of fear associated with introducing a catheter into the subclavian vein of a child. We believe this is inappropriate when such a procedure may be lifesaving in an emergency situation. In 103 subclavian catheterizations in infants aged between 6 months and 2 years, few complications were noted when the procedure was performed properly (93).

See the adult section for a full discussion of subclavian catheterization.

TECHNIQUE
Preparatory Steps

1. Place the child in 15 to 30 degrees of Trendelenburg (103). Restrain the infant and have the head turned to the opposite side.
2. Ipsilaterally elevate the shoulder in a "shrug" to straighten the angle between the subclavian vein and thus the superior vena cava.
3. Select a catheter. Although a 16- or 17-gauge catheter can be used in larger children, we prefer to use a 19-gauge, 1-inch Bardic or Deseret type catheter in the smaller infant. This size fits well between the infant's clavicle and first rib (93).

Procedural Steps

1. Insert the needle attached to a tuberculin syringe into the site. The site of insertion is somewhat different from that advocated for the adult. In addition, the direction in which the needle should be passed is slightly different because of the more horizontal position of the clavicle in the infant than in the adult. The site is the midclavicular region; direct the needle in a straight line between the first rib and the clavicle, 1 to 1.5 cm above the suprasternal notch (70, 93, 156).
2. Aspirate and advance.
3. Remove the syringe, and insert the catheter. Place thumb or index finger over the orifice of the needle. It is often necessary to manipulate the catheter into the superior vena cava, in contrast to the situation in an adult, where the catheter goes in easily (93). This manipulation of the catheter is by backward and forward motion as well as slight rotation, because the catheter tends to proceed into the opposite subclavian or internal jugular vein when being passed. This displacement, in our experience, has been more common in the infant than in the adult. If the catheter bends, then withdraw the needle and catheter together as a single unit.
4. Lower the intravenous bottle to check proper position of catheter in the vein.
5. Secure and dress in the routine fashion.

Subclavian Vein Catheterization in Children

Cannulate the subclavian vein percutaneously via the infraclavicular route in children (93, 100). Place the child supine with restraints on the extremities. Place a cylindrical roll of gauze longitudinally in the infrascapular region to allow the patient's shoulders to fall downward to improve access to the infraclavicular region. Maintain the head in the midline position with 1-inch tape across the forehead. A Trendelenburg position produces venous distention to improve access and prevent air embolism. After positioning the child, prepare the infraclavicular area with povidone–iodine.

Use an 18-gauge Intracath (Argyle Intramedicut). With this needle, puncture the skin in the deltoid–pectoral groove 2 cm from the clavicle so that the catheter is tunneled beneath the skin and enters the subclavian vein at a gradual angle. A topical groove is formed at the point where the clavicle and the first rib cross. At this point, the subclavian vein consistently passes beneath the clavicle and above the first rib. This minimizes inadvertent cannulization of the subclavian artery. Once this medial groove is located, place the Intramedicut needle with the bevel down at the inferior edge of the clavicle. Because the subclavian vein is located immediately beneath the clavicle, continuous gentle aspiration of the catheter is necessary to prevent inadvertent passage of the catheter through the vein (100). The course of the vein becomes parallel to the deltoid–pectoral groove, if the arm is gently pulled downward along the patient's side. The course of the subclavian vein becomes less cephalad with increasing age and weight. In older children, direct the syringe more medially and toward the sternal notch.

Catheterization of the Straight Sinus in the Infant

This procedure was introduced by Kunz (127) and is used only in a dire emergency. It is not advocated as a routine procedure, although in Kunz's article, there was a very low incidence of complications. We cannot find reports testing the procedure elsewhere in the literature. It can be used for emergency transfusions of blood or fluids.

TECHNIQUE

1. Place the infant on one side with the back toward the operator. An assistant

immobilizes the head and body in a position similar to that in which one places an infant when performing a lumbar puncture.

2. Palpate the center of the posterior fontanelle, and prepare the skin.
3. Introduce a 2.5-cm short-bevel, 20- to 22-gauge needle (Angiocath) 3 to 4 mm. Direct the point toward the uppermost part of the forehead in the sagittal plane.[1]
4. Aspirate blood from the straight sinus. For transfusions, place the needle 1 to 1.5 cm below the skin in the straight sinus.
5. Inject blood very carefully with as little pressure as possible and frequently check the proper needle placement. Because the catheter gauge is very small, inject blood slowly rather than administering it by drip, as one would with a 16-gauge catheter.

Saphenous Vein Cutdown at the Ankle in the Infant

For a detailed discussion of this procedure, refer to the adult section on cutdowns. Although the procedure described here is for the saphenous vein at the ankle (the most commonly used site), use the same procedure in other accessible veins, including the basilic and cephalic.

TECHNIQUE

Preparatory Steps

1. Select a catheter. Use a 4-French catheter for most full term newborns. Have other catheters available, and select a catheter one size larger than the appearance of the vein.
2. Immobilize the leg and foot on an armboard.
3. Prepare and drape in the routine fashion.

[1]The coronal plane separates anterior from posterior, the sagittal plane separates right from left, and the transverse plane separates superior from inferior.

Procedural Steps

1. Make a transverse incision 0.5 cm long directly over the site of the vein (221), which lies just superior and anterior to the medial malleolus.
2. With a mosquito forceps, open the wound widely. Wipe the blood out of the field with a swab held in the forceps. With a *scooping motion,* using closed curved hemostat inserted directly anterior to the medial malleolus, lift the entire tissue beneath the skin incision upward onto the closed hemostat. Then dissect this tissue to find the vein (221). Make certain that the vein is not left behind and is accompanied by the saphenous nerve (221).
3. With forceps held under the vein, place two pieces of catgut under the vein (distal and proximal), and ligate the distal end (221).
4. With a mosquito forceps under the vein to stabilize it, make a small transverse incision in the vein with a no. 11 blade or a nick with an Iris scissors.
5. With the bevel of the catheter directed downward (221), insert the catheter. To do this, remove the mosquito from under the vein to relax the proximal end, and tense the distal ligature placed in step 3 distally by gentle traction. The catheter is usually passed easily with this technique (221). An introducer also can be used; insert it into the vein to dilate the puncture site.
6. Tie the proximal stitch around the catheter. We prefer 4-0 chromic to silk (3) in children. Do not tie the catheter too tightly.

Aftercare

Immobilize the catheter with tape after securing it with a suture.

Saphenous Vein Cutdown in the Infant Groin

Although this procedure is infrequently used in the child, it is commonly used in the adult who has had a traumatic arrest and is severely hypovolemic. A very large-bore cannula can be introduced with ease into the saphenous vein, where it enters the femoral vein at the groin. We recommend this site in the child in a similar situation or in any circumstance in which large volumes of fluid must be administered very rapidly. In situations in which a cutdown is needed for other than such a dire circumstance, we prefer the saphenous cutdown at the ankle.

TECHNIQUE

Preparatory Steps

1. Identify the femoral pulse below the inguinal ligament (96).
2. Select the catheter. Even the neonate will admit a 16-gauge catheter at this site. In large children, pass a 12- or 14-gauge catheter. When large volumes of fluid are needed in large children, pass the intravenous tubing itself, approximately 8 gauge.
3. Prepare and drape.

Procedural Steps

1. Make an incision at the upper thigh over the femoral pulse parallel to the groin crease (3). Dissect through the subcutaneous tissue and identify the saphenous vein.

   In the pulseless infant, begin the incision at the point where the scrotal (or labial) fold meets the medial thigh. Extend the incision laterally to approximately the midposition of the inguinal ligament. The saphenous vein lies just beneath the subcutaneous tissue one or two finger breadths lateral to the scrotal or labial fold.
2. Insert the catheter after incising the vein. Make a small nick with an Iris scissors transversely into the vein, and insert the catheter into the femoral vein.
3. Advance the catheter into the inferior vena cava.
4. Pass a suture ligature around the vein at the puncture site proximally and distally; tie the catheter in place proximally; then ligate the distal end of the saphenous vein. Because this is an emergency, do not perform this step until this point in the procedure. If bleeding is a problem, pass and constrict the ligatures as needed for visualization during step 2.

Aftercare

1. Suture the skin wound closed loosely with 4-0 nylon.
2. Secure the catheter in position with tape, and dress the wound with an antibiotic ointment and gauze.
3. Restrain the infant if necessary.

Catheterization of the Femoral Vein in the Infant

Another technique that has reported success for the intravenous access in the infant is catheterization of the femoral vein. This approach has been avoided because of its reported risk of septic arthritis of the hip (138). In 1996, 44 neonates that lacked other sites for venous access were all successfully catheterized by the femoral vein (186). Complications such as catheter-related sepsis, bacteremia, or thrombophlebitis did not occur. In situations in which all other routes of venous access have been exhausted, this technique is a viable option.

TECHNIQUE

Preparatory Steps

1. Prepare and drape the femoral area.
2. Insert a 19-French introducer needle at a point 1 cm below the inguinal crease and 5 mm medial to the femoral artery pulse.

Procedural Steps

1. Insert the needle at a 45-degree angle until venous return is obtained. Do not advance beyond 1 cm.
2. Then insert the femoral vein catheter into a predetermined length. Measure

the predetermined length from the side of insertion to the xiphoid area. The tip of the catheter should lie just below the diaphragm within the inferior vena cava.

Aftercare

1. Coil the remaining external portion of the catheter around the insertion site, and secure to the skin with an adhesive dressing (i.e., Opsite).
2. Confirm the catheter position radiographically.

INTRAOSSEOUS INFUSION IN THE INFANT

It may be difficult to secure an intravenous line in an infant. An approach that can be used for the infusion of drugs, fluid, and blood is to place a needle into the bone marrow space of the tibia of the child. Use standard bone-marrow needles, 18- to 22-gauge short, spinal needles, or standard 14- or 16-gauge hypodermic needles (201). A comparison of four techniques involving the use of different needles has recently been made (213). The spinal and bone marrow needles were the most successful for establishing this line. This is due to the harder nature of these needles and their stylets, which allow easy boring. Hollow bone needles may occasionally be obstructed by small plugs of bone.

Perform the procedure by placing a small sandbag behind the knee for support and cleansing the tibia with antimicrobial solution. The preferred site along the tibia is in the midline of the flat surface of the anterior tibia approximately 1 to 3 cm below the tibial tuberosity. Infiltration of a local anesthetic is preferable but may be omitted when time is of the essence. Direct the needle either inferiorly at approximately 60 degrees or perpendicularly at 90 degrees and advance it until marrow contents are aspirated (Fig. 12.31). Confirm intermedullary placement by the "give" after the needle passes through the cortex and after aspiration of marrow contents and free-flowing fluids after infusion is begun. To obtain free-flow fluids through a line, attach a pressure bag to the intravenous fluids (89, 169).

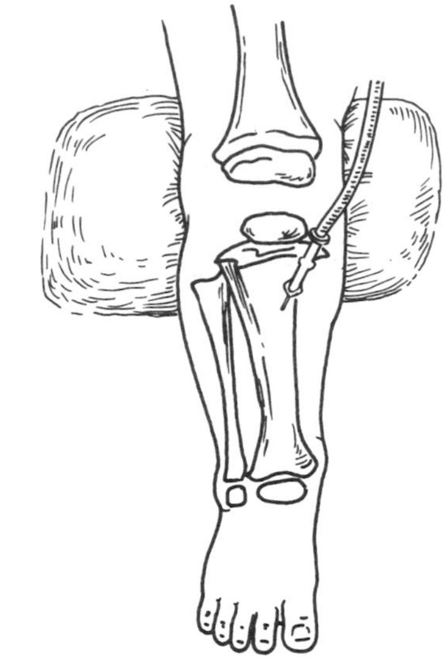

Figure 12.31. The placement of an intraosseous line just below the tibial tuberosity and the flat surface of the tibia of a child. See text for discussion.

Intraosseous infusion is contraindicated in diseases of the bone or ipsilateral fractures of an extremity (71). The most common complications of intraosseous infusion are subcutaneous and subperiosteal infiltration of fluid or leakage from the puncture site (3, 9, 23, 38, 40, 107, 181). Compartment syndrome has been reported, with resultant amputation, after intraosseous infusion (158). Bilateral tibia fractures also were reported in a 3-month-old infant after using this technique (128).

The original concerns for osteomyelitis, local abscesses, and systemic infections after intraosseous infusion have proven unfounded (201). A study of the risk of fat or bone marrow emboli through the lungs after this procedure demonstrated that although fat embolisms can complicate resuscitation, there is no evidence that this technique increases the incidence of such embolisms (166).

Intraosseous infusion can be performed whenever it is difficult to establish an intravenous access in a child or infant. Do not delay obtaining intravenous access in a critically ill or injured child by repeated attempts at central or peripheral line placement. Intraosseous infusion has been proven to be an effective modality for initiating intravenous therapy and providing drugs intravenously (85, 102, 116, 139, 178). Even succinylcholine has been given as a muscle relaxant through the intraosseous line before endotracheally intubating a patient (116).

It is important to point out that one may not be able to aspirate marrow, even though in the proper space. If fluid runs freely and one has checked that one is not in the subcutaneous space, then one can safely assume that one is in the proper location.

Intraosseous Infusion in the Adult

Intraosseous infusion in adults was recently described (107). In 22 adult patients who arrived in cardiac arrest, intraosseous needles were inserted along the medial malleolus, using 13-gauge Kormed–Jamshidi needles. These needles were then connected to standard intravenous tubing with a pressure bag delivering 300 mm Hg to the solution. The result was a flow rate of 5 to 12 mL/min.

With this technique, insert the needle to within 2 cm above the medial malleolus at a 90-degree angle to the tibia in the sagittal plane in the midline, and the more anteriorly placed saphenous vein thus is not compromised. This position is picked because it is a relatively flat location and is easily penetrable. Introduce the needle with a downward pressing and twisting motion, similar to that used for bone marrow biopsy (108). Then connect the needle to standard intravenous tubing. Flow is ascertained by one of the following techniques:

1. Rigid fixation of the needle.
2. Flow under pressure without progressive edema of surrounding tissues.
3. Loss of resistance on entering the bone marrow space.
4. Aspiration of bone marrow contents.

Interestingly, the last method was the least useful for confirming proper placement of the needle.

UMBILICAL VESSEL CATHETERIZATION

Umbilical vessel catheterization is a useful procedure for establishing an intravenous line in a newborn who is in distress. Occasionally the vein is mistaken for an artery, but this is not common. The vein is a single, thin-walled vessel, and there are two smaller, thick-walled arteries adjacent to one another that are usually constricted. The umbilical artery is the preferred vessel (15); venous catheterization also can be used when arterial catheterization is not successful (59, 124). It is usually still possible to insert the catheter for the first time in neonates at 48 to 72 hours old (94, 124); some catheters have been passed successfully up to 10 days after birth. The orifices of the umbilical artery are easily identifiable after 72 hours of age only if the umbilical cord stump is sterile (94). Within a few minutes of birth, the umbilical arteries constrict. This process is delayed with hypoxia and acidosis (124). In newborns who require umbilical artery catheterization for management of cardiorespiratory distress, successful catheterization is almost always possible in the first 15 to 30 minutes of life. The vast majority can be catheterized in the first day of life (124) with relative ease.

Catheterization can be performed by one person. Unless the infant is limp or the procedure is done as an extreme emergency, restrain the baby loosely before the procedure.

Because of obstructions, the catheter will not advance beyond 2 cm, or 6 to 8 cm, in 10% of cases. If this does pose a problem, then proceed to another vessel (38).

INDICATIONS

1. Administration of fluids and blood (94, 124) in a newborn infant.
2. Repeated arterial blood pH and gas determinations (187). Repeated specimens for blood gas analysis can be obtained by direct arterial puncture. With this procedure, however, peripheral vasoconstriction in the ill infant may result in inaccurate measurements (94). If the child cries during the procedure, this lowers the P_aCO_2 (94). It is not practical to obtain repeated samples by percutaneous puncture, so we prefer sampling of arterial blood through the umbilical artery catheter (94, 124).

   Try to keep the aortic PO_2 between 55 and 70 mm Hg. Excessively high O_2 tensions may injure the retina, resulting in retrolental fibroplasia (124). If an arterial catheter cannot be placed, then, in the healthy infant, determine the central venous pH, because it is usually 0.02 to 0.03 pH units lower than arterial values. Central venous PCO_2 is 5 to 6 mm Hg higher than respective arterial values (124). These values do not hold for blood from the portal system. The O_2 tensions in venous blood are lower, but do not correlate well with corresponding arterial samples. Therefore, venous samples cannot be used to guide oxygen therapy (124).

   Samples should not be obtained while the infant is straining or crying. The technique for obtaining a sample is as follows (124):

   a. There should be a constant inspired O_2 level.
   b. The infant should not be crying.
   c. Remove flushing fluid from catheter so it does not contaminate the specimen. Withdraw a volume equal to 3 times the capacity of the catheter system (usually 0.2 mL). A 0.4-mL sample should be removed if withdrawn from the stopcock port.
   d. Withdraw a sample in a heparinized syringe (see Arterial Puncture, later).
   e. Administer alkali (124). We recommend an arterial, not a venous, route to administer bicarbonate, because bicarbonate is diluted by the aorta and also by capillary vessels. Bicarbonate administered in a vein, especially if the catheter is in a portal vessel, decreases blood flow, and thrombosis and phlebitis may develop (124). If the catheter tip is in the inferior vena cava or atrium, alkali may irritate the sinoatrial node and cause cardiac arrhythmias.
3. Measure blood volume and cardiac output (124).
4. Perform exchange transfusion (124, 187) through an umbilical venous or arterial catheter or both, with the venous catheter tip placed in the portal circulation. Attempt to pass the catheter through the ductus venosus and into the inferior vena cava because citrated blood is alkalotic and may produce hypokalemia and chelate calcium, causing hypocalcemia. Rapid infusion of blood into the inferior vena cava can cause arrhythmias. Buffer the blood before administration. The best way to perform exchange transfusion is with two catheters that are of the end-hole type (hole at the end rather than on the side of the catheter); use the venous catheter for transfusion and the arterial catheter to withdraw blood samples for pH and blood gas determination (124). In placing a catheter from the umbilical vein to the inferior vena cava, some authors (124) advised an end-hole catheter so that suction during exchange transfusion does not perforate the very thin-walled inferior vena cava.

EQUIPMENT

Kitterman et al. (124) stated that the ideal catheter should have the following characteristics:

1. It should be flexible and not kink as it follows the curves of the vessels.
2. It should be made of nonwettable material so clots do not form on its surface.
3. The single end-hole variety is preferred to avoid clotting in the tip, which is a problem with the side-hole catheters.
4. It should be radiopaque.
5. Its capacity should be small so that only small amounts of blood need be withdrawn before samples are taken. The best catheter at present is the Argyle umbilical artery catheter, 3.5 French for infants less than 1.5 kg and 5 French for larger infants.

Circumcision drape with 2 × 2-inch hole in center
Four small towels
Straight Iris scissors
Large sharp scissors
Two mosquito forceps
Two curved eye-dressing forceps
Two umbilical cord tape ties
Two small needle holders
Gauze sponges
Syringes (2 or 5 mL)
No. 18 needle (blunt)
Three-way stopcock
3-0 silk on atraumatic noncutting needle
Medicine glass (a heparin solution is made by adding 250 units of heparin to a 250-mL bottle of isotonic saline to fill the medicine glass)

TECHNIQUE

Preparatory Steps

1. Keep the infant warm in an incubator (94, 187). Place babies on an ambient warmer with supplemental oxygen because it is hard to maintain the sufficiently high oxygen tension in the incubator (90). Place infants under a radiant heat source when not in an incubator (187).
2. Prepare the infant and catheter. Rinse the gloves with sterile water to remove talcum powder (124). This avoids introduction of talcum into the vessel. To facilitate sampling, fill the catheter with a heparinized solution with a concentration of 0.3 U/mL. This concentration prevents thrombus formation (59, 187). First empty gastric contents with a pediatric feeding tube to avoid vomiting and aspiration during the procedure. In a newborn infant, the aspiration of meconium from the stomach is a serious problem, leading to severe pneumonitis (187).

   Attach a three-way stopcock to the catheter filled with heparinized saline (124).
3. Prepare the umbilical cord with povidone–iodine followed by alcohol to prevent any iodine burns (59, 94, 124, 203). Drape with a circumcision drape with a hole cut out of the center.
4. Sharply transect the cord 0.5 to 1 cm from the abdominal wall after antiseptic preparation (59, 94, 124, 187, 203). Identify the vessel to be catheterized, and carefully dilate the lumen (187) with the tip of a mosquito forceps.

NOTE

When blotting the cut surface, one will see a single, large, thin-walled oval vein and two smaller, thick-walled arteries that are rounded. After birth, the arteries constrict to the size of a pinpoint. They can be dilated by gently inserting the closed tip of a small curved Iris forceps into the lumen (59, 124). The forceps can be opened to dilate the artery farther (203).

Hold the cord stump upright with 2 × 2-inch gauze. Tie either a cord ligature or preferably umbilical tape loosely around the base of the umbilical cord to prevent brisk arterial bleeding or venous oozing (94). Tie it loosely with a single knot (124), but tight enough to prevent bleeding during the procedure. Loosen the knot later if needed to permit passage of the cannula.

Procedural Steps

1. Insert catheter into umbilical artery or vein (Fig. 12.32): Gently thread a 3.5- or 5-French catheter. Once within the arterial orifice, advance the catheter (94).

NOTE

Obstruction can occur at two points: at 1 to 2 cm where the vessels suddenly course downward at the level of the anterior abdominal wall and at 5 to 6 cm at the level of the urinary bladder (124), where the umbilical artery may go into spasm as it enters the iliac vessel. The first site of obstruction often can be overcome by pulling the stump upward toward the baby's head (94, 203). The second site of obstruction may be overcome with 30 to 60 seconds of gentle steady pressure. Do not repeatedly attempt to thread the catheter past the point of obstruction. At 6 to 10 cm, blood easily can be withdrawn from the catheter (94). If unsuccessful at relieving the obstruction, do the following:

a. Fill the tip of the catheter with 0.1 to 0.2 mL of sterile 2% lidocaine without epinephrine.
b. Reinsert to the point of obstruction.
c. Inject the lidocaine. Do not try to pass the catheter; wait 1 to 2 minutes for the artery to relax, and then advance (124).
d. If this fails, use the other umbilical artery.

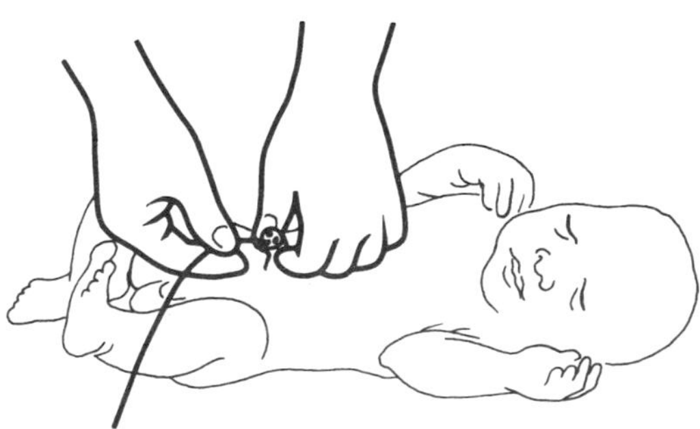

Figure 12.32. Umbilical artery catheterization. In the emergency center, perform this procedure only in the newborn infant who requires neonatal resuscitation. See text for discussion.

2. Position the catheter tip. Place the umbilical artery catheter in the aorta (59, 187). Advance the catheter until approximately 2 cm past the point where blood is obtained (124). Here the tip is usually at the aortic bifurcation. Radiographs should be obtained in the anteroposterior and lateral projections to check the position of the catheter (chest and abdominal films). Place it with tip at T7–T8. It has been found that with the tip at this level, there is half the complication rate as with catheter tip at L3–L4 (155).

   When the umbilical vein catheter is passed, it should go through the ductus venosus and into the inferior vena cava to the level of the right atrium (59, 124, 203), or, preferably, it should remain in the inferior vena cava.

NOTE

Table 12.2 will help guide the distance estimated for the size of the infant (94).

   After positioning the catheter, attach a three-way stopcock and withdraw blood and return the sample to the infant.

3. Fix the catheter and connect. With a purse-string suture of fine silk, suture

Table 12.2.
Distance Catheter Must Be Inserted to Reach the Diaphragm in a Neonate

Weight of neonate (g)	Distance (cm)
1,000	8–10
1,000–1,500	10–11
1,500–2,000	10–12
2,000–2,500	12–13
2,500+	14–15

the catheter in position. Tape it to the abdomen (Fig. 12.33) (94, 187). Place antibiotic ointment at the junction of the catheter and the umbilical cord (187, 203).

NOTE

The catheter volume is 0.2 mL. Each time a sample is drawn, flush with 0.3 mL heparinized saline (0.3 U/mL) (94). This is not necessary with constant infusion, which flushes the catheter (94).

Connect to infusion pump. If a Harvard constant infusion pump is not available (59), then the solution infused should be at a pressure sufficient to overcome arterial pressure (187), when the umbilical artery is used.

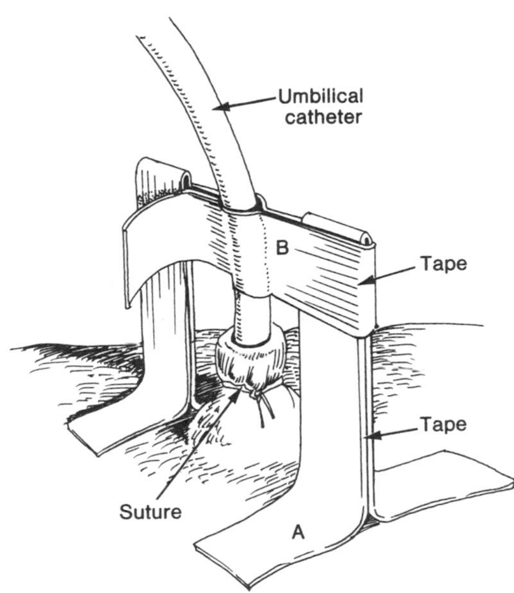

Figure 12.33. A method for securing an umbilical catheter to the abdomen. *A:* Fold a strip of adhesive tape back over itself in the middle. Two strips of the folded tape are then secured on either side of the infant's umbilicus. *B:* While holding the catheter in place, apply two strips of tape on either side of the catheter. This secures the catheter in place. In addition, secure the catheter with a suture placed around the umbilical cord as shown.

NOTE

Keep the catheter free of blood to prevent formation of clots (124). Each time blood is withdrawn from the catheter, flush with enough heparinized saline (3 times the capacity of the catheter) to clear the blood. Flush the catheter every hour when a constant infusion is not used. If using a continuous infusion, add 1 unit of heparin per milliliter of parenteral fluid.

NOTE

Treat all infants with umbilical catheters with penicillin, 50,000 U/kg/day, and with kanamycin, 5 mg/kg/day, intramuscularly for the duration of catheterization plus an additional 48 hours (203).

4. Remove the catheter slowly over 30 to 90 seconds. Tie the purse-string suture (187, 203), which allows the vessel to constrict and minimizes bleeding.

Complications

The mortality associated with exchange transfusion through umbilical veins is less than 1% in major centers (187). Umbilical artery catheters carry an overall complication rate of 10%, according to some authors (187). The use of umbilical venous catheters was associated with a twofold increase in the overall complication rate, as compared with that of umbilical arterial catheters, and a fourfold increase in pathologic changes demonstrated at necropsy (203). At autopsy, thrombi were noted in 6% of those with umbilical artery catheters and in 44% of those with umbilical venous catheters. The incidence of complications with umbilical artery catheters is related to the length of time the catheters are left in place, whereas the complications associated with umbilical venous catheters are unrelated to length of time the catheters are in place (203). Although the ease of placement of venous catheters has resulted in their common use, the greater complication rate should result in reserving their use to those cases in which the arterial route has proved impossible and catheterization is needed (203).

1. **Vasospasm.** Vasospasm of the umbilical artery (187) and blanching of an extremity occur in infants. Occasionally in infants, the leg will blanch during the procedure, and this is attributed to vasospasm (124). Leg blanching is relatively frequent with the umbilical artery cannulation (94).
2. **Loss of pulse and development of gangrene.** This complication has occurred in some infants after umbilical artery catheterization (59, 124, 187, 220), leading some authors to recommend its use only in those patients in whom other routes cannot be used.
3. **Extravascular catheter placement.** Perforation of the colon has been reported (35). Thus radiographs are needed to exclude pneumoperitoneum and to determine catheter placement. It is rare for this to occur with catheters that have rounded tips; thus do not use catheters with sharp, beveled tips (124). Large-bowel perforation can occur (59, 124, 187). In addition, position venous catheters in the inferior vena cava and not in the portal system through the ductus venosus.
4. **Cardiac arrhythmias** (187). A short PR interval without Wolf–Parkinson–White syndrome has been reported; bigeminy and prolonged sinus bradycardia also have been observed (59).
5. **Thrombosis and phlebitis** (187). The most commonly reported complication of umbilical vessel catheterization is thrombosis (124). The incidence of thrombosis varies from 3% to 5% at autopsy (124). In one study, 12.5% of patients who came to autopsy with umbilical catheters had thrombosis (220). These thrombi vary from small fibrin thrombi to thrombi of the renal arteries or aorta (124). Umbilical venous catheter thrombosis varies from 3% to 33%, as determined by autopsy or clinical examination (64, 220). Portal vein thrombosis may occur as a result of injection of hypertonic solutions (124) into the portal vein. Hypertonic dextrose, bicarbonate, and trihydroxymethylaminomethane (THAM) all can cause thrombosis (124). Portal vein thrombosis occurs more commonly when the venous catheter tip is in the portal system itself (12, 93, 220).

Necrotizing phlebitis and aortitis also have been reported (38). If the catheter is used for blood transfusion, then there also is an increased incidence of thrombosis (38). Hepatic necrosis secondary to the administration of undiluted bicarbonate also can occur (220). In 16% of infants of diabetic mothers, thrombosis develops with umbilical catheters (164). Neonatal hypertension secondary to renal infarct has been reported (19). Transverse myelitis and paraplegia secondary to spinal artery infarct have been reported from umbilical vessel catheterization (12). For venous catheters, no correlation exists between the length of time the catheter is in place and thrombosis (86). With umbilical artery cannulation, the risk of thrombosis is present almost exclusively during the first 12 hours, with the highest risk being shortly after catheterization.

To prevent thrombi, keep the catheter size small and the duration of catheterization and length of the catheter as short as possible. Avoid manipulating the catheter (187). Infuse hypertonic solutions into large vessels with a rapid flow rate (124) to reduce the risk of thrombosis in vessels such as the aorta or inferior vena cava. Reduce the rate of infusion with bicarbonate to 2 mEq/kg/min (124). If a catheter is clotted and the clot cannot be removed, then a new catheter should be inserted and may be inserted into the same artery (38).

6. **Embolism.** Catheters in the umbilical vessels may cause emboli from clots formed on the catheters or from air injected through the catheter tip (124). Emboli from the umbilical artery are lodged at the tip of the lower abdominal aorta and will go to the lower extremity, with infarction occurring most commonly in the toes. If infarction occurs, remove the catheter. Emboli from venous catheters are lodged in the portal system. If the catheter is passed through the ductus venosus, the emboli infarct lung tissue (124, 220). In the presence of a patent foramen ovale or a patent ductus arteriosus, venous emboli may be widely disseminated throughout the systemic circulation (124).

   For air embolism to occur in the arterial catheter, the air must be injected at a higher pressure than that of the systemic circulation (124). Venous air embolism can occur during inspiration, when the chest develops a more negative intrathoracic pressure, and can "suck" not only the fluid in the catheter but also air into vessels in the chest. When this complication occurs in the large vessels, it can be fatal (124). Thus never open the umbilical veins to atmospheric pressure (see Complications discussion under Infraclavicular Subclavian Vein Cannulation, earlier).
7. **Hemorrhage.** Umbilical artery catheters in the aorta have a constant risk of hemorrhage and must be observed for this complication (59, 94, 124, 220). Observe the catheter for disconnection, which may produce exsanguination. The infant may pull or kick the catheter and, to prevent this, should be restrained. If bleeding is significant, restore volume as soon as possible (124).
8. **Infection.** The catheter is a frequent source of infection, especially in infants who have received bicarbonate via the catheter (124). Gram-negative bacteremia may occur in some infants (59). Omphalitis is not uncommon (94). The infection rate is higher with umbilical vein than with umbilical artery cannulation (15). There is no difference in the infection rate with the administration of antibiotics (220); therefore, some authors do not support the prophylactic administration of antibiotics. There is reportedly a lower incidence of cord colonization with pathogens in infants receiving systemic antibiotics (15).

   To decrease the risk of infection, change umbilical dressing daily, and apply an antibiotic ointment. Remove the catheter as soon as possible and adhere to aseptic technique during handling (15).

SPECIAL PROCEDURES RELATED TO INTRAVENOUS CANNULATION

Central Venous Pressure Monitoring

CVP monitoring is a simple method of assessing the status of blood volume. Although it has considerable value in acutely ill patients for regulation of fluid or blood replacement, one must be aware of its shortcomings (198). Inaccurate measurements often are obtained by aberrant lodging of the venous catheter tip in addition to other problems (see Technique, later). Radiographic identification of the location of the catheter tip is essential to the elimination of some of these problems (84, 206). Patients with hypovolemia may have an elevated CVP, particularly when the cause of the hypovolemia is concomitant with pulmonary contusion or other injuries that elevate the CVP (76). The important parameter in measuring the CVP is not the isolated value per se, but the response to a sudden fluid infusion. The response of CVP is a more reliable indicator of the patient's volume status than the actual CVP. If, after rapidly infusing 200 to

300 mL of crystalloid, one notes no change or a decrease in CVP, one can safely assume the patient is volume depleted.

INDICATIONS

When a Swan–Ganz catheter is available and the skill and equipment necessary for insertion are at hand, this catheter is the preferred method to monitor CVP.

1. Sepsis.
2. Management of shock syndromes.

NOTE

More specifically, if a hypotensive patient does not respond to a volume infusion or responds, but subsequently becomes hypotensive again, then CVP measurements are important. In addition, CVP monitoring is useful in patients who are hypotensive but in whom volume infusion is prohibitive (e.g., patients with renal failure or congestive heart failure). In patients with probable hypovolemia, initially attempt to observe neck vein distention carefully and obviate CVP monitoring, provided that the neck veins are flat and easily visualized.

---

3. Massive hemorrhage.
4. Severe blunt chest trauma.
5. Evaluation of cardiac tamponade.

TECHNIQUE

The technique presented here is that of obtaining a CVP reading after a catheter has been inserted into the superior vena cava by any of the routes discussed in the chapter.

1. Place the patient in a supine position.
2. Place the zero point of the manometer in the midaxillary line at the fourth intercostal space. Hold the column vertically. Mark this point with a skin pen so that an accurate and reproducible measurement can be subsequently obtained for comparisons (Fig. 12.34).

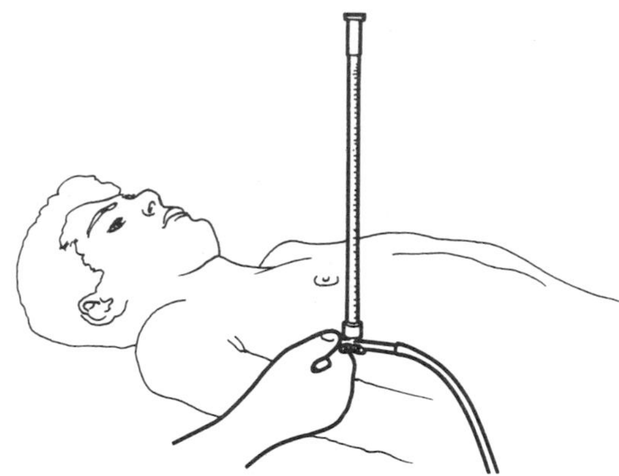

Figure 12.34. Place the zero point of the manometer at the midaxillary line of the fourth intercostal space. This provides more accurate central venous pressure readings.

3. Fill the manometer with intravenous fluid by opening the three-way stopcock to the intravenous solution. Remove all air bubbles from the tubing and manometer.
4. Open the three-way stopcock to the patient so that the channel that is open is that between the patient and the fluid-filled manometer.
5. Observe for respiratory fluctuations in the column of fluid in the manometer. With a patent channel (and a properly positioned catheter tip), the fluid level should rise with expiration and fall with inspiration. There is generally a 2.5-cm variance between the inspiratory and expiratory levels. A Valsalva maneuver also will increase the fluid level in the column.
6. Measure the CVP reading, and then open the line from the patient to the intravenous bottle so that a clot does not form in the catheter.

Transvenous Cardiac Pacemaker

Electrical pacing of the heart can be instituted rapidly at the bedside with the introduction of a transvenous electrode by a percutaneous route. Temporary cardiac pacemakers have been used for some time in the management of heart block and bradycardia associated with low cardiac output (180). Fluoroscopic control, although optimal, is generally not available in emergency centers, and a number of authors have documented excellent results with bedside cardiac pacing (13, 114, 153, 180). In the past, prolonged unsuccessful catheter insertion was attributed to soft pliable catheters and indirect approaches to the central venous system. A number of catheters have been used; these can be divided into three types: unipolar, bipolar, and dipolar. Although some authors reported a high success rate with unipolar electrodes (180), the latter two types are the best for use in the emergency center (194), because unipolar catheters require direct endocardial contact, which may be difficult to achieve. The Elecath semifloating bipolar pacemaker catheter has resulted in a very high percentage of successful insertions (13, 122, 180).

Three techniques have been described for placement of percutaneous transvenous pacemakers into the right ventricle: fluoroscopic positioning, electrocardiographic positioning, and blind positioning. Transfer of the severely ill patient to another unit may be hazardous, and bedside cardiac pacing is often preferred, making electrocardiographic and blind positioning the only two methods of importance to the emergency physician, and therefore, the only two that are discussed here. Electrocardiographic positioning is the preferred technique; however, it requires that cardiac activity be present. It is especially useful for the patient who is in complete heart block with bradycardia after an anterior myocardial infarction. In patients without spontaneous cardiac action, use the blind technique.

A number of venous routes have been advocated by various authors, each having their favorite site, including the antecubital vein (180, 183), external jugular vein (194), femoral vein (36, 145, 194), and subclavian and internal jugular veins (153, 180). Although any of these approaches can be used to gain access to the right atrium and thence to the ventricle, it would appear that three sites offer the advantages of ease of access and rapidity with which the veins can be cannulated (36, 39, 122, 145, 153, 180, 183, 194). These sites, preferred by us, are the *right internal jugular vein, left subclavian vein* and either femoral vein. The right internal jugular vein proceeds directly into the superior vena cava. The left subclavian vein is preferred to the right subclavian vein, because the natural curve of the catheter follows that of the left subclavian vein, permitting entrance into the superior vena cava more easily than with the right, where the catheter must make a sharper bend. When introducing the electrode using the blind technique for positioning, by far the most rapid and preferred approach is through the femoral vein (36, 145, 194). In one study involving 31 patients, the catheter could be introduced via the femoral vein in less than 30 seconds, and cardiac pacing initiated in 1 to 3 minutes (145).

INDICATIONS FOR PACEMAKER IN THE EMERGENCY CENTER

Asystole or bradycardia (<60 beats/min) with altered hemodynamic state or ventricular irritability (escape beats) that is unresponsive to atropine or isoproterenol (58, 114, 153). In the presence of myocardial infarction, isoproterenol is contraindicated for bradycardia, but not for asystole.

NOTE

In patients who enter the coronary care unit with a myocardial infarction, 6% to 8% will develop the complication of heart block, with 85% of such cases occurring in the first 48 hours (109).

EQUIPMENT

Monitor and ECG machine
Skin preparation
Alligator clips and connecting wire
Four towels
Towel clips
Gloves
Anesthetic prep
Elecath catheter (packaged in a kit) or any semifloating bipolar catheter. For a femoral route, a 100-cm long no. 5 bipolar catheter in which the distal 10 cm is in a "J" configuration is recommended.
Skin suture
Dressing
14-gauge Angiocath or Cordis catheter

ELECTROCARDIOGRAPHIC POSITIONING TECHNIQUE

Preparatory Steps

1. Select the catheter. The 4-French Elecath semifloating catheter, which is packaged in a kit and fits through a 14-gauge needle, yields the best results with either technique and is our preferred electrode catheter for cardiac pacing (122, 180, 183, 194). The catheter is 100 cm long and is bipolar, with two platinum ring electrodes at the distal tip, separated 1.5 cm by a balloon (93).

   For the femoral approach, the somewhat different 5-French bipolar catheter in which the distal 8 to 10 cm is in a "J" configuration is preferred (145).
2. Select the site. The basilic vein in the upper extremity, cannulated through a cutdown approach, was more commonly used in the past (180), but most authors do not recommend it (36, 153). There is a high frequency of dislocation of the electrode tip when the extremity is raised over the patient's head. There is as much as 2.5 cm displacement of the electrode tip from the right ventricular wall with such motions as elevation of the arm (36, 153). The subclavian and internal jugular venous routes are commonly recommended (153, 180). We recommend that the right internal jugular vein be used because this is a direct route into the superior vena cava (73). When the subclavian vein route is selected, we prefer the left because the catheter follows a natural curve, and cannulation into the superior vena cava is more easily achieved when this side is used (153). The femoral vein is less commonly used than either of these routes; however, many authors believe that it is the preferred route for emergency pacing because of the rapidity and success of the procedure, as discussed earlier. Our preferred approach is the right internal jugular vein initially; if rapid catheterization is not achieved, we recommend the femoral vein route.
3. Position the patient.

   Internal jugular or subclavian site: Place the patient in 10 to 20 degrees of Trendelenburg. Place a roll under the shoulders. Turn the patient's head to the opposite side of the entrance site.

   Femoral vein site: Place the patient supine.
4. Prepare and drape the patient.

Procedural Steps

1. Cannulate the vein. Cannulation of the vein is performed in the routine fashion, as discussed in other sections of this chapter. Use a 14-gauge Angiocath or a Cordis catheter.
2. Introduce the electrode catheter and position by ECG (in the patient with cardiac activity):

   Electrocardiographic positioning (13, 180, 183): Attach the limb leads of the ECG to the patient in the routine fashion. Attach the precordial lead (V_1) to the distal end of the electrode catheter, and record the electrical activity on the V lead as the catheter is advanced. Attach the catheter to the precordial V lead by the use of an alligator clamp. The ECG recorded from this electrode tip localizes the position of the electrode tip (Fig. 12.35).

As the catheter is passed, one will see a recording similar to that seen normally in AvR. Advance the catheter into the right atrium, where the recording will show a large negative P wave on the precordial lead. At this point, inflate the balloon, which then will "float" the catheter into other locations. Advance the catheter across the tricuspid valve into the right ventricle. If an obstruction is met, counterclockwise rotation and forward–backward motion help pass the catheter across the tricuspid valve. When the catheter tip is in the right ventricle, one will notice a wide QRS pattern of left bundle branch block.

Deflate the balloon. Advance 3–5 cm until premature beats or ST elevation in the intracardiac V lead is noted. This finding indicates firm contact with the right ventricular endocardial surface. With the J-shaped catheter, pull it back against the endocardial surface. One is now ready for pacing.

At this point, connect the pulse generator; adequate positioning can be definitely ascertained before connecting a pulse generator, if a current of injury is noted on the ECG.

Femoral approach (145): Introduce the catheter 15 cm into the vein. Inflate the balloon. Connect the distal terminal of the electrode to the V lead of the ECG, and attach the limb leads to the patient in the routine fashion. Float the electrode tip into the right ventricle. Entrance into the right ventricle and across the tricuspid is signaled by abrupt appearance of large negative intraventricular complexes, as noted earlier.

3. Establish pacing. Connect the catheter to the generator.

   Bipolar: Connect the distal end to the negative terminal, and the proximal end to the positive terminal.

   Unipolar: Connect the subcutaneous needle to the positive terminal electrode and then to the negative terminal.

   Pacing generator settings: Demand mode; rate of 70 beats/min; 2.5- to 6-mA output until pacing established.

   Turn generator on. Slowly increase milliamperage output until generator shows pacing spikes followed by a wide QRS. Decrease generator output to threshold (where pacing ceases), and then resume pacing at 2 mA above threshold.

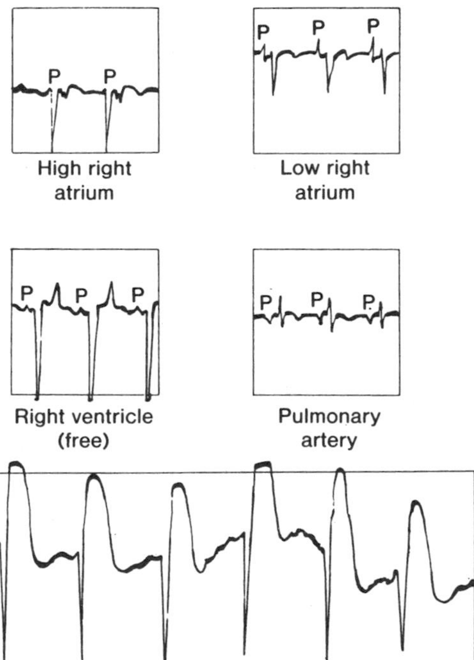

Figure 12.35. ECG tracings taken from the precordial lead attached to the pacemaker catheter at various levels in the heart.

AXIOM

Good positioning is indicated in part when the pacing threshold is less than 1.5 mA (36, 180). The 12-lead ECG should show a pattern during pacing. If a right bundle branch block is demonstrated, then the electrode is positioned in the pulmonary outflow tract or in the left ventricle because of septal perforation by the electrode.

NOTE

An alternative method of establishing pacing is to turn the pacemaker generator to maximal output (mA) and, once pacing is established, then to decrease the output slowly.

Aftercare

1. Secure the catheter. Place two loops of the catheter next to the side of the puncture site, and suture catheter in place.
2. Obtain anteroposterior and lateral chest films. An overpenetrated radiograph may be helpful to visualize the electrode wire.
3. Ask the patient with a femoral catheter to cough, breathe deeply, or shift position to be certain the catheter is well lodged.

BLIND POSITIONING TECHNIQUE

1. Slide the catheter into the superior vena cava, via the right internal jugular vein.
2. Attach the external end of the pacemaker catheter to the generator.
3. Set the generator to maximal output (mA), and a rate of 70 beats/min.
4. Turn the generator on.
5. Advance the catheter until ventricular pacing occurs.
6. Confirm position by anteroposterior and lateral chest radiographs.

FEMORAL APPROACH (PREFERRED) (146)

The usual routes for blind passage of a pacing catheter have many well-known disadvantages. The technique indicated here for the insertion of a "flow-directed" bipolar pacing catheter through the femoral vein is optimal. A 5-French catheter is used with a balloon located between the two electrodes, which are 1 cm apart and in which the distal 8 cm of the catheter is preformed into a J configuration. A stiffer wire with a balloon can be used when there is no cardiac activity, rather than a flow-directed catheter. The technique is similar to that indicated in the section on insertion through the femoral route under Electrocardiographic Positioning Technique, earlier. The inverted J-shaped tip predisposes to attainment of a stable position in the right ventricular apex.

COMPLICATIONS

1. **Myocardial perforation.** This occurs at the free wall of the right ventricle or atrium with hemorrhagic pericarditis or pericardial tamponade as a consequence. This complication may be secondary to excessive advance of a stiff electrode. One will note a transient pericardial rub with the catheter tip rubbing against the epicardial surface. In one case, a diaphragmatic twitching was noted with perforation (13).

   No *therapy* is generally needed, other than the withdrawal of the catheter. Pericardial tamponade secondary to continued hemorrhage is unusual.
2. **Catheter dislodgement or excessive loops in the catheter.** Frequently there is failure to sense or detect an increase in the pacing threshold. This dislodgment or looping occurs as a result of the catheter being inadequately anchored. This may cause arrhythmias, with the paced beats having the same configuration as the ectopic beats, because they are produced by the same section of myocardium (79, 211). Some catheter arrhythmias produced by the dislodged catheter will be

bizarre and uninterpretable, and others will occur during inspiration only (79, 211). Ventricular bigeminy may occur, but the coupling interval may vary. Even high doses of antiarrhythmics will be ineffective (79, 211). Atrial arrhythmias also may occur (136, 194). With excessive loops, each atrial systole thrusts the catheter tip against the myocardium, causing aberrant beats (136, 194). The beats will be preceded by P waves, and occasionally there may be fusion beats (136, 194).

The *treatment* is to remove or reposition the catheter (79, 211). When redundant loops are the problem, withdraw the loops carefully.

3. **Perforation of the interventricular septum or ventricular wall.**

   Septum: This results in the catheter tip's being displaced into the left ventricle. There are a number of clues to this occurrence:

   a. The pacer shows a change from a left to a right bundle branch block pattern (197).
   b. The chest radiograph shows the catheter tip in the left ventricle (197).
   c. There is an increase in the pacing threshold.

   Ventricular wall: In one study, when the right ventricle was perforated without tamponade, the patients had no signs of perforation (77). It was discovered incidentally at thoracotomy. In other cases, the only manifestation was failure to capture (77).

4. **Movement of the catheter tip** across the tricuspid into the hepatic vein, inferior vena cava, or coronary sinus with resultant loss of positioning for optimal pacing.
5. **Failure to obtain capture or sense the QRS complex.** This may occur as a consequence of a massive myocardial infarction, extreme electrolyte imbalance, hypoxemia, low oxygen transport, or a faulty generator. This complication is seen frequently (45% of cases) (77), especially in cardiac arrest. It was successfully managed in one third of cases by repositioning of the catheter tip, replacement of the generator, catheter removal and replacement, tightening of the electrode connections, or adjusting the amperage (77). In pacemaker malfunctioning, 75% of episodes occur in the first 24 hours (77).
6. **Phlebitis.** This complication may occur at the catheter puncture site. The treatment is warm soaks and antibacterial cream applied to the site. If dressings are changed frequently, the catheter may remain in place 1 to 2 weeks.
7. **Arrhythmias.** Ventricular fibrillation or ventricular tachycardia may occur (77, 79, 123, 211). These arrhythmias may occur during insertion, making the diagnosis easy, or may occur after insertion. There is 6% incidence of catheter-associated arrhythmias (123, 194, 211), and the emergency physician should have a defibrillator immediately available.
8. **Diaphragmatic pacing.** This complication is caused by faulty insulation or myocardial perforation.
9. **Muscle spasm.** Muscle spasm results from faulty insulation and stimulation of muscles by electrical current. The antebrachial site of pacemaker insertion could lead to muscle contractions at the same rate as the setting on the pacemaker impulse generator. To diagnose this entity, vary the pacing rate on the generator to see if the muscle contractions will vary in a like manner.

Transthoracic Cardiac Pacemaker

This is not the preferred approach for placement of a pacemaker. It is used only in emergencies. Transthoracic pacemakers have been used most frequently in the emergency center in patients who have had a cardiac arrest and are in asystole. One must discontinue cardiopulmonary resuscitation during insertion of the catheter; thus the procedure should be done rapidly. The femoral route offers quick access into the heart, even in the patient who has had a cardiac arrest, without having to stop cardiopulmonary resuscitation; however, the transthoracic approach is more reliable, and one is more certain of accurate placement in the patient with cardiopulmonary arrest. Tintinalli and White (208) reported that in brady-asystolic arrest, ultimate outcome was unaffected by transthoracic pacing despite 40% of patients having good capture.

INDICATIONS

1. Cardiac arrest in which the transvenous approach is not feasible either because of inability to pass a central catheter or a lack of skill or equipment.
2. Unsuccessful transvenous approach and existence of an emergency situation in a deteriorating patient (see Indications and Transvenous Approach).

EQUIPMENT

Anesthetic prep
Skin prep
Transthoracic pacemaker kit
6-inch, no. 18 spinal needle with obturator
Monitor and ECG

TECHNIQUE

Preparatory Steps

1. Monitor the patient.
2. Prepare the left chest over the fourth intercostal space or the area around the xiphoid process (should be done quickly in the patient in cardiopulmonary arrest).
3. Anesthetize area if indicated.

Procedural Steps

1. One may use the subxiphoid approach; this is discussed in more detail in Chapter 4, Cardiothoracic Procedures.

   Alternatively, introduce a 6-inch, no. 18 spinal needle with obturator into the fourth intercostal space at the region of the apical impulse. Aim the needle toward the tip of the right scapula.
2. Remove the obturator and attach a syringe. A brisk flow of blood indicates entrance into the ventricle.
3. Pass a bipolar electrode through the needle.
4. Attach to the pacing unit. The lead marked distal is attached to the negative pole and the proximal lead to the positive pacing unit.
5. Set the current at 1.5 mA, and observe for ECG capture. Increase the intensity of the current until capture occurs.

Aftercare

Suture the catheter in place.

COMPLICATIONS

1. **Pericardial hemorrhage and tamponade** results from cardiac injury or injury to the coronary arteries. This is a very serious complication, and there is no method of preventing it, because of the "blind" technique of insertion.
2. **Arrhythmias.**

Swan–Ganz Catheterization of the Pulmonary Artery

This procedure is commonplace in intensive care units. It may be useful in the emergency center, when, because of circumstances beyond the physician's control, the patient may have a prolonged stay in the emergency center or in a "holding unit." The Swan–Ganz catheter is a triple-lumen tube, with one lumen at the tip for pulmonary artery pressure and pulmonary artery blood sampling, one 30 cm farther back for CVP and central venous blood sampling, and one for inflating and deflating the balloon that has a thermistor at the tip. This catheter measures pulmonary artery pressure (PAP), pulmonary capillary wedge pressure (PCWP), right ventricular pressure (RVP), right atrial pressure (RAP), CVP, and cardiac output by using a thermal dilution technique. The PCWP correlates well with left atrial pressure, when PCWP is <15 mm Hg or positive end expiratory pressure is <10 cm of water.

The cardiac output usually is measured by a transducer after 0°C to 4°C water is injected into the central venous port rapidly. The temperature of the blood as it reaches the thermistor correlates with cardiac output and is computed and usually provided as a digital value on ancillary equipment. The measurement of the pulmonary artery wedge pressure and cardiac output is useful in patients who have hypotension and subclinical, chronic, or acute congestive heart failure or renal failure, in whom one wishes to administer large volumes of fluids (e.g., the patient who is hypovolemic after acute trauma). It also is useful in the patient who is in shock of undetermined etiology, and in monitoring the volume status and effects of therapy in patients with cardiogenic shock (7, 34, 74, 190, 199, 202). Several excellent articles give a detailed discussion of Swan–Ganz catheters (30, 115, 199, 202).

INDICATIONS

1. Measurement of pulmonary artery wedge pressure.
2. Measurement of cardiac output.

EQUIPMENT

Skin prep
Anesthetic prep
Four towels
Towel clips
Setup for subclavian or internal jugular vein cannulation with a 16-gauge Angiocath and guidewire
Balloon flotation catheter kit with introducer: 5-, 6-, or 7-French double-lumen catheter or 7-French triple-lumen catheter. In the adult, use a 6-French catheter with the introducing cannula one size larger. One needs a 12-gauge needle to pass a 7-French Swan–Ganz catheter. In the Seldinger technique, a smaller needle is used because a dilator is then inserted.
Monitors:
- Pressure transducer
- ECG monitor
- Pressure recorder

Connecting tubing and a three-way stopcock
Heparinized saline (1,000 units/100 mL)
Defibrillator

TECHNIQUE

Preparatory Steps

1. Introduce a no. 16 Angiocath via the right internal jugular or left subclavian vein approaches, as discussed in Central Intravenous Techniques, earlier.
2. Attach the Swan–Ganz catheter via a three-way stopcock to monitor the pressure.
3. Connect the pressure monitor to the other limb of the stopcock.
4. Calibrate the recorder (technician).

Procedural Steps: Modified Seldinger Technique (30, 115)

1. Slide the guidewire through the no. 16 Angiocath.
2. Remove the Angiocath, and replace with the introducer and sleeve. One may have to puncture the skin with a no. 11 blade to provide a hole large enough for the introducer.
3. Remove the guidewire.
4. Remove the introducer, and leave the sleeve in position.
5. Occlude the hub of the sleeve with the thumb to prevent air embolism (see Complications discussion under Infraclavicular Subclavian Vein Cannulation, earlier).
6. Slide the Swan–Ganz catheter (7 French) through the introducer.

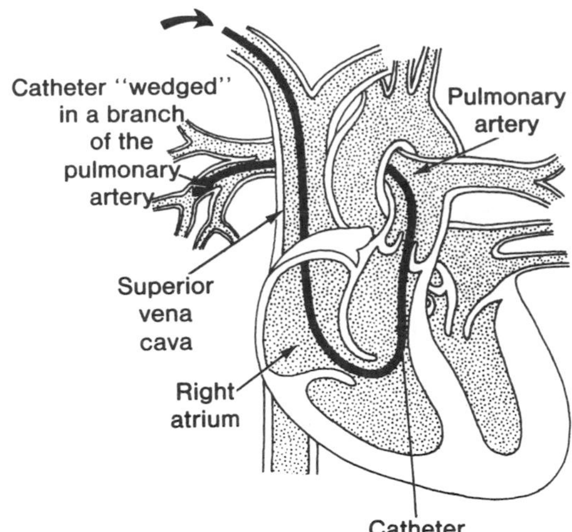

Figure 12.36. Swan–Ganz catheter wedged in a branch of the pulmonary artery.

7. Advance the catheter into the right atrium. When the catheter tip reaches the superior vena cava, inflate the balloon on the syringe with 0.7 to 0.8 mL of air to take advantage of the buoyancy of the balloon and "flow-direction."
8. Advance the catheter. Inflate the balloon, and pass the catheter into the pulmonary artery (Fig. 12.36). Follow the pressure tracings to determine catheter location (Fig. 12.37). Normal pressures are listed in Table 12.3.

NOTE

Pass the catheter smoothly to prevent vasospasms. Once the catheter occludes the pulmonary artery and a wedge pressure tracing is observed, deflate the balloon (Fig. 12.36), and obtain the pulmonary artery pressure tracing.

---

9. Pulmonary artery diastolic pressure usually approximates pulmonary artery wedge pressure and often may be used to monitor the clinical course of a patient, when the wedge pressure is no longer obtainable.

CAUTION

Watch the ECG closely for ventricular irritability. Persistent irritability requires that the catheter be withdrawn.

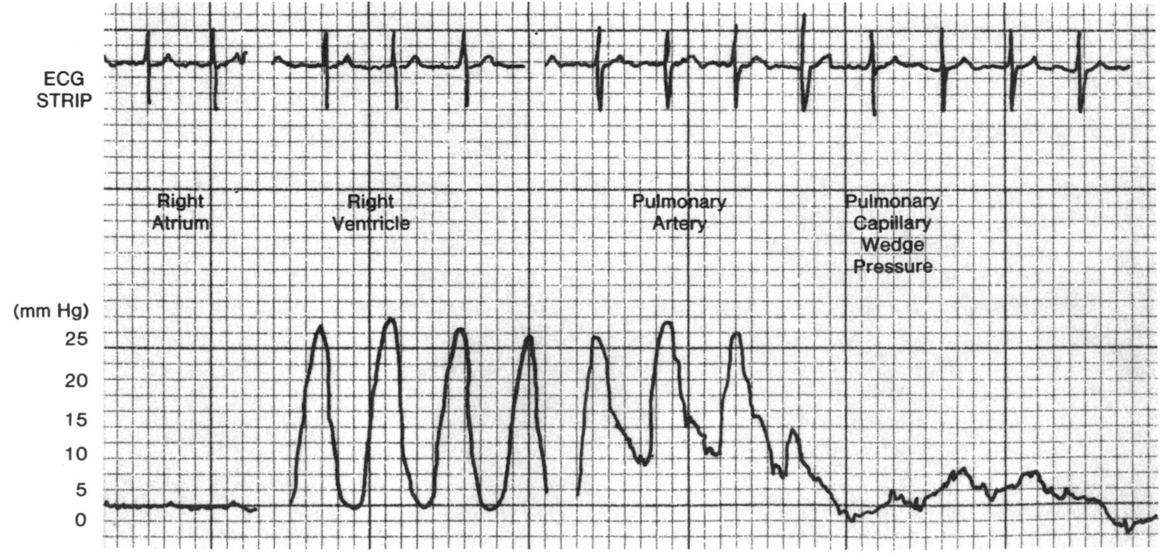

Figure 12.37. Cardiac and pulmonary artery pressures with a concomitant ECG tracing.

Table 12.3.
Normal Pulmonary and Cardiac Pressures

Region	Systolic (mm Hg)	Diastolic (mm Hg)	Mean (mm Hg)
Central venous			1–6
Right atrium			1–6
Right ventricle	20–30	<5	
Pulmonary artery	20–30	<10	<20
Pulmonary capillary wedge pressure			4–12

CAUTION

Inflate the balloon only when the wedge pressure is needed.

10. Check proper positioning of the catheter. With proper positioning, the pulmonary artery wedge pressure is lower than the mean PAP and, in most patients, is equal to the pulmonary artery diastolic pressure. Note the characteristic pressure waves obtained, indicating RAP, RVP, PAP, and PCWP (30, 110).

NOTE

To deflate the balloon, remove the syringe. Manual deflation of the balloon may cause inversion of and damage to the balloon.

11. Suture the catheter to the skin, and dress the wound. Record data from the catheter, and tape this to the catheter.
12. Attach heparin flush. The concentration used is 100 U/100 mL saline. Infuse at a rate of 2 to 3 mL/h.
13. Always obtain a radiograph to ensure proper positioning.

COMPLICATIONS (147, 185)

1. **Balloon rupture.** This is due to overinflation or frequent deflation of the balloon, damaging the balloon wall. It is heralded by a "damped" pulmonary wedge pressure. Prevent this complication by adding only 0.8 to 1.0 mL of air to the balloon and avoiding unnecessary deflation.
2. **Septic phlebitis** (91, 219). To prevent this complication, use sterile technique, change the tubing every 24 to 48 hours, and remove the catheter every 4 days.
3. **Traumatic endocarditis.** The catheter may injure the tricuspid or pulmonary valve or the right ventricular myocardium, resulting in thromboembolization. To prevent, see Septic Phlebitis.
4. **Catheter kinking or knotting.** This results from placing too much catheter in the ventricle, producing redundant loops. Looping in the atrium may produce atrial waveforms, then ventricular, and then atrial waveforms again because of the catheter tip "flipping" into the ventricle as the catheter is withdrawn.
5. **Arrhythmias.** These occur when the catheter is advanced into the right ventricle, which may be irritated by the catheter tip. Periodic arrhythmias may occur during looping of the catheter in the right ventricle. Avoid positioning the catheter in the right ventricle, and remove it from this location as soon as possible.
6. **Pulmonary infarction** (34, 74). This complication occurs when the balloon remains inflated too long or the uninflated catheter tip becomes wedged in

a small pulmonary artery. To treat continuous wedging, aspirate blood from the catheter; if wedged firmly, blood will withdraw with difficulty. Always deflate the balloon if this is suspected. If still wedged, inject heparinized saline to help dislodge the catheter tip. If wedged continuously, withdraw the catheter slowly until PA waveform appears. If this fails, check catheter replacement on chest radiograph.

7. **Damped waveform or high waveform.** This complication may be due to the catheter being up against a wall of a vessel, a clot at the tip of the catheter, or air bubbles in the transducer. To treat this complication, flush the catheter with a large volume of fluid after blood withdrawal from the catheter. If these procedures do not improve the waveform, obtain a radiograph to check the catheter position. If air bubbles are in the transducer, flush rapidly through the transducer.
8. **Abnormally low or negative pressure.** This complication is due to improper transducer level or incorrect zeroing and calibration of the monitor. To correct, recalibrate the transducer at midchest level and register zero.
9. **No pressure.** This complication is due to the transducer not being open to the catheter or to the amplifier being on calibrate, zero, or off. Treatment is to recalibrate.

Arterial Puncture

A number of sites, including the radial, ulnar, brachial, and femoral arteries, are commonly used for arterial puncture. The radial is perhaps the most commonly used site and is the one we recommend. The radial pulse is medial to the radial styloid where the artery courses over the distal end of the radius.

EQUIPMENT

Skin prep
Anesthetic prep
Heparin (concentration, 100 U/mL)
Ice and container
Cap for syringe
Glass syringe
(All of these, with the exception of the skin prep and anesthetic, are contained in commercially available kits.)
Butterfly needle, 23- or 25-gauge (preferred)
Alternative: 23-gauge, 5/8-inch needle

NOTE

We prefer the butterfly needle because of its ease of handling in regard to entering the artery, especially the radial artery. For larger deeper arteries, we prefer a 22-gauge, 1.5-inch needle.

TECHNIQUE

Preparatory Steps

1. Prepare the selected site.
2. Coat the syringe with the heparin solution (0.1 mL of heparin at a concentration of 1,000 U/mL). Draw heparin into the syringe, connecting the butterfly needle, and eject all of the heparin through the needle. The amount retained in the butterfly needle and tubing is enough to provide adequate heparinization.

   Alternative method: When using a larger vessel, draw 1 to 2 mL of heparin into a syringe, connect a 22-gauge, 1.5-inch needle to it, and eject all of the heparin; the amount retained on the sides of the syringe is all that is needed to prevent the arterial blood from coagulating.

Procedural Steps

1. Palpate the arterial pulse. Careful palpation is mandatory before needle puncture. Delineate the longitudinal course of the artery between the tips of the second and third fingers (Fig. 12.38). With a butterfly or a straight needle, puncture the skin at a 60-degree angle at the midpoint between these two fingers. One can feel the

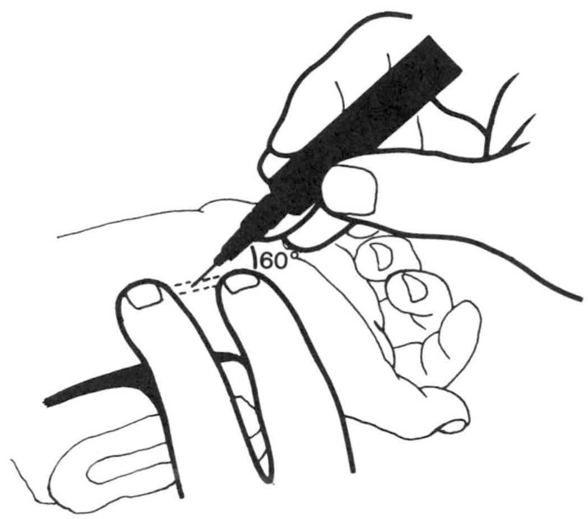

Figure 12.38. Radial artery puncture. See text for discussion.

pulse through the needle as the needle rests on top of the artery.

2. Puncture the artery; a pulsatile flow will raise the plunger of the syringe. A nonpulsatile but steady flow may occur in patients with high CVPs. If bone is contacted, slowly withdraw the syringe; one may still retrieve a sample on withdrawal through the back wall of the artery. Do not pierce or "spear" the artery because, occasionally, osteomyelitis or large hematomas have occurred in this fashion.
3. Remove air bubbles from the syringe. To remove air bubbles without disseminating drops of blood, apply an alcohol wipe over the needle tip and eject the bubbles onto the alcohol wipe.
4. Apply a cap to the tip of the needle or a rubber cap over the syringe (supplied in kits). Place the sample on ice and send it for analysis.

Alternative Technique

Thrombosis has been described as a significant complication of radial artery cannulation. Significant digital ischemia may ensue from such thrombosis. To use a recently described technique, palpate the radial artery pulse where the vessel emerges from the anatomic snuffbox, dorsally between the proximal heads of the first and second metacarpals (175). Insert a 20-gauge catheter percutaneously, and advance it until a brisk blood flow returns. This procedure avoids the full risk of digital ischemia, because the entire hand is not dependent on circulation at this point of the radial artery.

Aftercare

Apply pressure to the site for 5 minutes. Patients taking anticoagulants must have pressure applied to the site for 10 minutes. These times should not be estimated, but actually timed.

COMPLICATIONS

1. **Compression neuropathy.** The median nerve at the antecubital fossa may be injured during the puncture of the brachial artery. This complication can occur with an antecubital brachial artery puncture as a result of bleeding and nerve compression; pain and paresthesias in the distribution of the median nerve are noted. This is more likely to occur with patients taking anticoagulants (135). Discontinue anticoagulation if possible, elevate the extremity, and observe for 6 to 12 hours. Definitive treatment involves fascial decompression and hematoma removal. When nerve compression occurs in the leg, the results are poor (133).
2. **Pseudoaneurysm.** This condition can occur especially with femoral punctures. The patient has a "pulsating tumor," with a bruit anterior to the artery. These occur more often when the hematoma is large. Treatment is by removal of the pseudoaneurysm.
3. **Arteriovenous fistula.** An arteriovenous fistula may form after femoral puncture. This complication is another reason for advocating the use of the radial artery, because there is no accompanying major vein.
4. **Arterial spasm.** Arterial spasm occurs after puncture and may lead to vascular compromise. This complication is

fivefold more common with brachial than with femoral artery puncture (196).

5. **Hematoma formation.** Maintain pressure over the punctured artery for 5 minutes to avoid this complication. There is an overall 10% incidence of complications with arterial punctures (143). In patients who are taking anticoagulants, there is a fourfold increase in the overall complication rate.
6. **Septic arthritis.** This is a complication after puncture of the femoral artery. We do not advocate penetrating to the bone in performing arterial punctures at this site.

Arterial Cannulation

Two methods of arterial cannulation are used: percutaneous cannulation, in which the radial artery is the site most commonly used, and the cutdown approach (110). Both of these are discussed later.

INDICATIONS

1. Arterial pressure monitoring.
   a. Difficulty in obtaining cuff blood pressure in a critically ill patient who is severely hypotensive.
   b. Monitoring a patient who requires potent dilators or pressors for accurate pressure management (e.g., nitroprusside).
2. Repeated arterial blood sampling.

CONTRAINDICATIONS

1. Severe injury to the extremity.
2. Positive Allen's test.
3. Injury to the site proximal to the vessel to be cannulated.

EQUIPMENT

Percutaneous Technique

Armboard
Folded towel
1-inch wide adhesive tape
Skin prep
Sterile field
Local anesthetic
10-mL syringe
18-gauge Angiocath or Medicut cannula
Stopcock
Heparin, 1 mL, 100 U/mL
30-mL vial injectable saline
Dressing
Arterial pressure transducer
Pressure tubing
Calibrated oscilloscope

Cutdown Technique

Sterile sponges
No. 3 knife handle
No. 15 scalpel blade
Curved Iris and suture scissors
Fine-toothed forceps
Two curved mosquito clamps
One small self-retaining retractor
Needle holder
3-0 silk ligatures
10-mL plastic syringe
Angiocath, 18-gauge, or Medicut cannula, 18-gauge needle
Three-way stopcock
Heparin, 1 mL, 1,000 U/mL
30-mL vial injectable saline
4-0 nylon sutures for skin

TECHNIQUE

This method is for percutaneous cannulation of the radial artery or for cannulation of the radial artery by the cutdown method.

Preparatory Steps

1. Select site. We prefer the radial artery. Alternate sites include the brachial artery (although thrombosis may occur at this site) and dorsalis pedis. Do not use the femoral artery.
2. Perform the Allen's test (5, 161). Compress both the ulnar and the radial arteries at the wrist, and ask the patient to squeeze the fist several times to drain venous blood from the hand. Have the patient relax the hand with no flexion or extension at the wrist, and note the blanching (90). Release the ulnar artery, and observe the effect on blanching. In the hand with a

patent ulnar artery, the palmar surface should return to normal color (pink). Repeat by using radial artery occlusion, and note the return of pink color to the palm on release of the radial artery. If either artery is occluded, as demonstrated by delay of return or by no return of normal skin color, then do not cannulate either vessel.

3. Place the wrist in a supine position, with the arm abducted. Dorsiflex the wrist over a folded towel placed between the wrist and the armboard to make the artery more prominent. Tape the hand to the armboard to maintain the position shown in Fig. 12.39.
4. Anesthetize the skin over the site.
5. Prepare and drape.
6. Prepare the syringe with heparin. Use a 10-mL heparinized syringe. Attach a stopcock to the syringe. Adequate heparin concentration is 500 U/10 mL saline.

Procedural Steps

1. *Percutaneous approach:* Puncture the skin first with the 18-gauge needle to produce a small skin incision and avoid a skin plug. Through the skin puncture site, advance the 18-gauge Angiocath at a 30-degree angle to the skin and parallel to the artery. Insert the Angiocath into the artery at a 45-degree angle to the axis of the vessel.

   Cutdown approach: Make a transverse incision proximal to the flexion increase at the wrist. Mobilize the artery, exposing 1 to 2 cm of the length of the vessel. Ligate the distal end with a 2-0 suture. Place an elevating clamp beneath the artery. With an Angiocath, puncture the artery proximal to the elevating clamp.
2. Cannulate the artery.

   Percutaneous approach (our preferred method): Transfix the artery between two fingers. Puncture the artery and advance the cannula after pulsatile blood flow is noted (Fig. 12.38).

   Alternative method: When the artery is punctured through its back wall, it is transfixed. Arterial flow confirms entry into the artery. Remove the needle, leaving the cannula in place. Slowly withdraw the cannula until arterial blood is noted to "spurt out." Advance the cannula into the artery.

   Cutdown approach: Slide the needle and cannula into the artery until the tip lies in the arterial lumen. Remove the needle and advance the cannula.
3. Attach a three-way stopcock with a heparinized syringe used to prevent thrombosis in the arterial cannula. Flush the cannula after aspirating to confirm good blood flow. After flushing with heparinized saline, close the stopcock to the cannula, and remove the syringe from the stopcock.

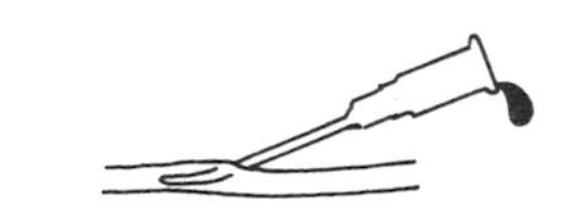

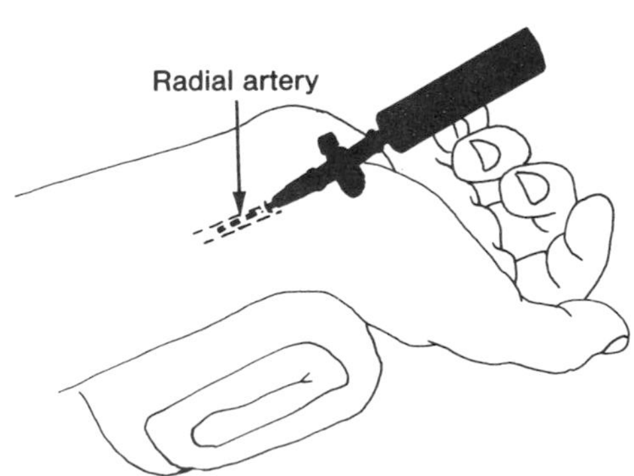

Figure 12.39. Radial artery cannulation. Secure the hand and wrist to the armboard, with the wrist placed in extension as shown. See text for discussion.

Aftercare

1. Connect the transducer.
2. Control bleeding with pressure dressing. Apply pressure over the artery at the tip of the cannula for 5 minutes to

stop bleeding. Release the tape on palms, remove the towel, and tape the hand to the armboard.

COMPLICATIONS

1. **Local infection or sepsis** (195).
2. **Hematoma.** This is due to lack of pressure to the cannulated artery for a sufficient time.
3. **Vasculitis.**
4. **Nerve damage.**
5. **Embolism.** Retrograde arterial embolism can occur from retrograde flushing of the cannula, and emboli may enter the cerebral circulation (53, 195). This danger is greater with smaller patients. To maintain patency of the artery in children, use volumes of heparinized solution smaller than 3 mL, or maintain a slow continuous flushing, because thrombi may be dislodged (53, 134).
6. **Tissue necrosis with distal ischemia** (108, 222). This complication is due to excessive arterial trauma, resulting in thrombosis. Avoid several consecutive punctures at the same site. Certain arteries, especially the brachial and femoral arteries, are more prone to ischemic complications and should be avoided. Finger ischemia occurs commonly in patients in shock and in those with poor ulnar artery flow. Perform the Allen's test before cannulating the radial artery; if the patient is in shock, the benefits must be weighed against the potential complications.

Intramuscular Injections

The upper outer quadrant of the buttocks is the site of choice for intramuscular injection. In this quadrant, the muscle is maximally thick so that one may inject deeply. This area avoids the blood vessels and nerves that are present in the inner quadrants. No other quadrant of the buttocks is acceptable (224). Zelman (224) believes that injections in the deltoid and other muscles are less satisfactory because of the greater sensitivity of these muscles, their smaller mass, and their proximity to nerves.

From the anatomy of the gluteal muscle and the distribution of the intramuscularly injected substances, it has been shown that injection into the lower central portion of the buttocks endangers the great sciatic nerve, if the injection extends through the gluteus maximus. More commonly, a temporary sciatica-like pain extends down the back of the leg; this pain is attributed to irritation of the small sciatic nerve, which overlies the great sciatic nerve in this area.

TECHNIQUE

Give the intramuscular injection with the patient in the prone position with the toes facing inward and heels outward.

After retracting the skin and subcutaneous tissue, introduce the needle. When the needle is later withdrawn, the return of these superficial tissues to their normal position breaks the direct needle track and decreases the likelihood of subcutaneous seepage of the injected material from within the muscle belly.

Remember to aspirate the syringe to exclude entry into a blood vessel. If blood or any other fluid is obtained, withdraw the needle, choose another site, and discard the inoculum (215).

Pass the needle through the skin and muscle in a single movement to a depth of 3 to 4 cm. Inject the medication slowly to allow time for distention of the accommodating space within the muscle to decrease the pain of injection. Deep firm massage of the muscle favors spread of the medication through a wider area of tissue and more rapid absorption.

Alternate Site

An alternate site, suggested by Grey Turner (92), is the region on the outer side of the thigh over the vastus lateralis muscle. He believes this is the ideal place for intramuscular injections. The area does not contain any important nerves or large blood vessels and is a large muscle mass. Introduce the needle at the middle of the outer side of the thigh. If the bone is reached, slightly withdraw the needle before making the injection.

AN EMERGENCY INTRAMUSCULAR SITE FOR DRUG ADMINISTRATION

Lidocaine and other local anesthetics can be injected lingually (173). Periorally injected lidocaine has been shown to produce peak blood levels rapidly. An intravenous bolus of lidocaine is the most rapid method of achieving peak blood levels (2 minutes); however, when an intravenous site is not available, intralingual injection of lidocaine without epinephrine produces peak blood levels in 10 minutes (173). In such a patient, if an endotracheal tube is in place, the administration of the drug by this route is probably the second most rapid method of achieving peak levels; however, the time varies widely from 5 to 25 minutes. In another study (160), in which epinephrine or aminophylline was injected along the lateral ventral surface of the tongue, it was found that an effect was noted within 35 seconds, both on the electrocardiogram and in the depth and rate of respiration.

REFERENCES

1. Acalovschi I, Corbaciu D, Paraianu I, et al: Cortical blindness after subclavian vein catheterization. J Parenter Enter Nutr 12:5, 526–527, 1988.
2. Adar R, Mozes M: Fatal complications of central venous catheters. Br Med J 3:746, 1971.
3. Adelman S: An emergency intravenous route for the pediatric patient. JACEP 5:596, 1976.
4. Ahmed N, Payne RF: Thrombosis after central venous cannulation. Med J Aust 1:217, 1976.
5. Allen EV: Thromboangiitis obliterans: Methods of diagnosis of chronic occlusive arterial lesions distal to the wrist, with illustrated cases. Am J Med Sci 178:237, 1929.
6. Allsop JR, Askew AR: Subclavian vein cannulation: A new complication. Br Med J 4:262, 1975.
7. Archer G, Cobb LA: Long-term pulmonary artery pressure monitoring in the management of the critically ill. Ann Surg 180:747, 1974.
8. Ashbaugh D, Thomson JWW: Subclavian-vein infusion. Lancet 2:1138, 1963.
9. Asimacopoulos PJ, Bagley FH, McDermott WF: A modified technique for subclavian puncture. Surg Gynecol Obstet 150:241, 1980.
10. Asnes RS, Arendar GM: Septic arthritis of the hip: A complication of femoral venipuncture. Pediatrics 38:837, 1966.
11. Aulenbacher CE: Hydrothorax from subclavian vein catheterization [Letter]. JAMA 214:372, 1970.
12. Aziz EM, Robertson AF: Paraplegia: A complication of umbilical artery catheterization. J Pediatr 82:1051, 1973.
13. Baird CL: Transvenous pacemaking: A bedside technique. Br Heart J 33:191, 1971.
14. Baker CC, Petersen SR, Sheldon GF: Septic phlebitis: A neglected disease. Am J Surg 138: 97, 1979.
15. Balagtas RC, Bell CE, Edwards LD, et al: Risk of local and systemic infections associated with umbilical vein catheterization: A prospective study in 86 newborn patients. Pediatrics 48: 359, 1971.
16. Band JD, Maki DG: Safety of changing intravenous delivery systems at longer than 24 hour intervals. Ann Intern Med 91:173, 1979.
17. Bansmer G, Keith D, Tesluk H: Complications following use of indwelling catheters of inferior vena cava. JAMA 167:1606, 1958.
18. Barenholtz L, Kaminsky NI, Palmer DI: Venous intramural microabscess: A cause of protracted sepsis with intravenous cannulas. Am J Med Sci 265:355, 1973.
19. Bauer SB, Feldman SM, Gelli SS, et al: Neonatal hypertension: A complication of umbilical-artery catheterization. N Engl J Med 293:1032, 1975.
20. Bentley DW, Lepper MH: Septicemia related to indwelling venous catheter. JAMA 206:1749, 1968.
21. Bergentz S-E, Hansson LO, Norback B: Surgical management of complications to arterial puncture. Ann Surg 164:1021, 1964.
22. Bernard RW, Stahl WM: Subclavian vein catheterizations: A prospective study, I: noninfectious complications. Ann Surg 173:184, 1971.
23. Bogen JE: Local complications in 167 patients with indwelling venous catheters. Surg Gynecol Obstet 110:112, 1960.
24. Borja AR, Masri Z, Shruck L, et al: Unusual and lethal complications of infraclavicular subclavian vein catheterization. Int Surg 57:42, 1972.
25. Bosch DT, Kengeter JP, Beling CA: Femoral venipuncture. Am J Surg 79:722, 1950.
26. Bower EB: Choosing a catheter for central venous catheterization. Surg Clin North Am 53: 639, 1973.
27. Braux E: Cardiac tamponade following penetrating mediastinal injuries. J Trauma 19:461, 1979.
28. Brinkman AJ, Costley DO: Internal jugular venipuncture. JAMA 223:182, 1973.
29. Brown HI, Burnard RJ, Jensen J, et al: Puncture of endotracheal-tube cuffs during percutaneous subclavian-vein catheterization. Anesthesiology 43:112, 1975.

30. Buchbinder N, Ganz W: Hemodynamic monitoring: Invasive techniques. Anesthesiology 45: 146, 1976.
31. Burgess GE, Marino RJ, Penler MJ: Effect of head position on the location of venous catheters inserted via the basilic vein. Anesthesiology 46:212, 1977.
32. Burns S, Herbison GJ: Spinal accessory nerve injury as a complication of internal jugular vein cannulation. Ann Intern Med 125:8, 700, 1996.
33. Buxton AE, Highsmith AK, Garner JS, et al: Contamination of intravenous infusion fluid: Effect of changing administration sets. Ann Intern Med 90:764, 1979.
34. Calvin MP, Savage TM, Lewis CT: Pulmonary damage from a Swan-Ganz catheter. Br J Anaesth 47:1107, 1975.
35. Castor WR: Spontaneous perforation of the bowel in the newborn following exchange transfusion. Can Med Assoc J 99:934, 1968.
36. Cheng TO: Percutaneous transfemoral venous cardiac pacing. Chest 60:73, 1971.
37. Christensen KH, Nerstrom B, Baden H: Complications of percutaneous catheterization of the subclavian vein in 129 cases. Acta Chir Scand 133:615, 1967.
38. Cochran WD, Davis HT, Smith CA: Advantages and complications of umbilical artery catheterization in the newborn. Pediatrics 42:769, 1968.
39. Corman LC, Levison ME: Sustained bacteremia and transvenous cardiac pacemakers. JAMA 233:264, 1975.
40. Corso JA, Agostinelli R, Brandriss MW: Maintenance of venous polyethylene catheters to reduce risk of infection. JAMA 210:2075, 1969.
41. Corwin JH, Moseley T: Subclavian venipuncture and central venous pressure: Technic and application. Am Surg 32:413, 1966.
42. Crenshaw CA: Prevention of infection at scalp vein sites of needle insertion during intravenous therapy. Am J Surg 124:43, 1972.
43. Crossley K, Matsen JM: The scalp-vein needle: A prospective study of complications. JAMA 220:985, 1972.
44. Daily PO, Griepp RB, Shumway NE: Percutaneous internal jugular vein cannulation. Arch Surg 101:534, 1970.
45. Daly BDT, Berger RL: Antecubital approach for intravascular monitoring. Surg Gynecol Obstet 135:434, 1972.
46. Daniell HW: Heparin in the prevention of infusion phlebitis: A double-blind controlled study. JAMA 226:1317, 1973.
47. Davidson JT, Ben-Hur N, Nathen H: Subclavian venipuncture. Lancet 2:1139, 1963.
48. DeFalque RJ: Percutaneous catheterization of the internal jugular vein. Anesth Analg 53:116, 1974.
49. Defalque RJ, Fletcher MV: Neurological complications of central venous cannulation. J Parenter Enter Nutr 12:406, 1988.
50. Defalque RJ, Fletcher MV: Neurological complications of central venous cannulation. J Parenter Enter Nutr 12:4, 406–409, 1988.
51. Doering RB, Stemmer EA, Connolly JE: Complications of indwelling venous catheters: With particular reference to catheter embolus. Am J Surg 114:259, 1967.
52. Dosios TJ, MacGovern GJ, Gay TC, et al: Cardiac tamponade complicating percutaneous catheterization of subclavian vein. Surgery 78:261, 1975.
53. Downs JB, Chapman RL, Hawkins JF, et al: Prolonged radial artery catheterization. Arch Surg 108:671, 1974.
54. Durant TM, Long J, Oppenheimer MJ: Pulmonary (venous) air embolism. Am Heart J 33: 269, 1947.
55. Durant TM, Oppenheimer MJ, Webster MR, et al: Arterial air embolism. Am Heart J 38:481, 1949.
56. Edelstein J: Atraumatic removal of a polyethylene catheter from the superior vena cava. Chest 57:381, 1970.
57. Edin MB, Dudley HAF: The local complications of intravenous therapy. Lancet 2:365, 1959.
58. Effert S, Skykosch J: Emergency pacing techniques. Ann N Y Acad Sci 167:614, 1969.
59. Egan EA, Eitzman DV: Umbilical vessel catheterization. Am J Dis Child 121:213, 1971.
60. Eichelberger MR, Rous PG, Hoelzer DJ, et al: Percutaneous subclavian venous catheters in neonates and children. J Pediatr Surg 16:547, 1981.
61. Emerman CL, Bellon EM, Lukens TW, et al: A prospective study of femoral versus subclavian vein catheterization during cardiac arrest. Ann Emerg Med 19:59, 1990.
62. English ICW, Frew RM, Pigott JF, et al: Percutaneous catheterization of the internal jugular vein. Anaesthesia 24:521, 1969.
63. Epstein EJ, Quereshi MSA, Wright JS: Diaphragmatic paralysis after supraclavicular puncture of subclavian vein [Letter]. Br Med J 1: 693, 1976.
64. Erkan V, Blankenship W, Stahlman MT: The complications of chronic umbilical vessel catheterization [Abstract]. Pediatr Res 2:317, 1968.
65. Falcone RE, Hickman DM, Rophie R, et al: The complication rate of elective subclavian vein puncture by the novice. J Parenter Enter Nutr 9: 379, 1985.
66. Farhat K, Nakhjavan FK, Cope C, et al: Iatrogenic arteriovenous fistula: A complication of percutaneous subclavian vein puncture. Chest 67:480, 1975.
67. Feliciano DV, Mattox KL, Graham JM, et al: Major complications of percutaneous subclavian vein catheters. Am J Surg 138:869, 1979.
68. Fenn JE, Stansel HC Jr: Certain hazards of the central venous catheter. Angiology 20:38, 1969.
69. Ferguson RL: Complications of heparin lock needles. Ann Intern Med 85:583, 1976.
70. Filston HC, Grant JP: A safer system for percutaneous subclavian venous catheterization in newborn infants. J Pediatr Surg 14:564, 1979.
71. Fiser DH: Intraosseous infusion. N Engl J Med 322:1579, 1990.
72. Fisher RG, Ferreyro R: Evaluation of current techniques for nonsurgical removal of intravas-

cular iatrogenic foreign bodies. AJR Am J Roentgenol 130:541, 1978.

73. Fletcher GF: Insertion of a temporary transvenous pacemaker. In: Cardiac Procedures. New York: Appleton-Century-Crofts, 329, 1974.
74. Foote GA, Schabel SI, Hodges M: Pulmonary complications of the flow-directed balloon-tipped catheter. N Engl J Med 290:927, 1974.
75. Formanek G, Frech RS, Amplatz K: Arterial thrombus formation during clinical percutaneous catheterization. Circulation 41:833, 1970.
76. Forrester JS, Diamond G, McHugh TJ, et al: Filling pressures in the right and left sides of the heart in acute myocardial infarction: A reappraisal of central venous pressure monitoring. N Engl J Med 285:190, 1971.
77. Fort ML, Sharp JT: Perforation of the right ventricle by pacing catheter electrode. Am J Cardiol 16:610, 1965.
78. Fry WR, Clagett GC, O'Rourke PT: Ultrasound-guided central venous access. Arch Surg 134:7, 738–741, 1999.
79. Furman SD, Escher JW: Transvenous pacing: A seven year review. Am Heart J 71:408, 1966.
80. Gallitano AI, Kondi ES, Deckers PJ: A safe approach to the subclavian vein. Surg Gynecol Obstet 135:96, 1972.
81. Garcia JM, Mispireta LA, Pinho RV: Percutaneous supraclavicular superior vena caval cannulation. Surg Gynecol Obstet 134:839, 1972.
82. Getzen LC, Erich WP: Short-term femoral vein cannulation. Am J Surg 138:875, 1979.
83. Gibson T, Norris W: Skin fragments removed by injection needles. Lancet 8:983, 1958.
84. Gilday DL, Downs AR: The value of chest radiography in the localization of central venous pressure catheters. Can Med Assoc J 101:363, 1969.
85. Glaeser PW, Losek JD, Nelson DB, et al: Pediatric intraosseous infusions: Impact on vascular access time. Am J Emerg Med 6:330, 1988.
86. Goetzman BW, Stadalnik RC, Bogren HG, et al: Thrombotic complications umbilical artery catheters: A clinical and radiographic study. Pediatrics 56:374, 1975.
87. Goldbloom RB, Hillman DA, Santulli TV: Arterial thrombosis following femoral venipuncture in edematous nephrotic children. Pediatrics 40: 450, 1967.
88. Goldman LI, Maier WP, Drezner AD: Another complication of subclavian puncture: arterial laceration [Letter]. JAMA 217:78, 1971.
89. Goldstein B, Doody D, Briggs S, et al: Emergency intraosseous infusion in severely burned children. Pediatr Emerg Care 6:195, 1990.
90. Greenbow DE: Incorrect performance of Allen's test: Ulnar artery flow presumed inadequate. Anesthesiology 37:356, 1972.
91. Greene JF, Fitzwater JE, Clemmer TP: Septic endocarditis and indwelling pulmonary artery catheters. JAMA 233:891, 1975.
92. Grey Turner G: The site for intramuscular injections. Lancet 2:819, 1920.
93. Groff D: Subclavian vein catheterization in the infant. J Pediatr Surg 9:171, 1974.
94. Gupta JM, Roberton NRC, Wigglesworth JS: Umbilical artery catheterization in the newborn. Arch Dis Child 43:382, 1968.
95. Hall DM: Percutaneous catheterization of the internal jugular vein in infants and children. J Pediatr Surg 12:709, 1977.
96. Haller JD, Cerruti MM, Silver W: A simple method for arterial and venous monitoring of neonates. Surg Gynecol Obstet 134:489, 1972.
97. Harford FJ, Kleinsasser J: Fatal cardiac tamponade in a patient receiving total parenteral nutrition via a Silastic central venous catheter. J Parenter Enter Nutr 8:4, 443–446, 1984.
98. Harken DE, Zoll PM: Foreign bodies in and in relation to the thoracic blood vessels and heart, III: indications for the removal for intracardiac foreign bodies and the behavior of the heart during manipulation. Am Heart J 32:1, 1946.
99. Hart GB: Treatment of decompression illness and air embolism with hyperbaric oxygen. Aerospace Med 45:1190, 1974.
100. Haynes BE, Carr FJ, Niemann JT: Subclavian catheterization in children. Ann Emerg Med 12: 606, 1983.
101. Henzel JH, DeWeese MS: Morbid and mortal complications associated with prolonged central venous cannulation. Am J Surg 121:600, 1971.
102. Hoelzer MF: Recent advances in intravenous therapy. Emerg Med Clin North Am 4:487, 1986.
103. Holland AJ, Ford WD: Improved percutaneous insertion of long-term central venous catheters in children: The "shrug" manoeuvre. Aust N Z J Surg 69:3, 231–233, 1999.
104. Hoshal VL Jr, Asuse RG, Hoskins PA: Fibrin sleeve formation on indwelling subclavian central venous catheters. Arch Surg 102:353, 1971.
105. Indar R: The dangers of indwelling polyethylene cannulae in deep veins. Lancet 1:284, 1959.
106. Irwin GR Jr, Hart RJ, Martin CM: Pathogenesis and prevention of intravenous catheter infections. Yale J Biol Med 46:85, 1973.
107. Iserson KV: Intraosseous infusions in adults. J Emerg Med 7:587, 1989.
108. James PM, Myers RT: Central venous pressure monitoring: Complications and a new technique. Am Surg 39:75, 1973.
109. Jernigan WR, Gardner WC, Mahr ME: Use of the internal jugular vein for placement of central venous catheters. Surg Gynecol Obstet 130:520, 1970.
110. Johnson CL, Lazarchik J, Lynn HB: Subclavian venipuncture: preventable complications: Report of two cases. Mayo Clin Proc 45:712, 1970.
111. Johnson RW: A complication of radial artery cannulation. Anesthesiology 40:598, 1974.
112. Johnston AOB, Clark RG: Malpositioning of cardiovascular catheters. Lancet 2:1395, 1972.
113. Joynt GM, Kew J, Gomersall CD, et al: Deep venous thrombosis caused by femoral venous catheters in critically ill adult patients. Chest 117:1, 178–183, 2000.
114. Kaltman AJ: Indications for temporary pacemaker insertion in acute myocardial infarction. Am Heart J 81:837, 1971.

115. Kaplan JA, Miller ED: Insertion of the Swan-Ganz catheter. Anesthesiol Rev 22, 1976.
116. Katan BS, Olshaker JS, Dickerson SE, et al: Intraosseous infusion of muscle relaxants. Am J Emerg Med 6:353, 1988.
117. Kawamura R, Okabe M, Namikawa K, et al: Techniques, materials and devices. J Parenter Enter Nutr 11:505, 1987.
118. Keeri-Szanto M: The subclavian vein: A constant and convenient intravenous injection site. Arch Surg 72:179, 1956.
119. Kellner GA, Smart JF: Percutaneous placement of catheters to monitor "central venous pressure." Anesthesiology 36:515, 1972.
120. Kerber RE: Electrocardiographic indications of atrial puncture during pericardiocentesis. N Engl J Med 282:1142, 1975.
121. Khalil KG: Thoracic duct injury: A complication of jugular vein catheterization. JAMA 221: 980, 1972.
122. Killip T, Kimball JT: Percutaneous techniques for introducing flexible electrodes for intracardiac pacing. Ann N Y Acad Sci 167:597, 1969.
123. Kimball JT, Killip T: A simple method for transvenous intracardiac pacing. Am Heart J 70: 35, 1965.
124. Kitterman JA, Phibbs RH, Tooley WH: Catheterization of umbilical vessels in newborn infants. Pediatr Clin North Am 17:895, 1970.
125. Knopp R, Dailey RH: Central venous cannulation and pressure monitoring. JACEP 6:358, 1977.
126. Krausz MM, Berlatzky Y, Ayalon A, et al: Percutaneous cannulation of the internal jugular vein in infants and children. Surg Gynecol Obstet 148:591, 1979.
127. Kunz HW: A technique for obtaining blood specimens and giving transfusions in small infants. J Pediatr 42:80, 1953.
128. LaFleche FR, Slepin MJ, Vargas J, et al: Iatrogenic bilateral tibial fractures after intraosseous infusion attempts in a 3-month-old infant. Ann Emerg Med 18:125, 1989.
129. Land RE: The relationship of the left subclavian vein to the clavicle. J Thorac Cardiovasc Surg 63:564, 1972.
130. Larsen HW, Lindahl F: Lesion of the internal mammarian artery caused by infraclavicular percutaneous catheterization of the subclavian vein. Acta Chir Scand 139:571, 1973.
131. Lee Y-H, Kerstein MD: Osteomyelitis and septic arthritis: A complication of subclavian venous catheterization. N Engl J Med 285:1179, 1971.
132. Lefrak EA, Noon GP: Management of arterial injury secondary to attempted subclavian vein catheterization. Ann Thorac Surg 14:294, 1972.
133. Leonard MD: Sciatic nerve paralysis following anticoagulant therapy. J Bone Joint Surg Br 54: 152, 1972.
134. Lowenstein E, Little JW, Lo HH: Prevention of cerebral embolization from flushing radial artery cannulae. N Engl J Med 285:1414, 1971.
135. Luce EA, Futrell JW, Wilgis EFS, et al: Compression neuropathy following brachial arterial puncture in anticoagulated patients. J Trauma 16:717, 1976.
136. Lumia FJ, Rios JC: Temporary transvenous pacemaker therapy: An analysis of complications. Chest 64:604, 1973.
137. McConnell RY: Experience with percutaneous internal jugular innominate vein catheterization. Calif Med 117:1, 1972.
138. McKay RJ: Diagnosis and treatment: risks of obtaining samples of venous blood in infants. Pediatrics 38:5, 906–908, 1966.
139. McKay RJ: Diagnosis and treatment: risks of obtaining samples of venous blood in infants. Pediatrics 38:906, 1966.
140. McNamara RM, Spivey WH, Unger HD, et al: Emergency applications of intraosseous infusion. J Emerg Med 5:97, 1987.
141. Maki DG, Goldman DA, Rhame FS: Infection control in intravenous therapy. Ann Intern Med 79:867, 1973.
142. Marlon Am, Cohn LH, Fogarty TJ, et al: Retrieval of catheter fragments: Report of two cases. Calif Med 115:61, 1971.
143. Massumi RA, Ross AM: Atraumatic, nonsurgical technic for removal of broken catheters from cardiac cavities. N Engl J Med 277:195, 1967.
144. Matensen JD: Clinical sequelae from arterial needle puncture, cannulation, and incision. Circulation 35:1118, 1967.
145. Mattox KL, Fisher RG: Persistent hemathorax secondary to malposition of a subclavian venous catheter. J Trauma 17:387, 1977.
146. Meister SG, Banka VS, Helfant RH: Transfemoral pacing with balloon-tipped catheters. JAMA 225:712, 1973.
147. Meister SG, DeVilla M, Banka VS, et al: An improved method for temporary transvenous pacing without fluoroscopy [Abstract]. Circulation (suppl II) 45, 46: II181, 1972.
148. Meister SG, Engel TR, Fisher HA, et al: Potential artifact in measurement of left ventricular filling pressure with flow-directed catheters. Cathet Cardiovasc Diagn 2:175, 1976.
149. Merk EA, Rush BF: Emergency subclavian vein catheterization and intravenous hyperalimentation. Am J Surg 129:266, 1975.
150. Michenfelder JD, Terry HR Jr, Daw EF, et al: Air embolism during neurosurgery: A new method of treatment. Anesth Analg 45:390, 1966.
151. Mitchell SE, Clark RA: Complications of central venous catheterization. Am J Radiol 133:467, 1979.
152. Miyamoto Y, Kinouchi K, Hiramatsu K: Cervical dural puncture in a neonate: A rare complication of internal jugular venipuncture. Anesthesiology 84:5, 1239–1242, 1996.
153. Mitty WF, Nealon TF: Complications of subclavian sticks. JACEP 4:24, 1975.
154. Mobin-Uddin K, Smith PE, Lombardo C, et al: Percutaneous intracardiac pacing through the subclavian vein. J Thorac Cardiovasc Surg 54: 545, 1967.
155. Mogil RA, DeLaurentis DA, Rosemond GP: The infraclavicular venipuncture: value in various clinical situations including central venous pressure monitoring. Arch Surg 95:320, 1967.
156. Mokrohisky ST, Levin RL, Blumhagen JD, et al: Low positioning of umbilical-artery catheters

increases associated complications in newborn infants. N Engl J Med 299:561, 1978.
157. Moran JM, Atwood RP, Rowe MI: A clinical and bacteriologic study of infections associated with venous cutdowns. N Engl J Med 272:554, 1965.
158. Morgan WW, Harkins GA: Percutaneous introduction of long-term indwelling venous catheters in infants. J Pediatr Surg 7:538, 1972.
159. Moscati R: Compartment syndrome with resultant amputation following intraosseous infusion. Am J Emerg Med 8:470, 1990.
160. Mostert JW, Kenny GM, Murphy GP: Safe placement of central venous catheter into internal jugular veins. Arch Surg 101:431, 1970.
161. Nichols WA, Cutright ED: Intralingual injection site for emergency stimulant drugs. Oral Surg 32:677, 1971.
162. Norden CW: Application of antibiotic ointment to the site of venous catheterization: a controlled trial. J Infect Dis 120:611, 1969.
163. Northfield TC, Smith T: Physiologic significance of central venous pressure in patients with hemorrhage. Surg Gynecol Obstet 135: 267, 1972.
164. Nowak RM, Tomlanovich MC: Venous cutdowns in the emergency department [Letter]. JACEP 8:245, 1979.
165. Oppenheimer EH, Esterly JR: Thrombosis in the newborn: Comparison between infants of diabetic and nondiabetic mothers. J Pediatr 67: 549, 1965.
166. O'Reilly MV: The technique of subclavian vein cannulation. Can Med Assoc J 108:63, 1973.
167. Orlowski JP, Julius CJ, Petras RE, et al: The safety of intraosseous infusions: Risks of fat and bone marrow emboli to the lungs. Ann Emerg Med 18:73, 1989.
168. Palm T: Evaluation of peripheral arterial pressure in the thumb following radial artery cannulation. Br J Anaesth 49:819, 1977.
169. Parrish GA, Turkewitz D, Skiendzielewski JJ: Intraosseous infusions in the emergency department. Am J Emerg Med 4:59, 1986.
170. Paskin DL, Hoffman WS, Tuddenham WJ: A new complication of subclavian vein catheterization. Ann Surg 179:266, 1974.
171. Phillips PJ, Pain RW, Brooks GE: The pain of venipuncture [Letter]. N Engl J Med 294:116, 1976.
172. Phillips SJ, Okies JE: Inexpensive simple monitoring techniques. Surg Gynecol Obstet 139: 761, 1974.
173. Plaus WJ: Delayed pneumothorax after subclavian vein catheterization. J Parenter Enter Nutr 14:414, 1990.
174. Pomeroy GLM, Loehr MM: Intralingual injection of lidocaine. JACEP 6:163, 1977.
175. Prince SR, Sullivan RL, Hackel A: Percutaneous catheterization of the internal jugular vein in infants and children. Anesthesiology 44:170, 1976.
176. Pyles ST, Scher KS: Cannulation of the radial artery in the anatomic snuffbox. Surg Gynecol Obstet 156:227–228, 1983.
177. Qureshi GD, Lilly EL: Complications of CVP catheter insertion in cubital vein. JAMA 209:1906, 1969.
178. Randolph J: Technique for insertion of plastic catheter into saphenous vein. Pediatrics 24: 631, 1959.
179. Redmond AD, Plunkett PK: Intraosseous infusion. Arch Emerg Med 3:231, 1986.
180. Rose SG, Pitsch RJ, Karrer WF, et al: Subclavian catheter infections. J Parenter Enter Nutr 12: 511, 1988.
181. Rosenberg AS, Grossman JL, Escher DJW, et al: Bedside transvenous cardiac pacing. Am Heart J 77:697, 1969.
182. Rosetti VA, Thompson BM, Miller J, et al: Intraosseous infusion: An alternative route to pediatric intravascular access. Ann Emerg Med 14:885–888, 1985.
183. Schapira M, Stern WZ: Hazards of subclavian vein cannulation for central venous pressure monitoring. JAMA 201:111, 1967.
184. Schnitzler RN, Caracta AR, Damato AN: "Floating" catheter for temporary transvenous ventricular pacing. Am J Cardiol 31:351, 1973.
185. Segall M: Infraclavicular subclavian venous catheterization. Surg Gynecol Obstet 148:925, 1979.
186. Serrao PR, Jean-Louis J, Godoy J, et al: Inferior vena cava catheterization in the neonate by the percutaneous femoral vein method. J Perinatol 16:129–132, 1996.
187. Shin B, Ayella RJ, McAslan TC: Pitfalls of Swan-Ganz catheterization. Crit Care Med 5: 125, 1977.
188. Silva YJ: In vivo use of human umbilical vessels and the ductus venosus arteriole. Surg Gynecol Obstet 148:595, 1979.
189. Simon RR: A new technique for subclavian puncture. JACEP 7:409, 1978.
190. Sink JD, Comer PB, James PM, et al: Evaluation of catheter placement in the treatment of venous air embolism. Ann Surg 183:58, 1976.
191. Sketch MH, Cale M, Mohinddin SM, et al: Use of percutaneously inserted venous catheters in coronary care units. Chest 62:684, 1972.
192. Smith BE: Complications of subclavian vein catheterization. Arch Surg 90:228, 1965.
193. Smith H, Freedman LR: Prolonged venous catheterization as a cause of sepsis. N Engl J Med 276:1229, 1967.
194. Smyth NPD, Rogers JB: Transvenous removal of catheter emboli from the heart and great veins by endoscopic forceps. Ann Thorac Surg 11: 403, 1971.
195. Solomon N, Escher DJW: A rapid method for insertion of the pacemaker catheter electrode. Am Heart J 66:717, 1963.
196. Stam WE, Colella JJ, Anderson RC, et al: Indwelling arterial catheters as a source of nosocomial bacteremia. N Engl J Med 292:1099, 1975.
197. Stephenson HE: Treatment of ruptured abdominal aorta. Surg Gynecol Obstet 144:855, 1977.
198. Stillman MT, Richards AM: Perforation of the interventricular system by transvenous pacemaker catheter. Am J Cardiol 24:269, 1969.

199. Sukigara M, Yamazaki T, Hatanaka M, et al: Ultrasonic real time guidance for subclavian venipuncture. Surg Gynecol Obstet 167:239, 1988.
200. Sulek CA, Gravenstein N, Blackshear RH, et al: Head rotation during internal jugular vein cannulation and the risk of carotid artery puncture. Anesth Analg 82:1, 125–128, 1996.
201. Swan HJC: Balloon flotation catheters: Their use in hemodynamic monitoring in clinical practice. JAMA 233:865, 1975.
202. Swan HJF: Guidelines for use of balloon-tipped catheter. Am J Cardiol 34:119, 1974.
203. Swanson RS, Uhlig PN, Gross PL, et al: Emergency intravenous access through the femoral vein. Ann Emerg Med 13:244, 1984.
204. Symansky MR, Fox HA: Umbilical vessel catheterization: indications, management and evaluation of the technique. J Pediatr 80:820, 1972.
205. Taylor FW, Rutherford CE: Accidental loss of plastic tube into venous system. Arch Surg 96: 177, 1963.
206. Thomas CS, Carter JW, Lowder SC: Pericardial tamponade from central venous catheters. Arch Surg 98:217, 1969.
207. Thomas TV: Location of catheter tip and its impact on central venous pressure. Chest 61:668, 1972.
208. Thurer RJ: Chylothorax: A complication of subclavian vein catheterization and parenteral hyperalimentation. J Thorac Cardiovasc Surg 71: 465, 1976.
209. Tintinalli JE, White BC: Transthoracic pacing during CPR. Ann Emerg Med 10:113, 1981.
210. Tofield JJ: A safer technique of percutaneous catheterization of the subclavian vein. Surg Gynecol Obstet 128:1069, 1969.
211. Torres DP: Massive hemothorax complicating subclavian venipuncture. JACEP 3:259, 1974.
212. Verghese ST, McGill WA, Patel RI, et al: Comparison of three techniques for internal jugular vein cannulation in infants. Paediatr Anaesth 10:5, 505–511, 2000.
213. Voukydis PC, Cohen SI: Catheter-induced arrhythmias. Am Heart J 88:588, 1974.
214. Wagner MB, McCabe JB: A comparison of four techniques to establish intraosseous infusion. Pediatr Emerg Care 4:87, 1988.
215. Walters MB, Stanger HAD, Rotem CE: Complications with percutaneous central venous catheters. JAMA 220:1455, 1972.
216. Ward ME, Lee PFS: Pneumothorax and contralateral hydrothorax following subclavian vein catheterization. Br J Anaesth 45:227, 1973.
217. Warden GD, Wilmore DW, Pruitt BA: Central venous thrombosis: A hazard of medical progress. J Trauma 13:620, 1973.
218. Wax PM, Talan D: Advances in cutdown technique. Emerg Med Clin North Am 7:1, 1989.
219. Webre DR, Aren JF: Use of cephalic and basilic veins for introduction of cardiovascular catheters. Anesthesiology 38:389, 1973.
220. Weinstein RA: Pressure monitoring devices: Overlooked source of nosocomial infection. JAMA 236:936, 1976.
221. Wigger HJ, Bransilver RR, Blanc WA: Thromboses due to catheterization in infants and children. J Pediatr 76:1, 1970.
222. Wright JE: Cut-down technique for intravenous infusion in infants. Med J Aust 37:1203, 1972.
223. Wyatt R, Glova I, Coopa EJ: Proximal skin necrosis after radial artery cannulation. Lancet 1:1135, 1974.
224. Yoffa D: Supraclavicular subclavian venipuncture and catheterization. Lancet 2:614, 1965.
225. Zaidi NA, Khan M, Naqvi HI, et al: Cerebral infarct following central venous cannulation. Anesthesia 53:2, 186–191, 1998.
226. Zelman S: Notes on techniques of intramuscular injection. Am J Med Sci 241:563, 1961.
227. Zinner SH, Denny-Brown BC, Braun P, et al: Risk of infection with intravenous indwelling catheters: Effect of application of antibiotic ointment. J Infect Dis 120:616, 1969.
228. Zollinger RW II: A useful intravenous access route. Surg Gynecol Obstet 154:725, 1982.

SUGGESTED READINGS

Atkinson JB, Bagnall HA, Gomperts E, et al: Investigational use of tissue plasminogen activator (t-PA) for occluded central venous catheters. J Parenter Enter Nutr 14:3, 310–311, 1990.

Banks DC, Yates DB: Infection from intravenous catheters. Lancet 1:443, 1970.

Berg RA: Emergency infusion of catecholamines into bone marrow. Am J Dis Child 138:810, 1984.

Brereton RB: Incidence of complications from indwelling venous catheters. Del Med J 41:1, 1969.

Coppa GF, Gouge TH, Hofstetter SR, et al: Air embolism: A lethal but preventable complication of subclavian vein catheterization. J Parenter Enter Nutr 5:2, 166–168, 1981.

Greenblatt DJ, Koch-Weser J: Intramuscular injection of drugs. N Engl J Med 29:542,1976.

How to give an intramuscular injection. Anesth Analg 45:205, 1966.

Harford FJ, Kleinsasser J: Fatal cardiac tamponade in a patient receiving total parenteral nutrition via a Silastic central venous catheter. J Parenter Enter Nutr 8:443, 1984.

Hunt LB, Olshansky B, Hiratzka LF, et al: Cardiac tamponade caused by pulmonary artery perforation after central venous catheterization. J Parenter Enter Nutr 8:711, 1984.

Iserson KV, Criss E: Intraosseous infusions: A usable technique. Am J Emerg Med 4:540, 1986.

Krauss AN, Albert RF, Kannan MM: Contamination of umbilical catheters in the newborn infant. J Pediatr 77:965, 1970.

Kravitz AB: Osteomyelitis of the clavicle secondary to infected Hickman catheter. J Parenter Enter Nutr 13:426, 1989.

Lewis ES, Freund HR, Rimon R, et al: Delayed pneumothorax: A complication of subclavian vein catheterization: The “all-in-one” system for TPN causes increased rates of catheter blockade. J Parenter Enter Nutr 10:542, 1986.

Manley L, Haley K, Dick M: Intraosseous infusion: Rapid vascular access for critically ill or injured infants and children. J Parenter Enter Nutr 14:63, 1988.

Meola F: Bone marrow infusions as a routine procedure in children. J Pediatr 25:13, 1944.

Mofenson HC, Tascone A, Caraccio TR: Guidelines for intraosseous infusions. J Emerg Med 6:143, 1988.

Neal WA, Reynolds JW, Jarvis CW, et al: Umbilical artery catheterization: Demonstration of arterial thrombosis by aortography. Pediatrics 50:6, 1972.

Rubenstein RB, Alberty RE, Michels LG, et al: Catheter separation. J Parenter Enter Nutr 6:754, 1985.

Simon RR: A new technique for subclavian puncture. JACEP 7:409, 1978.

Smith RJ, Kesg DP, Manley LK, et al: Intraosseous infusions by prehospital personnel in critically ill pediatric patients. Ann Emerg Med 17:491, 1988.

Stuart RK, Shikora SA, Akerman P, et al: Incidence of arrhythmia with central venous catheter insertion and exchange. J Parenter Enter Nutr 14:2, 152–155, 1990.

Zenk KE: Therapy consultation. Clin Pharm 9:90, 1990.

Index